OXFOR

Tho
Ana

Oxford Specialist Handbooks published and forthcoming

Oxford Specialist Handbooks in Anaesthesia
Thoracic Anaesthesia

Edited by

Jonathan N. Wilkinson

Consultant in Intensive Care and Anaesthesia
(past Fellow in Thoracic Anaesthesia
Nottingham University Hospitals)
Northampton General Hospital
Northampton, UK

Stephen H. Pennefather

Consultant Anaesthetist
Liverpool Heart & Chest Hospital
Liverpool, UK

Robert A. McCahon

Consultant Anaesthetist
Queen's Medical Centre
Nottingham, UK

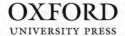

OXFORD
UNIVERSITY PRESS

OXFORD
UNIVERSITY PRESS

Great Clarendon Street, Oxford OX2 6DP.

Oxford University Press is a department of the University of Oxford.
It furthers the University's objective of excellence in research, scholarship,
and education by publishing worldwide in

Oxford New York

Auckland Cape Town Dar es Salaam Hong Kong Karachi
Kuala Lumpur Madrid Melbourne Mexico City Nairobi
New Delhi Shanghai Taipei Toronto

With offices in

Argentina Austria Brazil Chile Czech Republic France Greece
Guatemala Hungary Italy Japan Poland Portugal Singapore
South Korea Switzerland Thailand Turkey Ukraine Vietnam

Oxford is a registered trade mark of Oxford University Press
in the UK and in certain other countries

Published in the United States
by Oxford University Press Inc., New York

British Library Cataloguing in Publication Data
Data available

Library of Congress Cataloging-in-Publication-Data
Data available

Typeset by Glyph International, Bangalore, India
Printed in Great Britain
on acid-free paper by
Ashford Colour Press Ltd, Gosport, Hampshire

ISBN 978–0–19–956309–8

10 9 8 7 6 5 4 3 2 1

Foreword

Providing safe perioperative management for thoracic surgical patients remains one of the most consistently challenging areas, both technically and intellectually, within the specialty of anaesthesia. This excellent up-to-date handbook on Thoracic Anaesthesia by Drs. Wilkinson, Pennefather, McCahon and associates is a major advance in the information available to the practitioner working in this field.

The practice of thoracic anesthesia is continually evolving. The large majority of thoracic surgical patients in the first half of the last century presented for treatment of pulmonary processes secondary to infection. These patients are now infrequent in an adult practice in the developed world. However, complications such as empyema and broncho-pleural fistula still occur and the anaesthesia practitioner needs to know the principles of management which allow for maintenance of ventilation and protection of healthy lung regions in these difficult cases.

The majority of major pulmonary surgery now is for lung cancer and this surgical volume continues to increase as the cohort of the population with a high incidence of cigarette-smoking ages. Surgery has progressed from the first pneumonectomies in the 1930s to more complex operations such a segmentectomies and sleeve-lobectomies and more complex techniques such as video-assisted resections. These advances continually challenge the anaesthetist's ability to provide reliable lung isolation and to maintain oxygenation during one-lung anaesthesia.

Most recently thoracic surgery has been extended to treating a variety of end-stage lung diseases with lung transplantation and, in selected circumstances, lung-volume reduction. This extension now means than many severely disabled patients, previously considered inoperable, require safe anaesthetic management during prolonged surgery.

This handbook offers the trainee a comprehensive preview of perioperative management for all types of non-cardiac intra-thoracic surgery. It also offers the consultant a chance to review the specific anaesthetic considerations for all of these procedures, some of which occur infrequently, even in the busiest thoracic practices.

Even in centres which do not have a large volume of elective thoracic surgery, thoracic trauma cases present for surgery, often on very short notice. I believe the comprehensive section on anaesthesia for thoracic trauma in this handbook will be a valuable reference to anyone practicing in a surgical center that manages trauma.

I congratulate the Editors on this outstanding addition to the literature in thoracic anaesthesia and I thank them for allowing me to contribute a small portion of the text.

Peter Slinger MD, FRCPC
Professor of Anesthesia
University of Toronto, Canada

Acknowledgements

Medical artwork
Many thanks to our medical artists for their help with the book.

Mr Giles Barnwell
Nottingham, UK

Mr John M. Ross
Northampton, UK

Dr Polly Davies
Northampton, UK

Dr Jonathan N. Wilkinson
Northampton, UK

Contents

Major contributors

Dr Kan Alagesan
Consultant Anaesthetist and
Intensivist
Nottingham University Hospitals
City Hospital Campus
Nottingham, UK

Dr Victoria Banks
Specialist Registrar in Anaesthesia
Nottingham University Hospitals
Queens Medical Centre Campus
Derby Road
Nottingham, UK

Dr Jonathan Burch
Specialist Registrar in Anaesthesia
Queens Medical Centre
Nottingham, UK

Dr Alison Chalmers
Consultant Anaesthetist
Queen Victoria Hospital
Holtye Road
West Sussex, UK

Dr Myles Dowling
Consultant Anaesthetist
Nottingham University Hospitals
Nottingham, UK

Dr Helen Fenwick
Specialist Registrar in Anaesthesia
Nottingham University Hospitals
Nottingham, UK

Dr Alistair Glossop
Consultant in Intensive Care
and Anaesthesia
Sheffield Teaching Hospitals
NHS Foundation Trust
Sheffield, UK

Dr Christopher Harber
Consultant Anaesthetist
Queens Medical Centre
Nottingham, UK

Dr Simon Leach
Specialist Registrar in
Anaesthesia
Northampton General Hospital
Northampton, UK

Dr Martin Ma
Consultant Anaesthetist
Toronto General Hospital
Toronto, Canada

Dr Thomas McCarthy
Specialist Registrar in
Anaesthesia
Northampton General
Hospital
Northampton, UK

Dr Nicola Moores
Consultant Anaesthetist
Lincoln County Hospital
Lincoln, UK

Dr Gayle Rutherford
Consultant Radiologist
Sheffield Teaching Hospitals
NHS Foundation Trust
Sheffield, UK

Dr Michael Scanlan
Specialist Registrar in Anaesthesia
Sheffield Teaching Hospitals
NHS Trust
Sheffield, UK

Dr Peter D. Slinger
Consultant Anaesthetist
Toronto General Hospital
Toronto, Canada

Dr Paul Smith
Consultant Anaesthetist
and Intensivist
Sherwood Hospitals
NHS Foundation Trust
Sutton-In-Ashfield, UK

Dr Hannah Sycamore
Consultant Anaesthetist
Queens Medical Centre
Nottingham, UK

Dr Paul Townsley
Specialist Registrar in Anaesthesia
Nottingham University Hospitals
Nottingham, UK

Dr Patrick Waits
Consultant Anaesthetist
North Manchester General
Hospital
Oldham, UK

Dr Matthew Wiles
Consultant Anaesthetist
Sheffield Teaching Hospitals NHS
Foundation Trust
Sheffield, UK

Other contributors

Dr Alison Brewer
Consultant Anaesthetist
Leicester, UK

Dr David Castillo
Research Fellow in Anaesthesia
Liverpool, UK

Dr Melanie Davies
Consultant Anaesthetist
Lincoln, UK

Dr Polly Davies
Consultant Anaesthetist
Northampton, UK

Dr Chloe Fairbairns
Specialist Registrar in Anaesthesia
York, UK

Dr Nicola Hames
Consultant Anaesthetist
Northampton, UK

Dr Jonathan Hardwick
Consultant in Anaesthesia
and Intensivist
Northampton, UK

Dr Senthil Kumaran
Consultant Anaesthetist
Northampton, UK

Dr Ruffa Mustaq
Research Fellow in Anaesthesia
Liverpool, UK

Dr Suresh Paranjothy
Research Fellow in Anaesthesia
Liverpool, UK

Dr Darshan Pathak
Research Fellow in Anaesthesia
Liverpool, UK

Dr Som Sarkar
Consultant Anaesthetist
Sutton-In-Ashfield, UK

Dr Vyacheslav Seppi
Research Fellow in Anaesthesia
Liverpool, UK

Dr Vishal Thanawala
Specialist registrar in Anaesthesia
Leicester, UK

Dr Madan Thirugnanam
Specialist Registrar in Anaesthesia
Leicester, UK

Dr Liana Vele
Specialist Registrar in Anaesthesia
London, UK

Dr Pamela Wake
Consultant Anaesthetist
Nottingham, UK

Mr Richard Warwick
Specialist Registrar in
Cardiothoracic Surgery
Liverpool, UK

Symbols and abbreviations

❶	proceed with caution
❶❶	extreme caution
⚠	warning
♂	male
♀	female
📖	cross-reference to sections in this book
↔	normal
↓	decreased
↑	increased
→	leading to
►	important
►►	very important
∴	therefore
±	plus/minus
☛	controvertial
☠	extreme warning
ABC	airway, breathing, circulation
ABCDE	airway, breathing, circulation, disability, exposure
ABG	arterial blood gas
ACC	American College of Cardiology
ACh	acetylcholine
AChR	acetylcholine receptor
ADH	anti-diuretic hormone
AEC	airway exchange catheter
AED	accident and emergency department
AF	atrial fibrillation
AFOI	awake fibreoptic intubation
AHA	American Heart Association
AIC	Aintree Intubation Catheter
ALI	acute lung injury
ALS	advanced life support
AMPLE history	Allergies/airway, Medication, Past medical history/pregnancy, Last meal, Event (what happened)
ANP	atrial natiuretic peptide
Anti-AChR	acetylcholine receptor auto-antibodies
APTT	activated partial thromboplastin time

APUD	amine precursor uptake decarboxylation
ARDS	acute respiratory distress syndrome
ASD	atrial septal defect
ATLS	advanced trauma life support
AV	atrio-ventricular
AVNRT	atrio-ventricular nodal re-entry tachycardia
BAL	broncho-alveolar lavage
BMI	body mass index
BP	blood pressure
BPF	broncho-pleural fistula
BPn	bacterial pneumonia
Br	bromine
BTS	British Thoracic Society
BUN	blood urea nitrogen
BV	blood volume
C	carbon
CAP	chronic aspiration pneumonia
CBG	arterialized capillary blood gas
CEI	continuous epidural infusion
Cl	chlorine
CNS	central nervous system
CO	cardiac output
COPD	chronic obstructive pulmonary disease
CP	chemical pneumonitis
CPAP	continuous positive airway pressure
CPB	cardio-pulmonary bypass
CPR	cardiopulmonary resuscitation
CRP	c-reactive protein
CRT	capillary refill time
CT	computed tomography
CTZ	chemoreceptor trigger zone
CVP	central venous pressure
CVS	cardiovascular system
CVVH	continuous veno-venous haemofiltration
CXR	chest x-ray
DCCV	DC cardioversion
DLCO	lung diffusion capacity for carbon monoxide
DLT	double lumen endobronchial tube
DNR	do not resuscitate
DPH	dynamic pulmonary hyperinflation

E'PEEP	extrinsic peak end expiratory pressure
EBB	endo-bronchial blocker
ECG	electrocardiogram
ECLS	extra corporeal life support
ECMO	extra corporeal membrane oxygenation
ECV	extracellular volume
EEG	electro-encephalogram
ENT	ear, nose and throat
EPAP	expiratory positive airway pressure
ESR	erythrocyte sedimentation rate
ET	end tidal
$ETCO_2$	end tidal Carbon dioxide
ETT	endotracheal tube
EVSG	endo vascular stent grafting
F	fluorine
F/U	follow-up
FAST scan	Focussed Assessment Sonography in Trauma scan
FBC	full blood count
FDG	2-(18F)fluoro-2-deoxy-D-glucose
FEV_1	forced expiratory volume (in 1 second)
FFP	fresh frozen plasma
FiO_2:	fractional inspired oxygen concentration
FOB	fibreoptic bronchoscope
FOS	fibre optic scope
FRC	functional residual capacity
FVC	forced vital capacity
GABA	gamma amino butyric acid
GCS	Glasgow Coma Scale
GOJ	gastro-oesophageal junction
GTN	glycerine tri-nitrate
Hb	haemoglobin
HB	heart block
HCC	hepatocellular carcinoma
HDU	high dependency unit
HFFI	high frequency flow interruption
HFJV	high frequency jet ventilation
HFOV	high frequency oscillation ventilation
HFPPV	high frequency positive pressure ventilation
HHM	humoral hypercalcaemia of malignancy
HME	heat and moisture exchange

HPOA	hypertrophic pulmonary osteoathropathy
HR	heart rate
hrs	hours
I	iodine
I:E	inspiratory:expiratory ratio
ICD	intercostal drain
ICP	intracranial pressure
ICU	intensive care unit
ID	internal diameter
IJV	internal jugular vein
ILV	independent lung ventilation
iNO	inhaled notric oxide
IPAP	inspiratory positive airway pressure
IPPV	intermittent positive pressure ventilation
ITU	intensive therapy unit
IV	intravenous
IVC	inferior vena cava
IVI	intravenous infusion
JVP	jugular venous pressure
LA	local anaesthetic
LAP	left atrial pressure
LBBB	left bundle branch block
LE	limbic encephalitis
LEMS	lambert-eaton myasthenic syndrome
LFT	liver function tests
LI	lung isolation
LiDCO	lithium dilution cardiac output monitoring
LMA	laryngeal mask airway
LMWH	low molecular weight heparin
LoS	length of stay
LOS	lower oesophageal sphincter
LV	left ventricle
LVF	left ventricular failure
LVH	left ventricular hypertrophy
LVRS	lung volume reduction surgery
MAC	minimum alveolar concentration
MAOI	monoamine oxidase inhibitor
MG	myasthenia gravis
MGFA Score	myasthenia foundation of america score
MI	myocardial infarction

mls	milliliters
MR	mitral regurgitation
MRI	magnetic resonance imaging
MWD	minute walk distance
NG	naso-gastric
NHL	non-hodgkin's lymphoma
NICE	National Institute for Clinical Excellence
NIV	non-invasive ventilation
NMB	neuro-muscular blockade
NMDA	n methyl D aspartate
NSAIDS	non-steroidal anti-inflammatory drugs
NSCLC	non-small cell lung cancer
OGD	oesophago-gastroduodenoscopy
OLV	one lung ventilation
PAFC	pulmonary artery flotation catheter
$PaCO_2$	partial pressure of arterial Carbon Dioxide
PAFC	pulmonary artery flotation catheter
PAH	pulmonary artery hypertension
PaO_2	partial pressure of arterial Oxygen
PAP	pulmonary artery pressure
PAW	airway pressure
PAwP	peak airway pressure
PCA	patient controlled analgesia
PCD	paraneoplastic cerebellar degeneration
PCEA	patient controlled epidural infusion
PCP	pnuemocystis carinii pneumonia
PCV	pressure-controlled ventilation
PCWP	pulmonary capillary wedge pressure
PDA	patent ductus arteriosus
PE	pulmonary embolism
PEEP	positive end expiratory pressure
PEFR	peak expiratory flow rate
PET/CT	positron emission tomography/computed tomgraphy
PFO	patent foramen ovale
PFTs	pulmonary function tests
PGI_2	prostaglandin I2
PICC	peripherally inserted central catheter
PIP	peak inspiratory pressure
PM	pneumomediastinum
PO	oral administration

PONV	post operative nausea and vomiting
POP	post-operative pneumonia
PPH	primary pulmonary hypertension
PPPO	post-pneumonectomy pulmonary oedema
PRN	as required
PT	prothrombin time
PVA	paravertebral analgesia
PVB	paravertebral block
PVR	pulmonary vascular resistance
Q	perfusion
QDS	quarter die sumendus (four times daily)
QOL	health-related quality of life
RAP	right atrial pressure
RBBB	right bundle branch block
RBC	red blood cell
RCC	renal cell carcinoma
RCT	randomized control trial
ROW disease	Rendu-Osler-Weber
RSI	rapid sequence induction
RUMB	right upper lobe main bronchus
RV	right ventricle
SaO_2	arterial oxygen saturation
SCLC	small cell lung cancer
SCM	sternocleidomastoid
SE	subcutaneous emphysema
SIADH	syndrome of inappropriate antidiuretic hormone secretion
SIR	standardized incidence ratio
SLE	systemic lupus eyrthematosus
SLT	single lumen tube
SO_2	saturation of oxygen
SPD	surfactant protein D
SpO_2	pulse oximeter Oxygen saturation
SVC	superior vena cava
SVCO	superior venae caval obstruction
SVR	systemic vascular resistance
TB	tuberculosis
TCI	target controlled infusion
TEA	thoracic epidural analgesia
TIVA	total intravenous anaesthesia

TLC	total lung capacity
TLCO	transfer factor for Carbon Monoxide
TLV	2 lung ventilation
TOD	transoesophageal Doppler monitoring
TOE	transoesophageal echocardiography
TPN	total parenteral nutrition
TV	tidal volume
U&E	urea & electrolyte
UAO	upper airway obstruction
UE's	urea & electrolytes
V/Q	ventilation perfusion
V	ventilation
VAP	ventilator acquired pneumonia
VATS	video assisted thoracic surgery
VC	vital capacity
VCV	volume-controlled ventilation
VE	ventricular ectopics
VILI	ventilator induced lung injury
VSD	ventricular septal defect
V_T	tidal volume
WHO	World Health Organization
X match	cross match
XM	cross matched

Chapter 1

Basic physiology for thoracic anaesthesia

Abnormalities in the distribution of Q and V, diffusion of gases and hypoxic pulmonary vasoconstriction

Introduction
- Much of the physiological effects of OLV are due to changes in ventilation and perfusion matching.
- The ratio of pulmonary ventilation to pulmonary blood flow (V/Q) for the whole lung at rest is about 0.8.
  - Alveolar ventilation 4 L/min: pulmonary blood flow 5l/min.
- There are regional differences in the ventilation-perfusion ratio within the normal lung parenchyma.
- Differences can largely be explained by the effect of gravity on blood flow and alveolar compliance.
- V/Q mismatching leads to impairment in the transfer of gases between alveolar space and blood stream within the lung.
- Local changes in the V/Q ratio are very common in disease states.
- Although hypoventilation, diffusion abnormalities and shunts can all contribute to the development of hypoxemia in patients ventilated via one lung, understanding V/Q mismatching is central to the understanding of hypoxaemia and the necessary steps to correct it.

Factors affecting V/Q ratio in thoracic anaesthesia
- One lung ventilation.
- Lateral decubitus position.
- Hypoxic pulmonary vasoconstriction (HPV).
- Attenuation of HPV response by volatile agents.
- Ventilation strategies during OLV.
- Cardiac output.
- Surgical technique.
- Chest wall compliance.
- Lung disease.

Clinical relevance
- One-lung ventilation should still provide the ability to oxygenate the entire cardiac output.
- The role of the thoracic anaesthetist is to identify factors contributing to the impaired gas exchange and then corrected them in a stepwise manner from major to more minor.

One lung ventilation

The non ventilated lung

- The non-ventilated lung is perfused but, obviously, not ventilated.
- Surgical manipulation and hypoxic pulmonary vasoconstriction reduce what might otherwise be a substantial right-to-left shunt.

The ventilated lung

- In the lateral position, gravity usually ensures preferential perfusion of the dependent lung. (Increased shunt seen during OLV in the supine position as this gravity effect is not present).
- The alveolar compliance curve is shifted down and to the left for alveolar in the dependent lung. Abnormal V/Q ratios result. Alveolar collapse results in atelectasis.
- Without an increase in F_iO_2 hypoxaemia will occur.
- Due to greater solubility of carbon dioxide and its more linear dissociation curve, $PaCO_2$ is less affected by V/Q mismatch.

Lateral positioning of the patient

Upper lung now lies on the steep part of the compliance curve and the lower lung on the flatter part.

The non-dependent lung

- The upper lung receives a smaller percentage of the blood flow as a result of gravity.
- The upper lung now lies on the steep part of the compliance curve and thus receives a greater percentage of the ventilation.

The dependent lung

- The lower lung receives a greater percentage of the cardiac output as a result of gravity.
- The lower lung now lies on flat part of the compliance curve and thus receives a lower percentage of the ventilation.
- Malpositioning of a DLT in the dependent lung can further impair gas exchange eg misplaced right DLT resulting in the exclusion of the right upper lobe from ventilation.

Hypoxic pulmonary vasoconstriction (HPV)

- This important regulatory mechanism diverts blood flow away from hypoxic to better oxygenated areas of the lung.
- When changing from two-lung ventilation to OLV, HPV diverts blood flow from the non-ventilated to the ventilated lung, thereby reducing venous admixture and ameliorating the decrease in PaO_2.
- It involves the constriction of small arterioles (and to a lesser degree, venules and capillaries) in response to alveolar hypoxia.
- HPV occurs with seconds, reaches an initial plateau after 15 minutes but the maximum effect only occurs after about 4 hours.
- Alveolar (P_AO_2) is the primary stimulus (80%) to HPV although mixed venous P_VO_2 also exerts an effect (See Table 1.1 for other factors).
- The effect occurs in the physiological range (PaO_2 5.5–13kPa) and is mediated in part via inhibition of nitric oxide synthesis.

- HPV reduces the blood flow through the non ventilated lung by about 40%, some blood flow remains.
  - This is why insufflation of 100% O_2 into this lung via a catheter/CPAP circuit is effective in reducing hypoxia.
- HPV is more efficient if pulmonary artery pressure and mixed venous oxygen saturation are normal; very high and very low values greatly reduce the effect of HPV.
- Hypocapnia reduces HPV, potentially leading to an increase in shunt.

Volatile anaesthetic agents

- HPV is inhibited by all volatile anesthetics.
- In theory this would allow a right to left shunt causing venous admixture and hypoxaemia. However, clinically this does not happen because:
  - Degree of HPV is inversely proportional to cardiac output. Volatile agents inhibit HPV directly but also indirectly augment it by decreasing cardiac output.
  - Inhalational agents are bronchodilators. This will cause more uniform ventilation in the dependent lung and improve V/Q matching.
  - Haemodynamic stability and ventilation strategies are far more important than choice of anaesthetic to maintain oxygenation.
  - The relative effect in humans in vivo is: Halothane> enflurane> Isoflurane and sevoflurane> desflurane.
  - IV anesthetic techniques have not been shown to provide better oxygenation than the newer volatile anesthetics in <1MAC concentrations.
- Reduction in HPV may occur due to the direct vasodilatory effects of volatiles.
- Glyceryl trinitrate, sodium nitroprusside, isoprenaline, dobutamine and nitric oxide have also been shown to inhibit HPV.

Table 1.1 Factors affecting HPV

Anaesthetic agents—inhaled	All inhaled agents inhibit HPV but have a minimal clinical effect at levels of 1 MAC.
	1 MAC of isoflurane reduces HPV by 21%, increasing the shunt fraction from 20% to 24%.
	N2O reduces HPV by approximately 10%.
Anaesthetic agents—intravenous	Propofol, Thiopentone, Fentanyl, Remifentanil & Ketamine have no effect on HPV.
Anaesthesia—regional	Thoracic epidural anaesthesia has no significant effect on PVR and may enhance HPV.
Vasodilators	GTN, β agonists, nitroprusside, nitric oxide, calcium channel antagonists, prostcyclin & dobutamine all inhibit HPV.
	Aminophylline and hydralazine have only minimal effects.
Vasoconstrictors	Norepinephrine, epinephrine and phenylephrine constrict blood vessels in the ventilated lung, diverting blood flow to the non-ventilated lung, thereby having a HPV inhibiting effect.
Oxygen	Increasing the inspired oxygen concentration to the dependent lung decreases pulmonary vascular resistance and increases pulmonary blood flow to the ventilated lung.
	HPV is maximal when the percentage of the lung that is hypoxic is between 30–70%.
Carbon dioxide	Hypercapnia during OLV tends to increase PVR by acting as a direct vasoconstrictor, thereby diverting blood flow to the non-ventilated lung. Hypocapnia directly inhibits HPV, through the development of a respiratory alkalosis.
Acid-base balance	Acute respiratory or metabolic alkalosis reduces the effect of HPV, whilst metabolic acidosis enhances HPV.

Ventilation strategies during OLV

- Applying high peak inspiratory pressure and high end-expiratory pressure pressures to the ventilated lung can increase pulmonary vascular resistance, divert blood flow to the non-ventilated lung and decrease the cardiac output. Oxygen delivery may be impaired.
- In contrast, particularly in the relatively normal lung, modest PEEP can improve the compliance of the dependent lung, improve oxygenation and improve oxygen delivery.
- There is the potential, particularly in patients with severe COPD for PEEP, excessive ventilation or short expiratory times to lead to incomplete expiration with the "breath stacking" causing increased airway pressure. It may be necessary to accept a degree of hypoventilation in some patients with severe COPD.

- But the increases in $PaCO_2$ and decreases in pH may increase pulmonary artery pressure and thus potentially increase the V/Q mismatch.
- Pressure controlled ventilation is often the mode of choice during OLV.
- 5–7 ml/kg tidal volume, (ideal body weight), with inspiratory airway pressure limited to 25cm H_2O are useful initial parameters for OLV in the majority of patients.
- The high solubility of nitrous oxide may lead to increased dependent lung atelectasis.

Cardiac output
- A reduction in cardiac output will decrease the mixed venous PvO_2 and in the presence of a significant shunt decrease the PaO_2.
- Reduced perfusion to the dependent (ventilated) lung may increase V/Q mismatching in this lung.
- Overzealous infusion of crystalloids to improve the cardiac output may lead to impaired gas exchange in the ventilated lung (pulmonary oedema).
- Cardiac failure and RV dysfunction is common post-pneumonectomy (particularly after R pneumonectomy).
  - 2° to ↑RV afterload as a result of ↓size of pulmonary vasculature
  - ↓O_2 and/or ↑CO_2 further increases pulmonary arterial pressure via HPV.

Surgical technique
- Early ligation of the appropriate branch of the pulmonary artery to the operated lobe or lung will reduce/stop the shunt through the operated lung and improve oxygenation.
- Surgical manipulation can reduce venous return, cardiac contractility and cardiac output and thus impair oxygenation and oxygen delivery.
- Uncorrected bleeding may lead to impaired cardiac output, oxygenation and thus oxygen delivery.

Increased chest wall compliance
- Poor chest wall compliance will require an increase P_{insp} to achieve the necessary tidal volume.
- High P_{insp} may lead to an increased V/Q mismatch.
- Muscle relaxation results in upward movement of the abdominal contents, reducing the FRC of the ventilated lung.
- Conversely, poor muscle relaxation may lead to high airway pressures by a patient as the patient 'fights' the ventilator. Bronchospasm may be induced.

Lung disease
- The pathology of the patient may be a contributor to V/Q mismatch.
- Pathology (e.g. tumour) in the non-dependent lung may limit the perfusion to this lung. Thus paradoxically the shunt may be larger in patients without lung pathology undergoing OLV.
- Pulmonary fibrosis

- Oxygenation may be difficult due to a reduced diffusion capacity in the dependent lung.
- PE (discussed at length, see 📖 Pulmonary embolism, p. 664).

Further reading

Ganong WF. *Review of Medical Physiology*. 22nd ed. St Louis: Mosby Elsevier; 2005. Chapters 34&35, pp. 647–69.

Aitkenhead AR, Smith G, Rowbotham DJ, editors. *Textbook of Anaesthesia*. 5th ed., London: Churchill Livingstone; 2007. Chapter39, pp. 703–9.

Johnson LR, editor. *Essential Medical Physiology*. 3rd ed. New York: Academic Press; 2003. Chapter 21, pp. 299–315.

Normal pulmonary ventilation and perfusion

Introduction

The thoracic anaesthetist requires a working knowledge of pulmonary ventilation and perfusion in order to anticipate, prevent and when necessary treat hypoxaemia during one lung anaesthesia. Thoracic surgery and anaesthesia alter normal pulmonary mechanics and perfusion in several ways:

- Lateral decubitus position.
- The open chest.
- One-lung ventilation.

Normal pulmonary ventilation (V)

- Ventilation—process by which gas reaches the alveoli with each breath.
- May be quantified as alveolar minute ventilation (V_A ml/min). Thus:

$$V_A = (V_T - V_D) \times RR \rightarrow AND \rightarrow V_A \, \alpha \, VCO_2/PaCO_2$$

V_T = Tidal volume (ml)
V_D = Dead Space (ml)
RR = Respiratory rate (breaths/min)
VCO_2 = CO_2 production

For example $PaCO_2$ will double if V_A is halved and VCO_2 remains constant.

Regional differences in pulmonary ventilation

- Distribution of ventilation is affected by gravity and the resting volume of alveolar in different regions of the lung.

Table 1.2 Effect of patient position during spontaneous ventilation (in an awake subject), on the distribution of alveolar ventilation in a normal lung

Patient position	Greater ventilation	Lesser ventilation
Upright	Lung base	Lung apex
Supine	Posterior lung	Anterior lung
Lateral decubitus	Dependent lung	Non-dependent lung

Factors that impact on pulmonary ventilation

Dead space

- ~2 ml/kg.
- Anatomical:
  - Measured using Fowler technique i.e. measurement of expired N_2.
  - Essentially measures volume of the conducting airways.
- Physiological:
  - Measured using Bohr equation:

$$V_D/V_T = PaCO_2 - PECO_2/PaCO_2$$

  Where $PaCO_2$ = arterial CO_2 (kPa) and $PECO_2$ = expired CO_2 (kPa).
  - Essentially measures the volume of lung not involved in gas exchange i.e. does not eliminate CO_2.
- In normal subjects, anatomical and physiological dead spaces are almost identical.
- In lung disease, physiological dead space may be greatly increased e.g. chronic obstructive lung disease. ∴ V_A will be decreased.

Respiratory system compliance

$$\delta V/\delta P$$

- Represented by the slope of the p-v curve for the respiratory system.
- Two components:
  - Lung compliance (C_L).
  - Chest wall compliance (C_W).
- Respiratory system compliance (C_R):

$$1/C_R = 1/C_L + 1/C_W = 100 \text{ ml}/100 \text{ cm } H_2O$$

- ↓ at the extremes of the p-v curve. Thus greater pressures are required for alveolar ventilation.
- ↑ in:
  - Pulmonary emphysema.
  - Non-dependent lung during one-lung ventilation.

- ↓ in:
  - Dependent lung during one-lung ventilation,
  - Elderly patient,
  - Reduced surfactant,
  - Pulmonary fibrosis,
  - Pulmonary oedema,
  - Pulmonary atelectasis e.g. 2° hypoventilation,
  - ARDS.

Airway resistance

- Predominantly occurs at the medium-sized bronchi.
- As resistance increases, greater pressures are required to ventilate the alveoli.
- ↑ resistance:
  - Low lung volumes e.g. dependent lung during one-lung ventilation.
  - Bronchospasm.
  - Upper & lower airway obstruction e.g. foreign body/tumour/extrinsic compression.
  - Anaesthesia. i.e. ↓ FRC.

Normal pulmonary perfusion (Q)

- Low pressure and resistance system.
- ~ 80% lower than pressures within the systemic circulation.
- Pulmonary artery pressure (PAP) = 25/8 mmHg.
- Mean PAP = 15 mmHg.
- Two components:
  - Pulmonary arteries perfuse the parenchyma distal to the respiratory bronchiole i.e. the alveolar involved in gas exchange.
  - Bronchial arteries (1% of CO) perfuse the lung tissue proximal to the respiratory bronchiole (conducting airways). Their origin is variable but usually from the aorta or intercostal arteries. Contributes to anatomical shunt.
- R output slightly less that L output due to bronchial circulation.

Factors that impact on pulmonary circulation

Pulmonary vascular resistance (PVR)

- 10 times less that systemic vascular resistance.
- 1.7 mmHg/L/min.
- Pulmonary factors that alter PVR:
  - Recruitment of closed or underperfused pulmonary capillaries with rising arterial or venous pressure decreases PVR.
  - Distension of perfused pulmonary capillaries with rising arterial or venous pressure decreases PVR.

- At low or high lung volumes PVR increases due to collapse of extra-alveolar vessels and stretching of pulmonary capillaries respectively.
- Acute or chronic lung disease may cause raised PVR and resultant right ventricular failure.
- Positive pressure ventilation may increase PVR when alveolar pressure exceeds that within the pulmonary capillaries, causing them to collapse.
- Low pH raises PVR.
- Drugs that alter PVR:
  - Prostacyclin & nitric oxide both reduce PVR.
  - Vasoconstrictors e.g. serotonin, norepinephrine, histamine all↑ regional pulmonary vascular resistance in normoxic lung.

Distribution of pulmonary blood flow

- Blood flow is increased to dependent areas of lung, e.g. basal flow is greater than apical flow in the upright lung.
- This is explained by considering the upright lung as 3 zones:
- Apical zone:
  - PA > Pa > PV ∴ blood flow is absent. Under normal conditions this does not occur. However, it may occur in severe haemorrhage or during positive pressure ventilation.
- Mid zone:
  - Pa > PA >PV ∴ blood flow is dependent on the arterio-alveolar pressure difference.
- Basal zone:
  - Pa > PV > PA ∴ blood flow is dependent on the usual arterio-venous pressure difference.
- In the basal zone, increases in blood flow occur by recruitment and distension of pulmonary capillaries.
- At low lung volumes, collapse of extra-alveolar vessels due to atelectasis causes a reduction in blood flow.
- During exercise, the mid and apical zones behave more like the basal zone.

Hypoxic pulmonary vasoconstriction

(See 📖 Abnormalities of Q and V, the diffusion of gases and hypoxic pulmonary vasoconstriction, p. 2).

Ventilation-perfusion matching (V/Q)

To ensure adequate gas exchange it is important to match perfusion and ventilation in the alveoli. (See Fig. 1.1).

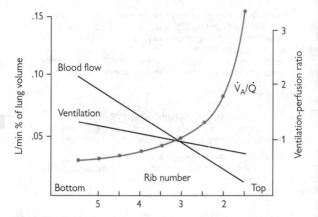

Fig. 1.1 Distribution of ventilation and perfusion and their relationship in the upright lung.

- The ideal V/Q relationship equally matches ventilation and perfusion.
- V/Q increases towards the lung apex.
  - ↑ V/Q = High P_ACO_2 & low P_ACO_2 (apex).
  - ↓ V/Q = Low P_AO_2 & high P_ACO_2 (base).
  - Note that the change in P_ACO_2 associated with changes in V/Q matching is much less than the change in P_AO_2.
- The regional differences in V/Q matching give rise to an alveolar-arterial O_2 difference = 4 mm Hg in normality.
- Increased V/Q mismatch in disease may give rise to:
- Hypoxaemia and/or hypercarbia.
- Increased alveolar-arterial difference.
- Increased shunt fraction.
- Increased physiological dead space.

Further reading

West JB. Respiratory physiology. *The Essentials*. Baltimore, United States: Lippincott Williams & Wilkins; 2004.

One lung ventilation and the lateral decubitus position

Upon moving the anaesthetized patient from the supine to the lateral decubitus position there are numerous changes to the ventilation and perfusion of both lungs, both before and after the thoracic cavity is opened.

Closed chest

Ventilation

- After induction of general anaesthesia both lungs take up lower positions on the pressure-volume curve (See Fig. 1.1).
- The *dependent (bottom) lung* falls onto the lower, flatter portion of the pressure-volume curve, with a subsequent decrease in FRC and compliance. This is caused by compression of the dependent lung by:
  - Cephalic movements of the abdominal contents, pushing on the paralysed hemi-diaphragm,
  - The weight of the mediastinal contents,
  - Placing the patient in a jack-knife or flexed position.
- The *non-dependent (top) lung* is now on the steep part of the pressure-volume curve, with an improved FRC and compliance, and is therefore preferentially ventilated.
- Gravity has no effect on the distribution of ventilation during IPPV.

Perfusion

- In the lateral decubitus position, blood flow is primarily determined by gravity with 60% going to the dependent lung.
- The net result is the production of a V/Q mismatch.

Open chest

Ventilation

- Upon opening the thoracic cavity, the differential ventilation between the lungs becomes more pronounced.
- As the non-dependent lung is no longer restricted by the chest wall, its compliance increases. This results in a further increase in ventilation of the non-dependent lung at the expense of the dependent lung.
- Compression of the dependent lung also results in areas of atelectasis, producing a degree of shunt.

Perfusion

- Blood flow remains unchanged with the majority still going to the dependent lung.
- This results in the dependent lung being poorly ventilated but well perfused, and the non-dependent lung, well ventilated but poorly perfused.
- This combination of V/Q mismatching and shunt produces an increase in the alveolar-arterial oxygen gradient and impaired oxygenation.

Collapse of the non-dependent lung
Ventilation
- After the institution of one lung ventilation (OLV), the non-dependent lung is no longer directly ventilated.
- This produces an obligatory shunt through this lung, in addition to any existing shunt in the dependent lung.
- A tidal ventilation of approximately 150 ml does occur in the non-dependent lung as a result of the transmitted pressure changes from the ventilated hemithorax.
- The compliance of this lung however, is markedly reduced due to direct pressure from surgical retraction and handling.

During OLV $PaCO_2$ is affected to a lesser extent than PaO_2. Blood flowing through the non-ventilated lung will carry a larger amount of CO_2. Due to the linear shape of the CO_2 dissociation curve, this is offset by the blood flowing through ventilated alveoli releasing a greater amount of CO_2. This compensation is not complete and a gradual increase in end-tidal CO_2 occurs.

Perfusion
- The collapse of the non-dependent lung would be expected to produce a shunt fraction of 40–60% (depending on whether it is the left or right lung that is collapsed), which could not be rectified by an increase in the FiO_2.
- Blood flow however is reduced in the non-dependent lung by several mechanisms, thereby reducing the degree of shunt (discussed below).

Pulmonary vascular resistance (PVR)
Hypoxic pulmonary vasoconstriction (HPV) (See 📖 Abnormalities of Q and V, the diffusion of gases and hypoxic pulmonary vasoconstriction, p. 2).

PEEP
- + The addition of positive end expiratory pressure to the dependent, ventilated lung results in an increase in the pulmonary vascular resistance of the lung
- + The addition of PEEP may improve lung compliance and prevent atelectasis thereby preventing increases in PVR in the dependent lung
- −This may result in the diversion of blood to the non-ventilated lung and may worsen the shunt.

Lung volumes
- During positive pressure ventilation PVR is lowest at FRC.
- At lung volumes above FRC, PVR increases due to the excess stretching of the capillaries and at low lung volumes PVR increases due to the loss of traction holding capillaries open.
- Thus ventilation of the dependent lung with high airway pressures may increase PVR and divert blood flow to the non-ventilated lung.

Cardiac output

Variations in cardiac output either affect HPV via changes in the pulmonary artery pressure or mixed venous oxygen saturation.
- High cardiac output—may attenuate HPV via directly increasing pulmonary artery pressure and increasing blood flow to the non-ventilated lung, or by an increase in mixed venous oxygen saturation inhibiting PVR by reverse diffusion of oxygen.
- Low cardiac output—will also attenuate HPV. Low cardiac outputs produce a decrease in the mixed venous oxygen partial pressure and thus a decrease in the alveolar oxygen tension in the dependent lung. This results in an increase in HPV in the dependent lung that offsets the HPV in the non-dependent lung. The net result is that less blood flow is diverted away from the more hypoxic collapsed lung.
- Balanced anaesthesia (usually consisting of general and epidural anaesthesia) can result in lower than normal cardiac output. In this situation, increasing the cardiac output back to normal levels will result in an improvement in the mixed venous oxygen saturation, thereby improving arterial oxygen saturations. This occurs despite a small increase in the amount of blood diverted to the non-ventilated lung by the increased pulmonary artery pressure.

Non-dependent lung effects

- The collapse of the non-dependent lung, in tandem with surgical handling, retraction and vessel ligation, causes a direct mechanical obstruction to blood flow through the lung.
- In addition, the underlying pathology of the operative lung may have already caused a reduction in lung blood flow prior to the collapse of the lung.

Basic anatomy for thoracic anaesthesia

Anatomy of the trachea and bronchial tree

Embryology
- 3rd week.
  - Lung buds start to develop.
- 4th week.
  - Endodermal and mesochymal elements begin to separate from foregut.
- 6th week.
  - Separation has taken place; carina descends to level of T4.
- 17th week.
  - 70% of alveoli are formed.

Tracheal anatomy
Position
- Begins at inferior border of cricoid cartilage (C6/7) extending to the carina.
- Carina is at T4/5 or T6 on deep inspiration (manubrio-sternal notch in adults). It is at the 3rd costal cartilage in children.
- It is 11–13 cm long (5 cm being above the suprasternal notch).
- In 33% of population it has an elliptical cross section with the transverse diameter > AP.
  - It is equal in dimensions in 25%.
  - Funnel shaped in children/cylindrical in adults.

Rings
- Incomplete rings are approx 4 mm wide 1 mm thick.
- They range from 12 to 22 in number.
- They calcify with age leaving them more susceptible to trauma.

Blood supply
- Blood supply is segmental from a lateral longitudinal anastomosis.
- Fed by branches from the inferior thyroid and bronchial arteries.
- Perforating branches feed a rich submucosal plexus that feeds the cartilage from the luminal surface.

- Bronchial arterial supply ends at the terminal bronchioles leaving the alveoli relatively sparsely supplied during single lung ventilation.
  - ❶ Therefore alveolar are at risk of ischaemia during OLV.
- ❶ Over inflation of a tracheal cuff can readily impair capillary perfusion leading to ischaemic damage to the mucosa and ultimately the cartilage.

Relations

Important relationships are:
- Anterior.
- Brachiocephalic artery.
- Thyroidea ima artery (particularly relevant if performing a percutaneous tracheostomy).
- Azygos vein.

Posterior
- Recurrent laryngeal nerves.
- Oesophagus.

Lateral
- Thyroid gland.
- Carotid sheath.
- Anterior jugular arch.
- Deep cervical fascia.

Physiology

- Inspiration.
  - Diameter increases reducing resistance.
- Expiration.
  - Diameter decreases increasing velocity.
- Cilia beat 160–1500 times/min moving mucous 166 mm/min (impaired muco-ciliary escalator with smoking).

Bronchial anatomy

See Fig. 2.1.

Divisions

Right main bronchus
- Wider, shorter (2cm), steeper and in line with the trachea.
- Gives rise to 10 segments:

Right upper lobe bronchus
- Divides into:
  - Posterior/Anterior/Apical segments.

Right middle lobe bronchus
- Divides into:
  - Medial/Lateral segments.

Right lower lobe bronchus
- Divides into:
  - Superior/Posterior basal/Anterior basal/Lateral basal/Medial basal segments.

Left main bronchus
- Narrower, longer (5cm) and more horizontal.
- Gives rise to 8 segments:

Left upper lobe bronchus
- Divides into:
  - Apical posterior/Anterior segments and Superior/Inferior lingular segments (remnant of LML).

Left lower lobe bronchus
- Divides into:
  - Superior Apical/Anterior basal/Lateral basal/Posterior basal segments.

Lymph drainage
- Drains inward from pleura to hilum.
  - 1st to bronchopulmonary nodes.
  - 2nd to tracheobronchial nodes found at the bifurcation of the trachea.
  - 3rd to paratracheal and mediastinal lymph trunks.
  - Finally to brachiocephalic veins.

Nerve supply
- Glossopharyngeal nerve.
- Superior laryngeal nerve.
- Inferior laryngeal nerve.

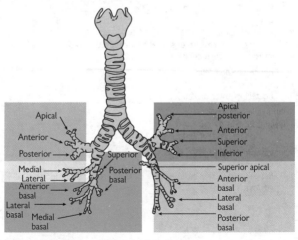

Fig. 2.1 The sub-divisions of the tracheobronchial tree.

Special points

- Adult male trachea diameter 2.3cm, female trachea 2/3 diameter.
- Blood supplies to cartilage via vulnerable submucosal plexus, remember endobronchial cuffs can cause ulceration!
- Trachea is enveloped in connective tissue sheath facilitating descent of infections.
- Cervical trachea susceptible to direct injury and deceleration injury.
- Thoracic trachea susceptible to compression and barotrauma.
- Right endobronchial tube more difficult to place due to RULMB
- Tubes and aspirated material tend to go down the right bronchus.
- Anomalous tracheal origin of RULMB in 0.5% (frequently only apical segment).
- RLLMB is susceptible to flooding when a prone patient aspirates.
- Right pneumonectomy is a risk factor for a bronchopleural fistula.

Anatomy of great vessels of the chest and neck

Aorta
Ascending aorta
LOCATION
- Lying in the middle mediastinum, approximately 5 cm long, beginning at the base of the left ventricle and curving forwards and right behind the sternum to the 2nd right costal cartilage.

RELATIONS
- Anterior.
  - Pulmonary trunk.
- Posterior.
  - Right pulmonary artery/left atrium/right main bronchus.
- Anatomical left.
  - Pulmonary trunk/left atrium.
- Anatomical right.
  - SVC/right atrium.

BRANCHES
- Right and Left coronary arteries.

Aortic arch
LOCATION
- In continuation with the ascending aorta, lying in the superior mediastinum.
  - Arches backwards and to the left behind the manubrium, over the right pulmonary artery and left main bronchus, ending at the level of the 2nd left costal cartilage.

RELATIONS
- Anterior.
  - Left vagus nerve/left phrenic nerve.
- Posterior.
  - Left recurrent laryngeal nerve (loops from vagus)/trachea/ oesophagus.

BRANCHES
- Brachiocephalic artery.
- Left common carotid.
- Left subclavian artery.

Descending thoracic aorta
LOCATION
- In continuation with the arch, beginning at the level of the 4th thoracic vertebra and lying in the posterior mediastinum.
  - Initially lying to the left of the vertebrae, it inclines medially lying anterior to 12th vertebral body as it passes behind the diaphragm becoming the abdominal aorta.

RELATIONS
- Anterior.
  - Left hilum/left atrium.
- Posterior.
  - Vertebral column/hemiazygous veins
- Anatomical right.
  - Azygous vein/thoracic duct/oesphagus.
- Anatomical left.
  - Pleura and left lung.

BRANCHES
- Pericardial.
- Right and left bronchial arteries.
- Oesophageal arteries.
- Nine paired posterior intercostal arteries.
- Paired subcostal arteries.

Thoracic systemic veins

Superior vena cava (SVC)
LOCATION
- Returns blood from all structures above the diaphragm except the lungs and the heart.
  - Formed from the union of the right and left brachiocephalic veins at the first right costal cartilage.
  - Terminates when it enters the right atrium at the level of the third costal cartilage.
  - The superior part lies in the right superior mediastinum while the terminal part is in the middle mediastinum.
  - The Azygous vein also drains into the SVC just prior to it entering the pericardium.

RELATIONS
- Anterior.
  - Pleura/right lung.
- Posterior.
  - Right pulmonary hilum.
- Anatomical right.
  - Right phrenic nerve/right lung.
- Anatomical left.
  - Trachea(posterior)/right vagus nerve.

Brachiocephalic veins
- The Brachiocephalic veins are formed by the union of the internal jugular and subclavian veins on each side.
  - Due to the SVC being right of the midline, the left brachiocephalic vein must pass obliquely and downward behind the manubrium sternum anterior to the branches of the aortic arch.

Inferior vena cava (IVC)
- Returns blood from all structures below the diaphragm.
  - It is formed by the union of the common iliac veins and ascends anterior to the vertebral bodies to the right of the aorta.
  - It pierces the tendonous part of diaphragm at the level of T8 vertebra and almost immediately enters the right atrium.

Azygous vein
- Origins vary but numerous tributaries exist with blood returning from the posterior thoracic and abdominal walls, oesophagus, bronchi and mediastinal lymph nodes.
  - The azygous vein connects the SVC and IVC which is of importance when there is obstruction of the vena cava.
  - It ascends in the posterior mediastinum, anterior and to the right of the vertebral bodies until the level of 4th vertebral body where it arches over the right pulmonary hilum to end in the SVC.

Hemiazygous and accessory hemiazygous veins
- These veins are analogous to the azygous vein but ascend and descend respectively to the left of the vertebral column, crossing posterior to the aorta at variable levels to drain into the azygous vein.

Pulmonary circulation

Pulmonary arteries
Pulmonary trunk
LOCATION
- Lying in the middle mediastinum, it begins at the upper part of the right ventricle and runs upwards, backwards and to the left for approximately 5 cm.
  - It then divides into the right and left pulmonary arteries in the concavity of the aortic arch.
  - It is enclosed in pericardium with the ascending aorta.

Right pulmonary artery
RELATIONS
- Anterior.
  - Aorta/SVC.
- Posterior.
  - Right main bronchus.
- Inferior.
  - Right pulmonary veins.
- Superior.
  - Azygous vein.

BRANCHES
- Truncus anterior (branch to upper lobe).
- Middle lobe artery.
- Superior segmental branch (to lower lobe).
- Distal to this the artery becomes the common basal trunk.

Left pulmonary artery
RELATIONS
- Anterior.
  - Phrenic nerve/pleura
- Posterior.
  - Aortic arch/descending aorta/left main bronchus
- Inferior.
  - Pulmonary veins
- Superior.
  - Aortic arch

BRANCHES
- Upper lobe branches.
- Lingular branch.
- Branch to superior segment of lower lobe.
- Distal to this the artery becomes the common basal trunk.

Pulmonary veins
- These drain blood from the lungs directly into the left atrium.
- Usually there are 2 pulmonary veins on each side, a superior and inferior vein.

Right pulmonary veins
- The superior vein drains the upper and middle lobes and at the hilum is anterior and inferior to the pulmonary artery.
- The Inferior vein is posterior and inferior to the artery, superior vein and bronchus at the hilum.
  - It drains the lower lobe.

Left pulmonary veins
- The superior vein drains the upper and lingular lobes, and at the hilum is anterior to the bronchus and anterio-inferior to the pulmonary artery.
- The inferior vein drains the lower lobe and lies inferio-posterior to the bronchus at the hilum.

Arteries in the neck
- The arterial supply to the head, neck and upper limbs originate from the three branches of the aortic arch and branch out from the root of the neck.
- The subclavian arteries (and veins) barely enter the neck but are classically considered with the neck vessels.

Brachiocephalic artery
- Arises posterior to the manubrium and passes superiorly and to the right, dividing into the right common carotid and right subclavian arteries behind the sternoclavicular joint.
- It usually has no branches.

Right common carotid artery
- Ascends within the carotid sheath (together with the internal jugular vein and vagus nerve) to divide at the level of C4 into the internal and external carotid arteries.

RELATIONS
- Anterior.
  - Skin, superficial fascia, sternocleidomastoid.
- Posterior.
  - Transverse processes of cervical vertebrae. Sympathetic trunk.
- Medial.
  - Pharynx, larynx, trachea, oesophagus.
- Laterally.
  - Internal jugular vein, vagus nerve (posterolateral).

Right subclavian artery
- Arches superiorly over the pleura and apex of the lung, then posterior to the midpoint of the clavicle and above the lateral border of the first rib posterior to the insertion of scalenus anterior on the rib. Following this it then becomes the axillary artery.

BRANCHES
- Vertebral.
- Internal thoracic.
- Thyrocervical.

- Costocervical.
- Dorsal scapular.

Left common carotid artery
- Second branch of aortic arch and ascends to the left behind the left sternoclavicular joint before entering the carotid sheath and dividing in the same manner and following the same course as the right common carotid.

Left subclavian artery
- Third branch of aortic arch it arches over the left lung following the same course as on the right side. It also has the same five branches as the right subclavian.

Right & left internal carotid arteries
- Main blood supply to intracranial contents and the orbit. No branches in the neck, only branching once they have entered the skull through the carotid canal in the petrous part of the temporal bone.

Right and left external carotid arteries
- Blood supply to neck, face, scalp tongue and the maxilla. Six branches are given off prior to bifurcating within the parotid gland.

Veins in the neck
As central venous access is often required in thoracic anaesthesia, an appreciation of the venous anatomy is necessary.

Internal jugular vein
- Receives blood from the brain, face and neck, beginning at the jugular foramen in the skull as a continuation of the sigmoid sinus.
- It is enclosed within the carotid sheath as it descend in the neck until it combines with the subclavian vein posterior to the medial end of the clavicle to become the Brachiocephalic vein.
  - The vein has a dilation or 'bulb' at either end.
  - Just above the distal bulb is a valve.

RELATIONS
- Anterior.
  - Skin/superficial fascia/SCM.
- Posterior.
  - Transverse processes/phrenic nerve.
- Medially.
  - Carotid artery (internal then common)/vagus nerve.

External jugular vein
- Drains the scalp and face.
- Begins behind the angle of the mandible and descends obliquely across the SCM before piercing the deep fascia just above the clavicle to drain into the subclavian vein.
  - Its size varies considerably but in an emergency it may be used as intravenous access.

Subclavian vein
- This is a continuation of the axillary vein as it drains the upper limb.
- It lies on the upper surface of the first rib in front of the subclavian artery, posterior to the clavicle.

Anatomy of lung and chest wall

Alveolar anatomy

- Terminal bronchiole → respiratory bronchioles → alveoli
- The alveolus is the main site of gas exchange
- There are between 150–400 million alveoli in the healthy adult lung
- Each alveolus is approximately 250 μm in diameter when inflated and consists of:
  - Alveolar air space
  - Alveolar wall—made up of type 1 and type 2 alveolar cells
  - Alveolar capillaries—direct contact with type 1 alveolar cells to facilitate gas exchange.

Alveolar cells

Type 1
- 40% of alveolar cells.
- 90% of the alveolar surface lining.
- Flat and thin.
- Few mitochondria and cytoplasmic organelles.
- Permit gas exchange.

Type 2
- 60% of alveolar cells.
- 10% of the alveolar surface lining.
- Rounded cells.
- Rich in mitochondria and DNA.
- Produce surfactant.
- Stem cell precursor of type 1 cells.

Anatomy of the chest wall

Skeletal anatomy
- The skeleton of the chest wall consists of the sternum, 12 pairs of ribs, costal cartilages and T1–T12 vertebral bodies.
- All ribs articulate posteriorly with the vertebral body of the relevant thoracic vertebra.

Ribs 1–7 (true ribs)
- Articulate anteriorly with the sternum via costal cartilages.

Ribs 8–10 (false ribs)
- Articulate with the costal cartilages of the 5th and 6th ribs.

Ribs 11–12 (floating ribs)
- No anterior articulation.
- Around 0.2% of the population has a cervical rib originating from C7 vertebra.

Typical ribs (ribs 3–10) consist of:
- The head
  - 2 articular surfaces with the vertebral bodies above and below via the costovertebral joints.
- The neck
  - Flat extension laterally from the head.
  - Lateral and medial tubercles lie posteriorly and articulate with the costotransverse ligament and transverse process of the vertebra.
- The angle
  - Most prominent posterior part of the rib.
- The costal groove
  - Runs inferiorly along the inside of the rib and carries the neurovascular bundle.

Atypical ribs (ribs 1, 2, 11 and 12)
- 1st rib
  - Widest and sharpest curve of all 7 true ribs.
  - Single articular surface on the head for T1 vertebra.
  - Grooves for the subclavian vessels.
- 2nd rib.
  - Tubercle for muscular attachments.
- 11th and 12th ribs.
  - Single articular surface on heads.
  - No necks or tubercles.
  - Both short and terminate in the abdominal wall.

Sternum
- The sternum forms the medial segment of the anterior chest wall
- It is around 18cm long in adults.
- Consists of:
  - The manubrium (superiorly).
  - Sternal body.
  - Xiphoid process (inferiorly).

Pleura
- Serous membrane arranged in the form of a closed invaginated sac surrounding each lung.
- Visceral pleura.
  - Covers the surface of the lung and dips into the fissures between its lobes.
- Parietal pleura.
  - Lines the inner surface of the chest wall, covers the diaphragm, and is reflected over the structures occupying the middle of the thorax.

- Different portions of the parietal pleura have nomenclature reflecting their position:
  - Costal.
  - Diaphragmatic.
  - Cervical.
  - Mediastinal.
- The two pleural layers are continuous with one another around and below the root of the lung.
- The potential space between them is known as the pleural cavity.
  - Contains approximately 10 ml of fluid representing a balance between (1) hydrostatic and oncotic forces in the visceral and parietal pleural vessels and (2) extensive lymphatic drainage.
  - Pleural effusions result from a disruption of this balance.

RELATIONS
Superiorly
- Clavicles
- Sternocleidomastoid muscles.

Laterally
- Costal cartilages of ribs 1–7
- The manubriosternal angle articulates with the 2nd costochondral cartilage.

Posteriorly
- Heart
- Trachea
- Major blood vessels (aorta, pulmonary artery, IVC, SVC).

Layers of the chest wall

From external to internal, the layers of the chest wall are:
- Skin and subcutaneous tissue
- Intercostal externus muscle
  - Inserts to the superior and inferior ribs, fibers run anteriorly from superior to inferior.
- Intercostal internus muscle
  - Inserts to superior and inferior ribs, fibers run posteriorly from superior to inferior.
- Neurovascular bundle
- Intercostal intimus muscle
- Parietal pleura

The mediastinum and lymph node stations

The mediastinum

- The mediastinum describes a group of structures in the thorax, surrounded by loose connective tissue. It is the central compartment of the thoracic cavity.
- Also described as the interpleural space.
- Contains all the thoracic viscera excluding the lungs.
- Divided into 2 parts:
  - Superior mediastinum, above the pericardium.
  - Inferior mediastinum, below the (upper) pericardium. Further divided into anterior, middle and posterior.

Relations
Anterior
- Sternum.

Posterior
- Vertebral bodies.

Inferior
- Posterior aspect of the diaphragm.

Lateral
- Pleurae.

Superior mediastinum

Relations
Anterior
- Manubrium of sternum.

Posterior
- Upper thoracic (to lower part of T4) vertebral bodies.

Inferior
- Oblique plane, from the angle of louis to the lower part of the 4th vertebral body.

CONTENTS
- Muscle
  - Sternohyoid and sternothyroid.
- Arterial
  - Aortic arch.
  - Inominate artery.
  - Left common carotid.
  - Left subclavian artery.
- Venous
  - Inominate veins.
  - SVC (upper left portion).

- Nervous
  - Vagus.
  - Phrenic.
  - Left recurrent laryngeal.
- Other
  - Trachea.
  - Oesophagus.
  - Thoracic duct.
  - Thymus remnants.
  - Lymph nodes.

Anterior mediastinum

Relations
Anterior
- Body of sternum.

Posterior
- Anterior aspect of pericardium.

Lateral
- Pleurae.
- Narrow superior aspect, widens slightly below.

CONTENTS
- Branches of the internal mammary artery.
- Loose areolar tissue.
- Lymph vessels and nodes.
  - NB. Only present on the left, due to slight deviation of the pleura from the midline.

Middle mediastinum
- Bounded by the pericardium.

CONTENTS
- Heart.
- Ascending aorta.
- Pulmonary artery and branches.
- Lower half of SVC and azygous vein.
- R+L pulmonary veins.
- Phrenic nerves.
- Trachea and bifurcation.
- R+L main bronchus.
- Bronchial lymph nodes.

Posterior mediastinum

Relations
Anterior
- Pericardium (posterior aspect).

Posterior
- Vertebral bodies T4–T12

Inferior
- Posterior aspect of diaphragm

Lateral
- Pleurae

CONTENTS
- Descending aorta
- Azygous and hemizygous veins
- Vagus and splanchnic nerves
- Oesophagus
- Thoracic duct and lymph nodes

Lymph node stations
- Mediastinal lymph node assessment is essential for staging of non-small cell carcinoma and directing treatment
- Lymph node stations are described below, and can be identified on CT and sampled by mediastinoscopy or endoscopic ultrasound with FNA
- There are 14 node stations:

SUPERIOR MEDIASTINAL NODES
- Highest mediastinal
  - Above left brachiocephalic vein.
- Upper paratracheal
  - Above aortic arch, but below brachiocephalic vein.
- Pre-vascular/pre-vertebral
  - Not adjacent to trachea
  - Either anterior to vessels (3A) or posterior to oesophagus (3P).
- Lower paratracheal
  - Below the upper level of the aortic arch to the level of the main bronchus.

AORTIC NODES
- Subaortic
  - Lateral to ligamentum arteriosum (i.e. not between the vessel and the pulmonary trunk).
- Para-aortic
  - Anterior and lateral to the arch and ascending aorta.

INFERIOR MEDIASTINAL NODES
- Subcarinal
- Para-oesophageal
- Pulmonary ligament

HILAR, INTERLOBAR, LOBAR, SEGMENTAL AND SUBSEGMENTAL NODES
- 10–14—external to the mediastinum.

Anatomy of the upper GI tract relevant to oesophageal surgery

Embryology

- Oesophagus is a foregut structure of endodermal origin.
- Developed from the primitive gut after around 16 days post-conception.
- Whole GI tract has four concentric layers.
  - Mucosa
  - Submucosa
  - Muscularis externa
  - Serosa
- The mucosa is further subdivided into epithelium, lamina propria (thin layer of connective tissue) and muscularis mucosa.

Structure & function

- Oesophagus is a smooth muscular tube connecting the oropharynx to the stomach.
- 25 to 30 cm long in the adult.
- Distance of approximately 45 cm exists between the teeth and cardia of the stomach.
- Lined with stratified squamous epithelium becoming columnar towards the gastro-oesophageal junction.
- Slight extrinsic compression can arise from the cricoid cartilage, the aorta and left main bronchus, an enlarged left atrium and the diaphragmatic hiatus.
- Divided into upper, middle and lower thirds with the gastro-oesophageal junction sometimes considered separately.
- Central sensorimotor supply is via both vagus nerves.
- Tiny contractions within the thin muscularis mucosa expel mucous from glandular crypts however, the muscularis externa contains well organized circular and longitudinal smooth muscle layers that provide peristalsis (although in the upper third striated muscle is present).
  - This is co-ordinated by the enteric nervous plexus that lies within the submucosal layer.

Blood supply & lymphatic drainage

- Upper third derives its blood supply from the inferior thyroid vessels and lymphatic drainage occurs via the deep cervical nodes.
- Middle third derives its blood supply from direct aortic branches and lymphatics drain into the mediastium.
- Lower third derives its blood supply from the left gastric vessels and lymph drains into gastric nodes.

- There is a rich sub-mucosal connection between lymphatic channels. This facilitates spread of cancer along the entire length of the oesophagus.

Relations

Anterior

- Trachea
- Recurrent laryngeal nerves
- Left main bronchus
- Left atrium and the diaphragm.

Posterior

- Vertebral bodies
- Thoracic duct (at T5)
- Hemiazygous vein
- Descending aorta
- First two intercostal arteries as direct branches of the aorta.

Lateral

- Anatomical left
  - Thoracic duct/aorta/left subclavian artery and pleura/lung
- Anatomical right
  - Azygous vein/pleural contents
- These anatomical considerations mean that low oesophageal tumours are readily approached from the left side, whereas upper lesions may be more easily reached from the right.
- Differing surgical approaches will depend to some extent upon local practice however the approach *per se* has not been shown to alter outcome.
- For benign tumours, minimally invasive resection via laparoscopy or thoracoscopy, appear to be gaining popularity.

Further reading

Moore KL, Dalley AF, (E editors.) *Clinically Orientated Anatomy*, 4th E ed. Philadelphia; Lippincott, Williams & Wilkins, 1999.

Suttie SA, Li AGK, Quinn M, Park KGM. The impact of operative approach on outcome of surgery for gastro-oesophageal tumours. *World Journal of Surgical Oncology* 2007; 5:95.

Palanivelu C, Rangarajan M, Madankumar MV, John SJ, Senthilkumar R. Minimally invasive therapy for benign tumours of the distal third of the esophagus – a single institute's experience. *Journal of Laparoendoscopic & Advanced Surgical Techniques*. 2008, 18(1):20–6.

Bronchoscopic anatomy

- Familiarity with bronchoscopic anatomy is fundamental to the practice of thoracic anaesthesia.
- There has been a reduction in anaesthesia-related morbidity and mortality since the advent of bronchoscopic confirmation of double lumen endotracheal tube placement.

Trachea

- Commences at lower end of larynx.
  - Level of C6 vertebral body.
- Bifurcates into left and right main bronchi.
  - Level of T4 vertebral body on full expiration.
  - T6 on full inspiration.
- 16–20 tracheal rings incomplete posteriorly.
  - A posterior muscle stripe can be traced to the main carina via the bronchoscope.
- Bifurcations to the left and right upper lobes and the left lower lobe DO NOT possess posterior muscle stripes.
- Average length of trachea varies between 10–15 cm
- Left-sided DLT depth (from upper incisors) for a 170 cm tall patient is 29 cm.
  - This increases or decreases by 1 cm for every 10 cm change in patient height.

Main bronchi

(See Fig. 2.2)
- Right main bronchus (RMB) arises from the trachea at the carina at a 30° angle to vertical.
  - It is 16 mm in diameter.
- Left main bronchus (LMB) arises from the trachea at the carina at a 45° angle.
  - It is 13mm in diameter.
- Hence RMB intubations/inhalations are far more common in the upright subject, i.e. it is closest to vertical.

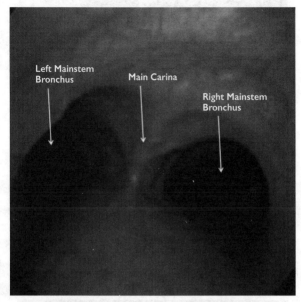

Fig. 2.2 Bronchoscopic view of the carina, right and left main bronchi.

Left main bronchus
(See Fig. 2.3)
- LMB bifurcates from the carina to supply the left upper (LUL) and left lower lobes (LLL)
  - At 6–8cm ♂.
  - At 5–6cm ♀
- LUL division also supplies the lingular lobe.

Right main bronchus
(See Fig. 2.4)
- The RMB usually gives off the bronchus to the upper lobe 2.5 cm from the carina and at 90°.
  - However, there is significant anatomical variation here.
  - In 1/250 individuals it arises directly from the trachea, while in others it arises at the level of the right middle and lower lobes.
- RMB then becomes the bronchus intermedius supplying the right middle and right lower lobes (RLL).
- RML bronchus arises from the anterior aspect of the bronchus intermedius.

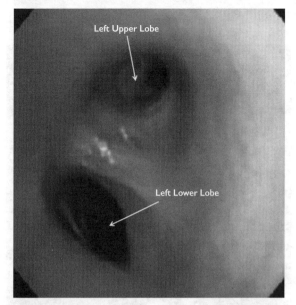

Fig. 2.3 Bronchoscopic view of the left main bronchus showing its divisions into upper and lower.

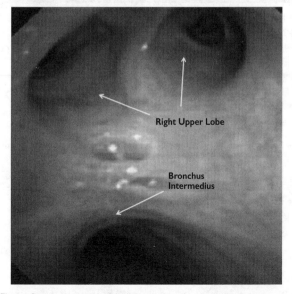

Fig. 2.4 Bronchoscopic view of the right main bronchus showing its divisions.

Bronchopulmonary segments

(See Table 2.1)

- 2nd order lobar bronchi divide into 3rd order bronchi.
- Each 3rd order bronchus supplies a bronchopulmonary segment.

Table 2.1 Bronchopulmonary segments and 3rd order bronchi

Lobe	Bronchopulmonary segment & bronchus
RUL	• Apical • Posterior • Anterior
RML	• Medial • Lateral
RLL	• Apical • Posterior basal • Anterior basal • Lateral basal • Medial basal
LUL (& lingula)	• *Apical/Posterior • Anterior • Superior lingual • Inferior lingual
LLL	• *Anterior basal/anterior medial • Posterior basal • Lateral basal • Superior

*These segments are often combined; therefore there are 8 bronchopulmonary segments on the left.

Top tips

- Orientate yourself first:
  - Tracheal rings lie anteriorly.
  - Posterior muscle stripe and cardiac pulsation.
- If you become lost, withdraw the fibrescope until you reach the carina and then re-orientate yourself.
- Practice!
- As you are scoping, ask an experienced surgeon to take you through the anatomy if you are unsure.

Epidural space

(See 🕮 Thoracic epidurals, p. 686 for discussion on epidural technique).
- The epidural space is potential space lying between the periosteum of the vertebral bodies and the dura mater of the spinal cord.
- Roughly triangular in cross-section.
- Extends from the foramen magnum to the sacral hiatus.
- The epidural space is widest posteriorly, especially in the midline, and narrows anteriorly.

Useful surface landmarks

C7 spinous process
- Vertebra prominens—most prominent spinous process in lower neck.

T7 spinous process
- At the level of inferior angle of the scapula.

L4 spinous process
- A line joining the highest points of iliac crests (Tuffier's line/Intercristal line).

Boundaries

Superior
- Foramen magnum; the meningeal and periosteal layers of the dura fuse here.

Inferior
- Sacral hiatus and sacrococcygeal membrane.

Anterior
- Vertebral bodies, intervertebral discs covered by the posterior longitudinal ligament.

Posterior (layers an epidural needle traverses in midline)
- Skin.
- Subcutaneous tissue and fat.
- Supraspinous ligament.
- Interspinous ligament.
- Ligamentum flavum:
  - Triangular in cross-section.
  - Extends between the laminae of adjacent vertebrae.
  - The distance between ligamentum flavum and dura mater decreases from lumbar to cervical regions (See Table 2.2).

Lateral
- The intervertebral foraminae and vertebral pedicles.

Table 2.2 Approximate distance between dura and ligamentum flavum

Level	Flavum-dura distance
Lower cervical	1.5–2 mm
Midthoracic	3–5 mm
Lumbar	5–7 mm

Contents of epidural space

- Fat in the form of loose areolar tissue.
- Dural sac containing the spinal cord:
  - Spinal cord terminates at L1 or L2 in 90% of adults.
  - Dural sac extends to S2.
- Spinal nerves traverse the epidural space within their dural sheaths.
- Lymphatics.
- Segmental arteries traverse the epidural space to supply the spinal cord.
- Valveless venous plexus of Bateson.
- Connective tissue.

- **❶** Increased intrathoracic and intra-abdominal pressures are transmitted into the epidural veins causing engorgement and decrease in the volume of epidural space.
- **❶** This can result in more extensive spread of local anaesthetics and increased susceptibility to needle trauma during epidural anaesthesia.

Unique features of thoracic epidurals

- Thoracic epidural space extends from lower border of C7 to upper border of L1.
- Epidural space is 3–5 mm deep in the midline and is much narrower laterally.
- Epidural pressure is negative (–1 to –9 cmH$_2$O).
  - The negative intrapleural pressure transmitted through the paravertebral spaces accounts for this.
- Ligamentum flavum is thinner than in the lumbar region.
- Thoracic vertebral laminae are broader and shorter.
- Spinous processes are close together and are angulated acutely.
  - The inferior border corresponds to the midpoint of lamina below.
- Thus, the paramedian approach is easier.

Thoracic paravertebral space

- The paraverterbral is a triangular space that lies on either side of the vertebral column.

Boundaries

Medial/base
- Vertebral body.
- Intervertebral disc.
- Intervertebral foramen.

Anterolateral.
- Parietal pleura.

Posterior
- Superior costo-transverse ligament.

Apex
- Continuous with the intercostal space.

Divisions

- The deep fascia of the thorax (endothoracic fascia) divides the thoracic paravertebral space into two compartments:
  - The anterior extrapleural paravertebral compartment
  - The posterior subendothoracic compartment.

Communications

Superior
- The paravertebral space above (cranial limit not well defined).

Inferior
- Adjacent space below (caudal limit is origin of psoas).

Medial
- Epidural space via the intervertebral foramina.

Contralateral
- Via paravertebral and epidural spread.

Contents of paravertebral space

- Fat.
- Thoracic spinal nerves:
  - The spinal nerves have no fascial sheath and divide into smaller bundles in the paravertebral space.
  - Therefore they are very susceptible to local anaesthetics.
- Intercostal vessels.
- Sympathetic trunk and the rami communicantes.

Further reading

Bromage PR. *Epidural Analgesia*. Philadelphia: WB Saunders. 1978. Chapter 2, Anatomy.

Richardson J, Groen GJ. Continuing Education in Anaesthesia Critical Care and Pain. *Applied Epidural Anatomy* 2005; 5: 99–100.

Richardson J, Lonnquist PA. Thoracic paravertebral block. *British Journal of Anaesthesia* 1998; 81: 230–8.

Neuroanatomy

The intra-thoracic contents are predominantly innervated by the autonomic nervous system, and by the vagus, phrenic and intercostal nerves.

The trachea

Sensory

● Recurrent laryngeal branch of the vagus and sympathetic branches of the middle cervical ganglion.

The tracheobronchial tree and lungs

Sensory

● Vagus and recurrent laryngeal nerves.

Motor

● Vagus → bronchoconstriction.
● Sympathetic fibres from T2 to T4 → bronchodilatation and minor vasoconstriction.

Pleura

Parietal sensory

● Phrenic (C3–5) and intercostal nerves.

Visceral sensory

● Phrenic and autonomic.

Diaphragm

Motor

● Phrenic nerve. (C3–5).

Sensory

● Phrenic nerve to the central tendon, lower thoracic nerves to muscular region.

The heart

Parasympathetic

● Cardio-inhibitor.
● The vagus innervates the nodal tissue and atrial musculature.

Sympathetic
- Cardio-accelerator fibres T1–T4.
- Cervical and upper thoracic ganglia give rise to superficial and deep cardiac plexi which are distributed alongside the coronary arteries to supply:
  - Myocardium.
  - Coronary arteries.
  - Conducting system of the heart.

Sensory
- Phrenic nerve (C3–5) supplies the pericardium.

Intercostal nerves
- Each spinal nerve has dorsal and ventral roots which join and then divide into dorsal and ventral rami.
- The intercostal nerves are derived from the ventral primary rami of T1 to T11 spinal nerves.
- The dorsal rami supply the extensor muscles and skin of the back.

Course
- After emerging from the intervertebral foramen, the ventral rami have small branches that communicate with the sympathetic ganglia (rami communicantes).
- The nerve passes posteriorly and then below the intercostal artery to run in the subcostal groove of the rib, lying between the innermost and internal intercostal muscle layers.

Innervation
- Sensory innervation to parietal pleura.
- Collateral branch arises at the angle of the rib.
- Lateral cutaneous branch arises at the mid-axillary line and supplies the skin and muscles of the posterolateral thorax and abdomen via anterior and posterior branches.
- Anterior cutaneous branch continues to the anterior chest wall to supply the skin and muscles of the anterior thorax and upper abdomen.
- The 1st intercostal nerve has no lateral or anterior cutaneous branches and supplies the lower part of the brachial plexus.
- The 2nd intercostal nerve gives rise to the intercostobrachial nerve which supplies the medial upper arm sensation.
- The 3rd to 6th intercostal nerves supply the muscles and skin of the thorax.
- The 7th to 11th intercostal nerves pass under the costal margin and supply the muscles and skin of the abdomen.

Sympathetic nervous system
Course
- The sympathetic trunk arises from the lateral horn of the thoraco-lumbar vertebrae.
  - Distribution is T1–L2.

- The trunk lies 2–3 cm lateral to the vertebral column.
- The trunk descends in the neck behind the carotid sheath and enters the thorax anterior to th e neck of the first rib.
- It passes over the head of the upper ribs and overlies the side of the lower four thoracic vertebrae.

Sympathetic ganglia
- Cervical ganglia.
- Stellate ganglion.
- Thoracic ganglia.
- Lumbar ganglia.
- Sacral ganglia.

Visceral innervation
- Cardiac plexus.
  - Deep cardiac plexus lies in front of the tracheal bifurcation.
  - Superficial cardiac plexus lies anterior to the pulmonary artery and under the aortic arch.
- Coeliac plexus.
- Hypogastric plexus.
- Acetylcholine is the neurotransmitter at the ganglia and the adrenal medulla.
- Norepinephrine is the neurotransmitter at the postganglionic nerve endings (except for sweat glands).

Further reading

Erdmann A. *Concise Anatomy for Anaesthesia*. Cambridge: Cambridge University Press; 2007.

Snell RS. *Clinical neuroanatomy for medical students*. 4th ed. Philadelphia: Lippincott-Raven; 1997.

Ellis H, Feldman S. *Anatomy for anaesthetists*. 7th ed. Oxford: Blackwell Scientific Publications; 1996.

Basic pharmacology for thoracic anaesthesia

Pre-medication

Pre-medication, pharmacological preparations given before surgery should be individually tailored according to the patient's anxiety, pre-existing pathology and nature of the planned surgery. For thoracic surgery pre-medication may be particularly important for short, highly stimulating procedures (bronchoscopy) and for patients with high reflux potential.

Objectives of pre-medication include:

- Anxiolysis
- Antacids (particularly oesophageal/anti-reflux surgery)
- Antisialogogue—dry secretions (bronchoscopy), sedation, anti-emesis
- Anti-autonomic (obtund response to intubation/rigid bronchoscopy)
- Analgesia
- Anti-emesis
- Amnesia

Anxiolytics

Aim

- Relieve psychological distress such that a calm, compliant and cardiovascularly stable patient arrives in the anaesthetic room.
- Provide amnesia.

Pitfalls

- Incorrect dose.
- Incorrect timing of dose.
- Inter-patient variability of required dose.
- Elderly may be very sensitive → apnoea (10–77%), un-responsiveness and delayed recovery.
- Care in COPD patients as risk of apnoea and desaturation (decreases response to hypercapnoea).

Patients given an adequate explanation of the anaesthetic process during the preoperative visit may experience less anxiety.

Suggested regime

- **Diazepam**
  - 5–10 mg PO 1 hour pre-op.

Or
- **Temazepam**
  - 10–20 mg PO 1 hour pre-op.

Or
- **Lorazepam**
  - 1–2 mg PO 2 hours pre-op.

If necessary these doses can be given the night before surgery and then repeated on the morning of surgery.

Antacids

Aim

- Minimize the risk of intra and post operative aspiration of caustic gastric contents, with the hope of minimizing post-operative pneumonitis.
- The thoracotomy position predisposes to reflux and risk of aspiration.
- Patients undergoing thoracotomy as part of surgery for gastro-esophageal disease are at particular risk of reflux.

Pitfalls

- Poor absorption.
- Mis-timing of dose.
- Inadequate duration of treatment (PPIs do not act immediately).
- Aspiration risk is NOT eradicated completely!

Suggested regime

Oral
- **Lansoprazole**
  - 30 mg night before surgery and 30 mg 2 hr pre-op.
Or
- **Ranitidine**
  - 150 mg night before surgery and 150 mg 2 hr pre-op..

IV
- **Omeprazole**
  - 40 mg night before surgery and 40 mg 2 hr pre-op.
Or
- **Ranitidine**
  - 50 mg night before surgery and 50 mg 2 hr pre-op.

Anti-sialogogues

Now rarely used.

Aim

- Dry secretions prior to instrumentation procedures e.g. bronchoscopy (Atropine++/hyoscine++/glycopyrolate+++).
- Bronchodilatation (Atropine++/glycopyrolate+++/Hyoscine+).
- Sedation (hyoscine+++ atropine ++/Glycopyrolate+).
- Anti-emesis (hyoscine+++/atropine++/Glycopyrolate+).

Pitfalls

- Secretions can become excessively viscid causing airway plugging.
- Anticholinergic side effects such as dry mouth, retention of urine and blurred vision can be unpleasant.

- Atropine/hyoscine can cause confusion in the elderly as it crosses the BBB and causes excessive sedation.
- Hyoscine and atropine can be antanalgesic.
- Excessive tachycardia. Care in those with IHD.

Suggested regime

- **Atropine.**
  - 5–10 mcg/kg IM 60 mins pre-op.
  - 5–10 mcg/kg IV 5 mins prior to instrumentation.

Or

- **Glycopyrolate** (not licensed for control of secretions).
  - 4–5 mcg/kg (max 400 mcg) IV 3 mins prior to start.

Anti-autonomic

Aim

- Reduce excessive circulating catecholamines preoperatively.
- Obtund CVS response to intubation/instrumentation of the airway.
- Minimize haemodynamic instability in patients with IHD.

Pitfalls

- Timing and variability of this effect cannot be relied upon.
- Drugs have variable onset/offset.
- Tendency to cause bradycardias.

Suggested regime

Although a variety of β blockers are available opiates are usually used and are described below.

Analgesia

Aim

- Provision of pre-emptive pain relief, particularly for patients undergoing short, stimulating thoracic procedures.
- N.B.—most patients undergoing thoracotomy will receive a combination of short acting opioid IV and placement of an epidural catheter for intra and post-op analgesia rendering pre-med analgesia unnecessary.
- Analgesia is given if the patient is in pain pre-operatively and a combination of opioid and simple analgesia should be titrated to effect.

Pitfalls

- Opiates may lead to undesired prolonged apnoea. Care in particular with remifentanil!
- Remifentanil can cause rapid and profound bradycardia.
- Wooden chest is rare but can be cumbersome if jet ventilating!

Suggested regime

- **Alfentanil**
  - 10 mcg/kg IV 90 sec prior to intubation/instrumentation.
Or
- **Fentanyl**
  - 1 mcg/kg IV 2–4 mins prior to intubation/instrumentation.
Or
- **Remifentanil**
  - 1 mcg/kg IV 1–2 mins prior to intubation/instrumentation.

Prevention of bradycardia

- Patients can receive vagolytic pre-medication as a means of preventing bradycardias at induction and during bronchoscopy.
- The route and timing of the administration however, mean an effective dose to prevent bradycardia may not be reached at the correct time.
- Bradycardia is better treated at anaesthetic/operation with faster acting intravenous vagolytics.

Anti-emetics

- Routine provision of anti-emetics pre-operatively is rare.
- These drugs can be given at the start of anaesthesia, to take effect for the post-op period.
- Dexamethasone should be considered for selected patients.
- Can cause burning/pain in groin if given awake or too rapidly. Cheap and effective drug.
- 8 mg IV given at the start of induction.

Further reading

Cucchiara S. *British National Formulary*. 55th ed. March 2008.

Agnew NM, Kendall JB, Akrofi M, *et al.* Gastroesophageal reflux and tracheal aspiration in the thoracotomy position: should ranitidine premedication be routine. *Anaesthesia and Analgesia.* 2002; 95: 1645–9.

Levack ID, Bowie RA, Braid DP, *et al.* Comparison of the effect of two dose schedules of oral omeprazole with oral ranitidine on gastric aspirate pH and volume in patients undergoing elective surgery. *British. Journal of Anaesthesia.* 1996; 76: 567–9.

Bronchodilators

β_2 agonists

Mechanism of action

- Stimulation of bronchiolar smooth muscle β_2-adrenergic receptors → ↑ intracellular (cAMP) → bronchodilatation.

Uses

- Acute asthma/bronchospasm.
- COPD.

System effects

- RS
  - ↑ PEFR and FEV_1.
  - Directly inhibit antigen-induced release of histamine and Slow Releasing Substance of Anaphylaxis from mast cells.
  - Attenuation of hypoxic pulmonary vasoconstriction → ↑ shunt and therefore oxygen should be co-administered to avoid hypoxaemia.
- CVS
  - High doses—β_1 effects predominate → positive inotropy & chronotropy
  - Low dose—β_2 effects predominate → SVR and ↓ diastolic BP.
- GI
  - Raises plasma glucose/fatty acid concentration → ↑ insulin secretion → ↓ plasma K^+.

Toxicity/side effects

- Anxiety.
- Insomnia.
- Tremor.
- Sweating.
- Palpitations.
- Tachycardia.
- Ketosis.
- Headache.
- Hypokalaemia.

Salbutamol

Dose

- 200–400 mcg (1–2 puffs)/INH/QDS.
- 2.5–5 mg/NEB/QDS.
- 0.5 mg/IM, SC/4Hrly.
- 0.5 mcg/kg/min/IV.

- Sympathomimetic amine.
- Onset 15 minutes lasts up to 4 hrs.
- Potentiates action of NDMR.
- x3 normal nebulized dose may be jetted down ET tube in at least 0.5ml diluents.

Terbutaline

Dose

- 0.25–0.5 mcg/INH/4Hrly.
- 2–5 mg/NEB/TDS.
- 0.25–0.5 mg/SC, IM, IV/ QDS.
- 1–5 mcg/min/IV/for 8–10 hrs.

Salmeterol

- Long acting β_2 agonist (duration of action approximately 12 hrs).
- Not useful in acute asthma attack due to relatively long onset of action.

Anticholinergics

Ipratroprium Bromide

Mechanism of action
- Competitive inhibition of cholinergic receptors on bronchial smooth muscle → antagonism of bronchoconstictor action of vagal efferent impulses.
- May also reduce mast cell degranulation by blocking cholinergic receptors.

Uses
- Chronic asthma (not acute).
- COPD (particularly chronic bronchitis).
- Onset 2 hrs, lasts 4–6hrs.

Dose

- 100–500 mcg/INH, NEB/QDS.

System effects
- CVS.
  - IV administration → ↑HR, ↑BP, ↑CO.
- RS
  - Bronchodilatation.

Phosphodiesterase inhibitors

Aminophylline

Mechanism of action

- Phosphodiesterase inhibitor—inhibits the breakdown of cAMP → ↑ intracellular (cAMP) → bronchodilatation.
- Synergistic effect with catecholamines that directly activate adenylate cyclase.
- Also interferes with influx of calcium ions into smooth muscle cells → bronchodilatation and stabilizes mast cells.

Uses

- Acute asthma.
- COPD.
- Heart failure.

System effects

- CVS
  - It has weak positive inotropic and chronotropic effects → ↑ CO and → SVR. It is arrythmogenic at upper extremes of the therapeutic range.
  - Decrease LVEDP (useful in acute heart failure) and PCWP.
- RS
  - Bronchodilatation, ↑ VC.
  - Sensitizes respiratory centre to CO_2.
  - ↑ diaphragmatic contractility.
  - Attenuation of hypoxic pulmonary vasoconstriction → ↑ shunt and therefore oxygen should be co-administered to avoid hypoxaemia.
- CNS
  - CNS stimulant lowering seizure threshold in epileptics.
- GU
  - ↑ renal blood flow and GFR → diuresis/kaleuresis → hypokalaemia (can be severe as also ↑ cellular uptake of K^+).

Toxicity/side effects

- GI disturbance.
- CNS disturbance (including convulsions).
- Cardiac dysrhythmias.

Special points

- Co-administration of drugs that inhibit cytochrome P450 enzymes such as barbiturates, alcohol and phenytoin will reduce the plasma concentration of aminophylline.
- Conversely drugs such as cimetidine, propanolol and erythromycin will elevate the plasma concentration of the drug.
- May speed onset of recovery from desflurane anaesthesia.

Dose

- 900 mg/PO/OD in 2–3 divided doses.
- 5 mg/kg/IV loading dose over 10–15 minutes.
- 0.5 mg/kg/hr maintenance infusion

- ❶Extreme caution during administration of loading dose to patients taking oral aminophylline as possesses very narrow therapeutic window.

Steroids (see 📖 Steroids, p. 68)

- Used for both acute exacerbations and maintenance therapy of patients with asthma and COPD because of their anti-inflammatory and membrane stabilising effects.
- Beclomethasone, budesonide and fluticasone are synthetic steroids commonly used in metered dose inhalers.
- IV hydrocortisone or methylprednisolone are used acutely for severe attacks.
- Usually require several hours to become effective.

Magnesium (see 📖 Magnesium, p. 64)

- BTS guidelines recommend a single dose of 1.2–2 g IV magnesium over 20 minutes for patients with acute severe asthma who have not responded to initial bronchodilator therapy, or have life threatening or near fatal asthma
- Multi-factorial effects of the Magnesium ion at a cellular level bring about bronchodilatation. It acts as a physiological antagonist of calcium and inhibits smooth muscle contraction
- Magnesium may also have a role in inhibiting mast cell degranulation, thus reducing inflammatory mediators such as histamine, thromboxanes, and leukotrienes
- It also inhibits the release of acetylcholine from motor nerve terminals and depresses the excitability of muscle fibre membranes.

Isoprenaline

- Can be used in acute asthma.
- Synthetic catecholamine with β adrenergic action.
- Potent bronchodilator → ↑ anatomical dead space → V/Q mismatch and potential decrease O_2 saturation if FiO_2 is not increased in conjunction with administration.
- Also inhibits SRSA and histamine release.
- ↑ inotropicity and ↑ chronotropicity and can ↓ BP.
- Can cause hyperglycaemia, angina, and dysrhythmias.

Dose
- 30mg/INH/TDS.
- 0.5–8mcg min-1/IV/Titrated to response.

Epinephrine
- Can be used in acute asthma.
- Nebulized formulation can cause increased viscosity of bronchial secretions.
- ↑ RR, ↑ Vt and potent bronchodilator.
- Obvious side effects of tachycardia and ↑ BP/arrhythmias.
- x3 normal nebulized dose may be jetted down ET tube in at least 0.5 ml diluent volume.

Dose
- 0.5 ml/kg of 1:1000 solution or 10–20 metered doses/NEB/Titrated to response.

Other agents
The bronchodilatory effects of ketamine and inhalational anaesthetics (halothane, sevoflurane) have also been utilized in certain cases of resistant bronchospasm.

Further reading
British National Formulary 2008. **56**: Royal Pharmaceutical Society, London (UK).

Leukotriene receptor antagonists

- Cysteinyl leukotrienes are synthesized from arachidonic acid via a pathway catalysed by 5-lipoxygenase enzyme within pro inflammatory cells such as eosinophils and mast cells.

Mechanism of action

Leukotrienes → bronchial smooth muscle $CysLT_1$ receptors → microvascular leakage + bronchoconstriction + eosinophil recruitment.

- Leukotriene receptor antagonists (LTRA) interrupt the pro-inflammatory effects of leukotrienes by inhibiting their effects at the above receptors, and thus have a role in prevention of asthma triggered by these mediators.

Uses

- Preventative therapy in Asthma:
  - As a single agent.
  - Additive effect when used together with inhaled steroids.
- Prevention of exercise induced asthma.
- Treatment of rhinitis.
- Less effective in patients with more severe or unstable asthma who are on high doses of other drugs (i.e. inhaled β_2—agonists, oral corticosteroids).
- Examples:
  - Montelukast.
  - Zafirlukast.

Toxicity/side effects

- Palpitations, bleeding disorders, thrombocytopaenia, oedema.
- Respiratory tract infection.
- Gastro-intestinal upset, dry mouth, excessive thirst, cholestasis, derangement of LFT's, hepatitis.
- CNS disturbance (dizziness, sleep disturbance, hallucinations, seizures).
- Arthralgia, polymyalgia, Churg Strauss Syndrome (see below).
- Allergy (inc. anaphylaxis, angioedema, cutaneous reactions).

Dose

- Montelukast.
  - 10 mg/PO/OD nocté.
- Zafirlukast
  - 20 mg/PO/BD.

Churg Strauss Syndrome (CSS)

- Might very rarely be precipitated by the use of LTRA.
- Especially in patients who have recently reduced or stopped oral corticosteroids.
- CSS is a systemic vasculitic disorder characterized by:
  - Asthma.
  - Systemic eosinophilia (often >10%).
  - Rhinitis and sinusitis.
  - Granulomatous skin lesions.
  - Poly and mononeuropathy.
  - Pulmonary infiltrates.
  - Cardiac and pulmonary complications tend to be more prominent than renal involvement.
- Treatment is with corticosteroids and in severe cases cytotoxic agents such as cyclophosphamide.
- Five year survival, if treated with corticosteroids, is 25%.

❶ Patients receiving LTRAs should be monitored for development of eosinophilia, vasculitic rash, worsening asthma symptoms and peripheral neuropathy.

Further reading

Joos S, Miksch A, Szecsenyi J, Wieseler B, Grouven U, Kaiser T, Schneider A. Montelukast as add-on therapy to inhaled corticosteroids in the treatment of mild to moderate asthma: a systematic review. *Thorax* 2008 63: 453–62.

Keogh KA, Specks U. Churg-Strauss syndrome. *Semin Respiratory Critical Care Medicine*. 2006 27: 148–57.

Magnesium

4th most common cation in the body, 2nd most common intracellular cation.

Normal physiology

- Essential co-factor in over 300 enzyme systems within the body.
- Physiological calcium antagonist.
- Stores:
  - 53% in bone.
  - 27% in muscle.
  - 19% in soft tissues.
- Present in serum 62% ionized, 33% protein bound to albumin and 5% associated with anions in plasma.
- Estimated average magnesium requirement 200 magnesium ♀, 250 magnesium ♂.
- Absorption is variable (roughly 25–65% absorbed) predominantly from colon and ileum.
- Excretion occurs via the kidney:
  - Aldosterone increases renal excretion.
  - PTH decreases renal excretion, whilst enhancing gut absorption of magnesium.

Measurement

- Notoriously inaccurate. One off serum measurements only indicated during acute setting and for monitoring magnesium therapy
- Normal range, 0.76–1.06mmol^{-1}. Normal 24hour urinary excretion, 3.6mmol ♀, 4.8mmol ♂.

Physiological effects of magnesium

CVS

- Direct Depression of myocardial contractility.
- Prolongs SA node conduction time, PR interval and AV node refractory period.
- Catecholamine receptor blockade.
- Inhibition of catecholamine release from adrenal medulla.
- Coronary artery vasodilatation.
- Reduced pulmonary and peripheral vascular resistance attenuates HPV.
- Required for the inotropic effects of adrenaline.

CNS

- Antagonizes release of pre-synaptic calcium → reduction of Ach release at the neuro-muscular junction.
- Decreases excitability of muscles and nerves.

- Decreased deep tendon reflexes (used to monitor treatment/ infusions).
- Suppresses epileptic activity.
- Reverses cerebral vasospasm.

RS
- Respiratory muscle depression.
- Bronchodilatation.

GIT
- Osmotic laxative.

Haematological
- Prolongs clotting time, decreases thromboxane B_2 synthesis and inhibits thrombin induced platelet aggregation.

Common causes of hypomagnesaemia
(See Table 3.1)

Table 3.1 Causes of low magnesium

Cause	Condition
Decreased intake	Dietary deficiency
	Malabsorption
	Inappropriate IV infusion
Intrinsic renal loss	Drug induced
	Bartters syndrome
	Intrinsic renal failure
	Hyperaldosteronism
	Other electrolyte imbalances
Extra renal loss	G.I losses
Redistribution	Primary hyperparathyroidism
	Insulin administration
	Excessive citrated blood transfusion

Manifestations of hypomagnesaemia
- Low magnesium may occur in up to 68% of ICU population.
- Commonly co-exists with hypocalcaemia/hypokalaemia and impairs release of PTH.
- Hypocalcaemia accompanying hypomagnesaemia inhibits normal release of PTH. Thus, administration of magnesium not only combats hypomagnesaemia, but also synergistically allows PTH release to combat the accompanying hypocalcaemia.
- The various clinical manifestations are shown (See Table 3.2).

Table 3.2 Manifestations of low magnesium

System	Manifestation
CVS	Hypertension
	Angina
	Dysrhythmias
	Torsades de pointes
	Re-entry tachycardia
	VT/VF
	ECG Changes
	Prolonged PR/QT
CNS	Psychiatric disturbance
	Convulsion
	Coma
	Myoclonus
	Tetany
RS	Stridor
GI	Dysphagia
Electrolytes	Hypocalcaemia
	Hypokalaemia

▶▶ Uses in thoracic anaesthesia

❶ Patients presenting with oesophageal tumours, Barrett's disease, and other upper G.I related diseases may have low Mg^{2+} levels due to chronic malabsorption/malnutrition/alcoholism. Always check Mg^{2+} levels pre-op.

Anti-arrhythmic
- Via calcium channel blocking effect, regulation of intracellular potassium and generation of ATP. Particularly useful in treatment of torsades de pointes.
- Dose
  - 2g/IV—over 10–15min.

❶ Mg^{2+} blunts the chronotropic (and vasoconstrictor) effect of adrenaline.

Vasodilator
- Decreases vascular tone. Blunts response of vessels to vasoconstrictors like noradrenaline and angiotensin II.
- Dose.
  - 30mg/kg/IV.

- Useful agent to decrease PA pressure during OLV and in cases with pulmonary hypertension.

Acute bronchospasm

- The increased IgE leads to increased intracellular calcium. This in turn causes histamine release; therefore administration of Mg^{2+} counters this effect.
- Dose.
  - 2g/IV—over 10–15min.

Suppression of suxamethonium pains

- A single dose of Mg2+ preceding suxamethonium may reduce K^+ release and reduce severity of muscle pain.
- Dose.
  - 40mg/kg/IV.

▶▶ Anaesthesia and the hypomagnesaemic patient

- Be vigilant, other electrolytes may be deranged.
- Avoid magnesium infusions in patients with AV block, myasthenia gravis (thymectomy) or muscular dystrophies.
- Hypomagnesaemia will exacerbate arrhythmias in those with pre-existing cardiovascular disease (common in the thoracic population).
- Standard drugs and pre-medicants are fine.
- Stridor is more common on manipulation of the airway (during rigid or flexible bronchoscopy in particular).
- Avoid hyperventilation as it shifts magnesium intracellularly; further amplifying hypomagnesaemia.
- Magnesium potentiates non-depolarizing neuromuscular blockade; particularly rocuronium. Therefore, reduce doses.
- When used with nifedipine (particularly patients with pulmonary hypertension) as an anti-hypertensive therapy, neuromuscular blockade may be profoundly prolonged.
- Suxamethonium is not potentiated. Plasma cholinesterase may be induced by magnesium.
- Twitch response may be reduced with no fade.
- May obtund HPV response to one lung ventilation. Unlikely to be of physiological significance in the fit patient.

Further reading

Watson VF, Vaughan RS. Magnesium and the anaesthetist. British Journal of Anaesthesia. *Continuing Education in Anaesthesia, Critical Care & Pain.* 2001; 1:16–21.

Fawcett WJ, Haxby EJ. Magnesium : physiology and pharmacology. *British Journal of Anaesthesia.* 1999; 83:302–20.

Steroids

Normal physiology

- Endogenous steroid hormones, i.e. mineralo- and glucocorticoids, are secreted by the adrenal cortex.
- Mineralocorticoid (aldosterone) secretion is controlled by the renin-angiotensin-aldosterone (RAA) system, the hypothalamic-pituitary-adrenal (HPA) axis, and changes in plasma Na^+/K^+. Aldosterone is responsible for water and electrolyte balance.
- Glucocorticoid (cortisol) secretion is controlled by the HPA axis via a negative feedback loop. Cortisol is responsible for carbohydrate and protein metabolism.
- Synthetic steroids show a much clearer separation of action especially the glucocorticoid, anti-inflammatory and immunosupressive actions.
- In a normal individual there is a daily secretion of 30mg of cortisol. In response to minor surgery there is a minimal increase in cortisol secretion (50mg) and a 2 to 3-fold increase (75–100mg) after major surgery.

Mode of action

- Lipid soluble steroid crosses cell membrane → binds to intracellular cytoplasmic/nuclear receptor → nuclear DNA exposed → RNA polymerase activation → production of mRNA ►► Protein synthesis. The new proteins formed are the effectors.

Glucocorticoids

Main actions
- Anti-inflammatory.
- Immunosupressive.
- Analgesic.
- Anti-emetic.

Common pre-operative indications
- Replacement in adrenocortical deficiency states.
- Interstitial lung disease.
- Numerous auto-immune diseases.
- Chemotherapy regimes.
- Asthma and chronic obstructive airways disease.
- Hypercalcaemia.
- Immunosuppression after organ transplantation.

Peri-operative considerations
Long term steroid therapy is associated with the following:
- Adrenocortical suppression.
- Hypertension.
- Obesity, diabetes, adrenal suppression, hypokalaemia.

- Proximal myopathy.
- Peptic ulceration, pancreatitis.
- Immuno-suppression.
- Poor wound healing.
- Depression, euphoria, psychosis.

Peri-operative steroid replacement

- Steroid therapy can cause suppression of the HPA axis with secondary adrenocortical insufficiency. These patients may develop post-operative complications related to an impaired stress response if steroid replacement is insufficient.
- Replacement should be considered in those on long-term corticosteroids via the oral, inhaled, topical or parenteral routes at a dose of >10 mg prednisolone daily (or equivalent; See Table 3.3). Patients who have stopped steroids at this dose within 3 months of surgery should be included also.
- (Table 3.4) summarizes peri-operative steroid replacement.

Features of acute adrenocortical insufficiency

- Malaise.
- Hypotension; patients remain refractory to usual therapies.
- Confusion.
- Fever.
- Severe abdominal pain.
- Weakness & tiredness.
- Hypokalaemia.
- Hypoglycaemia.

Table 3.3 Corticosteroid doses equivalent to Prednisolone 10mg

Steroid	Dose
Betamethasone	1.5mg
Cortisone acetate	50mg
Deflazacort	12mg
Dexamethasone	1.5mg
Hydrocortisone	40mg
Methylprednisolone	8mg
Triamcinolone	8mg

Table 3.4 Peri-operative steroid replacement regime for a patient taking >10 mg prednisolone or equivalent daily

	Minor surgery	Moderate surgery	Major surgery
Pre-operative	Usual steroid dose	Usual steroid dose	Usual steroid dose
Induction	Hydrocortisone 25 mg IV	Hydrocortisone 25 mg IV	Hydrocortisone 50 mg IV
Post-operative	Usual dose	Hydrocortisone 25 mg IV TDS for 24 hours	Hydrocortisone 50 mg IV TDS for 48–72 hours
		Recommence pre-operative steroid	Maintain IV replacement until light diet and normal pre-operative steroid recommenced

Further reading

Davies M, Hardman J. Anaesthesia and adrenocortical disease. *Continuing Education in Anaesthesia, Critical Care & Pain.* 2005; 5(4):122–6.

Nitric oxide

Endogenous nitrous oxide (NO) mediates vascular smooth muscle cell relaxation. When inhaled, NO has been shown to be an effective and selective pulmonary vasodilator with few systemic effects.

Uses

- Hypoxaemia in infants secondary to pulmonary hypertension, particularly associated with congenital disease.
- Severe acute respiratory distress syndrome (ARDS):
  - Inhaled NO selectively produces pulmonary vasodilatation and improves systemic oxygenation.
  - However, there is currently no evidence of improvements in mortality or duration of mechanical ventilation in this context.
- Prediction of response to vasodilator treatment in patients with pulmonary hypertension.
- Acute right heart failure 2° pulmonary hypertension:
  - NO inhalation can reduce RV afterload and improve its function during cardiopulmonary bypass.
  - Post-operative pulmonary hypertension is a cause of early death following cardiac transplantation.
  - It may also be used in the treatment of RV dysfunction following the placement of a LV assist device.

Mechanism of action and effects

- Synthesized from L- arginine by endothelial nitric oxide synthetase
- Intracellular 2nd messenger.
- Mediates vascular smooth muscle relaxation by increasing levels of intracellular cyclic GMP, which influences intracellular calcium.
- Rapidly inactivated by combining with oxyhaemoglobin to produce methaemoglobin and nitrate (NO_3^-) or binding with oxygen to form nitrite (NO_2^-). Methaemoglobin is subsequently reduced and the nitrates and nitrites undergo urinary excretion.

Administration

IVI

- Drugs that generate NO, e.g. sodium nitroprusside, glyceryl trinitrate are used as vasodilators in the treatment of hypertension and ischaemic heart disease.
- Such compounds can also be used in the treatment of pulmonary hypertension. However their efficacy is limited by systemic hypotension. These drugs can also cause pulmonary ventilation/perfusion mismatching, leading to arterial hypoxaemia.

Inhaled

- Inhaled NO causes a dose-dependent reduction in pulmonary artery pressure and pulmonary vascular resistance.

- Dose
  - 0.5–20 ppm—must have a scavenging system.
- NO has an intravascular half-life of only seconds.
- Abrupt discontinuation of inhaled NO should be avoided, as this can result in "rebound" pulmonary hypertension, causing a reduction in cardiac output and systemic hypotension.

Special note

- NO rapidly reacts with oxygen to form gaseous NO_2, which is highly irritant. Therefore, NO is stored in an inert gas such as nitrogen.
- Delivery of NO to the patient must ensure that NO exposure to oxygen is minimized.
- Equipment is available which permits safe administration of NO to both intubated and non-intubated patients.
- Continuous monitoring of NO and NO_2 levels must take place, as well as measurement of methaemoglobinaemia levels. Adjust the dose of inhaled NO accordingly.

Epoprostenol

Epoprostenol (prostacyclin, PGI2) is a metabolite of arachidonic acid metabolism, and is a potent vasodilator. It has an immediate onset of action, and has a half-life of approximately 5 minutes.

Uses

- Severe idiopathic pulmonary hypertension (New York Heart Association (NYHA) Class III and IV). Intravenous administration associated with:
  - Improvement in life expectancy is comparable to transplantation
  - Improved haemodynamics, 6 minute walk time, and quality of life.
- ARDS:
  - Equivalent improvement in oxygenation as NO, but there is no improvement in clinical outcome.
- Anti-coagulation, e.g. extracorporeal circuit for renal dialysis.
- Prediction of response to vasodilator treatment in patients with pulmonary hypertension.

Mechanism of action and effects

- Increases intracellular cyclic AMP.
- Potent pulmonary and systemic vasodilator.
- Most potent inhibitor of platelet aggregation.
- Inhibition of smooth muscle proliferation. This latter effect may have implications for beneficial remodeling of the pulmonary vascular bed.

Administration

IV

- 5 ng/kg/min via central venous catheter or extracorporeal circulation.
- Effects may persist for 30 minutes following cessation of infusion.

Inhaled

- 50 ng/kg/min delivered by jet nebulizer.

Alternative therapies

Iloprost

- Prostacyclin analogue commonly used in the UK for the treatment of pulmonary hypertension
- Administered via a Hickman line, or as nebulized therapy
- Short half-life 6 patients need to administer the nebulizer up to 6–9 times per day.

Trepostinil

- Prostacyclin analogue.
- Can be infused subcutaneously into the abdomen, thighs or arms.
- Pain at infusion site can be problematic.

NO vs. Epoprostenol in thoracic anaesthesia

- A recent randomized trial found no difference in cardiorespiratory. parameters when inhaled NO was compared to inhaled prostacyclin in patients who had undergone heart and lung transplant.
- However, inhaled prostacyclin does not require the same degree of monitoring as NO does.

Further reading

Khan TA, Schnickel G, Ross D, et al. A prospective, randomized, crossover pilot study of inhaled nitric oxide versus inhaled prostacyclin in heart transplant and lung transplant recipients. *Journal of Thoracic and Cardiovascular Surgery* 2009; 138(6):1417–24.

Surfactant

- A group of phospholipids and proteins produced by type II pneumocytes from approximately 24 weeks gestation.
- Surfactant decreases alveolar surface tension, thereby increasing lung compliance.
- The reduction in alveolar surface tension by surfactant is greatest at lower alveolar volumes. As an alveolus expands surface tension increases and the rate of alveolar expansion decreases. This is explained by the surfactant phospholipid molecules being pulled away from one another, thus reducing their ability to decrease surface tension.
- Surface tension encourages the movement of free water across cell membranes and this is limited by the presence of surfactant.
- Deficiency of surfactant contributes to the respiratory distress syndrome seen in pre-term neonates and may have a role in Adult Respiratory Distress Syndrome (ARDS).

Surfactant and COPD

- Patients with COPD have been noted in some studies to have lower level of phospholipoproteins in broncho-alveolar washings than healthy controls.
- Surfactant proteins in serum such as surfactant protein D (SPD) have been suggested as possible biomarkers in the monitoring of COPD.

Surfactant and ARDS

- Surfactant deficiency may contribute to hypoxia, poor lung compliance and high airway pressures in ARDS. This may be mediated by reduced production or by inactivation by serum proteins and inflammatory mediators present in the alveolus.
- Endogenous surfactant administration has not been demonstrated to reduce mortality in ARDS although it may improve oxygenation.

Surfactant and lung transplantation

- Administration of bovine surfactant has been demonstrated in small trials to improve oxygenation and decrease primary graft dysfunction in recipients.
- It can be administered to the donor before harvesting, or to the recipient intra- or post-operatively.

Administration of surfactant

- Surfactant replacement therapy is typically in the form of a preparation of porcine or bovine lung extracts; artificial surfactants have been used in trials but are not currently available in the UK.
- It is currently only licensed for use in respiratory distress syndrome in neonates.
- Surfactant is aerosolized and administered via the endotracheal tube
- ⚠ Caution must be taken to avoid hyperoxaemia or volutrauma as improvements in lung compliance may be rapid and dramatic.

Further reading

De Perrot M, Mingyao L, Waddell T, Keshavjee S. Ischemia–Reperfusion–induced Lung Injury. *American Journal of Respiratory and Critical Care Medicine* 2003; 167:490–511.

Kesecioglu J, Beale R, Stewart T, et al. Exogenous natural surfactant for treatment of acute lung injury and the acute respiratory distress syndrome. *American Journal of Respiratory and Critical Care Medicine* 2009; 180:989–94.

Davidson WJ, Dorscheid C, Spragg R, et al. Exogenous pulmonary surfactant for the treatment of adult patients with acute respiratory distress syndrome: results of a meta-analysis. http://ccforum.com/content/10/2/R41 (Accessed 6/3/10).

Volatile agents

Specific volatile usage in thoracic anaesthesia

- Halothane and enflurane have been superseded by agents with a more preferable side effect profile.
- Isoflurane remains the cheapest option but is very irritant to the airways. During prolonged anaesthesia/upper airway instrumentation, this may result in prolonged respiratory depression or excessive coughing.
- Sevoflurane offers the most cardio-stable anaesthetic, and permits relatively rapid changes in anaesthetic depth. It is non-irritant and easier to achieve spontaneous ventilation with during anaesthesia.
- Desflurane offers the benefit of more rapid emergence but is intensely irritant to the airway. It is not suitable for use as a gaseous induction agent.

Mechanism of action

- This is not yet clear.
- Possible mechanisms include potentiation of GABA and antagonism at NMDA receptors.
- Other theories revolve around the clathrate crystal hypothesis, cell membrane expansion and protein channel disruption.

Chemical structure

- Sevoflurane, isoflurane, desflurane & enflurane are halogenated ethers.
- Halothane is a halogenated hydrocarbon.

Pharmacokinetics

Absorption & onset of action

- The anaesthetic effect of volatile agents is dependent on their brain partial pressure, which is approximate to the expired concentration of volatile.
- Inhaled volatile diffuses down a concentration gradient across the alveolar membrane and into the pulmonary blood. Thus, the partial pressure of volatile in the alveoli, blood and the brain approach equilibrium.

Many factors influence the speed at which the volatile agents reach equilibrium:

Agent factors

- Blood:Gas (B:G) Partition Coefficient (See Table 3.5):
  - This represents solubility in blood. A low value indicates reduced solubility in blood. The partial pressure of poorly blood-soluble volatile agents rises rapidly in the alveoli, blood and brain. Thus, the onset/offset of anaesthesia is more rapid in volatile agents with a low B:G partition coefficient.
  - Using a high inspired concentration will result in a more rapid rise in alveolar concentration and therefore speed of induction.
  - Concentration and Second Gas effect if used with N_2O.

Equipment factors
- The inspired concentration of volatile set on the vapouriser may not represent the actual delivered concentration due to dilution by gases in the breathing circuit.

Patient factors
- Functional residual capacity (FRC);
  - The volatile agent is diluted in the alveolus
  - The greater the FRC the greater this dilution
  - Patients with a reduced FRC demonstrate a faster onset of anaesthesia.
- Hyperventilation results in faster onset
- Cardiac output:
  - When cardiac output is high, a concentration gradient is maintained between the alveolus and the blood, resulting in a slow build up of alveolar partial pressure.
  - Thus steady state is not achieved and onset of anaesthesia is slow. If cardiac output is low, alveolar and thus arterial partial pressure reach higher values more quickly.

Distribution
- Distribution follows cardiac output with 15% supplying the brain and resulting in anaesthesia. During prolonged anaesthesia, the more lipid soluble volatiles accumulate in fat resulting in prolonged emergence.

Metabolism
- The Carbon-halogen bond is metabolized by hepatic cytochrome P-450. The C-F bond is most stable with C-Cl, C-Br and C-I bonds becoming progressively less so. Free halogen ions and triafluroacetic acid are produced, which may cause renal and hepatic damage.

Elimination
- The volatiles are exhaled in a reverse physiological process of inhalation. Metabolites are usually excreted in the urine.

Potency
- The oil:gas (O:G) partition coefficient indicates CNS lipid solubility.
- The Meyer-Overton Hypothesis demonstrates a linear relationship between the potency of the volatile and its lipid solubility.
- The CNS concentration achieved at steady state is related to the end-tidal alveolar concentration.
- Minimum Alveolar Concentration (MAC) is a measure of potency, and is the concentration at steady state that prevents reaction to a standard surgical stimulus (skin incision) in 50% of subjects at sea level i.e. 1 atmosphere of pressure. (See Table 3.6).
- Different physiological states will alter MAC. Age is the most important with a peak MAC value in infancy. Pharmacological factors must also be taken into account when observing MAC values.

Pharmacodynamics of the volatile agents

- CVS
  - Dose-dependent reduction in myocardial contractility. Sevoflurane and Desflurane have minimal effect.
  - A reduction in heart rate associated with Halothane. No change is observed with Sevoflurane and reflex tachycardia is observed with the others.
  - Dose-dependent reduction in systemic vascular resistance
  - Resultant hypotension.
  - Halothane and to a lesser extent enflurane sensitize the heart to circulating catecholamines. Arrhythmias are possible and care should be taken if the surgeon administers adrenaline; <100mcg adrenaline per 10 minutes is advised.
  - Isoflurane causes coronary vasodilatation; coronary steal is possible.
- RS
  - All depress ventilation with a reduction in tidal volume.
  - Ventilatory response to hypercarbia or hypoxia is obtunded by all.
  - All cause bronchodilatation.
  - Isoflurane and desflurane are intensely irritant to the airway and likely to cause coughing. Halothane, sevoflurane and enflurane are non-irritant and can be used for gaseous induction.
  - All inhibit HPV in a dose-dependent manner with halothane the most significant. There is little difference exhibited between isoflurane, sevoflurane and desflurane. Shunt fraction is increased when volatile anaesthesia is compared to intravenous anaesthesia with propofol. Clinically, volatiles do not cause significant problems with oxygenation.
- CNS
  - Dose-dependent cerebral vasodilatation and resultant increase in cerebral blood flow and ICP. Halothane is the most potent.
  - Reduction in cerebral O_2 requirement.
  - Enflurane can induce epileptiform EEG changes. Avoid in epileptic patients.
  - Desflurane offers the benefit of rapid recovery even after prolonged anaesthesia. This is highly desirable in thoracic surgery so that spontaneous ventilation returns quickly. Sevoflurane may offer some benefit in short procedures, but this has not been proven in prolonged cases.
- GU/GIT
  - Halothane and enflurane reduce splanchnic blood flow.
  - Decreased renal blood flow related to associated hypotension.
  - Dose-dependent relaxation of the pregnant uterus.

Other issues
- All are triggers for malignant hyperpyrexia with Halothane the most potent.
- Halothane and to a lesser extent Enflurane are associated with hepatic damage with repeated exposure.

Nitrous Oxide (N_2O)

N_2O is used as an adjuvant to the volatile agents. It possesses analgesic properties, allows a dose reduction in the inspired volatile and permits a more rapid onset and emergence from anaesthesia.

Use of N_2O in thoracic anaesthesia
- Avoid when there is an abnormal gas filled space such as a pneumothorax or bulla.
- In patients with significant respiratory dysfunction, and particularly during OLV the need for high inspired O_2 concentration may make N_2O use impossible.
- In the frail, its use may reduce the dose-dependent side effects of volatile agents. However, this cannot be justified in the face of hypoxia.
- It is contraindicated in severe head injury, e.g. polytrauma patients.

Physical characteristics
- N_2O is an inorganic gas
- A very low B:G partition coefficient results in rapid onset/offset.
- 20 times more soluble in blood than O_2 and N_2, resulting in more N_2O leaving the alveoli and entering pulmonary capillary blood than other gases passing back into the alveoli. This causes a relative increase in the fractional concentrations of the alveolar gases (2nd gas effect).
- It has a very low O:G partition coefficient resulting in a low potency. It is therefore given at very high concentration (up to 70%).
- Because of these characteristics it will also rapidly diffuse into any air filled spaces in the body. Pressure or volume effects can then occur depending upon whether the space is of fixed volume or not.

Pharmacodynamics
- CVS
  - Decrease in myocardial contractility when combined with volatile agents or opioids
  - BP maintained by reflex increase in SVR.
- RS
  - Slight depression in respiration
  - Non-irritant to airway
  - Diffusion hypoxia may be an issue during emergence if high concentrations have been used. This is the reverse process of that which causes the 2nd gas effect.

- CNS
  - Analgesic in concentration above 20%
  - Profound CNS depression with possible loss of consciousness at higher concentrations alone
  - Increased intracranial pressure.
- GIT
  - Associated with increased incidence of PONV.

Other

- Toxicity is associated with prolonged exposure. N_2O oxidizes the cobalt ion in Vitamin B_{12}, which is then unable to act as a cofactor for methionine synthase. The result is a reduction in thymidine, tetrahydrofolate and DNA synthesis. This may result in bone marrow suppression and peripheral neuropathy.

Table 3.5 Physical properties of the inhalational anaesthetic agents

	MAC (100% O_2)	MAC (66% N_2O)	O:G Partition coefficient	B:G Partition coefficient	Metabolized (%)
N_2O	104	N/A	1.4	0.47	<0.01
Halothane	0.75	0.29	224	2.3	20
Isoflurane	1.17	0.5	91	1.4	0.2
Enflurane	1.63	0.65	96	1.91	2
Sevoflurane	1.8	0.66	91	0.59	3.5
Desflurane	6.6	2.8	18.7	0.42	0.02

Table 3.6 Factors affecting Minimum Alveolar Concentration

Factors increasing MAC	Factors decreasing MAC
Infancy	Neonatal period and the elderly
Hyperthyroidism	Hypothyroidism
Pyrexia	Hypothermia
Hypernatraemia	Pregnancy
Catecholamines/i sympathetic drive	α_2 agonists
Chronic use of alcohol or opioids	Acute use of alcohol, opioids or sedatives
Acute amphetamine use	Chronic amphetamine use
	Lithium

Further reading

Sasada, M, & Smith, S, editors (2003). *Drugs in Anaesthesia and Intensive care*. 3rd ed. Oxford. Oxford University Press.

Intravenous anaesthetic agents

Propofol

- 2,6-disisopropylphenol (phenol derivative).
- Prepared as a 1% emulsion in Intralipid, containing 10% soybean oil, 2.25% glycerol and 1.2% egg lecithin.
- As the emulsion readily supports bacterial growth, a bacteriostatic agent is added depending on the manufacturer.

Mechanism of action

- Unknown; most likely potentiates inhibitory neurotransmitters (glycine and GABA), leading to anaesthesia.
- No analgesic properties.
- Antiemetic properties via anti-serotinergic effect and antagonism of D_2 receptors?

Uses

- Induction and maintenance of thoracic anaesthesia.
- Sedation on ICU.
- Anti-emesis—particularly chemotherapy induced nausea and vomiting.

Dose

- For induction:
  - 1.5–2.5 mg/kg/IV.
- IV infusion for maintenance:
  - 3–6 µg/ml/IV via TCI pump for induction and maintenance of anaesthesia (titrated to effect).
- Sedation:
  - 0.5–1.5 µg/ml/IV via TCI pump for sedation (titrated to effect).
- Anti-emesis:
  - 0.5 mg/kg IV.

Pharmacokinetics

- Rapid onset <1 minute due to very high lipid solubility.
- Redistribution half life 1–2 minutes.
- Duration of action 3–4 half lives, or 3–8 minutes.
- Effect terminated by redistribution.
- Terminal elimination half life 4–6 hours.
- Metabolized by the liver/renal excretion.

Effects

- CNS.
  - Smooth and rapid induction of anaesthesia, primarily via the $GABA_A$ receptor.

- ↓ CBF, ICP and the $CMRO_2$.
- Intrinsic anti-emetic activity.
- Least incidence of PONV of any anaesthetic agent, IV or inhalational.
- Anticonvulsant.
- Appears to share the neuroprotective effect of thiopentone.
- CVS.
  - ↓ BP/SVR, probably due to systemic release of NO.
  - No compensatory ↑ HR seen due to blunting of baroreceptor response. Resultant 20% ↓ CO.
  - Bradycardia can occur.
- RS.
  - Dose dependent ↓ RR and ventilatory drive.
  - Bolus administration usually produces apnoea for a few minutes.
  - Obtunds upper airway reflexes, allowing LMA insertion/airway instrumentation.
  - Causes bronchodilatation.
  - No significant effects on hypoxic vasoconstriction. The clinical relevance of this to thoracic anaesthesia is controversial.

Adverse effects

- Pain on injection.
- Hypersensitivity reaction to egg lecithin product is very rare, as the product contains no egg albumin which is the usual causative agent.

Thiopentone

- Thiopentone sodium is a thiobarbiturate; first used in 1934.
- Supplied as the sodium salt in hygroscopic powder form, also containing 6% sodium carbonate; reconstituted with sterile water to make a 2.5% solution. Stored in atmosphere of nitrogen to prevent salt precipitation.
- Stable at room temperature for 24–48 hours after mixing.

Mechanism of action

- Damping of all post-synaptic impulses causing anaesthesia (particularly brainstem and ARAS).
- Decrease Na^+ and K^+ ion conductance within cells, similar to local anaesthetics; hence decreasing excitatory post-synaptic potentials.
- Enhances Cl^- conductance via $GABA_A$ receptors and may decrease excitatory Ca^{2+} conductance.

Uses

- Induction of anaesthesia only.
- Cessation of status epilepticus.

Dose

- 2–7 mg/kg/IV.

Pharmacokinetics

- Rapid onset of action, typically < 1 minute.
- Redistribution half life longer than propofol at 2–4 minutes.
- Duration of action 3–4 half lives or 6–16 minutes.
- Effect terminated by redistribution.
- Terminal elimination half life is 6–12 hours.
- Metabolized by oxidation in the liver at 10–15% per hour, a reaction catalyzed by cytochrome P450.

Effects

- CNS
  - Similar to propofol with smooth, rapid onset of anesthesia, primarily via the $GABA_A$ receptor.
  - ↓ CBF, ICP and the $CMRO_2$
  - In some circumstances may exhibit a "neuroprotective" effect.
  - Excellent anticonvulsant.
  - Dose dependent effect on the EEG to burst suppression and finally isoelectric (flat-line) activity.
- CVS.
  - ↓ cardiac contractility and vasodilatation → ↓ CO.
  - Compensatory tachycardia common.
- RS
  - Dose dependent decrease ↓ respiratory drive similar to propofol.
  - Bolus administration usually produces apnoea for a few minutes.
  - ↑ reactivity of airway with high incidence of coughing and laryngospasm during induction.
  - Causes bronchoconstriction.
  - Unsuitable for LMA insertion or airway instrumentation

Adverse effects

- Anaphylactic reaction is rare but can be fatal (1:14,000–1:30,000).
- Contraindicated in porphyria.
- Irritant to tissues if extravasates as pH of 10–11.
- Intra-arterial injection can cause vasospasm, thrombosis and limb loss unless treated rapidly with vasodilator (eg papaverine, GTN) and an anticoagulant (e.g. heparin).

Etomidate

- Etomidate is an imidazole derivative.
- Supplied either as a colourless 2 mg/ml solution in 35% propylene glycol or as a white lipid emulsion.

Mechanism of action
- Acts at $GABA_A$ receptors modulating fast inhibitory post synaptic potentials throughout the CNS.

Uses
- Induction of anaesthesia only.

Dose
- 0.3 mg/kg/IV.

Pharmacokinetics
- Loss of consciousness is rapid, <1 minute.
- Not as studied as propofol or thiopentone because of adrenal side effects (see below).
- Redistribution half life is 2–4 minutes.
- Duration of action is 5–10 minutes.
- Metabolised via hydrolysis by plasma and hepatic esterases.

Effects
- CNS.
  - Rapid induction via $GABA_A$ receptor.
  - Induction is frequently accompanied by myoclonic movements.
  - Changes in CMRO2, CBF and ICP similar to thiopentone and propofol.
  - ↓ ICP with cardiovascular stability may increase CPP.
- CVS.
  - Relative cardiovascular stability.
  - Minimal ↓ SVR or contractility with relatively little change in HR unless large dose given.
  - Significant anti-platelet activity.
- RS.
  - Less ventilatory depression than propofol or thiopentone.
  - Bolus dose is still likely to produce a period of apnea.
  - Transient hiccoughing and coughing is common.
- Endocrine.
  - Potent inhibitor of the 11ß-hydroxylation reaction in cortisol synthesis.
  - A single induction dose results in depression of cortisol synthesis and the normal response to ACTH for up to 24 hours.
  - The clinical relevance of this remains controversial.

Adverse effects
- Highest incidence of postoperative PONV (30–40% by some estimates).
- Propylene glycol can cause pain on injection and superficial phlebitis.
- The safety of etomidate in prophyria is questionable.

Ketamine
- Ketamine is a phencyclidine derivative.
- It is supplied as a clear colourless liquid containing a racemic mixture of ketamine hydrochloride (10, 50, 100 mg/ml).
- The S-isomer is available and is a more potent anesthetic with fewer adverse effects.

Mechanism of action
- Docks at the phencyclidine binding site on the NMDA receptor.
- Inhibits Ca^{2+} passage through the ion pore, thus decreasing excitatory post synaptic potentials.
- Muscarinic and opioid receptor action → analgesia?

Dose
- Induction—IM:
  - 10 mg/kg/IM onset 2–8 mins.
- Induction—IV:
  - 1.5–2 mg/kg/IV onset 30 secs.
- Maintenance infusion:
  - 50 µg/kg/min/IV.
- Analgesia:
  - 0.5 mg/kg or infusion 0.15–0.3 mg/kg/hr/IV.

Pharmacokinetics
- Rapid onset after an induction dose of 1–2 mg/kg.
- Redistribution half life of 11–17 minutes.
- Awakening is slower and hangover more prolonged than any other intravenous induction agent.
- Ketamine is metabolized in the liver by N-demethylation to norketamine.
- Norketamine is one fourth as potent and further metabolized to an inactive glucuronide which is excreted in the urine.

Effects
- CNS.
  - Produces a state of dissociative anesthesia by blocking NMDA receptors.
  - Patients may move, vocalize and open their eyes, but do not respond to noxious stimuli with marked amnesia.
  - Profound analgesia persists into the postoperative period.
  - ↑ CBF, $CMRO_2$ and ICP in contrast to other agents.
  - Causes dose dependent changes in the EEG making EEG based monitors of depth of anaesthesia unreliable.
- CVS.
  - ↑ BP, HR, contractility and SVR.
  - These are indirect effects caused by increased central sympathetic tone and centrally mediated release of catacholamines from the adrenal medulla.
  - Arrhythmias uncommon.

- RS.
  - Minimal effect on ventilatory drive with preservation of airway reflexes.
  - Profound bronchodilatation occurs.

Adverse effects

- PONV is common
- Copious salivation occurs so administration of an anticholinergic is often prudent
- Emergence delirium often accompanied by hallucinations is common, and must be balanced against the desire for a lack of CVS depression.

Uses in thoracic anaesthesia

Induction of anaesthesia

- *Propofol*
  - Commonest induction agent used for thoracic anaesthesia.
  - Cardiovascular stability is possible in most cases with careful dosage, influenced by the patient's medical condition.
  - It facilitates instrumentation of the airway as it obtunds upper airway reflexes well.
- *Etomidate*
  - Is considered a useful alternative if cardiovascular instability is expected, although the benefits must be balanced against the known risks of adrenal suppression.
- *Thiopentone*
  - Usage is classically associated with rapid sequence induction, as it is reported that it gives a clearer induction end point.
  - It does not obtund instrumentation of the airway, so is not the drug of choice for rigid bronchoscopy.
- *Ketamine*
  - Perhaps under-used in thoracic anaesthesia.
  - With its benefits of bronchodilatation, cardiovascular stability and analgesia, it can be a useful agent in the thoracic anaesthesia patient population (poor cardiac function, COPD etc.).
  - Emergence delirium is a potential problem, but is not reported as frequently as reputed.

Maintenance of anaesthesia

- Propofol TCI, often with remifentanil (combination = TIVA) is the technique of choice for rigid bronchoscopy and other procedures requiring jet ventilation.
  - Use of propofol TCI for maintenance of anaesthesia during one lung ventilation has theoretical advantages over volatile. agents regarding maintenance of hypoxic vasoconstriction.
  - However, the vasodilatation and the direct suppressant effect upon the myocardium, may result in shunt and decreased effective oxygen flux.

Analgesia

- Low dose ketamine is a useful adjunct for analgesia.
  - At low doses the unpleasant psychological effects are minimal, and it can produce good analgesia without the respiratory depressant effects of opioids.

Inotropes

- Increase the velocity and force of myocardial fibre shortening with a resultant increase in cardiac output and blood pressure
- Many inotropic agents also have effects on preload and afterload
- No definitive evidence to support one inotrope or combinations thereof over another with respect to clinical outcome
- Their effects on an individual patient are not easily predicted
- If necessary, the dose and/or agent should be changed if the desired effect is not achieved.

Mechanism of action

- Increase myocardial contractility by increased release of Ca^{2+} from the sarcoplasmic reticulum into the myocyte cytoplasm, mediated by intracellular 2nd messengers, i.e. cAMP, IP_3 (via α_1 adrenoceptor activation).

Catecholamine inotropes

- In the failing myocardium there may be significant de-sensitization and down-regulation of cardiac β adrenoceptors.
- Clinically, this may manifest as tachyphylaxis and an increasing inotropic requirement (β agonists). Therefore, the role of β agonists in severe myocardial dysfunction has been challenged.

Epinephrine

General

- β agonism at low dose → ↑ MAP, ↑ systolic pressure, ↓ diastolic pressure 2°:
  - ↑ HR.
  - contractility.
  - dromotropy.
  - Vasodilation.
- α agonism at high dose → ↑ SVR
- Coronary vasodilation predominates throughout the dose range 2° local metabolic changes in the coronary circulation induced by increasing myocardial work
- Dose dependent effect on renal and splanchnic perfusion i.e. ↑ with low dose infusion and vice versa
- Bronchodilation.

Uses

- Anaphylaxis.
- Cardiac arrest.
- Low cardiac output states.

Dose

- Anaphylaxis:
  - 0.5–1 ml aliquots of (1:10,000 mini-jet)/IV every 3–5 minutes.
  - 0.5–1.0 mg (0.5–1ml of 1:1000) IM every 5–10 minutes.
  - IV route is recommended by the RCOA. Particularly when profound CVS collapse.
  - IM route is preferred if no IV access or early stages of anaphlaxis and no CVS shut-down.
  - There is no harm in giving an initial IV dose, and following it with an IM dose.
  - ADRENALINE IS GIVEN TO STOP FURTHER MAST CELL DEGRANULATION.
- Cardiac arrest:
  - 1 mg IV bolus (10ml of 1:10,000 mini-jet) every 3–5 minutes.
  - 2–3 mg diluted to 10ml water for jetting down ET tube.
- Infusion via central vein (100 mcg/ml e.g. 5mg in 50ml saline) at 0.04–0.4 mcg/kg/min titrated to effect.

Norepinephrine

- Onset under 30sec, short half-life. Potent!
- Not suitable for bolus doses
- Predominant action due to indirect α-agonism
- Direct and indirect action at α- and β-adrenoceptors.
- Predictable increase in blood pressure and possible reduction in cardiac output.
- Coronary blood flow is increased.
- PVR increases.

Uses

- Refractory hypotension.
- Shock:
  - Less deleterious effects in septic shock than epinephrine and as such is currently considered a first line agent in this context.

Dose

- Administer via CENTRAL VEIN ONLY
- Typical doses range from 0.04–4 mcg/kg/min
- Control of intra-operative hypotension:
  - Re-constitute 4 mg (1 standard vial) into 50 ml N saline = 80 mcg/ml.
  - Start the infusion at 4 ml/hr (4–20 ml/hr) and titrate to MAP.
- Post-operative infusion:
- 1–30 mcg/min.
- Add 4 mg to 250 ml 0.9% NaCl or 5% dextrose to give 16 mcg/ml. Run at 0–20 ml/hr.

Special note
- ⚠ Can cause tissue necrosis after extravasation.

Dopamine
- Endogenous precursor of norepinephrine
- Low dose
  - Effects on peripheral D_1 receptors predominate causing renal vasodilatation and a moderate diuresis. β_2 effects lead to overall ↑ CO.
- Medium doses
  - Agonist action at β-adrenoceptors is seen with ↑ HR and cardiac contractility.
- High doses
  - α-adrenoceptor activity is seen with peripheral vasoconstriction. ↑SVR.

Uses
- Low cardiac output states.
- Septic shock.
- ☞Impending renal failure (2° to low CO) to promote diuresis.

Dose
- Administer via a CENTRAL VEIN ONLY.
  - Low dose (<5 mcg/kg/min).
  - Medium dose (5–10 mcg/kg/min).
  - High dose (15 mcg/kg/min).
- Infusion.
  - Add 3 mg/kg (body weight) to 50 mls 0.9%NaCl or 5% glucose.
  - 1 ml/hr = 1 mcg/kg/min.

Special note
- ⚠ Can cause tissue necrosis after extravasation.
- Marked nausea due to effects at CTZ.

Dobutamine
- Mainly acts at β_1 adrenoceptors (β_1: β_2 = 3:1).
  - ↑ HR.
  - ↑ contractility.
  - ↑ dromotropy.

- $\downarrow$ venous return 2° B_2 adrenoceptor venodilation → $\downarrow$ MAP especially in hypovolaemic patients.
- There is very little effect at A adrenoceptors.
- No effect on renal vasculature.
- $\triangle$ combination of $\uparrow$ HR & $\downarrow$ MAP may induce myocardial ischaemia in at-risk patients.
- No respiratory effects.

Uses
- Systolic heart failure e.g. post cardiac surgery/myocardial infarction.
- Sepsis; in combination with norepinephrine.

Dose
- Infusion via central vein:
  - 2.5–30 mcg/kg/min titrated to effect.
  - Add 3 mg/kg (body weight) to 50 mls 0.9% NaCl or 5% glucose.
  - 1 ml/hr = 1 mcg/kg/min.

Dopexamine
- There is little evidence to support its use in acute heart failure.
- No evidence to support a benefit over epinephrine or norepinephrine.

Dose
- 0.5–6 mcg/kg/min.

Non-catecholamine inotropes
Phosphodiesterase inhibitors (type III)
- Enhancement of diastolic relaxation (lusiotropy).
- Positive inotropy without a significant increase in myocardial O_2 consumption.
- Profound vasodilation → $\downarrow$MAPs:
  - $\downarrow$ preload.
  - venous return.
  - SVR.
- PVR
- Enoximone exhibits more inotropy than vasodilation.

Uses
- Advanced heart failure i.e. low cardiac output state with elevated SVR.
- During and after cardiopulmonary bypass.

Dose

- Enoximone (2 mg/ml e.g. 100 mg in 50 ml saline).
  - 90 mcg/kg/min IV for 10–30 minutes.
  - 5–20 mcg/kg/min thereafter.
  - Maximum dose = 24 mg/kg/day.
- Milrinone (0.2 mg/ml e.g. 10 mg in 50 ml saline).
  - 50 mcg/kg IV over 10 minutes.
  - 0.375–0.750 mcg/kg/min thereafter.
  - Maximum dose = 1.13 mg/kg/day.

Special note

- ⚠ Signifcant hypotension may accompany administration. Therefore, it is important that consideration is given to the concomitant administration of epinephrine or norepinephrine to maintain MAP.
- ⚠ Both agents have a prolonged elimination half-life and will accumulate in patients with renal impairment.

Glucagon

- No definitive role in cardiovascular support.
- Large doses required to produce positive inotropic effect.
- May be used in B-blocker or tricyclic overdose.
- ⚠ causes hyperglycaemia and hyperkalaemia.

Digoxin

- ↑ contractility.
- ↓HR 2°:
  - Depressed sino-atrial node discharge & atrio-ventricular conduction
  - Indirect vagotonic effect.
- ❶ Rapid IV administration may cause vasoconstriction and reduced coronary blood flow.

Mechanism of action

- Increases availability of bound intracellular Ca^{2+} via inhibition of Na^+-K^+-ATPase pump within the plasma membrane. The resultant increase of intracellular Na^+ causes displacement of bound intracellular Ca^{2+}
- The concomitant reduction of intracellular K^+ slows the cardiac pacemaker cells and atrio-ventricular conduction.

Uses

- Atrial fibrillation and flutter.
- Chronic heart failure.
- Role in acute heart failure is debatable with a poor response seen. where there is a high sympathetic drive.

Dose

- Loading dose:
  - 10–20 mcg/kg IV every 6 hours until desired effect achieved
  - Rate of injection <25 mcg/min.
- Maintenance dose:
  - 125–500 mcg/day.
- ⚠ ↓ dose in the elderly, and in patients with renal, electrolyte and acid-base abnormalities.

▶ Narrow therapeutic index; blood assay should be taken approximately 6 hours after IV dose. Acceptable plasma digoxin concentration is 1–2 ng/ml.

Levosimendan

- Positive inotropy without an increase in myocardial O_2 consumption.
- Non-arrhythmogenic.
- Coronary and systemic vasodilation.
- ↓ cardiac filling pressures in heart failure.

Mechanism of action

- Binds to cardiac troponin C which is Ca^{2+} dependent, thus sensitizing the myofilaments to Ca^{2+}. Therefore, the action of levosimendan is not dependent on agonism at β adrenoceptors.
- Also facilitates ATP-dependent K^+ channel opening:
  - Anti-ischaemic effects.
  - Vasodilation.

Uses

- Treatment of chronic, decompensated cardiac failure.
- Role in severe, acute heart failure remains unclear with no improvement in survival shown as yet.

Dose

- Loading dose: 6–12 mcg/kg IV over 10 minutes
- Maintenance dose: 0.05–0.2 mcg/kg IV over 2 days
- Active metabolite results in improved myocardial contractility for up to 1 month.

Further reading

Sasada M, Smith S, editors (2003). *Drugs in Anaesthesia & Intensive Care*. 3rd Edition. Oxford. Oxford University Press.

Overgaard CB, Dzavik V. Inotropes and Vasopressors. Review of physiology and clinical use in cardiovascular disease. *Circulation* 2008; 118: 1047–56.

Vasopressors

Vasopressors increase blood pressure through increases in vascular tone.

General considerations

- They increase blood pressure to the detriment of cardiac output and thus may paradoxically reduce oxygen delivery.
- Use with caution in:
  - Patients with severe hypertension.
  - Ventricular tachycardia with hypotension.
- Should be used with extreme caution in:
  - Geriatric patients, patients with hyperthyroidism, bradycardia, partial heart block or with other heart disease.
- Hypertension with bradycardia resulting from baroreceptor response to increased SVR, if severe, can be treated by the administration of phentolamine (an alpha blocking agent).
- △ Indirectly acting agents should be avoided in patients treated with MAOI or those with secretory neuroendocrine tumours.

Mechanism of action

- Induce venoconstriction, arteriolar constriction (and thus ↑ SVR) or both.
- Most commonly via agonism of α-adrenoceptors via:
  - A direct post-synaptic effect.
  - An indirect release of pre-synaptic norepinephrine.

Ephedrine

- Indirect action via norepinephrine release from sympathetic nerve terminals.
- Direct α and β adrenergic effects.
- Similar cardiovascular effects to adrenaline, but more prolonged.
- Positive inotropic and chronotropic effects →
  - ↑ MAP.
  - ↑ myocardial O_2 consumption.
  - Arrhythmia.
  - ↑ coronary perfusion.
- ↑ pulmonary artery pressure.
- Splanchnic and renal vascular vasoconstriction.

Uses

- Hypotension during general or regional anaesthesia.
- △ avoid in situations where hypotension is associated with tachycardia.

- Re-constitute 30 mg to 10 ml.
- Initial 3 mg (1 ml) bolus.
- ↑ to 6–12 mg if response not adequate.

Phenylephrine

- Onset within 1 min, duration 5 min.
- Post-synaptic α-adrenergic effects at therapeutic doses. Negligible β effects at normal dose, but β effects can occur at high doses.
- Peripheral vasoconstriction results in increased diastolic and systolic pressures, small decrease in cardiac output and an increase in circulation time.
- Reflex bradycardia (blocked by atropine) can occur.
- Most vascular beds are constricted (renal, splanchnic, pulmonary, cutaneous), but coronary blood flow is increased.
- PVR increases.

Uses

- Treatment of hypotension and shock (after adequate volume replacement), but often not favoured due to resulting bradycardia.
- Treatment of hypotension resulting from idiosyncratic hypotensive reactions to drugs such as phenothiazines, adrenergic blocking agents, and ganglionic blockers.
- Has been used to increase blood pressure to terminate attacks of paroxysmal supraventricular tachycardia associated with hypotension.

Dose

- 50–500 mcg IV or as a continuous infusion 20–50 mcg/min, titrated to effect.

Metaraminol

- Onset 30 sec–2 min, lasts 20–60 min.
- Predominant action due to indirect α-agonism.
- Direct and indirect action at α- and β-adrenoceptors.
- Peripheral vasoconstriction, resultant increase in diastolic and systolic blood pressures, small decrease in cardiac output and increased circulation time.
- Reflex bradycardia can occur but less so than with phenylephrine.
- Most vascular beds are constricted (renal splanchnic, pulmonary, cutaneous). Coronary blood flow increases via an indirect mechanism.
- PVR increases.

Uses

- Treatment of hypotension and shock.
- Treatment of intra-operative hypotension secondary to general anaesthesia and epidural analgesia.

Dose

- Re-constitute 1 mg vial to 20 ml (500 mcg/ml solution).
- Initial 0.5 mg bolus IV (1 ml of above solution).
- Titrate subsequent doses to effect, e.g. 0.25–1 mg IV.

Special note

- ⚠ Extravasation has been associated with local tissue necrosis.

Other agents

Vasopressin

- ADH is an endogenous peptide hormone formed in the hypothalamus and secreted by the posterior pituitary gland. Its main homeostatic function is to aid water reabsorption in the collecting ducts of the renal tubules; basal secretion increasing in response to increased plasma osmolality.
- Substantial release occurs in hypovolaemia and this stimulates vasoconstriction through activation of V_1 receptors.
- During established septic shock there may be relative vasopressin deficiency and this observation has led to the increasing use of vasopressin as an adjunct to norepinephrine or dopamine in vasopressor-resistant septic shock.
- It has also been used with some success as a fixed dose during cardiopulmonary resuscitation. Terlipressin is a synthetic prodrug of vasopressin and is used to treat bleeding oesophageal varices.

Dose

- 0.01–0.04 units/min IV. Should ideally be CENTRAL VEIN ONLY.
- 1–2 mg IV up to QDS for treatment of bleeding varices.
- *40 units stat* IV in cardiopulmonary resuscitation.

Methylene blue

- Aromatic dye compound.
- Inhibits both nitric oxide synthase and guanylate cyclase.
- Leads to indirect effects via suppression of the generation of endogenous vasodilators and may be used in the ICU setting for refractory septic shock.

Octreotide

- Synthetic (octapeptide) somatostatin analogue.
- Opposes the effects of growth hormone, glucagon and insulin and also appears to reduce serotonin and VIP release from carcinoid and VIPomas respectively.
- Can be used to minimize the hypotension and bradycardia seen during handling of these tumours and is given in doses of 50–200 mcg SC or by very slow IV injection prior to, and during, surgery.

Effect on hypoxic pulmonary vasoconstriction

Vasoconstrictors

- Normoxic lung vessels preferentially constrict.
- ↑ regional pulmonary vascular resistance in normoxic lung.
- → diversion of blood away from areas of normal ventilation to areas of absent or reduced ventilation.
- ↑ pulmonary shunt fraction.

Vasodilators

- ↑ pulmonary shunt fraction 2° inhibition of regional HPV.

Further reading

Sasada M, Smith S, editors (2003). *Drugs in Anaesthesia & Intensive Care*. 3rd Edition. Oxford. Oxford University Press.

Overgaard CB, Dzavik V. Inotropes and Vasopressors. Review of physiology and clinical use in cardiovascular disease. *Circulation* 2008; 118: 1047–56.

Blood products

- A blood product is defined as any therapeutic substance prepared from human blood.
- Blood components include red cells, platelets, fresh frozen plasma, cryoprecipitate, and white cells.
- Every donation is tested for:
  - Hepatitis B surface antigen.
  - Hepatitis C antibody and RNA.
  - HIV antibody.
  - HTLV antibody.
  - Syphilis antibody.

Red cells

- Indicated to increase oxygen flux where acute or chronic anaemia contributes to inadequate oxygen delivery to tissues.
- 4 ml/kg typically raises Hb by 1 g/dl, e.g. 1 unit transfusion in 70 kg patient.
- 250 ml bag:
  - Haematocrit of 0.6.
  - No platelets.
  - 2, 3-DPG levels remain normal for up to 14 days after donation
  - 35 day storage life with SAGM (saline, adenine, glucose, mannitol) or for up to 42 days with A-CPD (adenine, citrate, phosphate, dextrose).
  - Leucocyte depleted.
- Infusion should be complete within 4 hours of removal from cold storage.

> ### Transfusion trigger
>
> - Transfusion triggers are both institution and clinician dependent. The priority is to determine the patient's physiological reserve.
> - TRICC trial recommended 'a restrictive strategy of red-cell transfusion is at least as effective as and possibly superior to a liberal transfusion strategy in critically ill patients, with the possible exception of patients with acute myocardial infarction and unstable angina'.
> - The usual lower threshold chosen is a Hb of 7 g/dl in a pre-morbidly fit patient.
> - In patients with co-pathologies that reduce physiological reserve (heart failure or ischaemic heart disease, severe COPD, sepsis), this threshold is often raised to >8 g/dl.

Platelets

- Indicated for the prevention and treatment of haemorrhage $2°$ thrombocytopenia or platelet dysfunction.
- Storage for five days at $22 ± 2°C$ (optimal platelet function at $22°C$). Must be continually agitated to prevent clumping.

- ABO identical or compatible platelets are preferred.
- Rh compatibility is required in Rh negative children and women.
- Should be infused over 30–60 minutes.

Dosing guide

1 Adult therapeutic dose
- Pooled from 4–6 donors.
- 310 ml bag; contains 2.5–3.0×10^{11} platelets.
- ↑ platelet count by 20–40×10^9/ml in 70 kg patient.
- Can be administered with standard blood giving set; replace with each infusion of platelets.

Pre-operative targets
- Surgery in critical area.
  - Platelet count $\geq 100 \times 10^9$/l.
  - Infuse immediately prior to surgery and recheck count.
- Epidural.
  - Platelet count $>100 \times 10^9$/l; careful consideration of the risks and benefits of epidural analgesia should be made in those patients with platelet count 80–100×10^9/l.
- Central venous catheterization.
  - Platelet count $>50 \times 10^9$/l.

Fresh frozen plasma
- Used to:
  - Replace coagulation factors deficiencies associated with massive transfusion.
  - In the absence of specific product the treatment of isolated coagulation factor deficiencies, reversal of warfarin effect and the treatment of thrombin III deficient patients undergoing surgery requiring heparin.
  - Treatment of thrombotic thrombocytopenia.
- Should be ABO compatible, but does not need to be RhD matched.
- Each bag contains all clotting factors, albumin and gamma-globulin.
- Fibrinogen content = 20–50 g/l.

Dosing guide

- 10–15 ml/kg (equivalent to four packs of FFP for a 70 kg person) given at a rate of 10–20 ml/kg/hr. Anecdotally, rapid infusion rates have been associated with acute transfusion reactions.
- Should raise the coagulation levels by 12–15% and fibrinogen by 1 g/l.

- Must be used immediately after thawing.

Cryoprecipitate
- Treatment of plasma fibrinogen <0.8 g/l.
- One unit is 20–50ml and contains:
  - High levels of factor VIIIc (>70 IU/unit).

- Fibrinogen (>140 mg/unit) and von Willebrand factor.
- Stored at −30°C for up to 12 months and is thawed to 37°C immediately before use.
- ABO compatible units should be used.

> **Dosing guide**
>
> - Two 5-donor pools = 10 single donor units.
> - This contains 3–6 g fibrinogen in a volume of 200 to 500 ml.
> - 10 units cryoprecipitate should increase fibrinogen level by 1 g/l.

Recombinant factor VIIa (NovoSeven®)

- Recombinant factor VIIa complexes with tissue factor to activate factor X (Xa) and factor IX (IXa). Factor Xa acts on prothrombin to create thrombin, which converts fibrinogen to fibrin thus allowing formation of a haemostatic plug.
- Recombinant factor VIIa can only work if there are adequate functioning platelets and coagulation factors present.
- Licensed for use in haemophilia patients with inhibitors.
- Increasing unlicensed use in the management of major haemorrhage associated with trauma and surgery.
- Potential for thrombotic complications.

> **Administration of factor VIIa for traumatic/surgical haemorrhage**
>
> ♠ The use of factor VIIa in massive post-operative haemorrhage is an "off-label" use of a licensed drug. Therefore, the clinician takes ultimate responsibility for any adverse events related to it administration.
>
> *Suggested criteria for administration of activated factor VIIa in the absence of a local protocol.*
>
> - Consultant/senior trainee decision.
> - Liaise early with senior haematology staff.
> - Bleeding cannot be controlled surgically.
> - >8 units RBC transfusion.
> - PT & PTT < ×1.5 control.
> - Fibrinogen >0.5 g/l.
> - pH >7.2.
> - Temperature >36°C.
>
> *Factor VIIa dosage for catastrophic traumatic/surgical haemorrhage*
>
> - In the absence of a local guideline, consider:
> - <55 kg = 5 mg.
> - 55–75 kg = 7 mg.
> - 76–100 kg = 9 mg.
> - 100–120 kg = 11 mg.

Factor II, VII, IX and X concentrate (prothrombin complex concentrate; PCC)

- Used to reverse warfarin in life threatening haemorrhage or before emergency surgery, e.g. craniectomy for intracranial haemorrhage.
- Consider use when FFP is contraindicated.

Dosing guide

- Administer 1–5 mg vitamin K before PCC is given.
- Dependent on current INR and target INR.
- Dosing range = 30–50 iu/kg.
- Liaise closely with senior haematology medical staff.

Further reading

McClelland DB. *Handbook of Transfusion Medicine*. 4thed. London: The Stationary Office; 2007. Available at: http://www.transfusionguidelines.org.uk/index.aspx?Publication. (Accessed 25/4/10).

Intravenous fluids

Thoracic surgery spans from the more minor to major surgery. Cases are often associated with significant blood loss, fluid shifts and electrolyte disturbances. The thoracic anaesthetist must therefore be vigilant and choose replacement carefully, guided where possible by invasive monitoring.

Basic physiology

Fluid compartments

- % TBW water:
  - Female- 55%.
  - Male 60%.

Basic physiology fluid compartments in a 70kg male

- Total Body Water (TBW) = 42l.
  - Intracellular = 28L → (40%/2/3rd TBW).
  - Extracellular = 14L → (20%/1/3rd TBW).
  - Interstitial = 10.5L.
  - Intravascular = 3.5L.
  - ❶ Transcellular/3rd space—eg; CSF, Peritoneal fluid etc. normally ignored in calculations.
  - ❶ Significant fluid shifts within this space are often forgotten, however, there must be care with over prescription of IV fluids in certain post-operative thoracic cases. In particular:
  - Oesophagectomy.
  - Bi-lobectomy.
  - Pneumonectomy.
  - Patients with significant cardiac co-morbidity.

Fluid types

Crystalloids

- Water and electrolytes pass easily through the cellular semi-permeable membrane; the degree to which this occurs is down to tonicity.
- Infused sodium will remain in the ECF.
- Any free water expands the TBW.
- (Table 3.7) demonstrates overall intravascular volume expansion after 1000ml of IV fluid.

Hartmann's solution or Compound Sodium Lactate (CSL)

- Balanced salt solution, most commonly used fluid replacement therapy during the intra-operative period.
- Isotonic solution and can used to restore extracellular volume.
- Its use is limited in diabetic patients (lactate being gluconeogenic), hyperkalemic conditions and with citrated blood transfusions.

Normal saline 0.9%
- Use in UK as a sole intra-operative maintenance fluid has greatly declined because of the potential for hyperchloraemic metabolic acidosis.
- ECF Replacement Fluid.
- Its $[Na^+]$ is similar to that of the extracellular fluid and this effectively limits its distribution to the ECF (distributing between the ISF & the plasma in proportion to their volume ie 3:1).
- Plasma osmolality and tonicity will be unchanged because normal saline is isosmotic.
  - The *osmoreceptors* do not contribute anything to the excretion of normal saline.
  - Blood *volume* increases by 250 mls; 5% increase. This is below the sensitivity of the volume receptors. Neither osmoreceptors nor volume receptors are stimulated.

> - Blood loss of 1,000 ml requires about 3,000 to 4,000 ml volume of N saline to restore normal intravascular volume.

Dextrose 5%
- Mainly used in the post-operative period for administering free water as the glucose rapidly enters cells and is metabolized immediately.
- The net effect is of administering pure water, so it is distributed throughout the total body water.
- Each compartment receives fluid in proportion to its contribution to the TBW (i.e. 2/3rd to ICF and 1/3rd to ECF; the ECF fluid is distributed one quarter to plasma & three quarters to ISF).
- Thus, 1000 ml will only give a net rise in intravascular (desired) volume of 80 ml.
  - This volume increase of less than 2% which will not be sensed by the *volume receptors* (as it is below the 7–10% threshold).
- Osmolality of plasma (3,200 ml) will decrease by: $[287-(287 \times 3.20/3.28)]$ which is about 7mOsmol/l or a 2.5% decrease
  - This is enough to be detected by the *osmoreceptors*
  - ADH release will be decreased and renal water excretion will rise
- ❶ It should NOT BE USED AS A RESUSCITATION FLUID!

> • ❶ Blood loss of 1000 ml requires 12.5 litres of 5% dextrose to restore normal circulating volume.

Table 3.7 The distribution of 1000ml of infused IV solution

Fluid	Distribution of 1000 ml		
	ICF(ml)	ECF(ml)	
		Plasma	Interstitial
N Saline	0	250	750
5% Dextrose	670	80	250
Hartmann's	100	225	675

Dextrose 4% & saline 0.18%
• Normally used in paediatrics, this is relatively a hypotonic solution which is used in the post-operative phase to administer some free water and at the same time preventing hyponatraemia.

Dextrose 10%, 20% and 50%
• Used in hypoglycaemia to promote euglycemia. These are very rarely used routinely, because of the hyperosmolarity of these solutions.

Severe hypoglycaemia

• For a blood sugar <4 mmol/l.
• Dextrose 10% delivered in 5 g (50 ml) aliquots = 5g glucose.
• Dextrose 50% delivered in 5 g (10 ml aliquots = 5g glucose.

Research has demonstrated that 10% solution in larger volume aliquots results in better resolution of hypoglycaemia with lower post treatment blood sugar.

Colloids
• Larger molecules, do not readily pass through semi-permeable membranes, thus offer a greater theoretical plasma volume expansion.
• Colloids are often the preferred choice to offer as a fluid challenge, titrated to the patient's CVP, blood pressure and heart rate trends.

- The duration of action of colloids is dependent upon the type of solution infused, pharmacodynamics and pharmacokinetics.
- ❶ Can contain vast amounts of Na^+.
- ❶ Colloids are NOT FOR USE AS MAINTENANCE FLUIDS.

Gelatins
- Succinylated gelatins (Gelofusine 4%).
  - Derived from bovine collagen which is hydroxylated and succinylated.
- Urea cross linked gelatin solutions (Haemaccel 3.5%).
  - More balanced in terms of other electrolyte composition the use of which has declined in the U.K.

> - ❶❶ Histamine release may be associated with administration of colloids causing:
>   - Urticarial rash.
>   - Bronchospasm.
>   - Hypotension.
>   - Tachycardia.
> - In the worst cases, anaphylaxis may occur.

Hydroxyethyl starches (HES)
Non-ionic starch derivative, categorized by:
- Molecular size.
  - Typically 130 to 200kDa.
- Degree of molar substitution (the proportion of the glucose units on the starch molecule that have been replaced by hydroxyethyl units)— typically around 0.4 to 0.7.
  - Hetastarches (0.6).
  - Pentastarches (0.5).
  - Tetra starches (0.4).
- Concentration in % (i.e. grams per 100ml).
  - E.g. Voluven® is described as 6% HES 130/0.4.
- Their elimination depends on the degree of molar substitution.
  - Molecules smaller than the renal threshold (60–70 kDa) are readily excreted in the urine.
  - Larger ones are metabolized by plasma A–amylase before the degradation products are renally excreted.
  - The higher the degree of substitution, the longer the plasma expanding capacity.
- Known adverse effects:
  - Pruritis.
  - Clotting and bleeding abnormalities.
  - Renal impairment.
  - Anaphylactoid reactions.

Dextrans
- Complex, branched glucose polysaccharides which are derived by bacterial action on sucrose.
  - Dextran 40 (MW- 40000 Da).
  - Dextran 70 (MW- 70000 Da).
- Used for plasma volume expansion in the treatment of hypovolemic shock and as a component of the pump prime for cardiopulmonary bypass.
- Dextran solutions may have a role in prophylaxis of postoperative thromboembolism.

Human Albumin Solution (HAS)
- 4.5% and 20%; the former is used in plasma expansion and the latter for correction of hypoalbuminaemia.
- HAS 4.5% is isotonic, HAS 20% is hypertonic containing around 4 times normal plasma albumin and exerts osmosis.

Table 3.8 Composition of common IV fluids

| | Fluid | | | Electrolyte composition (mmol/l) | | |
	Na^+	K^+	Cl^-	Other	Osmolality (Mosm/l)	pH
N Saline	154	-	-		308	5.0
CSL	131	5	111	Ca^{2+} (2) Lactate (29)	279	6.5
5% Dextrose	-	-	-	Glucose 50 g/l	278	4.0
Gelofusine	154	-	154	Gelatin 40 g		7.4
HES	154	-	154	Starch 60–100 g		5.5
Dextran 70/40	154	-	154			4.5
Albumin	<160	<2	136	Albumin 45 g		7.4

Special considerations

- The lung is very susceptible for injury and may accumulate interstitial fluid especially, when manipulated during the operation. Hence, the type and amount of fluids administered during the peri-operative period is much debated.
- As always the much debated issue of crystalloids vs. colloids exist. Benefits proposed towards colloids are limited fluid administration with less fluid translocation from the intravascular compartment. Many studies have failed to delineate a significant better clinical outcome with either of the fluids.
- The total volume of fluid. seems to be a critical contributory factor for post-operative pulmonary oedema.
- Usually, a combination of crystalloids and colloids are administered. Crystalloids up to 1–2 liters are given with the understanding that most of the fluid will translocate to extravascular space. Further fluids could be colloids or blood to replace the ongoing losses.
- Hypotension during the intra-operative period could be multifactorial and not just hypovolemia.
- The total amount of fluids to be given can be guided COP monitoring and other indices like HR, BP, CVP and UOP.

☛ *Post-pnemonectomy pulmonary oedema (PPE) (See later section)*

- PPE is very poorly understood phenomenon, though excessive fluid administration is attributed as a cause. Many studies have failed to show this, but restrictive fluid management strategies have been followed and have been employed in various studies.
- The remaining lung during the post-pneumonectomy phase could sustain increased capillary permeability secondary to shear stress from increased capillary flow and ventilator associated lung injury.

Problems secondary to excess fluid administration

- Administration of excess fluid may cause several problems after surgery.
- The resulting increased demands on cardiac function, due to an excessive shift to the right on the Starling myocardial performance curve, may potentially increase postoperative cardiac morbidity.
- Fluid accumulation in the lungs may predispose patients to pneumonia and respiratory failure.
- The excretory demands of the kidney are increased, and the resulting diuresis may lead to urinary retention mediated by the inhibitory effects of anaesthetics and analgesics on bladder function.
- Gastrointestinal motility may be inhibited, prolonging postoperative ileus.
- Excess fluid may decrease tissue oxygenation with implications for wound (anastomotic) healing.
- Finally, coagulation may be enhanced with crystalloids, which may predispose patients to postoperative thrombosis.

Crystalloids vs. Colloids

- A recent randomized controlled trial of 5% human albumin vs. saline infusion showed in a heterogeneous population of adult ICU patients that albumin can be considered safe, without demonstrating any clear efficacy advantage over saline.
- There is no firm evidence that the use of any colloid solution is superior to any other or that colloid solutions are associated with better outcomes than crystalloids in patients with trauma or burns or following surgery.
- Some colloid solutions affect haemostatic function and so could contribute to a bleeding tendency. It is advisable to adhere to the maximum doses recommended by the manufacturers.

Local anaesthetics

Structure and classification of LA

Esters (-COO-)

Indication

- Rarely used in thoracic anaesthesia.

Examples

- Procaine, cocaine, amethocaine and chloroprocaine are examples.

Relevant pharmacology

- Readily hydrolysed by pseudo-cholinesterase.
- Relatively unstable in solution when exposed to heat and light.
- Metabolized to PABA → methaemoglobinaemia, allergy and hypersensitivity.

Amides (-NHCO-)

Indication

- Commonly used LA agent for central neuraxial and peripheral nerve blocks.

Examples

- Lidocaine, prilocaine, bupivacaine, levobupivacaine and ropivacaine.

Relevant pharmacology

- Stable in solution.
- Fewer hypersensitivity reactions.

Mode of action

- LA drugs are weak acids in solution prior to injection.
- Un-ionized base ('B') of LA is formed when it enters a more alkaline environment.
- 'B' enters the axon, becomes ionized (BH^+) and blocks the Na channel from the inside—hydrophilic pathway.
- 'B' also blocks the Na channel from the outside—hydrophobic pathway.
- Na channel blockade is reversible but leads to failure of depolarization and nerve conduction → analgesia.

Clinical properties of LA

(See Table 3.9 for more detailed LA information).

- Closer the pKa to the normal pH (7.4) more base will be released → faster onset.
- Potency of LA is directly proportional to its lipid solubility.
- Duration of action is directly proportional to its protein binding and vasoconstrictive properties (cocaine and ropivacaine)
  - Lidocaine and prilocaine are vasodilators → shorter acting.

Table 3.9 The comparative onset times, potency, duration of action and maximum doses

	pKa	Onset	Lipid solubility	Potency	Protein binding	Duration	Max Dose
Lidocaine	7.7	Fast	150	Medium	64%	Medium	3mg/kg 7mg/kg + Ep.*
Prilocaine	7.7	Fast	50	Low	55%	Medium	6mg/kg 8mg/kg +Fp *
Bupivacaine	8.1	Slow	1000	High	95%	Long	2mg/kg
Levobupi-vacaine	8.1	Slow	1000	High	95%	Long	2mg/kg
Ropivacaine	8.1	Slow	400	High	95%	Long	3mg/kg

*Ep—with added epinephrine *Fp—with added felypressin.

Modifying effects of LA

Onset of action
- For faster onset, select a drug with pKa closer to 7.4.
- Addition of 1 ml 8.4% $NaHCO_3$ for every 10 mls of LA = faster onset.
- Higher concentration of LA = faster onset.

Duration of action
- Effects of lidocaine, prilocaine and bupivacaine (field and nerve blocks only) can be prolonged by adding epinephrine 1:200,000. (See Table 3.10).
  - ⚠ Maximum dose is 200 mcg.
  - ⚠ Contraindicated in severe hypertension and dysrhythmias.
  - Felypressin 0.03 unit/ml is a suitable alternative but may induce coronary vaso-spasm.
  - Do not use epinephrine in epidurals or with long acting LA drugs—⚠ Risk of spinal artery spasm, ischemia and cord infarction.
- Clonidine can be added to LA drugs to prolong the analgesic effect and it is effective in epidural, paravertebral, spinal and intercostal nerve blocks.
- Addition of $NaHCO_3$ prolongs the duration of ropivacaine epidural block.

Table 3.10 Duration of action in minutes with epinephrine

		Chloropro-caine	Lidocaine	Ropivacaine	Bupivacaine
Infiltration	Plain		60–120		180–360
	+Ep		90–180		300–480
Spinal	Hyperbaric		60		120–360
	+Ep		60–90		120–360
Epidural	Plain	30–45	80–120	140–200	120–240
	+Ep	45–60	120–180	160–220	180–360

Selective blockade
- Order of conduction block by LA:
  - Pain → Cold → Warmth → Light touch → Deep Pressure → Motor.
- Motor blockade can be spared by using lower concentrations of LA. drugs, while analgesic potency is increased by adding synergistic agents:
  - Opiates—fentanyl, diamorphine, morphine.
  - Ketamine.
  - Clonidine.

Cocaine

- Only used topically and never injected.
- Potent vasoconstrictor and can induce arrhythmias.
- 10% paste applied intra-nasally will reduce the risk of bleeding and provide analgesia during awake nasal intubation.
- Maximum dose 1.5 mg/kg.

Bupivacaine

Preparations
- Plain 0.25 and 0.5% solutions.
  - For epidural, paravertebral, intrathecal, intercostal, phrenic nerve blocks, field blocks and local infiltration.
- 0.25 and 0.5% solutions with epinephrine 1:200,000.
  - For field blocks, nerve blocks and local infiltration.
- 0.5% with glucose 80 mg/ml (heavy).
  - For intrathecal injections eg. CSE before thoracotomy.

Maximum dose
- 2 mg/kg.

Toxicity
- Low therapeutic index. Blood levels needed to produce CNS and CVS toxicity are similar.
- High affinity binding with cardiac myosites.
- Cardiac failure and arrest are more intractable than after other LA.

Levobupivacaine

Preparations
- 0.25, 0.5 and 0.75% solutions
  - Epidural, CSE, paravertebral, intercostal, pleural and field blocks.

Maximum dose and toxicity
- Structurally an isomer of bupivacaine: similar toxicity profile but less cardiotoxic.
- Max dose during continuous infusion 400 mg/24 hours.

Lidocaine

Preparations
- 10% spray pump.
  - Surface analgesia before endoscopy and bronchoscopy.
  - Max dose 20 sprays—200 mg.
- 4% jet spray, 4ml vial (Laryngojet®)
  - Laryngoscopy, awake intubation.
- 4% solution—topical use only.
  - Bronchoscopy—max dose 5 ml.
- 2% gel—6 ml
  - For urinary catheter insertion.
- 0.5, 1 and 2% solutions.
  - Field, regional blocks, nerve blocks and local infiltration.

Maximum dose
- 7 mg/kg with epinephrine and 3 mg/kg without epinephrine.

Toxicity
- Better therapeutic index and less cardiotoxic than bupivacaine.

Ropivacaine

Preparations
- 0.75 and 1% solutions.
  - Surgical anaesthesia with field, regional and nerve blocks.
- 0.2% solution.
  - Pain relief with field, regional and nerve blocks.

Maximum dose
- 3 mg/kg.

Toxicity
- High therapeutic index.
- Convulsions, arrhythmias and CVS collapse rare.
- Relatively easy to resuscitate following an overdose.

Prilocaine

Preparations
- 3% with felypressin 0.03 u/ml
  - Field and nerve block.
- 1% solution
  - Nerve blocks.

Maximum dose 6 mg/kg.
Toxicity
- Same as other LA + methaemoglobinaemia.
- Hypersensitivity reactions more common due to PABA.

Toxic effects
- Accidental intravascular injection → CVS collapse.
- Over dosage from a correctly placed block (slower absorption) → CNS signs dominate.

☙ CNS signs
- With increasing blood levels excitatory signs give way to CNS depression
  - Circum-oral and tongue numbness, lightheadedness → tinnitus, visual disturbances, muscular twitching, convulsions, unconsciousness, coma, respiratory arrest and death.

☣ CVS signs

- Excitatory phase during convulsion → tachycardia & hypertension.
- ↓ cardiac output, vasodilatation = hypotension.
  - ▶▶ Acute collapse without convulsion can occur as a result of massive and inadvertent sub-arachnoid block from a misplaced thoracic epidural.
- AV block, bradycardia and asystole.

Management of neurological and cardiovascular collapse

- Basic resuscitation—100%O_2 ABC approach.
- If injecting, STOP.
  - +/– rhythm control.
  - +/– ETT and IPPV.
  - +/– CPR.
- Anticonvulsants—benzodiazapines, propofol, thiopentone.
- Unresponsive Cardiac arrest → Intralipid 20%, 500ml bag.
  - 1.5 ml/kg bolus stat 7100ml/70kg man.
  - Give the rest of the bag at 0.25 ml/kg/min i.e. over 20 mins.
  - If still unresponsive give two further boluses 5 mins apart.
  - Continue further infusion until stable circulation.
  - ▶▶ Prolonged CPR may be needed if bupivacaine toxicity.
- CPB as a last resort if available.
- Methaemoglobinaemia is treated with methylene blue 1 mg/kg/IV.

Prevention of severe LA toxicity

- Use the lowest concentration and volume needed.
- Aspirate before injection.
- Consider the use of ultrasound guidance when placing blocks where appropriate (See NICE guidance).
- Large volumes given in small aliquots.
- Observe for at least 30mins following injection.
- Facilities for resuscitation (and intralipid) must be available immediately.
- Always consider LA toxicity early rather than late!!

Further reading

Guidelines for the management of severe local anaesthetic toxicity. *AAGBI* 2007.

British National Formulary. September 2008.

http://www.lipidrescue.org (accessed 21/04/09).

Analgesics

- Thoracotomy is one of the most painful surgical incisions. It is associated with a high incidence of both acute and chronic post-operative pain, which delay recovery and cause long term disability.
- Inadequate analgesia causes:
  - Hypoventilation with hypoxaemia and hypercarbia.
  - Ineffective cough with retained pulmonary secretions.
  - Reluctance to mobilize/undergo physiotherapy.
- A multi-modal approach should be adopted to ensure adequate analgesia, while minimizing any potential side effects.
- Consider pre-emptive analgesia to reduce wind up and sensitization.
- The BEST analgesia regimen will be tailored to the unique needs of each patient.

Drug information at a glance (see Table 3.11)

Table 3.11 Common analgesics used in thoracic anaesthesia

Drug	Dose (adults)	Description	Cautions/Notes
Paracetamol	1 g qds, IV/PO/PR	Prostaglandin inhibitor	Overdose
Ibuprofen	400 mg tds PO	NSAID	Renal, GI, CVS
Diclofenac	50 mg tds PO		Asthma,
	75 mg bd IV		GI, bleeding
Ketorolac	10–30 mg IV qds		
Morphine	0.1 mg/kg IV titrate to effect	Opioid	Resp. depression
Fentanyl	1–5 mcg/kg IV	Short-acting opioid	Respiratory depression, More cardiac stable
Alfentanil	5–20 mcg/kg/IV	Short-acting opioid	Respiratory depression, bradycardia, hypotension
Remifentanil	Infusion 0–2.0 mcg/kg/min	Ultra short-acting opioid	Respiratory depression, bradycardia, hypotension, muscle rigidity
Tramadol	50–100 mg qds	Opioid and non-opioid analgesic	MAOI, Less respiratory depression

Non-opioid analgesics

Paracetamol
- Good analgesic and antipyretic; minimal anti-inflammatory effects.
- Inhibits central prostaglandin synthesis (mainly PG_E); minimal peripheral effects.
- Not associated with gastric or anti-platelet side effects.
- Available as Oral/IV/PR administration, and in combination preparations.
- Well tolerated by most patients.

Kinetics/dynamics
- Rapid oral absorption, bioavailability 80%.
- Peak plasma levels achieved within 60 minutes of oral administration
- Hepatic conjugation to form inactive metabolites:
  - < 10% are toxic; these are rendered harmless by conjugation with glutathione. In overdose, glutathione is exhausted and the toxic metabolite remains unconjugated.

NSAID's
- Effective anti-inflammatory and analgesic drugs.
- Ibuprofen has antipyretic action.
- Inhibit cyclo-oxygenase, and thus prevent PG and thromboxane synthesis which can cause gastro-intestinal, renal, and haematological side effects.
- Enhance analgesia when administered with opioid and non-opioid analgesics.

Cautions
- >65 years old.
- Peripheral vascular disease.
- Cardiovascular disease.
- Diabetes.
- Gastro-oesophageal reflux disease or peptic ulceration.
- Patients taking:
  - ACE inhibitors.
  - Diuretics.
  - Beta blockers.

Kinetics/dynamics
- Bioavailability varies from 60–80% depending on drug of choice.
- Peak plasma levels after oral administration in 1–2 hours.
- Predominantly renal metabolism for ibuprofen, hepatic for diclofenac.

Side effects

- RS:
  - By inhibiting the action of cyclo-oxygenase, there is increased production of leukotrienes by the action of lipoxygenase on arachidonic acid.
  - Leukotrienes can cause bronchospasm in asthmatics.
- CVS:
  - COX-2 inhibitors have been shown to be related to post-operative cardiovascular thrombotic events in CABG patients, and as such are contraindicated (VIGOR/CLASS trials).
- GIT:
  - Nausea, abdominal pain, peptic ulceration and bleeding.
  - Lower risk associated with COX-2 selective NSAID.
- Renal:
  - Renal hypoperfusion; patients most at risk include those who have pre-existing renal disease, are hypovolaemic, or are taking diuretics.
  - Acute interstitial nephritis.
  - Both the above can cause acute renal failure.
- Haematological:
  - ↓ thromboxane A_2 synthesis causes impaired platelet aggregation and vasoconstriction at the site of injury, which can result in prolonged bleeding.

Opioid analgesics

- Opioid receptors are found in high concentrations in the limbic system and spinal cord.
- Receptors are pre-synaptic and activate Gi-proteins, leading to ↑ intracellulear Ca^{2+}, which in turn ↑ K^+ conductance → hyperpolarization of excitable cell membranes.
- Leads to → nociception.
- May inhibit adenylate cyclase and Ca^{2+} channels, thus preventing 'wind-up'.

General effects

- CNS:
  - Analgesia.
  - Miosis.
  - Anxiolysis/euphoria/dysphoria.
  - Pruritis—may be reversed with naloxone.
  - Muscle rigidity.
- RS:
  - ↓ sensitivity of brain stem to CO_2 (CO_2 response curve shifted to right).
  - ↓RR and V_T.

- ↓cough reflex (profound with remifantanil).
- Bronchospasm is possible secondary to histamine release.
- Wooden chest phenomenon may be observed with remifantanil.
- CVS:
  - Vasodilatation.
  - Bradycardia; ↓ sympathetic tone, vagotonic effects, & direct action. on SA node: 20% reduction in HR possible with remifantanil.
  - Hypotension; → sympathetic tone, histamine release.
- GIT/GU:
  - ↑ resting tone of smooth muscle causes delayed gastric emptying and constipation.
  - Nausea & vomiting mediated by activation of chemoreceptor trigger zone by $5HT_3$ and Dopamine receptors.
  - ↑ ADH → urinary retention and hyponatraemia.
- Endocrine:
  - ↓ ACTH, prolactin, and gonadotrophic hormone release mediated by action on hypothalamic D_2 receptors.

Morphine

- Multiple routes of administration.
- Titrate dose to effect.

Kinetics/dynamics

- Peak effect 30 mins after IV injection.
- Duration of action 3–4 hours.
- Low lipid solubility:
  - Unreliable uptake from sub-cutaneous injection.
  - Delayed respiratory depression after intrathecal/epidural dose.
- pKa = 8.0. ∴ ionized in gastric environment, and absorption delayed until small bowel.
- Extensive first pass metabolism; oral bio-availability = 20–30%.
- Hepatic metabolism with active metabolites:
  - Morphine 3-glucuronide.
  - Morphine 6-glucuronide (analgesic properties).
- Renal excretion:
  - ❶ Morphine-6-glucuronide accumulates in renal failure.

Fentanyl

- Synthetic phenylpiperidine derivative.
- Dose varies according to desired effect:
  - 1–2 mcg/kg IV commonly used for minor procedures; duration of effect 30 minutes.
  - Larger doses needed to obtund CVS response to laryngoscopy.
  - Epidural 25–100 mcg.
  - Spinal 10–25 mcg.

Kinetics/dynamics

- Not administered orally as it may become trapped in acidic environment of stomach (99.9% is ionized).
- Rapid onset of action (1–2 minutes), due to very high lipid solubility.
- Peak effect after 4–5 minutes.
- Duration of action:
  - 20 minutes after 1–2 mcg/kg bolus
  - Tissues become saturated during infusion, thus prolonging the duration of action.
- Clearance and elimination similar to morphine.

Remifentanil

- Synthetic phenylpiperidine derivative
- Usually administered as initial IV bolus followed by infusion
- Provides effective obtundation of CVS response to laryngoscopy

Kinetics/dynamics

- Onset 1–3 mins
- Dose
  - Bolus 0.5–1 mcg/kg over 30–60 seconds.
  - Infusion 0.025–0.1 mcg/kg/min during spontaneous ventilation, or 0.05–2.0 mcg/kg/min during IPPV.
- Context-sensitive half-time = 3–5 minutes
- Rapidly metabolized by non-specific tissue and plasma esterases:
  - Unaffected by cholinesterase levels.
  - Anticholinergics do not alter its metabolism.
- Renal (unaltered by renal failure) and hepatic elimination.

Notes on remifentanil

- It must be borne in mind that due to its extremely short half-life, other forms of analgesia should be available for more painful procedures.
- Many ICU's now use remifentanil as part of a combined sedation regime. If the patient is to remain intubated post-operatively, contact the unit to enquire regarding continuation the intra-operative regime/dilution for post-operative use.
- Alternative pain relief must be initiated prior to stopping a remifentanil infusion as the patient will experience rapid rebound pain.
- ❶ Rapid bolusing can render a patient rapidly apnoeic. Profound bradycardia can also occur.
- Combine with volatile or intravenous anaesthesia.

Bolus for induction/obtundation of response to laryngoscopy or rigid bronchoscopy (authors recommendation)

- Dissolve remifentanil 2 mg in normal saline to a total volume of 40ml, i.e. 50 mcg/ml solution.
- Withdraw 2 ml (100 mcg) of this solution and dilute up to 10 ml, i.e.10 mcg/ml.

Dose
- 1 mcg/kg
  - (for a 70 kg male, = 70 mcg = 7ml)
  - Repeat at 0.5mcg/kg as necessary

TIVA induction schedule using TCI pump
Dose
- Aim for 4 ng/ml 30 seconds prior to stimulating intervention/intubation.
  - Reduce dose according to patient response.

Intra-operative use
Dose
- Infuse at 4–8 ng/ml via TCI pump according to patient response
- Ensure that a longer acting form of analgesia is established by the end of surgery, e.g. morphine, epidural, paravertebral.

Research has shown that the optimal time to administer morphine before terminating a remifentanil infusion is 45 minutes prior to the end of the procedure.

Other drugs
Tramadol
- Clohexanol derivative, with action at all opioid receptors
- Particular affinity for mu receptor.
- Inhibits noradrenaline and 5-HT re-uptake, and thus potentiates the descending, inhibitory pain pathways at spinal cord level.
- Similar effects to morphine, but in equi-analgesic doses has less respiratory depression.

Nefopam
- Centrally-acting non-opioid analgesic drug of the benzoxazocine chemical class.
- An alternative to opioid analgesic drugs, which is used in rheumatic disease and other musculoskeletal disorders in the UK.
- A Cochrane review in July 2009 concluded that there was no evidence to support the use of oral nefopam in post-operative pain.

Ketamine
- N-methyl-D-aspartic acid (NMDA) antagonist with analgesic properties.

- Blocks NMDA receptors on the post synaptic membrane of dorsal horn neurons which are activated by glutamate to stimulate ascending spinal pathways.
- Ketamine may be added in small doses (10–20 mg/h) to morphine PCA to avoid dysphoria, improve analgesia, and reduce the respiratory side effects associated with opioids.

Gabapentin/pregabalin

- These are anticonvulsant medications commonly used for chronic pain states.
- Growing evidence suggests that their anti-neuropathic pain properties may be ideal for post-thoracotomy pain.

OxyContin® and Oxynorm®

- Oxycodone hydrochloride is an opioid analgesic supplied 10 mg, 15 mg, 20 mg, 30 mg, 40 mg, 60 mg, 80 mg, and 160 mg tablet strengths for oral administration.
- It is predominantly an agonist at κ-opioid receptors; which may account for its better side effect profile as compared with morphine.
- 1.5–2 times as potent as morphine when administered orally
  • Therefore 120 mg oral oxcodone equates to 210 mg oramorph.
- OxyContin is a sustained ('contin'—continuous) oral formulation of oxycodone hydrochloride. It is indicated in cases where continuous analgesia is required, minimizing multiple top-up doses.
- Oxynorm however is an immediate release ('norm' = normal) formulation designed to be given frequently.
- ❶ OxyCodone should not be given immediately post-op, to anyone where the pain is classified as mild, or if their pain is expected to be brief.

Oxycontin dose

- 20–40 mg OD/PO
  • Peak onset 3 hours.

Oxynorm dose

- Oxycontin dose, divided QDS/PO.
  • From the above schedule 5–10 mg QDS/PO.
  • Peak onset 20–30 mins.

Muscle relaxants

Non-depolarising muscle relaxants

Mechanism of action

- Competitive antagonism of ACh at post-synaptic nicotinic receptors within the neuromuscular junction.

Uses

- To facilitate tracheal intubation for elective thoracic surgery and interventional procedures (e.g. bronchoscopy) requiring a secured airway.
- To facilitate emergent tracheal intubation in the obtunded patient, e.g. after trauma.
- To facilitate surgical access, especially for intra-abdominal procedures.
- To prevent movement and coughing during thoracic surgery.

Doses

- Rocuronium *(aminosteroid)*.
  - Intubation: 0.6 mg/kg/IV—onset 2 mins; duration 40 mins.
  - Modified RSI: 1 mg/kg/IV—onset 1 min; duration 60 mins.
  - Maintenance: 300–600 µg/kg/hr or boluses of 75–150 µg/kg/IV.
- Vecuronium *(bis-quaternary aminosteroid)*.
  - Intubation: 0.1 mg/kg/IV—onset 3.5 mins; duration 40 mins.
  - Maintenance: 50–80 µg/kg/hr or boluses of 20–30 µg/kg/IV.
- Pancuronium *(bis-quaternary aminosteroid)*.
  - Intubation: 0.1 mg/kg/IV—onset 3.5 mins; duration 45–60 mins.
- Atracurium *(benzyl-isoquinolium esther)*.
  - Intubation: 0.5 mg/kg/IV—onset 3 mins; duration 30 mins.
  - Maintenance: 300–600 µg/kg/hr or boluses of 100–200 µg/kg IV.
- Mivacurium *(benzyl-isoquinolium esther)*.
  - Intubation: 0.15 µg/kg IV—onset 2.5 mins; duration 15 mins.
  - Maintenance: 400 µg/kg/hr or blouses of 100 µg/kg IV.

Effects
- CVS
  - Rocuronium and pancuronium have a vagolytic effects → small increase HR and CO.
  - Atracurium and mivacurium may cause histamine release → dBP.
- RS
  - Atracurium and mivacurium may result in histamine release → bronchospasm.
  - All cause profound apnoea, duration discussed above.
  - HPV is unaffected by any of the neuromuscular blocking drugs.

Monitoring
- Neuromuscular monitoring is suggested by AAGBI guidelines, and TOF watch is most commonly utilized.
- Adductor pollicis and corrugator supercilii (eyebrow movement) both correlate well with the degree of diaphragmatic and laryngeal muscle paralysis.

Reversal
- Inadequate reversal of neuromuscular blockade is associated with an increased risk of postoperatively pulmonary complications.
- Sugammadex is more effective than neostigmine in the reversal of rocuronium induced neuromuscular blockade and avoids the need for anticholinergics (and their associated side effects, e.g. tachycardia).

---

❶ Difficult situations

- Clinical experience suggests that rocuronium has a rather abrupt offset so regular monitoring or infusion may be preferable.
- Neuromuscular blocking drugs can usually be avoided in patients with myasthenia gravis undergoing thymectomy; if required an 80–90% dose reduction is recommended.
- The degree of muscle relaxation may affect BIS monitoring
- Caution required in patients with muscular dystrophies (prolonged block results).

Depolarising muscle relaxants
- Suxamethonium is the only depolarising NMB in common usage
- It is the dicholine ester of succinic acid (2x ACh molecules joined back to back).

Mechanism of action
- Mimics the action of ACh at post-synaptic nictonic receptors within the neuromuscular junction.
- Initial prolonged depolarization of the motor end-plate is followed by profound relaxation.

Uses
- To facilitate tracheal intubation for elective thoracic surgery and interventional procedures in patients who are at risk of aspiration.
- To facilitate emergent tracheal intubation in the obtunded patient, e.g. after trauma.

Dose
- Intubation: 1–2 mg/kg/IV—onset 0.5–1 min; duration 3–5 mins.
- Emergency IM dose: 3 mg/kg—in the emergency where access is impossible.

Effects
- CVS
  - Repeated doses can result in bradycardia.
  - Histamine release may result in ↑ HR and ↓ BP (often mistaken for anaphylaxis).
- RS
  - Profound apnoea.

Monitoring
- Suxamethonium is rarely monitored in clinical practice, unless there are concerns regarding a prolonged duration of action.

Reversal
- Not necessary (unless phase II block), as the drug is metabolized by plasma cholinesterase.
- Plasma cholinesterase concentrations may be reduced in:
  - Pregnancy.
  - Liver disease, cardiac failure and renal disease.
  - Hypoproteinaemic states (ICU patients, burns).
  - Muscular dystrophy, carcinomatosis and thyrotoxicosis.
  - Scohne apnea (inherited condition).

❶ Difficult situations

- If using intermittent boluses of suxamethonium to maintain paralysis for short procedures (rigid bronchoscopy, oesophagoscopy), prophylactic atropine should be given to avoid bradycardia.
- Be wary that repeated dosing may result in a phase II block (poorly sustained tetanus, post titanic fasciculation, TOF ratio >0.3, reversal with anticholinesterases).
- Increase in serum K^+ concentration by 0.25–0.55 mmol/l (can cause cardiac arrest and fatal arrhythmias):
  - This may be significantly greater in conditions causing an increase in extra-junctional acetylcholine receptors, e.g. burns.
  - May be of significance in the critically ill patient on ICU (critical care myopathy) or those with renal failure and pre-existent hyperkalaemia.
  - Duchenne muscular dystrophy → increased K^+ release, rhabdomyolysis.
- Trigger agent for malignant hyperpyrexia. (Caution in patients with muscular dystrophies; particularly Duchenne variant as they are more prone to MH).
- Prolonged block in those with suxamethonium apnoea.
- Significant suxamethonium myalgia occurs in certain individuals.
- High dose rocuronium is an alternative for rapid sequence induction, but the risk of prolonged paralysis must be considered on a case to case basis.

Antibiotics

A detailed account of microbiology and the pharmacology of antimicrobial agents is beyond the scope of this chapter. This section will focus on commonly encountered anti-microbial agents in thoracic surgery, with a view to sensible and rationalized prescription.

Prophylactic antibiotics for surgery

Patients presenting for thoracic surgery risk developing wound infection, empyema and pneumonia. Studies have suggested that antibiotic prophylaxis may reduce wound infection after thoracic surgery. However, the antibiotic used and its duration is still debated. Antibiotics administered for prophylaxis in thoracic surgery may need to cover a broad spectrum of bacteria.

Skin commensals
- Most are gram + aerobes although *Mycobacteria*, *Propionibacterium* and *Corynebacteria* are also encountered.

Oral cavity commensals
- *Streptococcus*, *Neisseria*, *Lactobacillus*, and *Staphylococcus* species.

Upper respiratory tract commensals
- *Neisseria* sp., *Staphylococcus epidermidis*, *Micrococcus*, avirulant strains of *Streptococcus pneumoneae*, and *Corynebacteria*.

The lower respiratory tract is virtually free of bacteria in a healthy human. Prophylaxis should also take account of the upper alimentary tract flora when oesophageal surgery is undertaken.

Cephalosporins reduce infections in pulmonary surgery. The addition of metronidazole to cephalosporins for oesophageal surgery has been shown to reduce postoperative infections when compared to cephalosporins alone.

The recommendations may change if the patient is at high risk of endocarditis (i.e. the use of co-amoxiclav or teicoplanin).

Prophylactic antibiotic suggestion for thoracic cavity surgery

Doses

- Cephalosporin
  - Cefuroxime 1 g or Cephradine 1 g IV—at induction.
- Penicillin
  - Flucloxacillin 1–2 g or Co-amoxiclav 1.2 g IV—at induction.

For gram negative cover during G.I surgery add in:
- Metronidazole
  - 500 mg IV—at induction.

Bacterial infections of the lung

Known bacterial infections should be aggressively treated with guidance from microbiological cultures. (See Table 3.12).

Respiratory pathogens

Common

- *Streptococcus pneumonia* (G+).
- *Haemophilus influenza* (G–).

Less common

- *Staphylococcus aureus* (G+).
- *Klebsiella pneumoniae* (G–).
- *Pseudomonas aeruginosa* (G–).
- *Mycoplasma pneumoniae* (no stain).
- *Mycobacterium tuberculosis* (no stain).
- *Chlamydia pneumoniae* (no stain).
- *Legionella pneumophila* (no stain).
- *Aspergillus fumigates* (Fungus).

Table 3.12 Empirical treatment of respiratory infections

Condition	Antibiotic	Alternative
LRTI : infective exacerbation of COPD	Antibiotics not always indicated Doxycycline 100 mg BD for 1/7 then 100 mg OD for 4/7	Levofloxacin 500 mg OD 5/7
Community acquired pneumonia, non severe	Amoxicillin 500 mg—1 g TDS plus Erythromycin 500 mg QDS 7/7	Levofloxacin 500 mg OD 7/7
Severe	Co-amoxiclav IV 1.2 g TDS plus Clarithromycin IV 500 mg BD	Cefuroxime IV 1.5 g TDS plus Clarithromycin IV 500 mg BD
Hospital acquired pneumonia, non-severe	Co-amoxiclav 375 mg TDS plus Amoxicillin 250 mg TDS 7/7	Levofloxacin PO 500 mg OD 7/7 (or Cefuroxime IV 1.5 g TDS)
Severe	Co-amoxiclav IV 1.2 g TDS; plus stat Gentamicin IV 5 mg/kg	Ceftazidime 2 g TDS or Cefuroxime 1.5 g TDS 7/7; plus stat Gentamicin IV 5 mg/kg (Or Levofloxacin PO) 500 mg BD plus Vancomycin IV 1 g BD 7/7)

(Contd.)

Table 3.12 (Contd.)

Condition	Antibiotic	Alternative
Community acquired empyema	Cefuroxime IV 1.5 g TDS plus metronidazole IV 500 mg TDS	Clindamycin 600 mg PO QDS
Hospital acquired empyema	Tazocin® IV 4.5 g TDS and Vancomycin IV 1 g IV BD	

Tuberculosis

The surgical treatment of tuberculosis is mainly confined to the management of multi-drug resistant TB (MDR-TB). A patient with MDR-TB, who remains culture positive after many months of treatment, may present for lobectomy or pneumonectomy. Surgery may assist in diagnosis of extrapulmonary TB with lymph node excision, abscess drainage and tissue biopsy.

Table 3.13 The British Thoracic Society (BTS) recommended drug treatment of uncomplicated TB

2 Months of	4 Months of
Isoniazid	Rifampicin
Pyrazinamide	Isoniazid
Rifampicin	
Ethambutol	
(Streptomycin) subs. for ethambutol	

▶▶ Anaesthesia

- Give prophylactic antibiotics as directed by local microbiological advice.
- Aggressively treat pulmonary infections.
- Continue antibiotics intra-operatively.

Further reading

Wertzel H., Swobada L., Joos-Wurtemberger A., Frank U, Hasse J. Perioperative antibiotic prophylaxis in general thoracic surgery. *Thoracic and Cardiovascular Surgery*. 1992; 40:326–9.

Joint Tuberculosis Committee of the British Thoracic Society. Chemotherapy and management of tuberculosis in the United Kingdom: recommendations. *Thorax* 1998; 53:536–48.

Anti-emetics

At least five different receptor sites on the chemoreceptor trigger zone (CTZ) respond to various chemical emetogenic stimuli in the blood. These receptor sites are:

- Histaminergic.
- Serotonergic.
- Muscarinic.
- Opioid.
- Dopaminergic.

Risk factors for PONV are listed (See Table 3.14). The Apfel score may be used to quantify an individual's peri-operative risk.

Table 3.14 Risk factors for PONV

Risk class	Risk factor
Patient	Younger patients
	Female gender
	Previous PONV/motion sickness
	Non-smoker
	Obesity
	Anxiety
	Opioid use for pain
Surgery	Abdominal/gynaecological
	Strabismus/ENT
	Baseline risk iby 60% every 30 min increase of surgical time
Anaesthesia	Volatile agents/N_2O
	Opioids
	Neostigmine
	Dehydration

PONV prophylaxis

- Minimize anaesthetic risk factors.
- Use anxiolytic therapy & PONV prophylaxis if the Apfel score is high.
- Use combination therapy with 2–3 agents of different modes of action in those patients at moderate to high risk of PONV.

Apfel score and **PONV** risk

- Score 0 or 1 for each of the following:
- Female
- Previous PONV/motion sickness
- Non-smoker
- Opioid/volatile agent

Total Apfel Score	Risk (%)
0	10
1	21
2	39
3	61
4	79

Anti-emesis & thoracic anaesthesia.

- Pre-operative neo-adjuvant chemotherapy often predisposes patients to delayed phase emesis post-operatively.
- Many patients are taking opioids pre-operatively. These patients may require much larger doses of opioid post-operatively, which may lead to significant PONV.
- Remember, epidural infusions typically contain opioids.
- Post thoracotomy pain is a significant cause of PONV.

Oesophagectomy

- Retching and vomiting stress and compromise the integrity of the anastamosis. Therefore:
  - Avoid N_2O during anaesthesia.
  - Administer PONV prophylaxis before extubation.
  - Ensure adequate analgesia, i.e. thoracic epidural.
  - Adequate drainage and control of pressure of the anastamosis with an NG tube on free drainage.
- ❶ Prokinetic anti-emetic agents (metoclopramide) are contraindicated in the presence of recent G.I anastamoses.

Hiatus hernia repair

- ▶▶ Delicate endoscopic repair of hiatus hernia can be easily damaged by retching and vomiting.
- Need attention to detail to minimize PONV risk factors and use multimodal prophylaxis.

Anti-emetic agents

5-HT$_3$ antagonists

- Especially effective against chemotherapy induced (late phase). N+V (common in thoracic surgery patients with neoplasia).
- 1st line agent for PONV prophylaxis.
- At equi-potent doses all four 5-HT$_3$ antagonists currently available have comparable efficacy, but the duration of action differs.

Mechanism of Action

- Highly selective antagonists at central and peripheral 5-HT$_3$ receptors:
  - High density of 5-HT$_3$ receptors found in the CTZ
  - Peripheral 5-HT$_3$ receptors found on the vagus nerve in the gastrointestinal tract.

Effects

- 5-HT$_3$ antagonists have very little effect on the cardiovascular and respiratory systems and they do not have any sedative effects.

Special points

- Headache, flushing and dizziness have been reported.
- Reduce dose in liver impairment.

Doses

Ondansetron

- 4–8 mg/PO TDS; administer 1–2 hrs before surgery as prophylaxis.
- 4 mg/IV TDS; ideally administer 20 minutes prior to emergence.
  - If initial dose fails further doses are futile 2° to ceiling effect; try granisetron.
  - Duration of action 4–6 hours.
  - May control post-operative shivering.

Granisetron

- 1 mg PO/IV TDS; transdermal patch now available also.
  - Duration of action 12–14 hours.

Tropisetron

- 2 mg slowly/IV TDS
  - Duration of action 24 hours.

Dolasetron

- 100mg/PO TDS
  - Duration of action 16–24 hours.

Dopamine antagonists

Three main groups:
- Phenothiazines, e.g. prochlorperazine, chlorpromazine.
- Butyrophenones, e.g. haloperidol, droperidol.
- Benzamides, e.g. metoclopromide, domperidone.

Uses
- PONV prophylaxis.

Mechanism of action

Phenothiazines
- Main site of action is at D_2 and $5HT_3$ receptors in the CTZ.
- They also have moderate anti-histaminergic, antimuscarinic and anti-noradrenergic actions.

Butyrophenones
- Phenothiazines, e.g. prochlorperazine, chlorpromazine. Similar pharmacological and anti-emetic profile to the pheonthiazines.
- Main action via antagonism at D_2 receptors at CTZ.
- Post synaptic GABA antagonism.

Benzamides
- Central D_2 receptor blockade in the CTZ.
- Peripheral anti-dopaminergic action enhances gastric and upper intestinal motility.
- Decrease afferent impulses in peripheral visceral nerves to the vomiting centre.
- At high dose, metoclopramide also exhibits a weak $5HT_3$ antagonist effect. However, metoclopramide is a relatively weak anti-emetic.

Effects

Phenothiazines
- CVS.
  - α- adrenoceptor antagonism $\rightarrow$ peripheral vasodilatation & $\rightarrow$ BP.
- CNS
  - Sedation is common.
  - Can cause arrhythmias and ECG changes.
  - Extrapyramidal side effects occur due to central dopamine antagonism. This may manifest as akathisia (motor restlessness), acute dystonia (spasmodic contractures producing trismus, torticollis, opisthotonos and oculogyric crisis), or tardive dyskinesia.

- Anticholinergic side effects can occur, e.g. dry mouth, blurred vision.
- The neuroleptic malignant syndrome (catatonia, cardiovascular instability, hyperthermia and myoglobinaemia; mortality >10%) has been reported in association with prochlorperazine.

Butyrophenones
- Sedation may be an unwanted side effect at doses >5 mg.
- ☞ Droperidol was withdrawn in 2001, following an FDA warning about its potential to prolong the QT interval. This assertion has been challenged.

Benzamides
- Hypotension, tachycardia, bradycardia.
- Metoclopramide crosses the blood brain barrier → extrapyramidal side effects, e.g. oculogyric crisis, akathisia.
- Increase lower oesophageal sphincter tone.

Special points
- These drugs should be avoided in cases of intestinal obstruction or in the presence of recent bowel anastamosis.
- Domperidone does not cross the blood brain barrier and is therefore less likely to cause central effects and sedation. The intravenous preparation was withdrawn following serious arrhythmias during the administration of large doses.

Doses

Prochlorperazine
- 12.5 mg IM/IV TDS.
- 20 mg PO loading dose, then 5–10 mg PO TDS.
- 6 mg BUCCAL loading dose, then 3 mg Buccal TDS.

Haloperidol
- 0.6–1.25 mg PO/IM/IV OD.

Domperidone
- 10–20 mg PO QDS.
- 30–60 mg PR QDS.

Metoclopromide
- 10 mg PO/IM/IV TDS.

Antihistamines
Uses
- PONV prophylaxis.
- Effective against opioid induced nausea and vomiting.

Mechanism of action
- Block histamine at H_1 receptors in the VC.
- Block action of ACh on the vestibular apparatus.

Effects
- Mild tachycardia.
- Anticholinergic side effects include sedation, dry mouth, blurred vision, and urinary retention.

Special points
- Cyclizine should not be used in patients with heart failure or glaucoma Rapid IV injection is painful.

Doses

Cyclizine
- 50 mg IM/IV/SC TDS.

Promethazine
- 25–50 mg PO/IM TDS.

Hyoscine

Mechanism of action
- ACh blockade at muscarinic receptors within the vomiting centre
- Inhibition of transmission at cholinergic and muscarinic receptors in the cortex and pons.

Uses
- More effective in treating motion sickness than PONV.
- Rarely used as PONV prophylaxis.
- Use as drying agent prior to awake intubation.

Effects
- Mild tachycardia may be seen.
- Bronchodilatation and a marked decrease in airway secretions.
- Sedation and antisialogogue.

Special points
- May precipitate central cholinergic syndrome; characterized by excitement, ataxia, hallucinations, behavioral abnormalities and drowsiness.
- Avoid in thymic surgery.

Dose

- 200–600 mcg IM/IV/SC as a pre-medication.

Dexamethasone

Mechanism of action
- Inhibition of prostaglandin formation and/or membrane stabilizing effect may play a role in the anti-emetic action of corticosteroids.

Uses
- Effective in PONV if given prior to induction.

Effects
- There are no reports of dexamethasone related adverse effects in the doses used for the management of PONV.
- Patients may experience a minor 'burning' sensation in their groin on rapid IV injection.

Dose
- 5–10 mg IV QDS.

Miscellaneous

Neurokine receptor antagonists (NK₁)
- Antagonizes the effects of substance 'P' at many NK_1 sites around the body including CTZ and VC.
- Non-peptide drug Aprepitant was approved by FDA in 2003 and T-2328 is undergoing trials.
- Appear to be potent anti-emetics.

Cannabinoids
- Nabilone acts at the VC and has been used as an anti-emetic following chemotherapy.

Acupuncture/Acupressure
- Acupuncture applied to Chinese acupoint P6 causes a demonstrable decrease in the incidence of PONV.
- The acupressure (bilateral wrist bands with beads, 'Sea Bands®') is better than placebo when applied before the procedure and continued for several days post-operatively.
- There are no side effects associated with this method.

Further reading

Gan TJ, Meyer T, Apfel CC, *et al.* Consensus guidelines for managing postoperative nausea and vomiting. *Anesthesia and Analgesia* 2003; 97:62–71.

Pierre S, Benais H, Pouymayou J. Apfel's simplified score may favourably predict the risk of postoperative nausea and vomiting. *Canadian Journal of Anaesthesia* 2002; 49:237–42.

Chemotherapy

Patients presenting for thoracic surgery may have had previous chemotherapy or may subsequently undergo chemotherapy. A wide range of chemotherapeutic agents may be seen as many tumour types will be present in patients presenting for diagnostic biopsy, staging, curative or palliative surgery. Commonly seen tumours include non small cell lung cancer (NSCLC) and oesophageal cancer others include small cell lung cancer (SCLC), lymphoma, mesenchymal tumours, germ cell tumours, neurogenic tumours and 2° lung tumours.

Classification of anticancer drugs

Drugs are classified according to their mechanism of action.

Tumour antibiotics (bleomycin, mitomycin C)

Action
- Bleomycin inhibits DNA synthesis.

Side effects
- Potential for pneumonitis with bleomycin
  - ❶ Lung toxicity presents with hypersensitivity like reaction; fever, tachypnoea, ↓ DLCO and basal crackles.
  - Bleomycin induced pneumonitis occurs secondary to induced free radicals. High FiO_2 and radiotherapy will worsen its effects.

Anthracyclines (doxorubicin, daunorubicin, epirubicin)

- Also classified as antibiotics.

Action
- Topoisomerase II dependent DNA cleavage and intercalation with double stranded DNA.

Side effects
- Potential for cardiac toxicity
  - ❶ Acute effects include ECG changes (sinus tachycardia, ST changes, ectopic beats, low voltage QRS).
- Chronic use causes dose dependent cardiomyopathy.
- Risk factors for cardiomyopathy include mediastinal radiotherapy, pre-existing cardiac disease, concurrent cyclophosphamide/mitomycin, extremes of age.

Alkylating agents (cyclophosphamide, busulphan, carboplatin, cisplatin)
Action
- Alkylate DNA and interfere with mitosis.

Side effects
- May cause tumour lysis syndrome
- Metal salts may cause neurotoxicity (peripheral neuropathy, ototoxicity).
- Neuropathy may be sub-clinical particularly after cisplatin therapy.

Anti-metabolites (methotrexate, pemetrexed, 5FU, gemcitabine, capecitabine)
Action
- Enzyme inhibition or incorporation of wrong DNA code during cell synthesis.

Side effects
- Nitrous oxide may potentiate methotrexate toxicity.

Mitotic inhibitors (vincristine, vinblastine)
Action
- Inhibit the formation of microtubule complexes within the cytoplasm, thereby arresting cell growth in metaphase.

Side effects
- Inadvertent intrathecal administration of vincristine is invariably fatal.

Mitotic stabilizers/taxanes (docetaxel, paclitaxel)
Action
- Stabilize microtubule assembly once formed, thus preventing mitosis from proceeding.

Side effects
- Occasional severe hypersensitivity reactions.

Topoisomerase inhibitors (etoposide, teniposide)
- Inhibit unwinding of DNA during replication.

Hormonal agents (tamoxifen, anastrazole)
Action
- Diverse mechanisms of action incompletely understood.

Antibodies (trastuzumab, rituximab)
Action
- Trastuzumab is a targeted treatment to HER_2 receptors in breast cancer.
- Rituximab is used in the treatment of NHL.

Tyrosine kinase inhibitors (imatinib, erlotinib)
Action
- Cancer cells exploit tyrosine kinase to increase cell survival and proliferation.

(See Table 3.15 for side effects of anti-cancer drugs).

Chemotherapy in lung and oesophageal cancer
(See NICE guidelines)

Non squamous cell lung cancer
- Adjuvant chemotherapy is offered to all after complete resection.
- Neoadjuvant chemotherapy/chemoradiotherapy followed by surgery is one treatment option for Stage III disease.
- 3rd generation drug (docetaxel, gemcitabine, paclitaxel, vinorelbine) with addition of a platinum drug (cisplatin, carboplatin) for T3 +/or N1 and above as tolerated.

Squamous cell lung cancer
- All patients are offered multidrug platinum based chemotherapy.

Oesophageal cancer
- Preoperative chemo-radiation may improve long term survival.
- Neoadjuvant chemotherapy with cisplatin and 5FU followed by surgery improves short term survival over surgery alone.

Table 3.15 Side effects of anticancer drugs

System	Side Effect	Drugs
CVS	Cardiomyopathy	*anthracyclines, 5FU, trastuzumab*
	Cardiotoxicity	*capecitabine*
RS	Pneumonitis	*bleomycin, methotrexate, nitrosureas, cyclophosphamide*
	Pulmonary fibrosis	*bleomycin, busulfan, cyclophosphamide*
	SOB	*gemcitabine*
CNS	Peripheral neuropathy	*cisplatin, oxaliplatin, paclitaxel, vincristine*
	Confusion	*ifosfamide*
	Dizziness	*interferon, temozolamide*
	Headaches	*interferon*
	Insomnia	*temozolamide*
GIT	Nausea and vomiting	numerous
	Diarrhoea	*5FU, capecitabine, irinotecan*
	Constipation	*Vincristine*
	Stomatitis	*doxorubicin, epirubicin, methotrexate*
	Mucositis	*5FU*
	↑ bilirubin	*capecitabine*
Renal	Haemorrhagic cystitis	*cyclophosphamide, ifosfamide*
	↑ creatinine	*cisplatin*
	Fluid retention	*docetaxel, imatinib, tamoxifen*
Skin/ Musculoskeletal	Rashes	*bleomycin, docetaxel, gemcitabine, imatinib*
	Osteoporosis	*anastrazole, letrozole*
	Musculoskeletal pain	*anastrazole, paclitaxel*
Other	Fatigue	*platins, interferon, anthracyclines, taxanes*
	Gonadal failure/ dysfunction	*cyclophosphamide, ifosfamide, anthracyclines*

▶▶ Relevence to thoracic anaesthesia

- Bleomycin causes pneumonitis and pulmonary fibrosis.
- O_2 enhanced bleomycin toxicity may occur if prolonged exposure to $FiO_2 > 0.3$ especially in those with pre-existing bleomycin lung injury or bleomycin exposure within the past 2 months. FiO_2 should be minimized with PaO_2 monitoring.
- Anthracyclines may cause abnormalities of cardiac function which may exist even in those with normal resting function and only become apparent during anaesthesia and exercise.
- Anthracycline induced cardiomyopathy may be present years after treatment.
- Cisplatin causes peripheral neuropathy (primarily sensory) in 20–30% of cases in addition to a higher proportion of subclinical neuropathy. A detailed preoperative neurological examination is therefore warranted especially if regional anaesthesia is to be used.

Further reading

De Souza P. Cancer Drug Toxicities and Anaesthesia. *Australian Anaesthesia* 2007. 71–9.

Clinical Guideline 24: Lung Cancer: *The Diagnosis and treatment of lung cancer.* February 2005. www.nice.org.uk (Accessed 1/6/10).

Pre-operative assessment of the thoracic patient

History

Key aims:
- To assess the patients cardio-respiratory function.
- To identify those patients at higher risk of:
  - Intra-operative hypoxia.
  - Post-operative respiratory failure.
  - Post-operative cardiac complications.
- To allow focused examination and investigation of those patients at higher risk.
- To allow optimization of the patient pre-operatively.
- To identify potential contraindications to specific post-thoracotomy analgesic techniques.

> An accurate history allows for identification of potential problems, optimization of pre-existing co-morbidities, risk stratification and planning of anaesthetic technique.

- The history should begin as for a standard anaesthetic assessment:
  - Details of past anaesthetics, including intubation history and family history.
  - Available patient notes should be reviewed and further hospital notes requested if required.
- Patients presenting for thoracic surgery should be questioned about:
  - Pulmonary symptoms—cough, dyspnoea, haemoptysis, chest pain.
  - Extrapulmonary symptoms—chest wall pain, dysphagia, voice hoarseness, arm pain or weakness, facial weakness.
  - Extrathoracic symptoms—headaches, seizures, bony pain and fractures (relating to metastatic spread of bronchial Ca).
  - Non specific symptoms—weight loss, lethargy, malaise, thirst, oedema.
  - Evidence of ischaemic heart disease or congestive cardiac failure.

The following areas should be concentrated on:

Assessment of cardio-respiratory reserve

(See 📖 Cardio-pulmonary exercise testing, p. 208)
- An accurate patient history provides the most useful assessment of cardio-respiratory function.
- Assessment of oxygen consumption (See Table 4.1).
- The single most important clinical indicator of cardio-respiratory fitness is the ability to climb a flight of stairs at patient's own pace = >4 MET.

- This is associated with a low level of peri-operative cardio-respiratory complications.
- Further assessment of cardio-respiratory function by cardiopulmonary exercise testing or the 6 minute walk test is not necessary in ASA 1 or 2 patients with no limitation of activity and an exercise tolerance corresponding to >4 METS.
- British Thoracic Society regarding appropriate pre-operative investigations for thoracic surgical patients are discussed later (See 📖 BTS guidelines, p. 158).

Table 4.1 Metabolic equivalents

MET*	Activity	O_2 consumption
1	Resting	3.5 ml/kg/min
2	Walking 2 mph/Dressing	7 ml/kg/min
4–10	6 minute walk/1 flight stairs**	14–35 ml/kg/min
>12	Intensive running 8 min mile	>42 ml/kg/min

*1 MET = 1 kilocalorie per kilogram per hour (3.5 ml/kg/min) O_2 consumption (caloric consumption of a person while at complete rest).

**One flight of stairs = 20 steps 6" height.

Significant co-morbidities

Age
- 80–92 years.
  - 3% mortality.
- Associated morbidity however is common:
  - 40% incidence of respiratory complications.
  - 40% incidence of cardiac complications.
  - Higher mortality (22%) from right sided pneumonectomy.

Cardiovascular disease
Risks
- Cardiac complications are the second commonest cause of peri-operative morbidity and mortality in the thoracic surgical population. Patients with pre-existing cardiac disease are significantly more likely to develop cardiac complications.
- Most thoracic procedures are deemed intermediate risk procedures and therefore the most effective way of reducing cardiac morbidity is to identify high risk patients pre-operatively (See Table 4.2).

- Routine cardiac screening is not cost effective and therefore an accurate history is essential to identify those patients who require further investigation for accurate risk assessment and optimization prior to surgery.
- All patients should have an ECG (See 📖 ECG, p. 192).
- Echocardiography is not required unless deemed appropriate from the history (See 📖 Echocardiography, p. 204).

Who to refer on
- If the patient's exercise capacity is moderate or excellent, they are low risk.
- If their functional capacity is poor:
  - Non-invasive testing (→) HIGH RISK (▶) Coronary angiography.
- Refer the following patients to a cardiologist pre-op:
  - M.I within the last 6 months.
  - Unstable angina—significant angina at rest or on minimal exertion.
  - Severe CCF—orthopnoea/PND/significant dependent oedema and breathlessness on minimal exertion.
  - Syncopal episodes associated with palpitations.
  - Those with significant arrhythmias. (See 📖 Post-operative arrhythmias, p.670).
  - Newly diagnosed murmurs.

Delay non-urgent surgery
- 4–6 weeks after recent M.I.
- 4–6 weeks after recent metallic coronary stenting to allow a full course of anti-platelet therapy to be completed and for platelet function to return to normal.
- 12 weeks after drug eluting stent placement.

Table 4.2 Cardiovascular risk factor categorization

Major	Intermediate	Minor
Unstable coronary syndrome	Mild angina	Age over 80
Decompensated heart failure	Previous MI	Uncontrolled hypertension
Recent M.I (1/12)	Previous CHF	Previous cardiovascular accident
Significant arrhythmia	Diabetes	ECG—RBBB. LVH
Severe valvular lesion		Non-sinus rhythm
		Poor exercise tolerance (<2 flights of stairs)

Smoking

- Many patients requiring thoracic surgery have a significant smoking history, increasing the risk of cardiac disease and coexisting respiratory disease.
- Work out pack year smoking history:

(No. cigarettes smoked per day x No. years smoked) ÷ 20

- Counsel to stop smoking post-operatively.
- Assessment of cough, shortness of breath, orthopnoea, and wheeze should be made.
- Stopping smoking:
  - >12 hours pre-op reduces CO levels to normal/reduces broncho-spasticity.
  - >2 days pre-op reduces intra-op ST changes.
  - >4 weeks pre-op reduces wound complications and respiratory complications.
  - >8 weeks pre-op confers benefit with re-generation of muco-cilliary escalator/optimal sputum clearance.

Respiratory disease
Risks

- Many patients undergoing thoracic surgery will have significant COPD. It is important to identify them early and minimize further harm as a result of your anaesthetic/surgery.
- Degree of airway reversibility and response to steroid therapy can be established from a detailed history.
- As for cardiac disease, a good history identifies patients who will benefit from more detailed pre-operative investigation.

- Most will have seen, or will be under the care of a respiratory team already; liaison with them is important.
- Most patients undergoing thoracic procedures will have had basic lung function tests performed pre-operatively. Flow volume loops are not required as a routine test in patients who have no supine exacerbation of cough or shortness of breath. (See ☐ Assessment of respiratory mechanics, p. 186).

Who to refer on

- Consider discussion with respiratory team regarding further medication/bronchdilator therapy if uncontrolled symptoms.
- Refer high risk patients for pre-operative physiotherapy. Physiotherapy has various benefits:
  - Proven decrease in pulmonary complications in COPD patients especially if contemplating lung volume reduction surgery.
  - Particularly beneficial in patients with excessive secretions.

Renal disease

- Renal failure post lung resection is associated with a high mortality rate (19%).
- Risk factors for post-operative renal failure need to be identified pre-operatively.
- These include:
  - Pre-existing renal disease.
  - Hypertension/diabetes.
  - Patients receiving diuretic therapy.
  - Recent chemotherapy.
  - Ischaemic heart disease.
  - Those undergoing pneumonectomy.

Disease history

- Patients with lung tumours must also be assessed for the following:
  - **M**ass effects—obstructive pneumonia, abscess, SVC obstruction, tracheobronchial distortion, Pancoast's syndrome, recurrent laryngeal/phrenic nerve palsy, chest wall and mediastinal extension.
  - **M**etabolic effects—Lambert-Eaton syndrome, hypercalcaemia, hyponatraemia, Cushing's syndrome.
  - **M**etastases—particularly to bone, liver, brain, adrenals.
  - **M**edications—interactions and side effects of chemotherapy.

- For example, a recent history of increasing shortness of breath and facial swelling may indicate SVC obstruction which requires further pre-operative investigation.
- Any evidence of cor pulmonale must be investigated as a dysfunctional right ventricle will decompensate with increases in afterload caused by pulmonary resection.
- A recent history of weight loss of more than 10% strongly suggests advanced disease.

Drug history

- A history of drug allergies is of obvious importance.
- A history of chemotherapy agents may have importance. Recent exposure to bleomycin can exacerbate oxygen induced pulmonary toxicity.
- Drugs that affect coagulation such as heparin and warfarin may preclude certain post-operative analgesic options such as thoracic epidurals.

Other important factors in the patient history

- Factors that may make endobronchial intubation difficult:
  - Previous radiotherapy.
  - Massive tumour with mass effect.
  - Infection.
  - Previous thoracotomy and airway surgery.
  - Previous difficult intubation.

Further reading

Kaplan JA, Slinger PD. *Thoracic Anaesthesia* 3rd edition 2003. Churchill Livingstone. 1–23.

Examination

Pre-operative anaesthetic assessment for thoracic surgery should include a clinical examination in order to guide peri-operative investigation, risk stratification, and management. Particular attention should be paid to the airway and cardio-respiratory system.

Airway examination

Difficult airway management is likely to be compounded when using double lumen tubes which are more bulky and less maneuverable. Complete examination of the airway for thoracic surgery may include assessment of the sub-glottic airway by CXR and CT chest if clinically indicated.

- Perform a routine anaesthetic airway assessment. In addition, assess for the following features in thoracic surgical patients:
  - Signs of upper airway obstruction, e.g. breathlessness, audible stridor (may be positional), use of accessory muscles of respiration.
  - Tracheal deviation; tracheal or bronchial distortion/compression may affect tracheal intubation, tube positioning, and lung isolation.
  - Inspect for neck scars, e.g. tracheostomy (previous long stay on ITU?), previous neck surgery. Consider if the airway could be difficult due to tracheal stenosis.
- Careful planning and preparation are required for anticipated difficult airway/intubation.
- ❶ The majority of thoracic patients will require rigid bronchoscopy. This may be impossible if the patient requires an awake fibreoptic intubation. Discuss this with the surgeons.

Respiratory system

Consider whether the examination findings correlate with available investigations. If not, consider further/new investigations.

Extrapulmonary signs

- Central cyanosis, cachexia, clubbing, nicotine staining, muscle wasting (hands/globally), cervical lymphadenopathy, facial plethora (SVC obstruction), facial weakness (Horner's syndrome), hoarse voice (recurrent laryngeal nerve palsy).

Chest signs

- Inspection:
  - Respiratory rate.
  - Equal/unequal chest expansion.
  - Scars from previous thoracic surgery.
  - Intercostal drain; what is it draining and is it functioning adequately?

- Percussion note:
  - Dull = consolidation/atelectasis.
  - Stony dull = effusion/blood.
  - Hyper-resonant = pneumothorax.
- Auscultation:
  - Wheeze.
  - Focal crackles = infection/oedema/fibrosis.
  - Reduced air entry = collapse/effusion/consolidation/fibrosis.
  - Bronchial breathing = consolidation.

Cardiovascular system

- Assess rate, rhythm, volume and character of pulse.
- Measure blood pressure.
- Inspection:
  - Signs of heavy smoking, e.g. tar staining of fingers, cough which clears loose sputum.
  - Signs of peripheral vascular disease.
  - Raised jugular venous pressure, e.g. SVC obstruction, CC.
  - Peripheral oedema.
  - Sternotomy scar from heart surgery.
  - Pacemaker.
- Auscultate:
  - Assess for signs of heart failure, e.g. gallop rhythm, bibasal crepitations. Consider if treatment is optimized.
  - Most heart murmurs will require echocardiographic assessment.

General examination

- Examine intended cannulation sites to exclude unforeseen difficulties.
- Examine the thoracic spine if epidural/paravertebral block is planned.
- Assess volaemic state to guide fluid management/resuscitation.
- Measure the temperature. Sepsis will influence your anaesthetic technique and other peri-operative requirements.
- Examine for and consider the impact of other co-morbidities.

Emergency thoracic examination
- Adopting an ABC approach in conjunction with ATLS guidelines will provide a rapid assessment for any thoracic emergency.
- The examination is intended to identify and treat immediate threats to life (ATOMFC):
  - **A**cute severe haemorrhage.
  - **T**ension pneumothorax.
  - **O**pen pneumothorax.
  - **M**assive haemothorax.
  - **F**lail chest.
  - **C**ardiac tamponade.

Further reading

Gothard J, Kelleher A, Haxby E. Preoperative assessment of the thoracic surgical patient in Cardiovascular and Thoracic Anaesthesia. *Anaesthesia in a Nutshell*. Oxford. Butterworth-Heinemann; 2003 p.117–21.

BTS guidelines

Background

The British Thoracic Society and Society of Cardiothoracic Surgeons of Great Britain and Ireland published guidelines in 2001 (currently being revised) for the selection of lung cancer patients for surgery after recognition that operative mortality was higher in the UK than in Europe and the USA. The guidelines relate to two areas:

- Fitness for surgery.
- Surgical resectability.

Fitness for surgery requires assessment of:
- Age.
- Predicted postoperative lung function.
- Cardiovascular health.
- Nutrition and performance ability.

Age

- Elderly patients are more likely to require intensive care post-op.
- Age above 80 is an independent risk factor for mortality for patients undergoing pneumonectomy but NOT lobectomy.
- Patients aged 70–80 years have similar risks to patients aged below 70.

Pulmonary function

FEV_1

- The single most useful test.
- In the absence of interstitial lung disease or unexpected disability due to SOB a post bronchodilator FEV_1 of:
  - >1.5L for lobectomy—low mortality. No further tests required.
  - >2.0L for pneumonectomy—low mortality. No further tests required.

❶ If patient is not clearly operable, obtain diffusion capacity, blood gases and V/Q scan.

Blood gases and saturation

SpO_2

- <90% on air or <4% drop in SpO_2 on walking/shuttle testing = high risk.
- This test alone does not determine suitability for surgery.

Arterial blood gases

PaO_2

- Hypoxia alone does not increase the risk but hypoxia with increased PAP increases the risk.

$PaCO_2$

- $PaCO_2$ >6.0kPa has higher post-op morbidity but is not a contraindication to surgery *per se*.
- Hypercapnoea is usually associated with a low DLCO.
- CO_2 retention is unlikely if $FEV_1 > \rightarrow 1.0L$ or VO_2 >12 ml/kg/min.
- Always correlate blood gases with other tests.

> ❶ Hypercarbia with COPD contraindicates pneumonectomy.
>
> ❶ Expected 5 year survival with hypercarbia is <50%.

Diffusion capacity

- The single breath carbon monoxide diffusing capacity (DLCO) also called transfer factor (TLCO) is a measure of the lungs ability to transfer gases.

Predicted postoperative lung function

- Calculate the estimated post operative FEV_1 (ppoFEV_1) and the estimated post operative DLCO (ppoDLCO) and express both as % predicted post operative values (%ppoFEV_1 & %ppoDLCO).

Calculations

%ppoFEV_1 calculation (lobectomy)

- ppoFEV_1 = pre-op FEV_1 x number of segments remaining post surgery/total number of segments in lung.
- ppoFEV_1 = pre-op FEV_1 x (19—segments to be resected)/19.
  - Segments: RUL 3, RML 2, RLL 5, LUL 3, Ling 2, LLL 4.

Example:

- Male patient for RLL lobectomy has FEV_1 of 1.3L (2.5L predicted for his age and height)
- ppoFEV_1 = 1.3L x (19–3)/19 = 1.09L
- %ppoFEV_1 = 1.09/2.5 = 44%
  - Modify calculation if any segments obstructed.
  - Similarly calculate %ppoDLCO.

%ppoFEV_1 calculation (pneumonectomy)

- ppoFEV_1 = pre-op FEV_1 x (1-% perfusion to lung to be resected).

Example:

- Male patient for L pneumonectomy FEV_1 1.8L (2.5L predicted) 40% perfusion to L lung.
- ppoFEV_1 = 1.8 x (1-.4) = 1.08l
- %ppoFEV_1 = 1.08/2.5 = 43%
- Similarly calculate %ppoDLCO.

❶ Average risk

%ppoFEV$_1$ >40% and %ppoDLCO >40%.

❶❶ High risk

%ppoFEV$_1$ <40% and % ppoDLCO <40%.

Cardiopulmonary exercise testing (CPET)

(See also 📖 Cardio-pulmonary exercise testing, p. 208)

- CPET measures the maximum uptake of oxygen per unit time by spirometry and gas analysis when the patient exercises (stair climbing/ treadmill/bike/arm exercises; depending on institution).
- Of all of the pre-operative tests, cardiopulmonary reserve is probably the most useful test of functional reserve and quality of life.

VO$_2$ values

- >15 ml/kg/min.
  - no increased peri-operative mortality.
- <12 ml/kg/min.
  - increased risk.

- There is a strong association between maximum oxygen uptake achieved and survival after major surgery. (See Table 4.3)
- The literature suggests that a pre-op VO$_2$ max as % predicted was 83% vs. 55% for survivors vs. non-survivors after thoracic surgery.

Table 4.3 Oxygen consumption on CPET and implications for surgery

Oxygen consumption (mlO$_2$/kg/min)	Exertion equivalent	Interpretation
3.5	Rest	Resting metabolic rate or 1 MET
10	Walking on the flat	Not fit for surgery if this cannot be achieved
15	Walking up 3 flights of stairs without stopping	Average risk if this cannot be achieved

Stair climbing
- 'Flight' = 20 steps of 6" height
  - 3 flights at patient's own pace without stopping—VO_2 of >15ml/kg/min
- 2 flights—VO_2 of 12 ml/kg/min.

> ❶ Inability to climb 2 flights—increased risk.

6 minute walk test
- Good correlation with VO_2
- 6 min walk of <2000 ft (650 yards) would suggest VO_2 <15ml/kg/min.

> ❶ Fall in SpO_2 during exercise—**high risk.**
>
> ❶ >4% fall during standard exercise—**high risk.**
>
> ❶ $ppoVO_2$<10 ml/kg/min—**high mortality.**

Cardiovascular fitness
- All patients should have a pre-op ECG
- All patients with a murmur on auscultation should have a transthoracic Echo (particularly if symptomatic)
- Lung resection should not usually be performed:
  - Within 6 weeks of MI.

Management strategy for patients with CVS conditions (adapted from ACA/AHA Guidelines 2007)

Active cardiac condition within MAJOR category
- Cardiology opinion—would the patient benefit from bi-ventricular pacing/CABG/valve surgery?

No active cardiac condition + can walk up a hill (4METs)
- Proceed with surgery.

Cannot perform 4METs + 1 or more clinical risk factors
- Proceed with surgery, consider heart rate control.
- Refer to cardiology for non-invasive testing only if this would be needed anyway.

- Within 2–4 weeks after stenting.
- Patients with past stroke should have carotid Doppler studies.

Nutrition and performance status

- Recent weight loss >10%, poor nutrition and exertion ability limited to self care, are each associated with poor prognosis in lung cancer.
- Limited evidence of association between these markers and operative outcome because these patients do not often undergo surgery.
- Objective markers of poor nutrition.
  - Ideal body mass <90%.
  - BMI <18.5.
  - Albumin <27 g/L (late sign).
  - Triceps skin fold thickness <25th centile.

Operability

Selection criteria based on TNM staging are discussed (See 📖 Surgical resectability, p. 172).

Simple pre-op assessment tests (See Fig. 4.1)
- Mortality should not be in excess of:
  - 4% for lobectomy.
  - 8% for pneumonectomy.
- Sublobar resection is useful in patients with impaired pulmonary function, but recurrence is higher than lobectomy and long term survival is decreased by 5–10%.

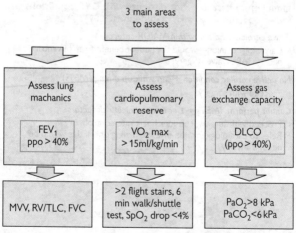

Fig. 4.1 Basic assessment strategy for thoracic patients who are to undergo thoracic anaesthesia.

The boxed text shows the most important tests and the ideal values permitting go-ahead for thoracic surgery. Other less important tests are shown below these.

Further reading

Guidelines on the selection of patients with lung cancer for surgery. British Thoracic Society and Society of Cardiothoarcic Surgeons of Great Britain and Ireland. *Thorax* 2001; 56:89–108.

Beckles. The physiologic evaluation of patients with lung cancer being considered for resectional surgery. *Chest*. 2003; 123:105–14.

American College of Cardiology/American Heart Association Guidelines on Perioperative Evaluation and Care for Noncardiac Surgery. 2007. http://circ.ahajournals.org/cgi/content/full/116/17/1971 (Accessed 2/2/10).

Pre-operative tests

Investigations should only be performed to inform management by:
- Confirming diagnosis.
- Determining what, if any surgery should be performed.
- Establishing co-morbidities and providing prognostic information.
- Identifying treatable risk factors.

After history and examination the following are common pre-operative investigations before thoracic surgery. The majority of these tests are discussed in more depth later in this section.

Radiology

CXR

(See CXR, PET, CT, p. 214).
- The primary investigation for the breathless patient with a persistent cough.
- When bronchogenic carcinoma is suspected postero-anterior and lateral radiographs are acquired.
- High voltage (>125 kV) is used to ensure penetration through tumour and mediastinum.
- Adenocarcinoma and large cell carcinoma, 30% and 20% respectively of lung cancers, will be peripheral on a CXR.
- Squamous cell and small cell carcinomas, 30% and 20% respectively of lung tumours, will be central on CXR.

CXR findings

Lung opacities
- Nodular (solid), reticular (fine lines) or alveolar ('fluffy').
- Nodules may be bronchogenic carcinoma, metastatic, infective or granulomatous (TB, sarcoid, Wegners).
- Reticular shadowing is interstitial fluid (cardiac or non-cardiac pulmonary oedema) or viral pneumonia.
- Alveolar shadowing is worsening pulmonary oedema, pneumonia, haemorrhage, ARDS.

Hila
- Equal size?
- Left higher than right?
- Enlarged hila = nodes, pulmonary hypertension (+/– enlarged pulmonary outflow tract—the notch below the aortic knuckle), calcification, old TB.

Widened mediastinum
- Retrosternal thyroid, lymph nodes, thoracic aortic aneurysm (stable and dissecting), pericardial cyst, oesophageal dilatation (hiatus hernia).

COPD
- Hyper-expanded chest, i.e. >7 anterior ribs and >10 posterior ribs.
- Bullae in emphysema.
- Consolidation with infective exacerbations.
- Areas of pulmonary fibrosis.

Pleural effusion
- Loss of costophrenic angle (CPA), only if patient erect.
- Uniform increased opacity, but clear CPA if supine.

CT
(See ⚏ CXR, PET, CT, p. 214).
- Tissue differentiation superior to plain radiography.
- Recommended as a staging procedure for patients with potentially resectable lung cancer. Spiral CT allows optimal contrast enhancement. Node staging with CT is poor with sensitivity and specificity of ~65% each.
- Will identify enlarged mediastinal lymph nodes (maximum short axis diameter = 10 mm) and determine the best approach for biopsy or aspiration cytology (bronchoscopy, mediastinoscopy or percutaneous needle pleural biopsy for pleural disease and effusions).
- Identification of pulmonary, hepatic or adrenal metastases, which are common sites of lung metastasis.

PET
(See ⚏ CXR, PET, CT, p. 214).
- Positron Emission Tomography maps glucose metabolism in the body. F-18-flourodeoxyglucose (FDG) has a short half life (110 minutes).
- Metabolism produces a photon which is detected. Neoplastic, inflammatory and granulomatous lesions have a high FDG uptake.
- High uptake in brain, liver, kidney, bladder cause false positive scans.
- For pulmonary lesions, when combined with CT, it has high sensitivity in differentiating benign from malignant lesions as small as 10 mm. (Note a lesion can be ~4cm before showing on CXR).

MRI
(See ⚏ Surgical resectability, p. 172).
- Not useful for lung parenchyma imaging.
- Indicated for tumour invasion of chest wall, root of neck or great veins.

Bone scintigraphy
- Uses bisphosphonates labeled with Tc^{99}.
- More sensitive than plain radiography for detecting metastases.
- Not used to screen for metastases before lung resection surgery, but it is indicated with advanced symptoms.

Bloods

Renal & hepatic function
- Renal impairment (eGFR<60 ml/min) is an independent risk factor for peri-operative morbidity & mortality following thoracic surgery.
- LFTs only increased with widespread liver metastases. Worth performing where there is significant nutritional deficit.

Full blood count
- Polycythaemia secondary to chronic hypoxaemia, e.g. COPD.
- Anaemia at presentation of lung cancer is a poor prognostic sign.
  - Hb <13.5 g/dl in men.
  - Hb <11.5 g/dl in women.
- Thoracic patients usually have a major peri-operative risk of serious cardiovascular complications. Therefore, a higher transfusion trigger may be appropriate in these patients.

ABG
(See 📖 Blood gases, p. 180).
- Blood gas results ALONE should not be used as a means to decide whether a patient is fit for surgery.
- Blood gases are not predictive of outcome. Resection and lung reduction surgery can proceed with PaO_2 >8.3kpa and $PaCO_2$ <6.3kPa.
- Refer to the appropriate section in this chapter for further detail.

Paraneoplastic syndromes & electrolytes

(Covered in more detail. See 📖 **The patient with: a paraneoplastic syndrome, p. 268**).
- Effects of malignancy not caused by the solid tumour.
- More common in small cell than non-small cell lung cancer, thus less likely operable.

SIADH
- Low serum sodium and osmolality (<260 mosmol/kg).
- Inappropriately high urine sodium (>20mmol/l) and osmolality (>500mosmol/kg) in a euvolaemic patient.

Ca^{2+}
- Elevated with boney metastases (also alkaline phosphatase) and with secretion of ectopic parathyroid hormone releasing peptide (PTHRp).
- More common in squamous cell carcinoma.

Cushing's syndrome
- Hypokalaemic metabolic alkalosis.
- Ectopic ACTH from small cell cancer (much less common than from pituitary adenoma) causes adrenals to release more cortisol and androgens.
- Other features include central obesity, glucose intolerance, hypertension, pigmentation.

Respiratory tests

Spirometry

(See 📖 Spirometry, p. 182).
- Measures functional lung volumes.
  - FEV_1 is the volume forcibly exhaled in 1 second after maximum inspiration.
  - FVC, forced vital capacity, is the total volume exhaled after a maximum inspiration. For 70kg man FVC = 4.5 litres. FEV_1/FVC = 75%.
  - FEV_1/FVC <75%, with normal FVC = obstructive deficit, e.g. asthma, COPD.
  - FEV_1/FVC ≥75%, with low FVC = restrictive deficit, e.g. lung fibrosis, sarcoid, connective tissue disease, pleural effusion, obesity.
- Total lung capacity and FRC are increased in obstructive airway disease. This means the oxygen reservoir at end expiration, or when apnoeic, is greater but despite this, V/Q mismatch leads to hypoxia faster than in healthy lungs.

> FEV_1 is the most informative of all of the tests, as it is a better predictor of outcome. Consideration of % predicted values carries more weight than volumes alone.

Transfer factor

(See 📖 Spirometry, p. 182).
- Measures the volume of carbon monoxide (CO) to diffuse across the lung/unit time/unit partial pressure difference of CO between alveoli and pulmonary capillaries.
- Normal = 25 ml CO/min/mmHg.
- Measured over a 10 second breath hold. The result is influenced by:
  - Area and thickness of gas exchange surface.
  - Volume of blood in pulmonary capillaries.
  - Alveolar volume as influenced by disease states.
- Indicated when predicted post-operative FEV_1 <40% normal.
- Predicted post-operative DLCO <40% normal is associated with a high peri-operative risk.

Cardiovascular tests

Cardio-pulmonary exercise testing and echocardiography are described elsewhere.

ECG

(See 📖 ECG, p. 192).
- Mandatory test for:
  - All patients >60 years.
  - Those with 1 or more cardiac risk factors.
  - Any cardiac history.
  - Intra-thoracic surgery.

- Look for:
  - Rhythm; atrial fibrillation is common post-operatively.
  - Ischaemic sequelae, e.g. Q waves, inverted T waves.
  - Right axis deviation and right ventricular hypertrophy; pulmonary hypertension confers a high operative risk.

Histology

Biopsy procedures to diagnose bronchogenic carcinoma or pleural disease are performed without general anaesthetic. Examples include:

- Fine needle aspiration of pleural fluid.
- Radiologically-guided fine needle biopsy of peripheral lung lesions.
- Cutting-needle pleural biopsy.
- Bronchoscopic biopsy and washings.

Further reading

Edward F, Patz J. Imaging Bronchogenic Carcinoma. *Chest*. 2000; 117:90s–95s.

Beckles M, Spiro S, Colice G, *et al*. Initial Evaluation of the Patient With Lung Cancer: Symptoms, Signs, Laboratory Tests, and Paraneoplastic Syndromes. *Chest* 2003; 123:97–104.

Chapter 3 Diffusion. In: J West, *Respiratory Physiology, The Essentials*. 7th edition. 2005. Baltimore: Lippincott Williams & Wilkins.

Assessment made easy

There is a lot to consider amongst the thoracic surgical population. This section aims to briefly summarize pre-operative assessment.

All patients—regardless of case complexity

- Exercise tolerance assessment.
  - Assess this crudely (question stair climbing ability. Asking a patient how far they can walk on the flat is useless!).
- Estimate their ppoFEV$_1$.
- Discuss the analgesia options with them.
- It is prudent to discuss smoking cessation; >8 weeks has the most benefit.
  - This is contentious as it may not be easy for a life-long smoker to quit.
  - The larger the operation, the more value there is in making this compulsory at all costs.
- If they are obese, counsel them regarding weight loss.
- If they are cachectic with significant nutritional impairment, refer them for dietitian advice.

Is their ppoFEV$_1$ <40%?

- They are high risk so they need to be considered for:
  - DLCO.
  - V/Q scanning.
  - CPEX.

Do they have malignancy?

- Thorough assessment of history and examination findings, followed by further tests is vital.
  - Do they have a paraneoplastic syndrome or metastases that may negate surgery?

Do they have COPD?

- How bad is it?
- How will this affect your anaesthesia; particularly from the intra-op hypoxia/hypercarbia angle and for their post-operative course?
- Assess:
  - ABG.
  - CXR.
- Optimize them:
  - Physiotherapy.
  - Steroids.
  - Further bronchodilator therapy.
  - Consult chest physicians.
  - Antibiotics if infection.

Renal function
- Renal failure comes with significant morbidity:
  - Assess U&E with creatinine clearance to further risk stratify.

What are they having done?
- Anatomical location of the surgery? As far as post-operative morbidity goes, the order of severity is:
  - Thorax/upper abdomen > lower abdomen > peripheral
  - Thoracotomy > sternotomy.
- Anaesthesia risk?
  - General anaesthesia > central neuraxial/regional.
- Will the length of operation lead to morbidity?

Will they cope on one lung?
- Those less likely to cope are:
  - Those where the V/Q demonstrates that the operative lung has a high degree of functionality.
  - Those struggling to saturate (maintain reasonable PaO_2 on TLV or in the lateral position).
  - Were a right sided thoracotomy is to be performed.
  - Those with any significant lung disease.
  - Those in the supine position for OLV.

Surgical resectability

The majority of lung resections are carried out for the treatment of primary malignant lung tumours.

Tumors of the lung may be subdivided:

- Epithelial tumors.
  - Small cell lung cancer.
  - Non-small cell lung cancer.
  - Carcinoid.
  - Bronchial gland carcinomas.
- Mesenchymal tumors.
  - Pulmonary hamartomas.
  - Carcinosarcomas.
  - Primary sarcomas.
  - Lymphoproliferative lesions.
- Lymphoproliferative disorders.

Diagnosis of a lung neoplasm

The initial clinical assessment of the potential lung cancer patient includes history, physical examination, chest radiography and CT scan.

Radiology

- **CXR**.
  - This is the first step in a cascade designed to determine the diagnosis, extent of disease and optimal treatment for the patient.
- **CT thorax and abdomen**
  - Primary lesions, size and location.
  - Satellite lesions.
  - Nodes, report of stations and size.
  - Metastases, lung (contralateral), liver, adrenals, bone, skin etc.
  - Nodes larger than 1 cm in long axis are more likely to be malignant.
- **CT/MRI brain**
- **PET scan**
  - Has a role in both diagnosis and staging of lung cancer.
  - High take up of fluror-deoxy-glucose by lung cancer cells.
  - Good for nodes that are not accessible by mediastinoscopy, or second intrapulmonary lesions.
  - Sensitivity of 95% and specificity of 80%.
- **MRI thorax or abdomen**
  - Enhanced anatomical detail may aid treatment decisions, eg. Invasion of local structures by primary lesion.
  - Distinguishing between adrenal mets. or benign growths.

Other
- **Percutaneous needle biopsy**
  - Can be used in patients with peripheral lesions who are unfit for surgery, having a high diagnostic success rate with acceptably low morbidity.
- **Sputum cytology**
  - Primarily when the tumours invade transmucosally.
- **Bronchoscopy**
  - Differentiate tumour type (T1,T2,T3).
  - Permits sampling of nodes.
  - Identifying lesions not seen on CT.
  - Samples from lavage, brushings, endobronchial/transbronchial biopsies.
- **Mediastinoscopy**
  - To distinguish between benign and metastatic enlarged nodes.
  - Able to sample several lymph node stations [1, 2 (R+L), 3, 4 (R+L), 5 6 and 7] with standard and left anterior approach.
- **Endobronchial ultrasound (EBUS)**
  - Relatively new technique.
  - Paratracheal and subcarinal nodes are localized and sampled under ultrasound guidance.
  - Also sampling of stations 7, 8 and 9.
- **Pleural aspiration**
  - Any pleural effusion present should be aspirated for cytology.
  - +/– CT/US guidance.

Staging

This process generates the clinical TNM grading (Table 4.4) which may further be refined with pathological data if resection is undertaken. (Table 4.5) shows separate classification of non-small cell lung cancer. This staging classification addresses three modalities:
- The primary tumour (T).
- The status of the mediastinal and intrapulmonary lymph node (N).
- The detection of distant metastases (M).

T status
- *Operability* is questionable in most T3 and virtually all T4 lesions.
- *Proximity* of tumour to the carina is assessed by bronchoscopy.
- *Size* of tumour can be evaluated by CT.
- *Invasion* of chest wall and mediastinal is important, but CT scan is not particularly accurate in differentiating contiguity from invasion.
- *Pleural effusion* can indicate pleural dissemination of malignant disease but may also represent an inflammatory reaction to pneumonia or consolidation secondary to bronchial obstruction of the tumour.

N status

- The topography of the pulmonary and mediastinal nodes is described according to a lymph node map.
- The relationship between involved node stations and long-term survival has been studied in detail.
- It is not practical to stage the intrapulmonary nodes by direct sampling prior to surgery.
- Mediastinal node sampling is achieved by different approaches.
  - Most require GA.
  - Often combined with rigid bronchoscopy.
- *Mediastinoscopy.*
  - Allows subcarinal, ipsilateral and contralateral paratracheal nodes to be sampled.
- *Mediastinotomy.*
  - Can assess nodes situated around the aortic arch.
- *Endobronchial ultrasound (EBUS).*
  - Relatively new technique.
  - Usually performed under local anesthesia.
  - Is rapidly replacing mediastinoscopy.
- *Video-assisted thoracoscopic surgery.*
  - Allows the surgeons to sample nodes lateral to the superior vena cava, the lower paraoesophageal nodes and pulmonary ligament nodes.
  - A useful method for obtaining a tissue sample in undiagnosed poor-risk patients with locally advanced bronchogenic carcinoma is the use of endoscopic ultrasound guided trans-oesophageal biopsy.

M status

- Detection of extrathoracic disease should include CT scan of head and abdomen.
- Ultrasound may be required to differentiate hepatic cysts from metastatic disease.
- Biopsy of palpable deposits such as cutaneous lesions or scalene lymph nodes.
- Bone marrow aspiration for small cell lung carcinoma may be warranted as metastases at this site are frequent.

Table 4.4 TNM classification

Classification	Description
T0	No Primary
Tis	Carcinoma in situ
T1	<3 cm diameter. No invasion to visceral pleura or to proximal lobar broncus
T2	>3 cm diameter. Main bronchus involvement >2 cm from carina. Invasion of visceral pleura. Atelectasis/obstructive pneumonitis to hilum
T3	Invasion of chest wall, diaphragm, mediastinal pleura, parietal pericardium. Main bronchus involvement >2 cm from carina (not involving carina). Atelectasis/obstructive pneumonitis entire lung
T4	Invasion of mediastinum, heart, great vessels, trachea, oesophagus, vertebra, main carina
	Malignant pleural or pericardial effusion satellite nodules within same lobe as primary tumour
N0	No nodal involvement
N1	Ipsilateral peribronchial, intrapulmonary
	+/– hilar nodes by direct invasion or metastasis
N2	Ipsilateral mediastinal +/– subcarinal nodes
N3	Contralateral hilar or mediastinal nodes. Ipsilateral or contralateral scalene or supraclavicular nodes
M0	No metastases
M1	Distant metastasis or satellite pulmonary nodules in separate lobe from primary

Table 4.5 Staging information for non-small cell lung cancer

Stage			
0	Tis	N0	M0
Ia	T1	N0	M0
Ib	T2	N0	M0
IIa	T1	N1	M0
IIb	T2	N1	M0
	T3	N0	M0
IIIa	T3	N1	M0
	T1-T3	N2	M0
IIIb	T any	N3	M0
	T4	N any	M0
IV	T any	N any	M1

Surgical management

- T1, T2/N0, N1 cancers:
  - Resection is generally regarded as the optimum treatment strategy.
- T3 cancers:
  - May be excisable, if there is confidence that all of the intrathoracic disease can be excised.
- T4 cancers without metastases or cancer with N3 nodes:
  - Not candidates for surgical resection.
  - The exception are carinal tumours where carinal resection and reconstruction may be possible.
- N2 cancers:
  - If surgically resectable, frequently require neoadjuvant or adjuvant therapy.
- M1 cancers:
  - With isolated cerebral metastases, combined pulmonary and cerebral resection could lead to prolonged survival.

> ❶ There is no role for 'palliative' resection. Survival is no higher, whilst the morbidity associated with a thoracotomy is considerable.

Extent of the lung to be resected
(See Pancoast tumour and resection, p. 338).

Lobectomy/bilobectomy
- For intralobar lesions which do not cross a fissure.

Limited sublobar resection
- Segmentectomy or wedge resection.
- A valid option in patients with very poor pulmonary function.
- Higher local recurrence rate.

Pneumonectomy
- Right pneumonectomy removes 55% of the lung tissue.
- Left pneumonectomy removes 45% of the lung tissue.
- Associated with higher morbidity in the elderly therefore age should be a factor in considering suitability.

Bronchoplastic resection
- Sleeve/carinal resection.
- May be appropriate in selective patients.
- Carinal resection is a technically demanding procedure with high rate of postoperative complications and an increased risk of local recurrence.

VATS resection
- For well delineated, minimally invasive peripheral tumours.

> If the lung to be resected is deemed non-functional via V/Q scanning, surgery will not affect residual lung function.

Assessment of fitness
The major concerns are:
- Advanced age.
- Poor pulmonary function.
- Poor cardiovascular fitness.
- Poor nutrition and performance status.
- Diagnosis and staging.
- Adjuvant therapy.
- Available operations.
- Local vs. advanced disease.
- Small cell lung cancer.

Pulmonary function
- If there is no evidence of interstitial lung disease or unexpected disability due to shortness of breath, no further respiratory function tests are required if the post-bronchodilator FEV_1 is:
  - >1.5 L for lobectomy.
  - >2.0 L for pneumonectomy.

- If spirometry is poor, patients should have:
  - Full pulmonary function tests including estimation of transfer factor (DLCO).
  - Measurement of oxygen saturation on air at rest.
  - Quantitative isotope perfusion scan if a pneumonectomy is being considered.
- These data should be used to calculate estimated ppoFEV$_1$ expressed as % predicted and the estimated ppoDLCO expressed as % predicted.
- Mild depression in arterial oxygen tension is not important but an elevated PCO$_2$ is a contraindication to surgical intervention.
- There should be formal liaison in borderline cases between the referring chest physician and the thoracic surgical team.

Further reading

Morris P, Wood W (2000). *Oxford Textbook of Surgery*, Oxford University Press.

Guidelines on the selection of patients with lung cancer for surgery. British Thoracic Society and Society of Cardiothoracic Surgeons of Great Britain and Ireland Working Party. *Thorax* 2001; 56:89–108.

Blood gases

Introduction

Thoracic pathology has a variable impact on pulmonary gas exchange and thus blood gases. Assessment of an individual's pulmonary gas exchange is a routine pre-operative investigation for many patients presenting for thoracic surgery.

Role of blood gas sampling

- The evidence base to support blood gas sampling as a predictive tool of outcome following thoracic surgery is limited.
- Blood gas results ALONE should not be used as a means to decide whether a patient is fit for surgery; (please refer to "Spirometry & Gas transfer factor).
- Blood gas analysis is not included in the British Thoracic Society algorithm for the selection of suitable patients for lung cancer resection.
- Blood gas analysis serves as a pre-operative baseline to guide and inform both pre- and post-operative management.

When is further action required?

The following should prompt further investigation and/or optimization prior to surgery:

- PaO_2 <8.3kPa
  - ❶ SpO_2 <90% (on room air) is considered a risk factor for increased peri-operative complications.
  - ✱ $\downarrow SpO_2$ >4% during exercise has been challenged as a risk factor for increased peri-operative complications.
  - ▶ Resection of diseased lobes/lung (low V/Q units) may actually reduce pulmonary shunt fraction, thus improving PaO_2 post-operatively.
- $PaCO_2$ >6.3 kPa
  - Hypercapnia is not an independent risk factor for increased peri-operative complications.

Types of blood gas sampling

- This section will not provide an in-depth discussion of blood gas analysis and interpretation as this can be found in any standard textbook of anaesthesia.
- Pre-operatively, the adequacy of alveolar gas exchange can be assessed by measurement of blood gas tensions in:
  - Arterial blood.
  - Arterialized capillary blood, i.e. it comprises blood from both capillary and venule.
- There is some evidence to suggest that COPD patients prefer capillary blood gas (CBG) sampling to arterial blood gas (ABG) sampling as it is less painful.

Arterialized CBG

- May be taken from the earlobe. Use a lancet.
- PO_2 gradient of approximately 8 kPa between the arterial and venous ends of the capillary bed. This difference may be reduced by inducing vasodilatation by the application of heat or a vasoactive cream
- Thus, CBG measurement may approximate ABG measurement
  - PO_2 typically 0.5–1.0 kPa <PaO_2
  - The lower the PaO_2, the greater the agreement between ABG and CBG.
  - There is greater divergence when PaO_2 >8–10 kPa.
  - PCO_2 ~ $PaCO_2$ (difference <0.1 kPa).
  - pH is essentially unchanged.
- CBG sampling can be easily performed during exercise.

Pitfalls of CBG measurement

- Training is required to take samples correctly.
- Sample needs to be anaerobic; record SpO_2 when the sample is taken and compare with measured SaO_2. Repeat sample if there is a difference of 2%.
- Do not use in hypo-perfused states.
- Do not use the first drop of blood, as this contains tissue fluid.

Further reading

Hughes JMB. Blood gas estimations from arterialized capillary blood versus arterial puncture: are they different? *European Respiratory Journal* 1996; 9:184–5.

British Thoracic Society Emergency Oxygen Guideline Group. Guideline for emergency oxygen use in adult patients. *Thorax* 2008; 63 (VI):31.

Colice GL, Shafazand S, Griffin JP, Keenan R, Bolliger CT. Physiological evaluation of the patient with lung cancer being considered for resectional surgery. *Chest* 2007; 132:161–77.

Spirometry

- An easily performed common test of pulmonary function involving the measurement of timed inspired and expired lung volumes.
- Useful in the pre-operative assessment of all patients, however in thoracic anaesthesia, spirometry plays a particularly important role in determining the suitability of patients for lung resective and lung volume reduction surgery.

Performance

- The procedure is usually performed during forced expiration after a maximal inspiration and measures:
  - Forced Expiratory Volume in one second (**FEV$_1$**)—the volume expired in the first second of forced exhalation from full inspiration.
  - Forced Vital Capacity (**FVC**)—the largest volume of air that can be expired during a forced exhalation from full inspiration.
- Three traces with good reproducibility should be obtained (the two highest values for both FEV$_1$ and FVC should agree to within 0.15 l).

Interpretation

- Absolute values (in liters) of FEV$_1$ and FVC are usually presented together with the percentage of the predicted value for the subject's age, sex, height and ethnicity.
- The **FEV$_1$/FVC ratio** is normally 75–80%—a reduction in this ratio indicates airflow obstruction.
- The FVC may be reduced when:
  - Lung compliance is reduced (reduced inspiration).
  - Inspiratory muscles are weak (reduced inspiration).
  - There is airflow obstruction (airway collapse in expiration causes gas-trapping).

Describing spirometry

Abnormal patterns of ventilation (See Fig. 4.2 and Table 4.6) may be described as:

- Obstructive.
  - FEV$_1$ reduced more than FVC.
  - Reduced FEV$_1$/FVC ratio.
- Restrictive.
  - FVC reduced.
  - Normal or raised FEV$_1$/FVC ratio.
- A reduced FEV$_1$/FVC ratio in combination with severe reduction in the FVC suggests a mixed obstructive and respiratory pattern.

Pitfalls

- Patients with interstitial lung disease may have normal spirometric values in the presence of significantly impaired pulmonary function.
- Volumes measured by spirometry in ambient conditions should be corrected for body temperature and allowance made for the saturated with water vapour pressure—otherwise the results may underestimate true volumes.

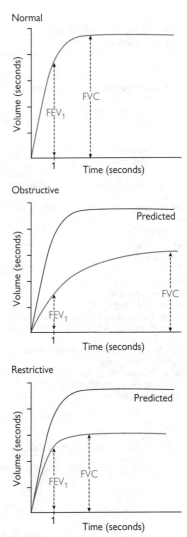

Fig. 4.2 Patterns of spirometry.

Gas transfer

- Measures the overall ability of the lungs to effectively transfer gas (in this test, the gas is carbon monoxide—CO).
  - Common misconception is that it merely concerns the alveolar-capillary membrane.
- CO and O_2 must pass through the alveolar epithelium → tissue interstitium → capillary endothelium → blood plasma → red cell membrane and cytoplasm → Hb.
- Useful to assess whether parenchymal lung disease is present when spirometry reveals reduced VC, RV, TLC.

The test

- The gas of choice is carbon monoxide; as it is completely taken up by Hb and closely resembles the behavior of oxygen.
- A VC breath is taken and held for 10 seconds, and then the patient exhales into a sample bag. 0.5–0.75 L is wasted to account for dead space.
- Gas transfer (DL_{CO}) is defined in ml/min/mmHg and is calculated as:

Volume of gas taken up/(P_AGas–P_cGas)
P_A—pulmonary alveolar gas
P_C—pulmonary capillary gas

Factors affecting DL_{CO}

- Epithelial-endothelial surface area.
  - Increases with size of subject.
- Pulmonary capillary blood volume and Hb concentration.
  - Increases in polycythaemia and pulmonary capillary distension.
  - Decreases with PE.
- Abnormal Hb levels require a correction factor to allow for normalization of diffusing capacity.
- Rate of reaction of CO with Hb.
- Thickness of alveolar-capillary membrane.
- Distribution of ventilation and ventilation-perfusion.

Test results

- DL_{CO} falls with:
  - Previous lung resection.
  - Thoracic cage abnormalities (e.g. kyphoscoliosis).
  - Small lungs.

Table 4.6 Examples of causes of abnormal ventilatory patterns

Obstructive	Restrictive
Asthma	Interstitial fibrosis
COPD	Pulmonary oedema
	Pneumonia
	Tuberculosis
	Kyphoscoliosis
	Pregnancy
	Respiratory muscle weakness

Emphysema
- DL_{CO} is reduced
  - But; due to poor distribution of inspired test gas, the V_A may be a gross underestimate of TLC
  - The resultant DL/V_A ratio may be normal.

Interstitial and pulmonary vascular disease
- A reduced DL_{CO} and a reduced DL: VA ratio suggest a true interstitial disease such as pulmonary fibrosis or pulmonary vascular disease.

Infiltrative disorders
- Pneumonia, interstitial infiltrative disorders, and alveolar proteinosis.

Interpretation of results
- Below the lower limit of normal, but >60% predicted = Mild.
- 40%–60% of predicted = Moderate.
- <40% = Severe.

❶ The patient MUST achieve the best possible VC result for the test to be correctly interpreted as accurate. Inability to achieve a VC of >90% of the largest VC measured that day must be noted on the report.

Assessment of respiratory mechanics

Ventilation is dependent on the balance between the mechanical properties and actions of the chest wall, the respiratory muscles, the conducting airways and the lungs themselves.

Components

Chest wall
- Elastic recoil stabilizes thoracic cage.
- Contributes to intra-pleural pressure.
- In equilibrium with elastic recoil of lungs at FRC, i.e. prevents further pulmonary atelectasis.

Respiratory muscles
- Inspiration:
  - Diaphragm.
  - External intercostal muscles.
  - Accessory muscles stabilize rib cage during deep inspiration.
- Expiration:
  - Typically passive.
  - Forced expiration uses abdominal wall muscles and internal intercostals muscles.

Conducting airways
- Contribute majority of airway resistance.
- Highest resistance in medium-sized bronchi.
- Site of dynamic airway compression during expiration.

Lungs
- Complex, heterogenous organ.
- Structure and function vary with age.

Determinants of respiratory mechanics

Compliance
- Defined as the volume change per unit pressure.
- Represents the gradient of the pressure-volume curve.
- Total compliance dependent on elastic properties of the lung and chest wall. Thus:

$$1/C_{total} = 1/C_{lung} + 1/C_{wall}$$

- Total compliance ~ 80–100 ml/cmH$_2$O.
- (See Table 4.7) summarising how compliance varies.

Airway resistance
- Majority of resistance at medium-sized bronchi.
- Very small bronchioles contribute little.

- Airway resistance varies:
  - Inversely with lung volume.
  - Directly with bronchial smooth muscle tone; ↑ by para-sympathetic stimulation, histamine, ↓ P_ACO_2, inhaled irritants; ↓ by β-agonists, sympathetic stimulation.
  - Directly with viscosity and density, e.g. Heliox.
  - Proportionally with the degree of airway obstruction.
- Therefore, general anaesthesia can easily increase airway resistance.

Table 4.7 Variation of total respiratory compliance

Factors that ↑ C_{total}	Factors that ↓ C_{total}
Emphysema	Extremes of age, pregnancy
Asthma	Alveolar infiltrates
(unclear pathophysiology)	(pneumonia, pulmonary oedema, haemorrhage)
Standing	Atelectasis
Resting lung volume = FRC	Bronchial obstruction
(C_{total} is maximum)	High/low resting lung volumes
	Supine position
	Chest wall disease
	Lack of surfactant

Dynamic airway compression
- Describes the mechanism that limits flow during forced expiration, i.e. flow is independent of effort
- Occurs secondary to the gradient between intra-pleural pressure and pressure within the airways
- Extreme positive pressure causes compression of proximal airways, increased airway resistance, and reduced gas flow
- Increased by the following:
  - ↑ airway resistance
  - ↓ lung volume
  - ↑ compliance, e.g. dynamic airway compression may be evident during tidal breathing in patients with severe emphysema.

Work of breathing
- Accounts for ~ 5% of O_2 consumption at resting conditions
- ↑ at rest by:
  - Interstitial lung disease (changes in compliance)
  - Chest wall disease
  - Diaphragmatic pathology
  - Increased airway resistance
  - Increased gas density + viscosity.

Clinical assessment

Forced expiratory volume in 1 second (FEV₁)

- Predicted post-operative FEV₁ (ppoFEV₁).
  - Most valid single assessment for pulmonary mechanics following thoracotomy.

    ppoFEV₁% = pre-op FEV₁% × (1 − % functional lung tissue removed/100)

- ppoFEV₁ >40%; few/minor respiratory complications following pulmonary resection.
- ppoFEV₁ <40%; major respiratory complications following pulmonary resection.
- ppoFEV₁ <30%; require post-operative ventilation following pulmonary resection.

Flow-volume loops

- May aid diagnosis of airway obstruction but inter-patient variability renders them less practical and difficult to interpret (See Fig. 4.3).
- The precise location of obstruction can be determined with CT, MRI and flexible fibreoptic bronchoscopy.
- More helpful as an intra-operative monitor of respiratory mechanics during one-lung ventilation.

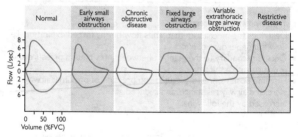

Fig. 4.3 Examples of pre-operative flow-volume loops.

Further reading

West JB. (2005) *Respiratory Physiology, the Essentials.* 7th ed. Baltimore: Lippincott Williams & Wilkins.

Pinnock C, Lin T, Smith T (2003). *Fundamentals of Anaesthesia.* 2nd ed. London: Greenwich Medical Media.

Oesophageal manometry

A means whereby oesophageal luminal and spincter pressures can be measured.

Normal values

- Lower oesophageal sphincter station analysis (wet swallows):
  - Resting pressure: 16.6–35.4 mmHg.
- Oesophageal body motility analysis (wet swallows):
  - Peristaltic performance as % of normal swallows: >90
  - Mean amplitude (distal): 64–154 mmHg.
  - Mean amplitude (proximal): 33–91 mmHg.
  - Mean duration (distal): 2.9–5.1 sec.
  - Mean duration (proximal): 2.0–3.6 sec.

Indications (British Society of Gastroenterology Guidelines)

- Surgical assessment of reflux symptoms prior to anti-reflux surgery. Oesophageal manometry differentiates between primary motility disorders (surgery not required) and actual gastro-oesophageal reflux.
- To diagnose and categorize suspected oesophageal motility disorders in patients with dysphagia or chest pain, in whom other investigations are negative or equivocal.
- Accurate placement of pH electrodes for 24 hour pH monitoring.
- ❶ Not be used to diagnose reflux, nor as first line investigation in patients with dysphagia or chest pain.

Contraindications

Absolute

- Suspected or confirmed pharyngeal or upper oesophageal obstruction
- Severe coagulopathy
- Bullous disorders of the oesophageal mucosa
- Cardiac conditions in which vagal stimulation is not tolerated
- Patients who are not able to obey simple instructions.

Relative

- Peptic strictures.
- Oesophageal ulcers.
- Oesophageal or junctional tumours.
- Varices.
- Large diverticulae.

Measurement devices

Water-perfused catheters

- A bundle of thin plastic tubes continuously perfused with bubble-free water. Each tube has an outward facing side-hole.
- Pressure in each tube monitored by a volume-displacement transducer.
- Allows simultaneous measurement of pressures at multiple locations.

Solid-state strain gauges
- Linear arrangement of miniature, solid-state strain gauges, each providing a direct measure of intraluminal pressure.
- Easy to use.
- More expensive than water-perfused catheters.

High resolution manometry
- Measures the dynamic movement and function of the pharyngeal swallow.
- Assesses the LOS and diaphragmatic components of the anti-reflux barrier.
- Allows measurement of gastric, pyloric and small bowel contractility.
- Facilitates positioning of the pH probe for reflux studies.
- Oesophageal function is easy to recognize on spatiotemporal plot.
- Inexperience with spatiotemporal plots increases the risk of over-diagnosis of functionally insignificant oesophageal dysmotility.
- Identifies the functional anatomy of the oesophagus and focal peristaltic dysmotility.
- Increases diagnostic yield and accuracy for achalasia.
- Differentiates true oesophageal spasm from rapid elevation of the intra-bolus pressure due to focal dysmotility or obstruction.
- Easy to position.
- Expensive.

Classification of primary oesophageal motility disorders

Inadequate LOS relaxation
- Achalasia
- Atypical disorders of LOS relaxation.

Uncoordinated contraction
- Diffuse oesophageal spasm.

Hypertensive contraction
- Nutcracker oesophagus
- Hypertensive LOS.

Hypotensive contraction
- Ineffective oesophageal motility.
- Hypotensive LOS.

Further reading

Fox M.R., Bredenoord A.J. Oesophageal high-resolution manometry: moving from research into clinical practice. *Gut* 2008; 57:405–23.

Pandolfino JE, Kahrilas PJ. American Gastroenterological Association medical position statement: Clinical use of esophageal manometry. *Gastroenterology* 2005; 128:207–8.

ECG

The ECG is a simple, non-invasive investigation that is readily available. Almost all thoracic patients should have a pre-operative ECG recorded.

Indications

- To provide a baseline record.
  - Post-op cardiac complications following major thoracic surgery.
- To detect un-diagnosed cardiac abnormalities e.g. conduction disorders.
- To help optimize cardiac conditions.
  - Coronary artery interventions.
  - Temporary pacemakers.
- To help determine risk for the patient.
  - Timing of surgery after MI.

Interpreting an ECG

- A systematic approach should be employed so as not to miss significant abnormalities.
- The classic approach of 'rate, rhythm, axis and morphology' is recommended.
- The following abnormalities relate to specific situations that may demand further investigation, indicate significant disease or require intervention prior to surgery.

ECG abnormalities

Ventricular hypertrophy
Right ventricular Hypertrophy

▶▶ ECG changes

- Right Axis Deviation >90°.
- Dominant R in V_1 (R wave height >7mm, exceeding depth of S wave in V_1, deep S wave in V_6).
- QRS <0.12 sec.
- Deep S wave in lead I, largest R wave in lead III.
- Peaked P waves if associated right atrial enlargement (P wave >2.5 mm).
- T wave inversion in leads V_2, V_3 in severe cases.

Causes
- Primary pulmonary hypertension.
- Pulmonary valve disease (rare).
- Intracardiac shunt e.g. ASD.
- Pulmonary hypertension secondary to respiratory disease.
  - Cor pulmonale (seen in 50% of COPD patients).

▶ Diastolic overload of RV (ASD, TR) may only produce incomplete RBBB.

Cor pulmonale

- Hypoxia → hypoxic pulmonary vasoconstriction → pulmonary arterial hypertension → ↑ RV afterload.
- RV systolic pressure increases to maintain forward flow gradient.
- At a point, further maintained increases in pulmonary arterial pressure → ↑ RV dilation, ↑ RVEDP.
- Combination of d RV output + ↓ LVEDV → ↓ LV output.
- ↓ LV output → ↓ aortic pressure ↑ ↓ RCA blood flow.
- Chronic hypoxia → renal stimulation → fluid retention → ↑ JVP and oedema.

Preoperative implications:
- **Warrants an echocardiogram**
  - To assess the valves, RV function, RV dimensions, intra-cardiac shunts and pulmonary arterial pressure.

For management and pre-operative implications (See below).

❶ OLV and hypoxia can precipitate RV failure if a patient has significant pulmonary hypertension and ventricular hypertrophy.

Left Ventricular Hypertrophy
Causes:
- Normal (athlete).
- Cardiomyopathies.
- Chronic arterial hypertension.
- Aortic valve disease (regurgitation or stenosis).
- Endocrine conditions causing high output failure.

▶▶ ECG changes

- Tall R wave >27 mm in V_{5-6}.
- S wave in V_{1-3} >30 mm.
- Sum of deepest S wave in V_{1-3} and tallest R wave in V_{5-6} >40 mm.
- T wave may be inverted in leads V_{5-6}.
- Left axis deviation may be present; deep S wave in lead III with dominant S wave in Lead II.
- May see U waves.

Preoperative implications:

❶ In the presence of LVH, myocardial O2 supply/demand may become imbalanced during OLV → ischaemia, and at worst peri-operative MI.

▶▶ ECG changes may be minimal when there is biventricular hypertrophy.
- **Warrants an echocardiogram.**
  - To assess the valves, LV dimensions and LV function.

Conduction disorders

First degree HB

▶▶ **ECG changes**

- PR interval >0.2sec.
- PR interval must be constant.

Causes:
- AV nodal dysfunction, IHD.
- Enhanced vagal tone in athletes.
- Myocarditis.
- Acute MI.
- Electrolyte imbalance.
- Drugs:
  - Digoxin, Calcium channel blockers, Cholinesterase inhibitors, β blockers.

Pre-operative implications:
- Identify and correct electrolyte imbalances.
- Identify and treat IHD.
- Withhold any medications that may slow AV conduction.
- Admission not required unless associated with myocardial infarction.
- Does not usually progress to higher forms of heart block.
  - 1° HB + any BBB may require outpatient follow up.

Second degree HB

▶▶ **ECG changes**

Mobitz type I (Wenchebach)

- Progressive lengthening of PR interval to a failed conduction of atrial beat.

Causes:
- AV nodal disease, IHD.

Pre-operative implications:
- Usually no further action needed.

▶▶ ECG changes

Mobitz type II
- Intermittent failure of excitation to pass through AV node, often at regular intervals (2:1, 3:1)

Causes:
- Disease of the His-Purkinje system.

Pre-operative implications:
- May progress rapidly to complete heart block.
- Patient may experience a Stokes-Adams attack, cardiac arrest, or sudden cardiac death.
- Definitive treatment for this form of AV Block is an implanted pacemaker.
- Discuss with cardiologist.

Third degree (Complete HB)

▶▶ ECG changes
- Failure of AV conduction.
- No relationship between P wave and QRS complexes.
- QRS is wide and escape rhythm is often slow.

Causes:
- Ischaemic heart disease.
- Rare congenital forms.
- Severe vagal stimulation.

Pre-operative implications:
- Will require referral for insertion of permanent pacemaker
- Pharmacological control of atrial fibrillation and or blood pressure may be required
- Treatment in emergency situations is atropine, isoprenaline IVI and an external pacer.

Right bundle branch block

▶▶ **ECG changes**

- Wide QRS >0.12 sec.
- RSR pattern in V_{1-3}.
- T wave inversion in V_{1-2}.
- Mnemonic **MaRroW** ('**M**' in V_1, **R**ight, '**W**' in V_6).

Causes:
- Normal phenomenon.
- Athletes.
- Post-cardiac surgery.
- ASD.
- PE.
- Blunt chest trauma.
- Polymyositis.

Pre-operative implications:
- None, as usually benign.
- If patient has new onset breathlessness or limited exercise tolerance, it may be associated with right heart strain/PE.

Left bundle branch block

▶▶ **ECG changes**

- Wide QRS >0.12 sec.
- M shape in leads V_{4-6}.
- q absent in V_{5-6}.
- Mnemonic **WiLliaM** ('**W**' in V1, **L**eft, '**M**' in V6).
- Further interpretation of ECG beyond rate and rhythm is not possible.

Causes:
- Myocardial infarction.
- Myocarditis.
- Cardiomyopathy.
- Haemochromatosis.
- Aortic valve endocarditis.
- Ostium primum ASD associated with Down's Syndrome.
- Rare autosomal bundle branch disease.

Pre-operative implications:

> ❶ LBBB is NOT normal. It signifies a pathological condition, in particular, recent MI if new.
>
> ❶ Acute MI cannot be reliably diagnosed in the presence of LBBB.

- Refer to cardiologist as soon as possible for further assessment and optimization.
- Consider admission if this is the first presentation.
- Can surgery be deferred?

Bi-fascicular block
- Combination of RBBB and either left anterior or posterior fascicle block.
  - Difficult to diagnose and seen as RBBB with left or right axis Deviation respectively.

> ❶ Any degree of AV block associated with syncope or symptomatic bradycardia should be considered for pacing. Bi-fascicular block is relatively stable and does not require temporary pacing
>
> ❶ Facilities should be in place in the theatre complex to provide temporary transcutaneous pacing, should it be required

Rhythm disturbances
Atrial fibrillation/flutter
Causes:
- Ischaemic heart disease.
- Cardiomyopathy.
- COPD.
- Valvular disease (particularly mitral valve disease).
- Ventricular hypertrophy.
- Hyperthyroidism.
- Alcohol intoxication/caffeine.
- Sepsis.
- Hypertension.

Pre-operative implications:
- Common in the elderly.
- The use of adenosine may aid diagnosis if AF slows revealing flutter waves.

- Check and correct electrolytes (magnesium and potassium in particular).
- Rate control should be achieved with a rate of <90bpm at rest.
- If onset is acute then ALS/NICE guidelines should be followed to control it prior to surgery.
  - Consideration of the need for synchronized DC shock or or pharmacological control. Beyond the scope of this topic.
- **Warrants echocardiogram**
  - If significant exertional dyspnoea or angina.
  - Assessment of LV function, left atrial size and mitral valve.
- Refer to cardiologist.
- Consider digoxin level. Watch serum potassium levels as hypokalaemia potentiates digitalis toxicity.

> ❶ May be chronic in which case the patient may be anti-coagulated. Do you need to admit them to convert from warfarin to heparin pre-op?

Wolff-Parkinson-White syndrome (AVNRT)

▶▶ **ECG changes**

- Short PR interval.
- Wide QRS complex.
- Slurred upstroke of the R wave (δ wave).

Causes:
- An accessory conduction pathway known as the bundle of Kent bypasses the AV node, thus allowing simultaneous conduction directly to the ventricles and to the AV node and the precipitation of a tachyarrhythmia.
- Type A tall R wave in V1.
- Type B QS complex in V1.

Pre-operative implications:
- Anti-arrhythmics must be continued peri-operatively.
- Efforts must be made to avoid sympathetic stimulation.
- Drugs must be available to treat any resulting tachydysrhythmias.
- Have a defibrillator at the ready in theatre.
- Consult a cardiologist regarding curative electrophysiological ablation therapy.

❶ Digoxin, Verapmil and Atropine should be avoided as these can trigger the accessory pathway by blocking normal conduction pathway.

Long QT Syndrome

▶ **ECG changes**

- A QT_C interval >0.45sec.

Causes:
- Genetic variations exist but are rare:
  - Jervell/Lange-Neilsen/Romano Ward/Andersen-Tawil/Brugada.
- Drugs; amiodarone, phenothiazines, tricyclics.
- Hypothyroidism.
- Hypocalcaemia.

Pre-operative implications:
- Potential for ventricular tachycardias, in particular torsade de pointes, which may be precipitated by sympathetic stimulation.

❶ Anaesthesia in untreated patients carries significant risk. An ECG should be performed in any patient with a family history of sudden cardiac death. β blockers form the mainstay of treatment. Cardiology advice should be sought.

Ventricular ectopics

- Frequent VE's including self-limiting runs of VT are not associated with increased risk of peri-operative death.
- Be aware that they are associated with an increased risk of other arrhythmias.
- Aggressive monitoring and treatment is not required.
- Institution of β blockade may reduce this risk.

Ischaemia and MI

▶▶ **ECG changes**

(See Table 4.8 for territories)

❶ STEMI
- Within hours acute ST elevation in leads:
  - II, III, aVF—inferior.
  - V3-4—septal.
  - V4-6, →, aVL anterolateral.
  - V1-6—anterior.
- Later:
  - Poor R wave progression across anterior leads.
  - Abnormal Q waves denote full muscle thickness M.I.
  - Inverted T waves—within days.
  - ST returns to normal, deep T inversion within weeks.
  - ST and T normal, Q and low R persist after months.

⚠ Normal Q waves are acceptable (<2 mm deep, <1 mm across or occuring in leads II, aVL and V_{5-6}).

❶ NSTEMI the classical features are not seen ... possible manifestations:
- ST depression (70–80%).
- T wave inversion (10–20%).
- Both ST depression and T wave inversion.
- Post MI NSTEMI.
  - ECG changes variable (Ironically, even a residual ST elevation may be present).
- Normal ECG.
- Inverse changes (ischaemic/depressed ST segments) in opposite. leads to MI territory may be seen.

❶ True posterior infarct is difficult to see!

Pre-operative implications:
- Pre-op ST depression
  - In a resting 12 lead ECG predicts adverse peri-operative cardiac events in moderate to major surgery.
- Consider postponing surgery if MI within 6 months.
- Pathalogical Q waves indicates an electrical window due to previous full thickness MI. Careful assessment should then be made of the patient's cardiovascular status.
- Residual IHD will need a cardiology review ± interventions.

Table 4.8 Territories of the heart involved in infarction according to ECG lead changes

Location of infarction	Leads showing primary change
Anteroseptal	V1–3
Anterior	V1–3 ± V4–6
Anterolateral	V4–6, I, aVL, ± II
Extensive anterior	V1–6, I, aVL
High lateral	aVL ± V4–6
Inferior	II, III, aVF
Inferolateral	II, III, aVF, V5–6, ± I, aVL
Inferoseptal	II, III, aVF, V2–3
Posterior infarction	V1–2 Inverse changes

Further points

Causes of right axis deviation

- Right ventricular hypertrophy.
- Normal in some tall and slim adults.
- Sometimes in Chronic lung disease.
- Antero-lateral MI.
- Left posterior hemiblock.
- PE.
- ASD.

Causes of dominant R in V$_1$

- Right ventricular hypertrophy.
- True posterior MI.
- Ventricular pre-excitation.
- Duchenne muscular dystrophy.
- RBBB.

Conditions that mimic MI on an ECG

- LBBB.
- LAHB.
- Ventricular pre-excitation.
- HOCM.
- LVH.
- Extreme clockwise rotation.
- PE.
- Hyperkalaemia.
- Intracranial haemorrhage.
- Left ventricular aneurysm.

Conditions producing prominent U waves

- Hypokalaemia.
- Hypomagnesaemia.
- Hypercalcaemia.
- Bradycardia.
- LVH.
- Hyperthyroidism.
- Mitral valve prolapsed.
- Drugs: digoxin, phenothiazine.

Pitfalls

❶ A normal ECG does not necessarily exclude serious cardiac disease and a positive cardiac history or signs should warrant a cardiology referral.

❶ Cardiac failure per se, does not cause any specific ECG changes—AF will be seen in 25% of cases.

❶ ECG morphology may mimic many abnormalities when the rhythm is implanted pacemaker dependent.

Further reading

Booker PD, Whyte SD, Landusans EJ. Long QT syndrome and anaesthesia. *British Journal of Anaesthesia* 2003; 90:349–66.

ACC/AHA guideline update on perioperative cardiovascular evaluation for non-cardiac surgery'. 2002. *The American College of Cardiology and American Heart association.*

NICE Clinical Guideline 36; *Atrial Fibrillation*: The management of Atrial Fibrillation. June 2006.

Echocardiography

The thoracic surgical patient is rarely entirely straight forward. With severe respiratory disease comes the potential for significant cardiac disease. Echocardiography provides qualitative and quantitative assessment of cardiac structure and function. Both transthoracic and transoesphageal approaches have a role in pre-operative diagnosis.

Advice

- It is always a grey area as to when to ask for an echo examination and advice is often conflicting.
- Echo is warranted if:
  - There is a suspicion of a lesion/condition that may pose significant risk to the patient, left unchecked.
  - If the results of the echo are likely to aid further treatment/ optimization a condition pre-operatively.
  - Overall, the aim is to minimize morbidity/mortality.
  - Ultimately, if in doubt, contact a cardiologist.

Echo assessment of the thoracic patient

Parameters measured vary in relevance and are numerous (Table 4.9). Pre-operative echo is of value in thoracic surgery for:

- Pulmonary hypertension assessment.
  - PA pressure and pulmonary valve status.
- Right ventricular performance assessment.
  - Particularly relevant if undergoing pneumonectomy as post-operatively, these patients are prone to right ventricular failure.
- Valvular assessment.
  - If relevant history (syncope, angina etc.).
  - If clinical examination (murmurs, other signs) point to a potential significant lesion.
  - Study should quantify valvular gradients.
  - Is there identifiable pathology leading to regurgitation/stenosis (Table 4.10 and 4.11).
- Global cardiac function assessment.
  - Fractional shortening and ejection fraction.
- Differentiation between cardiac and respiratory cause of symptoms.
- Comments on pleural effusions.

Transthoracic (TTE) vs. Transoesphageal (TOE)

TTE

- Non invasive
- Good images for most assessment/diagnosis.

- No absolute contra-indications.
- Poor images obtained in the presence of:
  - COPD, obesity, abdominal distension.
  - Pain, mechanical ventilation, pneumothorax, pneumopericardium.

TOE
- Semi-invasive.
- Sedation often required.
- Excellent image quality, especially of LA, Mitral and aortic valve.
- Contraindicated in oesophageal disease and untreated respiratory failure.

British Society of Echocardiography (BSE) indications for echo

- Heart Murmurs:
  - Murmur in the presence of significant cardiac or respiratory symptoms.
- Cardiomyopathy with presence of:
  - Heart failure.
  - SOB.
  - Persistent hypotension.
- Pulmonary disease to assess:
  - Cor pulmonale.
  - Pulmonary hypertension.
  - Pulmonary embolism.
  - Evaluation for surgical procedures for advanced lung disease.
  - Pulmonary artery pressure to evaluate response to vasodilators.
- Arrhythmia:
  - Determination as to whether structural heart disease is the cause.
- Hypertension:
  - Assessment of the degree of associated LV dysfunction.
- Pre-operative assessment:
  - Ischaemic heart disease with reduced functional capacity (<4 METS).
  - Unexplained SOB.

Focused Echo protocols

- **FATE**—Focused Assessed Transthoracic Echocardiography. This involves 5 standard views:
  - Subcostal 4C.
  - Apical 4C.
  - Parasternal LAX.
  - Parasternal SAX.
  - Both pleurae/lung bases.

- **FAST**—Focussed Assessed Sonography in Trauma.
  - Used to exclude a haemoperitoneum, cardiac tamponade, and haemothorax in trauma patients. This mainly involves abdominal views, as well as subcostal and pleural views.
- **FEER/FEEL**—Focused Echocardiography in Emergency Resuscitation, Focused Echocardiographic Evaluation in Resuscitation Management, or Focused Echocardiography Entry Level.
  - This mainly involves a single subcostal view during CPR for cardiac arrest, with minimal interruptions to diagnose cardiac tamponade, hypovolaemia, or myocardial failure, and differentiate the causes of PEA.

Table 4.9 Parameters recorded during echo examination

Structure	Measure	Calculate
Left Ventricle		
Size and function	LVIDd, LVIDs	Fractional shortening
LVOT	LVEDV, LVESV	Ejection fraction
LVOT outflow	LVOT diameter	LVOT area
LV Filling	V max	P max
	VTI	SV
	E, A	E:A Ratio
Right Ventricle		
RV diameter	RVOT diameter	RVOT area
RVOT	Vmax	Pmax
RVOT outflow	VTI	SV
Atria		
LA size	LA diameter, area, volume	
RA size	RA diameter, area, volume	
Aorta		
Aortic diameter	At 4 levels (annulus, root, ridge, ascending)	
Valves		
Valve stenosis	Vmax	Pmax
Valve regurg	Vmean	Pmean
	Vena contracta width	
Pulmonary artery	TR Vmax	RV or PA systolic pressure
	PR EVD	PA diastolic pressure

Table 4.10 Stenotic valve values (cm^2)

Valve	Normal	Mild Stenosis	Moderate Stenosis	Severe Stenosis
Aortic Valve	>2	1.5–2.0	1.4–1.0	<1
Mitral Valve	4–6	1.6–2	1.5–1	<1
Tricuspid Valve	>7			<1

Table 4.11 Fractional regurgitation grading

Valve	Mild Regurgitation	Moderate Regurgitation	Severe Regurgitation
Aortic Valve	<30	31–49	>50
Mitral Valve	<30	31–49	>50
Tricuspid Valve	<40	40–60	>60

Further reading

Jan Poelaert, Karl Skarvan. *Transoesophageal Echocardiography in Anaesthesia.* Wiley Blackwell 2000.

The British Society of Echocardiography (BSE) www.bsecho.org (accessed 8/7/09).

Cardio-pulmonary exercise testing

- Cardio-pulmonary exercise (CPEX) testing is considered to be the gold standard for the assessment of a combined risk of post-operative cardio-respiratory complications in thoracic anaesthesia.
- In the past, there have been scoring systems predicting the likelihood of single organ complications i.e., either cardiac, (Goldmann, Detsky, Lee), or respiratory (Arozullah), but they did not evaluate the overall cardio-respiratory risk.
- CPEX evaluates the functional capacity of patients through application of the knowledge of normal physiological responses to exercise and the patterns of change seen in a variety of disease states.

The test

- The test is performed in an adequately ventilated room with full resuscitation facilities.
- The patient pedals a cycle ergometer, initially against no resistance (unloaded cycling) and then against continuously increasing resistance at a pre-determined ramp rate.
- During the course of the test, the patient breathes through a mouthpiece or a tight fitting mask connected to a gas analyser which measures the oxygen consumption and carbon dioxide production by the patient.
- Other parameters monitored include a twelve lead ECG, NIBP, and SpO_2.
- The test can be terminated by the patient if they become breathless or exhausted, or by the technician if complications arise such as significant ST changes or new dysrhythmias.

Contraindications

- Before performing CPEX testing, absolute/relative contra-indications should be ruled out (the main factors) are:
  - Acute MI within 3–5 days.
  - Unstable angina.
  - Symptomatic uncontrolled arrhythmias.
  - Syncope.
  - Active endocarditis, myocarditis, pericarditis.
  - Symptomatic severe aortic stenosis.
  - Uncontrolled heart failure.
  - Acute severe asthma.
  - Desaturation on room air to a level of <85%.

Measurements

- Metabolic gas exchange parameters.
  - Oxygen consumption (VO_2), carbon dioxide production, respiratory exchange ratio and anaerobic threshold.
- Cardiovascular parameters.
  - Heart rate, 12 lead ECG, NIBP, Stroke volume (VO_2/HR).
- Ventilatory parameters.
  - Minute ventilation, tidal volume, respiratory rate, pulmonary gas exchange.

Computer software packages display the readings graphically in a standardized format called the nine panel plot (Table 4.12). Some of the panels, some relate to the cardiovascular system whereas others examine ventilation and ventilation-perfusion relationships. These panels (specific for a patient) are then compared with expected normal physiological variables according to height, weight, age and sex.

Table 4.12 Summary of the complex 9 panel plot

Panel number	x-axis	y-axis	Additional y-axis	Other comments
1	Time (min)	Minute ventilation (VE) (L/min)		
2	Time	Heart rate (HR)	Oxygen pulse (VO$_2$/HR) (ml/beat)	
3	Time	(VO$_2$) and (VCO$_2$)	Work rate (W)	The slope of the VO$_2$: time relationship will be parallel to the slope of the work rate : time relationship. For every 100 W increase in work rate, VO$_2$ should increase by approximately 1 L/min
4	(VCO$_2$)	(VE)		
5	(VO$_2$)	(HR)	(VCO$_2$)	Lactic acidosis threshold can be identified when the VO$_2$/VCO$_2$ axes relationship exceeds a slope of 1.0. A point is then marked, corresponding to the predicted maximum heart rate and VO$_2$ for the subject
6	Time	Ventilatory equivalents for oxygen and carbon dioxide (VE/VO$_2$ and VE/VCO$_2$)		

(Contd.)

Table 4.12 (Contd.)

Panel number	x-axis	y-axis	Additional y-axis	Other comments
7	Minute ventilation	Tidal volume (VT)		(VC), inspiratory capacity (IC) and (MVV) are measured at rest. They are then analysed during exercise and will reflect any changes resulting from diseases causing ventilation limitation during exercise
8	Time	Respiratory exchange ratio (VCO_2/VO_2) (R)		Because of changing gas stores during incremental exercise, the respiratory exchange ratio (R) is used
9	Time	End-tidal oxygen and end-tidal carbon dioxide ($PETO_2$ and $PETCO_2$) (mmHg). If ABG used, PaO_2 and $PaCO_2$ may be added. (SpO_2) vacan also be displayed.		

Anaerobic threshold (AT)
- The level of O_2 consumption where metabolic pathways shift from aerobic to anaerobic.
- The result is a rise in lactic acid production and an increase in carbon dioxide production.
- It is a marker of the combined efficiency of the lungs, heart and circulation and can be derived graphically from the nine panel plot.
- For most patients, the AT is normally reached about halfway through CPEX testing.

An AT of at least 11 ml/kg/min is required to safely undertake significant surgery.

Clinical implications

- CPEX provides a detailed evaluation of a patient's functional status before major surgery.
- It is particularly useful in patients undergoing thoracic surgery, in which the post-operative oxygen consumption may exceed 150 ml/m^2.
- CPEX represents a non-invasive simulation of the requirements of thoracic surgery, thus indicating the patient specific peak oxygen consumption and the AT.
- It also aids in decision making as to the appropriate post-operative care facility.

Institutions where CPEX is not available

6 minute walk test

- Measures how far a patient can walk in 6 minutes at their normal pace.
- Simple to perform needing relatively few resources and cheap.
- Measurements:
  - Distance achieved (median is around 500–600 m).
  - SPO_2.
  - Heart rate.
  - Borg scale (dyspnoea and fatigue measurement).

Shuttle testing

- Markers 10m apart.
- Patients start walking; the speed is increased by 0.17 m/sec in time with audible beeps.
- 25 shuttles approximates to 10 ml/kg/min VO_2 max.
- More difficult to perform.
- The test is stopped if the subject can't reach the cone by the next beep time, or if they get exhausted.
- Both correlate well with VO_2 and maximum work capacity that would have been calculated via the more complex CPEX testing.
- Both tests are dependent upon motivation of the patient, and when repeated, results can improve as the patient learns what is expected of them.
- CPEX gives a far more detailed look at a subject's functional ability, pin-pointing the cause of their functional capacity reduction far more clearly than the simple tests.

High risk patients

- CPEX
  - VO_2 max <10 ml/kg/min associated with significant post-operative morbidity and mortality. These patients WILL NEED CRITICAL CARE, and/or discussion as to whether surgery will be too much for them.
  - VO_2 max >15 ml/kg/min indicates average risk for surgery.
  - AT >11 ml/kg/min are less likely to require critical care.
  - Those with AT <11 ml/kg/min will benefit from post-operative critical care.
- 6MWT
  - <300 m = high risk for development of post-op morbidity.
  - >350 m = cut-off for consideration of LVRS for COPD and will predict a lower mortality post oesophagectomy.
  - <200 m = high 6 month mortality after major thoracic surgery/LVRS.
- Shuttle testing
  - <25 shuttles or desaturation of 4% = high risk.

Further reading

Agnew N. Preoperative cardiopulmonary exercise testing. Continuing education in Anaesthesia, *Critical Care & Pain* 2010; 10:33–7.

Win T, Jackson A, Sharples L, *et al.* Cardiopulmonary exercise tests and lung cancer surgical outcome. *Chest* 2005; 127:1159–65.

ATS/ACCP Statement on Cardiopulmonary Exercise Testing. *American Journal of Respiratory and Critical Care Medicine* 2003; 167:211–77.

CXR, PET, CT

Chest X Ray

Routine pre-operative CXR is usually performed in patients who are due to undergo thoracic surgery, and can provide valuable information regarding the patient's anaesthetic risk.

Cardiac assessment

Heart size
- Cardiac silhouette magnified on AP film, always assess PA film if available.
  - Useful for detection of cardiac enlargement and pulmonary congestion.
  - Cardiomegaly—↑ CTR >50% on PA film (ratio of maximal cardiac horizontal dimension to the maximal horizontal dimension of the lower thorax from inner aspect of ribs).
  - Interpret with caution in obese patients patients as epicardial fat deposition may give a false positive appearance.
- Chamber enlargement.
  - *R atrium*—prominent right heart border.
  - *R ventricle*—CTR may be normal. Uplifting of ventricular apex from diaphragm on PA CXR. Best assessed on lateral CXR with infilling of retrosternal space.
  - *L atrium*—Splaying of the carina, double right heart border.
  - *L ventricle*—prominent left heart border, downward displacement of cardiac apex, increased CTR.
- Cardiac failure.
  - Increased heart size.
  - Interstitial opacities (septal lines: look for small horizontal linear opacities in lower zones radiating to pleural surface). Note, similar appearance may also be present in patients with interstitial lung disease (look for volume loss or old films suggesting longstanding changes).
  - Alveolar opacity: fluffy ill-defined opacity, particularly in peri-hilar regions ('batwing' appearance).
  - Pleural effusions.
- Other signs of cardiac disease.
  - Previous median sternotomy.
  - Prosthetic valve.
  - Mitral valve ring calcification: may be due to rheumatic or degenerative valvular disease. Association with mitral stenosis.

Lung assessment
- Emphysema.
  - Hyper-expanded lungs (>7 anterior or 11 posterior ribs visible above the mid hemidiaphragm).
  - Bullous changes—areas of lucency with few vascular markings, predominantly upper zone distribution.

- Pulmonary fibrosis
  - Reduced lung volumes.
  - Reticular or nodular opacities—predominantly peripheries and bases.
  - Often longstanding changes on previous x-rays.
- Pneumothorax.
  - Pleural stripe that has fallen away from the chest wall.
  - Absence of lung markings beyond the stripe.
  - A very small pneumothorax may not be visible on x-ray.
  - Often related to recent biopsy of lung cancer/trauma/post CVP line insertion/blockage of ICD inserted blind or operatively.
- Pulmonary contusion.
  - Opacity in the peripheral lung near to the injured chest wall
  - Chest x-ray may lag 12–24 hours behind the clinical extent of the contusion.
- Pulmonary haemorrhage.
  - Upright or decubitus film is often necessary.
  - Area of opacity.
  - Up to a 1 litre of blood may be present, and not seen, on a standard portable supine chest x-ray.

The mediastinum
- Tracheal compression or displacement.
  - Superior mediastinal mass or benign retrosternal goiter.
- Hiatus hernia.
  - Rounded density containing air-fluid level in lower mediastinum (don't forget to look behind the heart!). Risk of aspiration.
- Pneumomediastinum.
  - From oesophageal or tracheal perforation in setting of trauma
  - Often a bad prognostic sign.
- Enlarged pulmonary arteries.
  - Due to primary or secondary pulmonary hypertension.

The diaphragm
- Diaphragmatic hernia or paralysis.
  - Unilateral diaphragmatic elevation. May increase risk of post-op respiratory failure.

Chest wall/spine
- Pectus excavatum/significant chest wall deformity.
  - May cause restrictive lung defect.
  - CXR signs of pectus excav.atum: ill defined right heart border, displacement of the heart to the left and downward pointing anterior ribs.

- Kyphoscoliosis.
  - Curvature of the thoracic spine and low position of the clavicles in patients on a frontal chest X-ray with a significant Kyphoscoliosis.
  - May affect ease of thoracic epidural or central line placement.
- Flail segment.
  - 3 adjacent rib fractures in 2 or more places
  - Chest drain advised.
- Rib fractures
  - Age >65 associated with higher mortality due to pulmonary sequelae such as atelectasis, pneumonia, and respiratory arrest
  - The presence of cardiopulmonary disease also significantly increases morbidity and mortality rates.

Cervical spine film

- Indicated in patients with possible atlanto-axial subluxation
  - Rheumatoid arthritis, Down's syndrome, diabetic patients.
- Single lateral flexion view should show any significant subluxation.

Computed tomography

In addition to assessment of above, also detects the following which may be relevant to anaesthetic risk assessment:

- Coronary artery calcification.
- Pericardial effusion/cardiac tamponade.
- Superior vena cava obstruction.
- Emphysematous and interstitial fibrotic changes with more sensitivity than CXR.
- Provides more accurate cross-sectional assessment of tracheal lumen if concern regarding compression (retrosternal goitre, tumour).
- Simple pneumothorax with greater sensitivity than CXR.
- Rib/vertebral fractures (particularly cervical spine injury which may require log rolling during anaesthesia).
- Pulmonary hypertension.
  - PA diameter of 2.72 cm is average in normal individuals
  - >3.32 cm = significant pulmonary hypertension (58% sensitivity, 95% specificity).

Positron emission tomography/CT

- May detect abnormalities in the oropharynx or larynx, which are not covered on a standard CT protocol for thoracic disorders.
- Detects neoplastic disease, determine extent of spread or recurrence.
- Used to assess the effectiveness of a treatment plan, such as chemotherapy.
- Can determine coronary blood flow in those unable to undertake CPET.
- Assess the effects of a myocardial infarction, on areas of the heart.
- Identify areas of the myocardium that would benefit from angioplasty or coronary artery bypass surgery (in combination with a myocardial perfusion scan).
- Otherwise, does not confer any additional benefit to contrast enhanced CT in the pre-operative assessment of patients in terms of anaesthetic risk.

Further reading

The Royal College of Radiologists. *Making the best use of clinical radiology services: referral guidelines.* London: The Royal College of Radiologists, 2007.

Ventilation perfusion scanning

A ventilation/perfusion (V/Q) scan is actually two tests that may be performed separately. The perfusion component of the scan involves the intravenous administration of technetium-radio-labelled-albumin. A gamma camera is the used to acquire quantitative images of the distribution of blood flow with in the lungs. Similarly for the ventilation component of the study, radioactive xenon is inhaled and a gamma camera used to acquire quantitative images of the distribution of ventilation.

Information

- Functional information:
  - Detects areas of reduced lung ventilation and/or perfusion, which can be correlated with anatomical imaging.
- Quantification:
  - Can be used to calculate percentage contribution of regions of the lung to the total percentage perfusion and ventilation in order to aid surgical planning.
  - Removing non-functioning lung tissue will have less of an impact on the post-operative cardio-respiratory function of the patient than removal of functioning tissue.

Indications

- Pre-operative assessment of patients for pneumonectomy with ppoFEV$_1$ <40% (BTS Guidelines).
- Pre-operative assessment of patients for lung volume reduction surgery.
- Diagnosis of pulmonary embolism (acute or chronic).

Although ventilation perfusion scintigraphy is not routinely recommended in the evaluation of patients with lung cancer being considered for lobectomy by the BTS guidelines, it may be of use in surgical planning, particularly in high risk patients with low/borderline lung function on spirometry.

Further reading

BTS Guidelines on the selection of patients with lung cancer for surgery. British Thoracic Society and Society of Cardiothoracic Surgeons of Great Britain and Ireland Working Party. *Thorax*. 2001; 56:89–108.

The patient with a lung transplant

Prevalence
- 122 lung transplants performed in UK between 2007–2008.
- 381 heart-lung transplants done between 1998–2008.
- 2168 lung transplants done worldwide by 2006.
- 80–90% will survive the first year after operation.
- 54% will survive for 5 years after operation.

Types of lung transplant
(See Table 4.13 for disease states and their corresponding requirement for transplantation).
- **Single Lung:**
  - Used in COPD and pulmonary fibrosis.
- **Bilateral Lung:**
  - Used in suppurative conditions, pulmonary vascular and bilateral emphysematous conditions.
  - Each lung is implanted separately and cardiopulmonary bypass is often required.
- **Heart/Lung:**
  - Used in pulmonary hypertension or Eisenmengers with uncorrectable cardiac abnormality.
- **Living-related lobar transplants.**

Table 4.13 Amenable to lung transplant

Condition	% requiring SLT	% requiring DLT
Emphysema	54.4	22.5
α_1 antitrypsin deficiency	8.7	9.9
1° pulmonary hypertension	1.3	8.3
Idiopathic pulmonary fibrosis	23.8	9.1
Cystic fibrosis	1.1	33
Re-transplantation	1.6	1.9

Problems associated with transplantation

Rejection

- Hyperacute.
  - Occurs from seconds to minutes due to pre-existing recipient antibodies.
- Acute
  - Occurs from 2 weeks to years if immunosupression fails.
- Chronic
  - With bronchiolitis obliterans: chronic fibrosis of the graft and vessels occurs from 6 weeks onwards.
- ❗❗ Transplanted lung rejection mimics URTI:
  - Fever, leucopenia, dyspnoea, hypoxaemia.
  - CXR may show peri-hilar infiltrates and graft opacification.
  - FEV, VC &TLC decrease significantly.
  - Rejection can be diagnosed using broncho-alveolar lavage and lung biopsy.
- Immunosuppressants are useless against hyperacute and chronic rejection.

The immunosuppressant drugs

- Common drugs include:
  - Cyclosporin.
  - Steroids.
  - Tacrolimus.
  - Mycophenolate mofetil.
  - Azothoprine.
- Involve transplant coordinator early.
- Involve pharmacist early.
- Maintenance doses MUST continue in the per-operative period.
- Cyclosporine
  - Daily levels are required.
  - Give PO cyclosporine 4–7 hours pre-op.
  - IV cyclosporine dose roughly 25% PO dose.
- Azathioprine.
  - PO/IV doses of are roughly equivalent.
- Prednisolone.
  - PO dose is roughly equivalent to same IV methylprednisolone dose.
- Tacrolimus.
  - Daily levels are required.

(See Table 4.14 for common side effects of immunosuppressant therapy. See Table 4.15 for common interactions).

Table 4.14 Common side effects of immunosuppresants

Azathioprine	Leucopaenia, pancytopenia
	Hair loss
	Hepatoxcity
Mycophenolate mofetil	GI upset
	Leukopaenia, thrombocytopaenia
Prednisolone	Osteoporosis
	Mood change
	Diabetes
	Easy bruising, thinning skin
	Infection
	Cushing's syndrome
Cyclosporin	Hirsuitism
	Gum hypertrophy
	Hypertension
	Hyperkalaemia
	Diabetes
	Reduced seizure threshold
	Nephrotoxicity
	Neurotoxcity
Tacrolimus	Hypomagnesaemia, hyperkalaemia
	CNS—seizures, tremor, headache

Table 4.15 Drug interactions of cyclosporin and tacrolimus

Serum concentration increases with:

Bromocriptine

Clarithromycin

Cimetidine

Co-trimoxazole

Diltiazem/Verapamil

Erythromycin

Metoclopramide

Fluconazole/Itraconazole/ketoconazole

(Contd.)

Table 4.15 (Contd.)

May cause renal dysfunction with:
Amphotericin
Cimetidine/ranitidine
Gentamicin/vancomycin
NSAIDS
Co-Trimoxazole

Serum concentration decreases with:
Carbamezapine
Phenobarbitone
Phenytoin
Rifampacin

The immunosuppressed state

- Infection
  - Significant cause of morbidity and mortality.
  - Involves typical & atypical organisms: CMV, PCP, toxoplasma, listeria, *Legionella pnuemophilia*, aspergillosis, *Candida*, herpes simplex
  - Clinical signs may be absent.
- Cancer
  - Squamous cell carcinomas, lymphoma, breast, lung, bowel, cervical., EBV related lymphopoliferative disease.

Physiological & pharmacological effects of lung transplantion

- Retained laryngeal sensitivity but loss of cough reflex below anastamosis.
- Abnormal mucous production and muco-cillary clearance.
- ↑ risk of silent aspiration.
- ↑ risk of bronchospasm.
- ↑ risk of pulmonary oedema due to disrupted lymphatic drainage.
- Respiratory rate & rhythm unaffected.
- Hypoxic pulmonary vasoconstriction unaffected.
- Central chemo receptors re-adjust to normal a month post transplant.
- LFTs normalize 6 months post transplant.
- Good response to inhaled beta agonists and ipratropium.
- Poor response to isoprenaline, aminophylline and adrenaline.

Immunosuppressants and anaesthesia

- Propfol infusion, isoflurane/N_2O anaesthesia are unlikely to affect cyclosporin concentrations; extrapolated from animal studies.
- Fentanyl and phenobarbitone action is prolonged by cyclosporin in mice.
- Muscle relaxant duration of action is prolonged by cyclosporin.
  - Especially vecuronium, pancuronium, atracurium.
- Azathioprine does not antagonize muscle relaxants.
- Take care with local anaesthetics and analgesia in patients with reduced renal function (lower doses required for toxic effects to occur).
- ⓧ Avoid NSAIDs as they augment the nephrotoxcity of cyclosporin.

Peri-operative care

Pre-operative assessment

- Early communication with transplant centre required for current information on:
  - Drug therapy, rejection status, graft function.
- Identify any ongoing infection, rejection or other organ dysfunction.

Investigations

Bloods.
- **FBC**.
  - **Look for pancytopenia, any other 'penia', anaemia etc**.
- **U&E, LFTs**
  - Chemotherapeutic agents can cause LFT derangement, as well as electrolyte imbalance and renal failure.
- **Clotting, glucose, calcium, magnesium, amylase**.
- **ABG's**.
  - As a baseline.
  - Type I or II failure picture may give clues to rejection.

Radiology
- CXR.

Other
- **ECG and Echo**.
- **Spirometry**.

☠ Elective operations MUST be postponed until rejection or infection have resolved.

Conduct of anaesthesia

- Choice of technique depends on general health and intended operation.
- Consider regional technique if no contra-indication so as to avoid pulmonary complications.
- Avoid intercostal and brachial plexus blocks as risk of pneumothorax.
- Insert invasive monitoring with strict asepsis (insert CVP line on side of native lung if possible).
- Administer standard prophylactic antibiotics.
- Consider supplemental steroids if major operation.
- Consider TOD/LiDCO® to guide IV fluid administration to avoid pulmonary overload.
- Aim for early extubation—avoid long acting benzodiazepines and high dose opioids.
- Avoid long acting muscle relaxants and use nerve stimulators.
- Avoid N_2O with bullous disease.
- Avoid high inspiratory pressures to protect the anastomosis.
- Extubate patient fully awake and able to cough with healthiest lung upper most to protect from aspiration.

Post operative care

- Consider HDU/ITU.
- Regular physio and incentive spirometry is required.
- Avoid fluid overload.
- Ensure adequate analgesia.
- Evidence of infection or rejection should be sought and treated.
- IV lines, drains, catheters should be removed ASAP.
- Immunosuppressants MUST be continued.

Further reading

Haddow GR. Anaesthesia for patients after lung transplantation. *Canadian Journal of Anaesthesia* 1997; 44: 182–97.

Kostopanagiotou G, Smyrniotis V, Arkadopoulos N, *et al.* Anaesthetic and peri-operatoive management of adult transplant recipients in non transplant surgery. *Anaesthesia and Analgesia.* 1999; 89: 613–7.

The patient with previous chemo-radiotherapy

As neoadjuvant (pre-operative) therapies for carcinoma are becoming first line, the anaesthetist must be familiar with the effects of chemotherapy and radiotherapy.

Pre-operative considerations

General

- Look for myelosuppression:
  - Anaemia.
  - Neutropaenia.
  - Thrombocytopaenia.
- Be aware of opportunistic infections.
- Cachexia/nutritional status.
- Radiation scarring.
- Difficult IV access.
- Pain control:
  - Opioid tolerance.
- Assess for cardiotoxicity:
  - ST alterations.
  - PVC's.
  - Tachycardia.
  - Low voltage complexes.
- Assess for pulmonary complications (fibrosis/infiltrates).

(See Table 4.16 for toxicity profiles)

Table 4.16 Major toxicity of chemotherapy agents

Class	Drug	Major organ Toxicity
Alkylating agents	Cyclophosphamide	CNS, N, R,D
	Busulfan	MS, CNS, GI, H, Ca
	Carboplatin	PN, MS, N
	Cisplatin	CNS, PN, R, MS
Antimetabolities	Methotrexate	MS, GI, D, R, N, Ca
	5-FU	GI, MS, CNS, C, D
	Gemcitabine	MS, GI, H
	Mercaptopurin	MS, GI, H, D
Vinca alcaloids	Vinblastine	CNS, MS, GI, C, D
	Vincristine	PN, GI, C, D
Taxanes	Paclitaxel	MS, PN, N, C
	Docetaxel	MS, R, CNS, GI

(Contd.)

Table 4.16 (Contd.)

Class	Drug	Major organ Toxicity
Antibiotics	Bleomycin	MS, D, R
	Doxorubicin	MS, GI, D, C
	Idarubicin	MS, GI, D, C
Modifier of biological responses	Interferon-α	H, MS, Coag
Epipodophylatoxins	Etoposide	MS, GI
Hormones	Tamoxifen	CNS, Coag, Ca
	Letrozole	Coag
	Flutamid	H, D

Abbreviations;
C: Cardiotoxic, Ca: Carcinogenic, CNS: Central nervous system, Coag: Coagulation, D: Dermatotoxicity, GI: Gastrointestinal, H: Hepatotoxicity, MS: Myelosuppression, N: Nephrotoxicity, PN: Perpherial nervous system, R: Respiratory system.

Chemotherapy

- Combination chemotherapy regimens of etoposide and a platinum compound (either cisplatin or carboplatin) are commonly used. Although all the drug classes listed below can be used.
- Adjuvant chemotherapy after surgery is now standard practice for patients with stage II or stage III disease, possibly also for patients with stage IB disease with tumors >4 cm.
- Clinical trials have shown an increase in 5 yr survival rates with the use of adjuvant chemotherapy.
- Most chemotherapy agents are metabolized by the P450 liver cytochrome enzyme system, as are many anaesthetic drugs.
- Nausea and vomiting will be more common.
- Remember, IV access may be difficult.

Radiotherapy

- Dysphagia:
  - May need rapid sequence Induction.
- Nausea and weight loss.
- Pneumonitis (made worse with concurrent bleomycin).
- Fibrosis and scaring (restricted movement):
  - Abnormal anatomy.
  - Caution with surgical positioning.
  - Technically difficult surgery.
  - Increased blood loss.
- Myocardial fibrosis, myopathy.

Investigations

Bloods

- **FBC** (mandatory).
- **U&E's, LFT's** and glucose.
  - To assess synthetic liver function.
- **Full septic screen**.
  - If febrile.
- **ABG**.

Radiology

- **CXR**.
  - Pneumonitis and fibrosis?
- **Echo**.
  - Consider if any suspicious clinical signs (arrhythmias may signify cardiac conduction pathway fibrosis; but it is important to exclude valvular abnormalities).
- **PFT's**.
  - Pulmonary fibrosis?
- **ECG**.
  - To exclude cardiac involvement/arrhythmias.

Anaesthesia

- Assess the airway for possible difficult intubation.
- Screen the patient for associated opportunistic infections.
- Avoid N_2O for patients on methotrexate, as may further worsen bone marrow toxicity.
- Limit oxygen concentration and crystalloids for patients on bleomycin.
- Cyclophosphamide inhibits plasma cholinesterase, thus caution with suxamethonium.

Further reading

Kloivk, S., Glavas-Obrova, L., Sakic, K. Anaesthetic implications of anticancer chemotherapy. *European Journal of Anaesthesiology* 2003; 20: 859–71.

Zaniboni, A., Prabhu, S., Audisio, R., Chemotherpay and anaesthetic drugs: too little is known. *Lancet Oncology* 2005; 6: 176–8.

The patient with severe emphysema

Emphysema forms part of the disease spectrum of COPD. It deserves separate consideration due to the potential benefit of Lung Volume Reduction Surgery (LVRS) and Lung Transplantation.

Definition

- Irreversible dilatation of the distal airways and destruction of alveolar space, resulting in cystic areas or 'bullae'.

Causes

- Smoking.
  - Causes neutrophil stimulation.
  - These neutrophils are retained → proteolytic enzyme damage to lung tissue.
- α1-antitrypsin deficiency.
  - Autosomal co-dominant condition.
  - Neutralizes neutrophil elastase normally, hence its deficiency results in elastase damage to the lung.
- Proteinase/anti-proteinase hypothesis.
  - Excess proteinases, deficiency of anti-proteinases, hence overall destruction.
- IV drug abuse.
  - 2% of users.
  - Attributed to pulmonary vascular damage from insoluble filler (e.g. cornstarch, cotton fibers, cellulose, talc) contained in methadone or methylphenidate.
- Immunodeficiency.
- Connective tissue diseases.
  - Marfans syndrome, cutis laxa and Ehlers-Danlos syndrome.
- Salla disease.
  - Storage disorder causing sialic acid accumulation.

Classification

Emphysema can be sub-classified depending on the site of lung damage:
- Centrilobular.
  - Affects respiratory bronchioles with preservation of the distal alveolar components, common in smokers.
- Panlobular.
  - Affects all air spaces distal to terminal bronchioles, predominantly due to α1-antitrypsin deficiency.
- Paraseptal.
  - Affects airspaces in the periphery of the lung next to the pleura.
  - Upper lobes more frequently involved.
- Irregular.
  - Damage to the lung is patchy and follows no pattern.

Pathophysiology

- Elasticity of the lung tissue is lost and there is a large increase in dead space.
- Expiratory airflow limitation and gas trapping occurs.
- Damage to the alveolus results in reduced gas transfer.
- In late stages, destruction of the pulmonary capillaries results in pulmonary hypertension and Cor Pulmonale.
- Patients rarely have pure emphysematous disease; elements of chronic bronchitis will usually co-exist.

Presentation and assessment

History and symptoms

- Commonest presentation is in 5th decade.
- Productive cough.
  - Usually worse in the morning.
  - Production of small amounts of colorless sputum.
- Breathlessness.
  - Does not usually manifest until the sixth decade of life.
- Wheezing.
  - In some patients, particularly during exertion and infective exacerbations.
  - Decreased exercise tolerance.

Signs

- Classically the 'pink puffer'.
- Cyanotic in severe disease with RHF.
- Thin/cachectic.
- Pursed lips, creating intrinsic PEEP.
- Tachypnoea.
- Using accessory muscles, leaning forward stabilising chest.
- Indrawing of intercostals.
- Hyper-inflated chest.
- JVP ↑.
- Hyper-resonance on percussion.
- Wheeze or diffusely decreased breath sounds.

Investigations

Bloods

- **FBC.**
  - ? Degree of polycythaemia.
- **α1-antitrypsin level.**
  - <3–7 mmol/L (protective value).
- **ABGs.**
  - PaO_2 normal or moderate decrease.
  - $PaCO_2$ normal in early disease. High in severe disease.

Radiology

- **CXR**
  - Hyperinflation with flat diaphragm.
  - Loss of peripheral lung markings.
  - Prominent hilar vessels.
  - Long narrow heart often with right ventricular enlargement.
  - Bullae.
- **CT chest**
  - Often not necessary, bullae more visible though.

Other

- **Sputum evaluation**
  - Stable disease → mucoid sputum with macrophages.
  - Severe disease → purulent with excessive neutrophils +/– organisms.
- **PFT's**—with assessment of response to bronchodilators (reversibility).
  - ↑ RV.
  - FRC.
  - TLC.
  - FEV_1.
  - VC.

Disease severity	FEV_1*
• Mild airflow obstruction	50–80% predicted
• Moderate airflow obstruction	30–49% predicted
• Severe airflow obstruction	<30% predicted

* Absolute values alone are a poor predictor of outcome or complication following anaesthesia and the functional ability of the patient must be assessed and given equal weight when assessing a patient's suitability.

Treatment

Preventative measures

- Smoking Cessation Aids.
  - Can even consider pharmacological therapy e.g. Varenicline (Chantix) new nicotinic receptor agonist.
- Regular vaccinations.
- Pulmonary rehabilitation.
- Mucolytic therapy.
- Nutritional support.

Maintenance therapy in stable disease (with increasing severity)

- Inhaled bronchodilator therapy; β_2 agonists (long and short acting), anticholinergics.
- Theophyllines.
- Inhaled corticosteroids.
- Phosphodiesterase IV inhibitors—e.g. cilomilast.
  - They cause a reduction of the inflammatory process (macrophages and CD8+ lymphocytes) in patients with COPD.
  - The preliminary clinical studies suggest a favorable clinical effect in COPD.
- Tamoxifen.
  - Stimulates release of α1-antitrypsin from the liver.
- Home nebulizers.
- Home O_2.
- Long term NIV.
- Treatment of Cor Pulmonale/pulmonary hypertension.

❶ Anti-tussive therapy, prophylactic antibiotics and α1-antitrypsin replacement therapy are not indicated in stable disease.

Management of acute exacerbations

- Early use of antibiotics if indicated (purulent sputum and cultured organisms, consolidation on CXR) as per regional microbiological guidelines.
  - S pneumoniae, H influenzae, and Moraxella catarrhalis are the most common organisms.
- Bronchodilators; inhaled and nebulized.
- Theophyllines.
- O_2 therapy guided by pulse oximetry and blood gas analysis.
- Physiotherapy.
- NIV.
- IPPV.

Surgical therapy

- Lung Volume Reduction Surgery (LVRS).
- Lung Transplantation.

NICE guidelines for consideration of LVRS

- Breathless, single large bulla on a CT scan and an FEV_1 less than 50% predicted → refer for consideration of bullectomy.
- Severe COPD with breathlessness and marked restrictions of activities of daily living despite maximal medical therapy (including rehabilitation) → refer for consideration of lung volume reduction surgery if they meet all of the following criteria:
  - FEV_1 >20% predicted.
  - $PaCO_2$ less than 7.3 kPa.
  - Upper lobe predominant emphysema.
  - DLCO more than 20% predicted.

NICE guidelines for consideration of lung transplantation

- Severe COPD with breathlessness and marked restrictions of activities of daily living despite maximal medical therapy (including rehabilitation) → refer for consideration of lung transplantation.
- Patients are considered to be within the transplant window if they fulfill the following criteria;
  - FEV_1<25% of predicted (without reversibility).
  - And/or $PaCO_2$ 7.3 kPa and/or elevated pulmonary artery pressures with progressive deterioration, e.g. cor pulmonale.
  - Preference should be given to those patients with elevated $PaCO_2$ with progressive deterioration who require long-term oxygen therapy, as they have the poorest prognosis.
- Age and degree of homogeneous distribution of emphysema on CT are also important factors when considering transplantation.

Pre-operative optimization

- Thorough assessment for any recent change in symptoms.
- Stop smoking; >8 weeks is beneficial in pre-op period.
- Physiotherapy/breathing techniques/pulmonary rehabilitation.
- Ensure that airway reversibility has been assessed and treatment is effective/appropriate.
- Culture sputum and treat any infection identified.
- Optimize treatment of co-morbidities especially right heart failure.
- Need to consider adrenal insufficiency if long term or regular oral steroid use.

Further reading

Chronic Obstructive Pulmonary Disease. National clinical guideline on management of chronic obstructive pulmonary disease in adults in primary and secondary care. *Thorax* 2004; 59 (1) 1–232.

The patient with pulmonary hypertension

Definition
- Mean pulmonary arterial pressure >22 mmHg.

or
- A systolic pulmonary arterial pressure >30 mmHg at rest with a normal left atrial pressure.

Causes
The disease was classically divided into primary/idiopathic (no cause found) and secondary (other known causes).
- The WHO (2003) classification based on aetiology is given in (Table 4.17).

Table 4.17 Venice 2003 revised classification system

WHO group I—pulmonary arterial hypertension	Idiopathic (IPAH)
	Familial (FPAH)
	Associated with other diseases (APAH): collagen vascular disease (e.g. scleroderma), congenital shunts between the systemic and pulmonary circulation, portal hypertension, HIV infection, drugs, toxins, or other diseases or disorders
	Associated with venous or capillary disease
WHO group II—venous hypertension	L sided atrial or ventricular disease
	L sided valvular disease (e.g. mitral stenosis)
WHO group III—associated with lung disease/hypoxia	Chronic obstructive pulmonary disease (COPD), interstitial lung disease (ILD)
	Sleep-disordered breathing, alveolar hypoventilation
	Chronic exposure to high altitude
	Developmental lung abnormalities
WHO group IV—associated with chronic thrombotic/embolic disease	Pulmonary embolism in the proximal or distal pulmonary arteries e.g. sickle cell disease
	Embolization of other matter, such as tumor cells or parasites
WHO group V	Miscellaneous

Pathophysiology

- WHO group I disease is thought to arise due to:

- Loss of normal NO-cGMP mediated vasodilatation
- blood flow + ishear forces → ↓ NO production by damaged endothelium → vasoconstrictive state
- Blood vessels undergo fibrosis → ↑ blood pressure within the lungs → impaired flow
- Resting PHT signifies loss of >70% of pulmonary vascular bed
- RV workload → RVH → R heart failure.

- WHO group II disease.
  - Results from venous congestion of the lungs as a result of forward pump failure.
- WHO group III disease.
  - Results from chronic hypoxia and chronic resultant hypoxic vasoconstriction.
- WHO group IV disease.
  - Results from chronic recurrent occlusion of the pulmonary vasculature by thrombi, with resulting increased resistance.

Presentation and assessment

- In the primary form, the disease is usually progressive and fatal (death from right heart failure) with a male:female ratio 1:2. and a overall incidence of two per million population per year.

History and Symptoms

- Fatigue
- Dyspnoea at rest (60%)
- Dizziness or syncope with little or no exertion
- Angina
- Cough
- Haemoptysis.

Signs

- Peripheral oedema, ascites.
- Cyanosis.
- Elevated JVP with accentuated V wave (TR).
- Parasternal heave.
- Hepatomegaly (pulsatile).
- Fixed splitting of second heart sound.
- Loud pulmonary component of second heart sound (often palpable).
- Pulmonary and or tricuspid regurgitant murmurs.
- Atrial S_3 or ventricular S_4 sound.
- Signs related to underlying secondary cause.

Investigations

- Investigations should be tailored based on the clinically suspected cause of the pulmonary hypertension.
- Below is a suggested list of investigations:

Bloods
- **FBC**.
  - Polycythemia.
- **Autoantibodies, HIV, TSH, thrombophilia and serum ACE**.
- **LFTs**.
  - Liver failure.
- **ABGs**.
  - Hypoxaemia.

Radiology
- **CXR**.
  - Right atrial and ventricular hypertrophy.
  - Right pulmonary artery >16 mm.
  - Hilar vessel enlargement; hilar: thoracic ratio >0.44.
- **V/Q scan**.
  - Identifies any thromboembolic causes.
- Pulmonary/CT angiogram.
  - Detailed structure of the pulmonary artery tree.

Others
- **ECG**.
  - Right axis deviation, right bundle branch block or right atrial and ventricular hypertrophy.
  - ST depression and T-wave inversions in the anterior leads.
  - Some patients have few or no abnormal ECG findings; thus, normal ECG results do not exclude a diagnosis of PAH.
- **Echocardiogram**.
  - Most useful of the tests.
  - Evidence of right heart hypertrophy ± failure.
  - Look for PFO with right to left shunting (33%).
- **Spirometry**.
  - If PAH is secondary to chronic lung disease.
  - Gas transfer factor (DLCO).
  - If interstitial lung disease or scleroderma is suspected.
- **Right heart catheterization**.
  - Measures RAP, PAP, PCWP and CO—gold standard in diagnosis.
  - Important to exclude left sided heart disease.

- Done in specialized centres along with vasoactivity studies (gauges response of vasculature to vasodilator drugs).
- **PFTs and CPEX**.
  - Assesses ventilatory efficiency and can differentiate intrinsic pulmonary vascular disease, cardiac disease and restrictive/obstructive lung disease.
  - In patients with PAH, values for peak exercise oxygen consumption, oxygen pulse, and ventilator equivalents (ratio of expired volume to carbon dioxide output at the anaerobic threshold) during exercise are abnormal to varying degrees.
- **Sleep studies**.
  - To exclude sleep apnoea as a cause.

Management options

- There is no known cure for primary pulmonary hypertension.
- Treatment is ultimately aimed at prolonging an active lifespan by reducing right ventricular strain via:
  - ↓ pulmonary arterial pressure.
  - ↑ right ventricular output.
- Secondary pulmonary hypertension usually benefits from treatment of the underlying cause.

Medical management

Vasodilator drugs
- Should only be given once good vasoactivity status is demonstrated (<25% of patients will demonstrate good response).
- These drugs may affect endothelial function and smooth muscle physiology.
- Their direct pulmonary arterial dilatation properties are only small
  - Prostacyclin receptor analogues e.g. Epoprostenol (See 📖 Nitric oxide, p. 72)
  - Nitric oxide therapy (See 📖 Nitric oxide, p. 72)
  - Endothelin receptor antagonists eg bosentan.
  - Phosphodiesterase-5 inhibitors eg sildenafil.
  - Calcium channel blockers eg nifedipine—should only be used in those found to be vaso-reactive on cardiac catheterization. Only those patients whose *mean* pulmonary artery pressure falls by more than 10 mm Hg with an unchanged or increased cardiac output when challenged with adenosine, epoprostenol, or nitric oxide are considered vaso-reactive. Of these, only half of the patients are responsive to calcium channel blockers in the long term.
- Anticoagulants:
  - Warfarin is usually used to reduce further thromboembolic episodes; (INR 1.5–2 x normal).

- Digoxin.
  - Has been used to improve those with severe right heart dysfunction (lack of evidence).
- Diuretics.
  - To manage peripheral oedema.
- Oxygen.
  - Caution if PFO with L → R shunt!

Specific Surgical management of PHT and complications

- Bronchoscopy ± CT embolization.
  - Consider if massive haemoptysis (See 📖 Bronchoscopy, p. 282).
- Lung biopsy to aid prognosis, e.g. Eisenmenger syndrome.
  - VATS biopsy is contraindicated—risk of massive bleeding.
- Transplantation.
  - In young patients with severe disease, a lung or heart-lung transplantation may rarely be considered.
  - CPB may be required if severe PAH and RV failure for anaesthetic management.
- Atrial septostomy.
  - Creates a right: left heart communication relieving R heart pressure but at the expense of arterial hypoxia.
  - Improved CO may however preserve O₂ delivery.
- Pulmonary thromboendarterectomy.
  - For chronic thromboembolic pulmonary hypertension.
  - It consists of removal of organized clot and the lining of the vessel to relieve the obstruction.
  - Need for CPB.

Anaesthetic management

❶ Patients with known pulmonary hypertension present a significant operative risk.

General anaesthetic considerations for thoracic surgery in patients with PHT

- Preoperative assessment and optimization of other co-morbidities driving PHT.
  - May be on immunosuppressants, steroids, anticoagulants, pulmonary vasodilators etc.
  - ❶ Pulmonary vasodilators should not be stopped pre-op.
  - Most patients from Group I & IV will be on warfarin.
  - ▶▶ dilemmas may arise in achieving optimal coagulation control and fluid filling.
- High PAP is associated from low survival and high risk of death and morbidity due to surgery and anaesthesia; consider the absolute need for surgery on an individual case basis.
  - 5 year survival if PAP >45 mmHg in COPD <10%.
- Peripheral oedema in cor pulmonale is due to fluid retention and ↑ permeability and not necessarily due to RV failure.
  - Echo to check PAP and RVH etc.

- Thoracic epidural anaesthesia may be safe but risk of RH decompensation due to ↓ RV preload.
  - Invasive monitoring as per GA needed.
  - Consider placing epidural early and build up the block slowly while manipulating haemodynamics.

Controlling PAP, systemic vasodilatation, CO, SaO_2 and SvO_2 during anaesthesia

- Establish invasive haemodynamic monitoring before induction; (CVP, SvO_2, arterial line, NICO, TOE if available.
  - TOE requires skilled operator, but best for guidance of fluid/inotrope/vasodilator therapy.
- Ensure adequate CVP by careful fluid challenge.
- Avoid factors that will increase pulmonary hypertension:
  - Hypertensive response to intubation—use remifentanil.
  - Hypoxia.
  - Acidosis.
  - High P_ACO_2.
  - Pain—epidural analgesia, continue to post-op phase.
  - Patients who are prone to alveolar hypoventilation (neuromuscular disorder) will probably need post-op ventilation.
- Judicious use of vasodilator therapy to control pulmonary hypertension.
  - NO has been used successfully, but delivery is cumbersome.
  - Epoprostenol should only be used as a last resort—affects platelets and ↑ risk of bleeding.
  - Trial of OLV—if excessive rise in PAP consider lobar isolation instead with a bronchial blocker. Alternatively abandon OLV.
- Judicious use of Inotropes (those that are also pulmonary vasodilators e.g. milronone, dubutamine).
  - Norepinephrine provides better control of low BP and CO than phenylepherine and has little effect on PAP.
- Avoid factors that will decrease ventricular function:
  - Hypovolaemia.
  - Excessive PEEP.
  - Arrhythmias.
  - Anaesthetic agent overdose (myocardial depression).
  - Excessive epidural dosing.

Avoid hypoxia during OLV

- Use SvO_2 in addition to SpO_2 or SaO_2 and maintain it close to 70%—better index of O_2 delivery.
- Volatile agents may ↑ hypoxia but ↓ PAP. Use haemodynamic monitoring and SvO_2 and <1MAC volatile agent.
- If DLCO<25% (interstitial lung disease or scleroderma) OLV will be impossible.
- HPV may be affected by the pulmonary vasodilators the patient is currently receiving. Use CPAP during OLV or abandon OLV.
- Almitrine at 8 mcg/kg/min is a useful adjunct to improve HPV and SvO_2 but in PHT can dangerously ↑ PAP.

Further reading

📖 Chapman, Robinson, Stradling, West (2005) *Oxford Handbook of Respiratory Medicine*, 391–406.

Rich S, Rubin LJ. *Executive summary from the World Symposium on Primary Pulmonary Hypertension*. Evian, France, September 6–10, 1998. Geneva: World Health Organisation, 1998.

Rich S, Dantzker DR. Primary Pulmonary Hypertension. A national prospective stusy. *Annals of Internal Medicine* 1987; 107:216–23.

The patient with cystic fibrosis

Pathophysiology of cystic fibrosis (CF)

- Commonest life threatening inherited disease in the UK.
- Gene mutation.
  - Long arm of chromosome 7, more than 1300 variants known to date.
- The normal gene codes for a protein; cystic fibrosis transmembrane regulator (CFTR).
- Defective CFTR results in:
  - Decreased secretion of chloride.
  - Increased reabsorption of sodium and water across epithelial cells.
  - Decreased hydration of mucus (becomes thick) → mucus stickier to bacteria → infection and inflammation.
  - Viscous secretions in the respiratory tract, pancreas, gastrointestinal tract, sweat glands, and other exocrine tissues.
  - Widespread dysfunction of exocrine glands occurs with damage to multiple organs.
- Lungs are particularly prone to damage.
- Average life expectancy is around 40 years.
- 95% of affected adults die from respiratory complications.

General considerations

Patients require anaesthesia for procedures directly related and unrelated to CF.

- Common non-thoracic procedures:
  - Venous access.
  - Parenteral feeding procedures.
  - Cholecystectomy.
  - ENT surgery eg. nasal polypectomy.
- Thoracic procedures may be diagnostic or therapeutic:
  - Bronchoscopy.
  - Pleurectomy.
  - Lobar resection.
  - Pneumonectomy.
  - Lung transplantation.
- Treatment is aimed at clearing viscous pulmonary secretions with physiotherapy and exercise programmes, control of chest infections, and providing nutritional support.
- There are conflicting studies assessing the effect of general anaesthesia on lung function in patients with CF.
  - In general, it is probably sensible to avoid general anaesthesia if possible.
- Surgery should be planned in advance if possible, and a multidisciplinary approach is required to manage these patients successfully.

Pre-operative assessment
- Assessment of severity of pulmonary and related systemic derangements.
- Should be anaesthetized by experienced staff in the patient's own base hospital.
- Management directed towards optimum clearance of pulmonary secretions to minimize the risk of post-operative respiratory complications.

Respiratory assessment
- Morphologically normal lungs at birth.
- Thick pulmonary secretions result in mucus plugging, bronchiolar obstruction and patchy atelectasis.
- Colonization and pulmonary infection causes further damage eventually resulting in bronchiectasis.
- Pulmonary assessment is often clinically difficult, and deterioration of lung function needs to be assessed by frequent lung function tests.

Other systems

Liver disease
- Increasingly common is adults with CF. Biliary cirrhosis occurs with progressive portal hypertension.
- Patients may have oesphageal varices, ascites and be at risk of hepatic decompensation post-operatively.

Pancreatic disease
- 85% have pancreatic insufficiency causing malabsorption. Enterohepatic circulation of bile salts is affected which can result in vitamin K deficiency.
- CF related diabetes mellitus is common, and should be assessed and managed as for other patients with diabetes.

Bowel disease
- 20% of adult patients suffer intermittent small bowel obstruction
- Gastrooesophageal reflux disease is common and may require alteration of anaesthetic technique.

Bone disease
- CF patients are prone to bone disease secondary to nutritional deficit and the effect of steroid treatment.

Investigations

Bloods
- **FBC**
  - Particular focus on WCC for signs of infection.
- **Clotting**
  - Detects vitamin deficiency induced coagulopathy.
- **U&Es**
  - To ensure electrolytes are not overtly deranged.
- **LFTs**
  - All patients should have LFT's pre-operatively; they may be normal until end stage disease.
- **Glucose**
  - Diabetes is common as a result of pancreatic damage.
- **ABG**
  - $PaCO_2$ is usually normal except in severe disease. $PaCO_2$ >6.7 kPa is associated with an 80% 2 year mortality.
  - PaO_2 declines as the disease progresses; <6 kPa is associated with cor pulmonale.
  - Some patients may rely on hypoxic pulmonary drive.

Radiology
- **CXR**.
  - Lobar collapse.
  - Thoracic kyphosis.
  - PA dilatation and RVH.
  - Bullae.
  - Air trapping and bronchiectasis in upper lobes.
  - Hyperinflation.
  - Infection.
  - Small pneumothoraces.
- **CT chest**.
  - Bronchiectasis (80%).
  - Peribronchial wall thickening (76%).
  - Mosaic perfusion (64%).
  - Mucous plugging (51%).
  - Enlarged lymph nodes.

Other
- **Echo**.
  - Clinical suspicion of right ventricular failure warrants a pre-operative echo, along with assessment and documentation of PA pressure.
- **ECG**
  - Is useful in all but the mildest of cases.
- **Sputum culture**
  - Essential to target antibiotic therapy.

- **PFTs**
  - FEV_1—most useful value; <30% of predicted is associated with a poor prognosis. Classical chest signs of infection are often absent.
  - ↑ (RV/TLC). TLC is also increased.
  - Advanced disease, extensive lung changes with fibrosis are reflected as restrictive changes characterized by declining TLC and vital capacity.

❶ Elective surgery should be postponed if respiratory symptoms are worse than usual.

Pre-operative optimization

Main aims: Reduce the chances of respiratory deterioration resulting from the physiological trespass from your anaesthetic.

- Involves close liaison with the patient's respiratory team and most importantly, the patient themselves. They have spent long periods of time in hospital and have detailed knowledge of their condition.
- Early admission gives an opportunity for the anaesthetist to build a rapport and fully answer questions the patient may have. Areas to consider:

Physiotherapy and sputum clearance

- Specific therapy such as nebulized dornase alpha may be instituted.
- Pre-op daily physiotherapy (postural drainage) and exercise is used to clear secretions, and encourage bronchodilatation.

Infection control

- Control of infection pre-op reduces the risk of post-operative chest infections.
  - Patients may be colonized with unusual microorganisms resistant to common antibiotics.
  - Common pathogens include *Pseudomonas aeruginosa* and *Staphylococcus aureus*.
- Do not prescribe pre-op antibiotics without prior discussion with the respiratory and microbiology team caring for the patient.

Nutritional status

- Nutritional status can be improved pre-operatively—dietiticians should be consulted for advice.
- Early admission allows time for correction of electrolyte and clotting abnormalities.

Peri-operative

Things to avoid

- Sedative pre-medication.
- Atropine.
  - Further increases viscosity of secretions.
- Inhalational induction.
  - May be slow due to V/Q mismatch.
  - Coughing and laryngospasm are more likely to occur on induction.

- Nitrous oxide.
  - Pneumothoraces are commoner, especially during one lung anaesthesia.

Things to consider
- Antireflux medication.
  - May be prescribed if needed.
- Intravenous access may be difficult.
  - Institutionalized patients will have thrombosed veins.
- Intubation allows flexible bronchoscopy and bronchoalveolar lavage.
- Suction.
  - At the start of the procedure, several times during procedure (with full relaxation) and at the end. This can be invaluable.
- A spontaneous breathing technique via a LMA may be used in patients undergoing flexible fibreoptic bronchoscopy to clear thick secretions.
- Regional anaesthetic techniques should be utilized where possible.
- Physiotherapy may be required intra-operatively.
- Effective analgesia is essential.

Post-operative
- Patients may benefit from a period of post-operative ventilation.
  - The aim would be to extubate as soon as possible to avoid the risk of development of ventilator associated pneumonia.
- Humidified oxygen and nebulized saline should be used.
- Patients being cared for on surgical wards post-operatively should be nursed in side rooms to avoid the risk of further lung colonization and infection.
  - ❶ CF patients should not be nursed together.
- The respiratory team should review the patient daily and advise on specific therapies needed.
- Aggressive physiotherapy will be required.
- Adequate nutrition is needed. Patients may benefit from a period of enteral feeding

Further reading
Hinder Della Rocca G. Anaesthesia in patients with cystic fibrosis. *Current Opinion in Anaesthesiology* 2002; 15(1):95–101.

Walsh TS, Young CH. Anaesthesia and cystic fibrosis. *Anaesthesia* 1995; 50:614–22.

Weeks AM, Buckland MR. Anaestheisa for adults with cystic fibrosis. *Anaesthesia and Intensive Care* 1995; 23(3):332–8.

The patient with a previous thoracotomy

An increasing number of patients are presenting for repeat thoracotomy. Some of these patients have tumour recurrence and resection of a new primary tumour or resection of a recurrence of the original tumour is planed.

- The risk of developing a second primary tumour is approximately 2% per year.
- Routine use of surveillance programmes for lung cancer patients increases the likelihood of second primary tumours being detected at an early stage when the tumour is potentially resectable.

Pre-operative assessment

General risk

- Patients should initially be assessed pre-operatively to identify those patients at increased risk.
- Previous medical notes, anaesthetic and HDU charts should be examined to anticipate and plan for any repeat of previous difficulties.
  - The size of the DLT used previously can usefully be noted.
- Increasing age and reduced lung tissue may increase the risk.
  - Patients who have previously undergone a pneumonectomy are a particular challenge.

Cardio-respiratory risk

- Patients who have previously undergone lung resection will usually have reduced pulmonary reserve.
  - This needs to be carefully assessed by means of a detailed history, lung function testing and if appropriate other investigations.

Intubation and isolation

- Providing OLV can be challenging.
  - Previous lung resection may have caused tracheal shift and more significantly bronchial distortion.
  - Patients should have their CXR and CT scans assessed by the anaesthetist to determine the degree of airway distortion and the probability that an endobronchial tube will provide adequate ventilation to the distorted lobes.
- Alternative means of providing OLV such as the use of bronchial blockers may be more appropriate.

Previous experience

- As for other patients it is important that adequate explanation and discussion occurs with the patient preoperatively.
  - This is particularly important for patients who have had difficulties (e.g. poor analgesia) with their original surgery.

The patient with suppurative lung disease

This section will focus heavily upon discussion of bronchiectasis and closely parallels the cystic fibrosis topic (as many CF patients will have bronchiectasis.

Definition

- Focal or diffuse disease of the lung resulting from chronic repeated respiratory infections → permanent irreversible dilatation of the airways distal to the terminal bronchioles (airways >2 mm diameter).
- Daily production of muco-purulent sputum with radiological changes.

Pathophysiology

- Infective exacerbations dominate the clinical picture and are associated with worsening of symptoms and signs of pneumonia.
- Once established, bacterial infections can become difficult or impossible to eradicate;
  - *H. influenza*, *Strep. pneumoniae*, *staph. aureus* and *Pseudomonas aeruginosa* being common pathogens.
- Multiple episodes of pulmonary infection: result from severely impaired clearance of secretions from the bronchial tree.
  - ↑ volume of sputum.
  - 10 ml/day = mild bronchiectasis.
  - 10–150 ml/day = moderate bronchiectasis.
  - >150 ml/day = severe bronchiectasis.
- ↑ viscosity of sputum.
  - +/− foul odour of sputum.

Causes

(See Table 4.18)

Table 4.18 Causes of bronchiectasis

Cause	Example
Post infection	TB
	Pertussis
	Non-tuberculous mycobacteria
Obstruction	Intrinsic—tumour/foreign body/right middle lobe syndrome
	Extrinsic—lymph node
Congenital	Defective bronchial walls
	Pulmonary sequestration
Pneumonitis	Aspiration of gastric contents
	Chemical inhalation

(Contd.)

Table 4.18 (Contd.)

Cause	Example
Immunogenic (Hyper)	Allergic bronchopulmonary aspergillosis
	Lung transplant rejection
	Chronic graft Vs. host disease
Immunogenic (Hypo)	Hypogammaglobulinaemia
	HIV
Poor mucous clearance	Immotile cilia syndrome (Kartagener's syndrome)
	Cystic fibrosis
	Young's syndrome (infertility and bronchiectasis)
Fibrosis	Cryptogenic fibrosing alveolitis
	Sarcoidosis
Inflammation	Pan-bronchiolitis (Japanese patients)
Co-association	Ulcerative colitis
	Crohn's
	Coeliac
Connective tissue	Rheumatoid arthritis
	SLE
Malignancy	ALL/CLL
Rare	Yellow nail syndrome (lymphoedema, yellow nails, pleural effusions, bronchiectasis)
	α1-antitrypsin deficiency

Presentation and assessment

Symptoms
- Chronic productive cough (90%).
- Dyspnoea (72%).
- Malaise.
- Intermittent haemoptysis can occur (50–90%); quantity of blood usually small.
- Pleuritic chest pain (46%).

Signs
- Findings are often non-specific and may be attributed to other conditions.
- General findings such as digital clubbing (3%) and weight loss.

- Physical stigmata of cor pulmonale may be observed in advanced disease, (peripheral oedema, pulsatile hepatomegaly and raised jugular venous pressure).
- Fever, particularly with active chest infection.
- Bounding pulse and fine hand flap indicates severe may indicate CO_2 retention.
- Nasal polyps and signs of chronic sinusitis may be present.
- Cyanosis and plethora secondary to chronic hypoxaemia and polycythaemia.
- Coarse inspiratory crackles (70%), rhonchi, wheezing and inspiratory squeaks heard on auscultation.
- Empyema.
- Chronic respiratory insufficiency of restrictive and/or obstructive pattern.

Investigations

Bloods
- **FBC**
  - May detect anaemia/polycythaemia (chronic hypoxaemia) and a raised white cell count with neutrophilia or eosinophilia, denoting infective exacerbation.
- **U&Es**
  - To ensure electrolytes are not overtly deranged.
- **Serum immunoglobulins**, α **1-antitrypsin** levels and **Rh Factor**.
- **ABG**.
  - Pre-operative hypoxia or carbon dioxide retention indicates the possibility of post-operative respiratory failure which may require a period of assisted ventilation on the Intensive Care Unit.

Radiology
- **CXR**.
  - Thickened bronchial walls (tramlining/ring shadows/ honeycombing) atelectasis, cystic shadows and pleural changes
- **HRCT chest**.
  - Internal bronchial diameters > adjacent pulmonary artery, lack of bronchial tapering, presence of bronchi within 1 cm of the costal pleura, presence of bronchi abutting the mediastinal pleura, and bronchial wall thickening.

Other:
- **Echocardiogram**.
  - Clinical suspicion of right ventricular failure warrants a pre-operative echocardiogram, along with assessment and documentation of PA pressure.
- **ECG**.
  - Useful in all but the mildest of cases.
- **Sputum culture**.
  - Gram stain & culture, smear for mycobacterium & fungi, presence of eosinophils.

- **PFT**.
  - Pulmonary function tests are useful in obtaining a functional assessment of the patient
  - Obstructive picture common
  - Obstruction is NOT usually reversible with bronchodilator therapy.
- **Bronchoscopy**.
  - Only performed if tumour suspected; may be useful for BAL.

Complications
- Mortality relates to progressive respiratory failure and cor pulmonale.
- Other complications:
  - Chronic bronchial infection.
  - Recurrent pneumonia.
  - Empyema.
  - Pneumothorax.
  - Pleural effusion.
  - Lung and cerebral abscess.

Treatment

General
- Patients should stop smoking.
- Patients should have adequate nutritional intake, supplemented if necessary.
- Influenza and Pneumococcal vaccinations.
- If the patient is requiring home O_2 therapy, it is likely that their bronchiectasis is end-stage. Look for cor pulmonale.

Pharmacological
- Antibiotics:
  - Treatment of acute exacerbations.
  - Prevent exacerbations.
  - Reduce bacterial burden.
  - In severe disease, the respiratory tract becomes chronically colonized.
- Mucolytics:
  - N-acetylcysteine targets the physiochemical characteristics of sputum seen in bronchiectasis, thinning it to enable expectoration.
- Anti-inflammatory agents:
  - Inhaled corticosteroids may reduce inflammation and improve airway obstruction, as in the treatment of asthma.

- Leukotriene receptor antagonists are a new class of drug that may be of benefit in bronchiectasis by inhibiting neutrophil mediated inflammation (See 📖 Leukotriene receptor antagonists, p. 62).
- Non-steroidal anti-inflammatory drugs may also be of use because they inhibit neutrophil function and the release of neutrophil elastase.
- Bronchodilators:
  - Patients often demonstrate bronchial hyper-reactivity and some reversibility of airflow obstruction with an inhaled or nebulized bronchodilator.

Non-pharmacological

- Physiotherapy and postural drainage with percussion and vibration help to reduce pulmonary secretions.
- Incentive spirometry may also be used.
- Pulmonary rehabilitation training.

Surgical

- Surgery is beneficial in a number of patients with advanced or complicated disease.
- In general, surgery should be reserved for patients who have focal disease that is poorly controlled by antibiotics.
- Patient selection plays an important role in peri-operative mortality, which may be as low as 1% in the surgical treatment of segmental or even multi-segmental bronchiectasis.
- The involved bronchiectatic sites should be completely resected for optimal symptom control. Alternative indications for surgical resection may include the following:
  - Reduction of acute infective episodes.
  - Reduction of excessive sputum production.
  - Massive haemoptysis (bronchial artery embolization may be an alternative option).
  - Foreign body or tumour removal.
- Single or double lung transplantation has been used as treatment for severe bronchiectasis, predominantly when related to CF.
- Complications of surgical intervention:
  - Empyema.
  - Haemorrhage.
  - Prolonged air leak.
  - Persistent atelectasis.

Pre-operative considerations

- The patient should be in optimal medical condition prior to elective surgery.
- Liaison with their respiratory physician, a course of IV antibiotics and chest physiotherapy for 3–10 days pre-operatively is useful.
- Convert inhaled bronchodilator therapy to the nebulized route
- For those patients taking long term oral steroids, the dose of oral prednisolone should be increased by 5–10 mg/day.
- Lung function tests and arterial blood gases should be performed.
- Recent sputum culture results should be used to guide antimicrobial therapy.
  - If not available, act on the assumption that the patient has *Pseudomonas aeruginosa* in their sputum and commence treatment with a combination such as ceftazidime and gentamicin or imipenem and gentamicin.
- Elective surgery should be postponed if deteriorating respiratory symptoms are present.

Post-operative considerations

- Regular physiotherapy should be continued until discharge.
- Adequate analgesia to facilitate effective physiotherapy.
- Oxygen should be prescribed and the patient's oxygen saturation levels monitored.
- Depending on the surgical procedure and/or the severity of the patient's disease, high dependency care may be more appropriate where monitoring of arterial blood gases may be useful.
- Intravenous antibiotics should be continued into the post-operative period or until discharge.
- Normal diet should resume as soon as possible. If not, adequate nutrition should be maintained by other means.
- The chest physician should be involved if the patient's respiratory status deteriorates.

The patient with myasthenia gravis

Introduction

- The incidence of myasthenia gravis (MG) is 1:10000–2000 adults.
- Typically, patients presenting for elective thoracic surgery with a diagnosis of MG are scheduled for thymectomy.
- 10–15% of patients have thymoma, while the remaining 85% have thymic hyperplasia.

A focused pre-operative assessment of the patient with MG is facilitated by knowledge of the presentation, pathophysiology, and treatment of the condition.

Presentation

- MG represents a spectrum of symmetrical, proximal, voluntary muscle weakness and fatiguability which improves with rest.
  - 85% patients describe generalized weakness.
  - 15% patients describe isolated extra-ocular weakness, e.g. ptosis, diplopia.
  - Respiratory failure to varying degree.
  - Bulbar palsy, e.g. dysarthria, dysphagia, nasal regurgitation.
  - Occasionally stridor, i.e. intrinsic muscles of larynx affected.
- 10% patients have a concomitant auto-immune disorder, e.g. hyper/hypothyroidism, rheumatoid arthritis, systemic lupus erythematosis.
- Peak onset:
  - ♀ = 2nd and 3rd decade.
  - ♂ = 6th and 7th decade.

Pathophysiology

- Acquired autoimmune disease.
- Histological evidence of thymic abnormality in 75% cases.
- Gives rise to nicotinic acetylcholine receptor antibodies (anti-AChR) which act at the neuromuscular junction causing:
  - ↑ receptor degradation.
  - Complement induced damage to neuromuscular junction.
  - Altered binding of ACh to receptors.
- Patients have approximately one third of the functional AChR that normal controls have.
- Net effect is voluntary muscle weakness and fatigue.

Management

Below are the medical options for the treatment of MG. Surgical therapy is discussed see ☐ Surgical resectability, p. 172.

Anticholinesterases
- Potentiate action of ACh at nicotinic receptors in neuromuscular junction.
- Pyridostigmine 60 mg PO QDS usual starting point for therapy.

Immunosuppression
Corticosteroids
- Effective in up to 70% cases.
- May require high dose prednisolone initially i.e. 50–100 mg per day.
- May exacerbate symptoms initially.

Azathioprine & cyclophosphamide
- Effective in up to 80% cases.

Plasma exchange
- Used for:
  - Pre-operative optimization of selected individuals.
  - Patients with severe respiratory failure.
- Produces significant improvements in vital capacity and maximal inspiratory pressure.
- Benefits last for a few weeks.

γ-Globulin
- Similar effects to plasma exchange.
- Unknown mechanism of action.

Pre-operative assessment
- Ideally, MG patients should be admitted at least 48 hours in advance of elective surgery.
- This allows adequate time for assessment and optimization of their respiratory and bulbar function.

History
The following should be considered:
- Duration of disease.
- Co-morbidity, especially respiratory disease.
- Respiratory function, i.e. exercise tolerance.
- Evidence of bulbar palsy, i.e. dysphagia, reflux.
- MG therapy and effects of missed anticholinesterase drugs.

Examination

Specifically for:
- Effectiveness of cough.
- Respiratory effort.
- Stridor.
- Chest infection.
- Cyanosis.
- Dysarthria.
- Ptosis.
- Myasthenic/cholinergic crises—refer to Chapter 8 for description.

Classification

- According to history, there are 2 main classifications of MG:

Osserman & Genkins classification

- Grade i=Ocular disease only.
- Grade ii=Generalized weakness.
  - (a) Mild.
  - (b) Moderate.
- Grade iii=Acute severe weakness with respiratory failure.
- Grade iv=Presence of Grade iii for >2 years.

Myasthenia Gravis Foundation of America score (MGFA)

Grade 0 Asymptomatic.
Grade I Ocular signs only.
Grade II Mild generalized weakness.
Grade III Moderate weakness.
Grade IV Severe weakness with respiratory failure.

Investigations

Bloods
- **ABGs.**
  - To quantify gas exchange and arterio-alveolar oxygen difference.

Radiology
- **CXR.**
  - Consolidation/atelectasis.
  - Tumour.
  - Tracheal deviation.
- **CT chest**
  - Tracheal compression by tumour?

Others:
- **Spirometry**
  - Maximal inspiratory pressure (ideally >25 cm H_2O).
  - FVC (ideally >50% predicted or >2.9L).
- **Supine/sitting flow-volume loop.**
  - If CT chest demonstrates large anterior mediastinal mass.
  - To assess for extrinsic, intra-thoracic compression of trachea by tumour.
  - May be dynamic or fixed.
  - If there is dynamic obstruction, i.e. when patient moves from upright to supine, awake fibreoptic intubation should be considered.

❶ The peri-operative management of MG patients presenting for elective surgery is summarized (See 📖 Surgical resectability, p. 172).

Post-operative planning
- The need for post-operative ventilation following general anaesthesia is more likely with the following patient factors:
  - Duration of MG >6 years.
  - Co-existing chronic respiratory disease.
  - Pyridostigmine >750 mg per day within 48 hours of surgery.
  - MGFA score III or IV.
  - FVC <50% predicted or <2.9L.
  - Use of the trans-sternal surgical approach.
  - Moderate to severe weakness and respiratory failure.
  - ♀ gender.

Except in the direst of circumstances, these patients should be optimized using the treatment options described above.

Further reading
(http://www.myasthenia.org/docs/MGFA_ProfessionalManual.pdf (Accessed 05/02/09).

Krucylak PE, Naunheim KS. Pre-operative preparation and anesthetic management of patients with myasthenia gravis. *Seminars in Thoracic and Cardiovascular Surgery* 1999; 11 (1):47–53.

Pullerits J, Holzman R. Anaesthesia for patients with mediastinal masses. *Canadian Journal of Anaesthesia* 1989; 36(6):681–8.

The patient with an implanted permanent pacemaker

- The implantation rate for permanent pacemakers (PPM), implantable cardioverter defibrillators (ICD), and cardiac resynchronization therapy devices (CRT) is increasing across Europe and the United Kingdom (UK).

Indications

- The following represents the main class I indications for PPM, CRT and ICD device implantation.

Permanent pacemaker

- Sinus node dysfunction (SND) with documented symptomatic bradycardia.
- Symptomatic chronotropic incompetence.
- Symptomatic sinus bradycardia 2° to necessary medical therapy.
- Third degree & second degree atrioventricular (AV) block associated with:
  - Symptomatic bradycardia
  - Documented periods of asystole in asymptomatic patients (≥3 seconds or escape rate <40 bpm).
  - Atrial fibrillation with bradycardia (1 pause ≥5 seconds).
  - Post-catheter ablation/cardiac surgery.
  - Neuromuscular disease e.g. muscular dystrophy.
  - Post-myocardial infarction.
- Asymptomatic third degree AV block (ventricular rate >40 bpm) associated with cardiomegaly or left ventricular dysfunction.
- Chronic bifascicular block associated with:
  - Type II second degree AV block.
  - Intermittent third degree AV block.
  - Alternating bundle branch block.
- Hypertensive carotid sinus syndrome.
- Prolonged QT syndrome.
- Sustained pause-dependent ventricular tachycardia.

Cardiac re-synchronization therapy

- Left ventricular ejection fraction (LVEF) ≤35% associated with NYHA functional class III or IV heart failure symptoms despite optimal medical therapy (QRS ≥0.12 seconds, and sinus rhythm).

Implantable cardioverter defibrillators

- Survivor of cardiac arrest 2° to ventricular fibrillation (VF) or haemodynamically unstable ventricular tachycardia (VT).
- Structural heart disease associated with spontaneous, sustained VT.
- Post MI (>40 days) with LVEF <35% in NYHA functional class II or III.
- Post MI (>40 days) with LVEF <30% in NYHA functional class I.
- Non-ischaemic dilated cardiomyopathy with LVEF <35% in NYHA functional class II or III.

Classification
- Based on the North American Society of Pacing & Electrophysiology and British Pacing & Electrophysiology Group alliance (NASPE/BPEG).

Pacemaker
- Described by 5 letters; (See Table 4.19)
  - 1st letter = Paced chamber.
  - 2nd letter = Sensed chamber.
  - 3rd letter = Response to sensing.
  - 4th letter = Programmable function.
  - 5th letter = Anti-tachycardia function.

Table 4.19 System for describing pacemakers

Paced	Sensed	Response	Programmability	Tachycardia
None = O	None = O	None = O	None = O	None = O
Atrium = A	Atrium = A	Inhibit = I	Communicating = C	Pace = P
Ventricle = V	Ventricle = V	Trigger = T	Simple programmable = S	Shock = S
D-Dual = A+V	D-Dual = A+V	D-Dual = I+T	Multi-programmable = M	D-Dual = P+S
S-Simple = A or V	S-Simple = A or V		Rate modulation = R	

Implantable cardioverter defibrillator
- Described by 4 letters; (See Table 4.20)
  - 1st letter = Shocked chamber
  - 2nd letter = Anti-tachycardia pacing chamber
  - 3rd letter = Tachycardia detection
  - 4th letter = Anti-bradycardia pacing chamber.

Table 4.20 System for describing internal cardioverter defibrillators

Shocked	Anti-tachycardia pacing chamber	Tachycardia detection	Anti-bradycardia pacing chamber
None = O	None = O	ECG = E	None = O
Atrium = A	Atrium = A	Haemodynamic = H	Atrium = A
Ventricle = V	Ventricle = V		Ventricle = V
D-Dual = A+V	D-Dual = A+V		D-Dual = A+V

- Common modes of pacing in the UK are summarized in (Table 4.21)

Table 4.21 Pacing mode at time of first PPM implantation in the UK (2005) as a proportion of total first implants

AAI (R)	VVI (R)	VDD (R)	DDD (R)	CRT-PM
1.41%	39%	0.8%	55%	3.72

Specific investigations
- **12-lead ECG.**
- **CXR.**
  - To confirm integrity of pacing leads and presence/absence of heart failure.
- **U&Es, Mg^{2+}, Ca^{2+}.**
  - Electrolyte abnormalities may cause loss of capture in PPM.

Peri-operative management

Considerations
- PPM/ICDs are highly tolerant of electrical and magnetic interference.
- Tolerance may be overcome by:
  - High energy fields close to device.
  - Frequency range of energy field similar to cardiac range.
- PPMs with impedance-based responsive pacing function (e.g. minute ventilation) may misinterpret signals from monitoring equipment causing an inappropriate rise in pacing rate.
- PPMs may be programmed to reduce the pacing rate at night.
- PPM/ICDs have a magnetic switch.
  - The response to placing a magnet over the device is dependent on how it has been programmed.
  - Magnet status should be confirmed by the implantation centre/follow-up team.

❶ Do not place a magnet over a PPM/ICD during surgery without reference to the patient's implantation centre/implantation team.

Pre-operative

- Key information may be obtained from the patient's follow-up team and includes:
  - Device model and serial number.
  - Date of implant.
  - Indication for implant.
  - Extent of any heart failure.
  - Degree of patient dependency on device.
  - Device complexity, e.g. DDD (R).
  - Whether device is nearing replacement.
- The following may be performed by a cardiac pacing/ICD physiologist:
  - Confirmation of device function/battery status.
  - Changes to pacing/sensing parameters if required.
  - Program ICD to "monitor only" to prevent inappropriate shock therapy.
  - Program PPM to avoid/minimize inappropriate inhibition/high rate pacing.
  - Program rate response to off (e.g. minute ventilation response).

Intra-operative

- Ensure the availability of resuscitation equipment and an external defibrillator.
- Risk of device malfunction is minimized where the surgical site is remote from the device.
- Risk of device malfunction is increased where the surgical site is close to the device and diathermy is required.
- If diathermy is required, bipolar mode is preferable
- Monopolar diathermy may:
  - Temporarily inhibit pacemaker output.
  - Temporarily increase pacing rate.
  - Cause device to enter safety mode (limited functionality).
  - Reset device to manufacturer default settings.
  - Stop the device completely if power source is near depletion.
  - Be misinterpreted as VT or VF, thus initiating shock therapy in patients with an ICD.

- Where diathermy is required:
  - Limit use to short bursts.
  - Ensure current pathway is as far away from device as possible.
  - Ensure diathermy cables kept clear from device site.
  - Consider external/transvenous pacing if device function significantly affected by diathermy.
- Connect patients to external defibrillator where an ICD has been deactivated to "monitor only".

Post-operative

- Device function should be confirmed by cardiac pacing/ICD physiologist.
- Reactivation of ICD shock therapy.

Magnets and pacemakers

- Magnets close internal reed switches within pacemakers; they enter asynchronous mode.
- Sensing is inhibited as a result.

Most pacemakers

- The pacemaker paces the heart at a continuous pre-set rate (which could be different than the rate pre-programmed).

ICD

- The pacemaker's ability to defibrillate is inhibited.
- Bradycardia pacing will remain.
- If the magnet is left on for approximately 30 seconds, the ICD is disabled and a continuous tone is generated.
  - To reactivate the device, the magnet must be lifted off the area of the generator and then replaced.
  - After 30 seconds, the beep returns for every QRS complex.
- Indications for ICD deactivation.
  - End-of-life care (after a discussion with the patient and family)
  - Inappropriate shocks.
  - During resuscitation.
  - With transcutaneous pacing (external pacing can cause an ICD to fire).
  - During procedures such as central lines or surgery with electrocautery.

Further reading

Epstein AE, DiMarco JP, Ellenbogen KA, *et al.* ACC/AHA/HRS 2008 guidelines for device-based therapy of cardiac rhythm abnormalities: Executive Summary. *Journal of the Americal College of Cardiology* 2008; 51:2085–105.

Diprose P, Pierce T. Anaesthesia for patients with pacemakers and similar devices. CEACCP 2001; 1(6):166–70.

Guidelines for the perioperative management of patients with implantable pacemakers or implantable cardioverter defibrillators, where the use of surgical diathermy/electrocautery is anticipated. *Medicines and Healthcare products Regulatory* Agency 2006.

The patient with a paraneoplastic syndrome

Paraneoplastic syndromes are a heterogeneous collection of non-metastatic disease manifestations caused by underlying neoplasms. Table 4.22 summarizes numerous paraneoplastic syndromes, some of which may be related to an underlying thoracic malignancy. A selection of syndromes relating to thoracic disorders will be discussed here.

Hypertrophic pulmonary osteoarthropathy (HPOA)

- Can occur months before diagnosis of malignancy.
- Symptoms may resolve following treatment of the primary tumour.

Features

- Periosteal new bone formation of the distal long bones.
- Soft tissue swelling of distal phalanges (digital clubbing).
- Arthralgia; typically of wrists and ankles.

Tumour associations

- Occurs in up to 31% lung cancer patients.
- Associated carcinomas.
  - Typically non-small-cell lung cancer (NSCLC).
  - Mesothelioma.
  - Oesophageal cancer.
- Pulmonary metastases from extrathoracic malignancy.
  - Melanoma, breast, renal cell carcinoma, osteosarcoma, nasopharyngeal carcinoma.

Benign associations

- Pleural fibroma.
- Bronchiectasis/cystic fibrosis.
- Pulmonary fibrosis.
- Cyanotic congenital heart disease.

Investigations

- **Plane x-ray of the wrists.**
  - Lamellar periosteal reaction in the diametaphyseal region of the distal long bones.
- **Bone scan.**
  - Symmetrical increased uptake along cortical margins of tubular bones in the diametaphyseal region.
  - Reported to be more sensitive for the detection and characterization of the extent of HPOA than radiography alone.

Dermatomyositis

Features
- Idiopathic inflammatory proximal myopathy.
- Pathognomonic Gottron's papules (violet-coloured inflammation over the knuckles).
- Periorbital heliotrope rash (brown discolouration of the eyelids).
- Increased risk of malignancy: several population-based cohort studies have demonstrated an excess cancer risk in patients with dermatomyositis. Standardized incidence ratios (SIRs) of up to 7.7 reported, with the excess cancer risk highest at the time of diagnosis and within the first 2 years of diagnosis.

(Polymyositis is a similar disease, but without the cutaneous signs).

Tumour associations
- Lung.
- Pancreas.
- Gastric.
- Colorectal.
- Ovary.
- Cervix.

Investigations
- Controversy exists as to the best way of investigating patients with dermatomyositis.
- In patients presenting with dermatomyositis, chest and abdominal CT in addition to routine clinical and laboratory screening is probably indicated to search for an underlying malignancy.

Syndrome of inappropriate antidiuretic hormone secretion (SIADH)

Features
- Hyponatraemia.
- Inappropriately elevated urine osmolality (>200 mOsm/kg).
- Excessive urine sodium excretion (Urinary Na^+ >30 mEq/L).
- Decreased serum osmolality.
- Occurs in euvolaemic patients in the absence of diuretic therapy, and in the setting of otherwise normal cardiac, renal, adrenal, hepatic, and thyroid function.
- May present clinically with neurological or psychiatric symptoms related to hyponatraemia or is detected on routine serum electrolyte measurement.

Tumour associations
- Small cell lung cancer (SCLC):
  - Most common (up to 11% of patients with SCLC).
  - Following chemotherapy for treatment of SCLC, rapid remission of clinical and biochemical features of SIADH (within 3–4 weeks) is achieved in the majority of patients, although they may relapse if the patient develops tumour recurrence.

- Note—some SCLCs also produce atrial natriuretic peptide (ANP), which also leads to hyponatraemia.
- Non-small cell lung cancer (NSCLC) rare.
- Head and neck tumours.
- Gastrointestinal tumours.
- Gynaecological malignancy.

Other associations
- Central nervous system disorders.
- Intrathoracic infection.
- Positive pressure ventilation.

Hypercalcaemia

Features
- Diagnosis of exclusion in cancer patients.
- Known as Humoral hypercalcaemia of malignancy (HHM).
- Hypercalcaemia in the *absence* of bone metastases.
- Multifactorial aetiology:
  - Due to a combination of increased bone resorption and decreased renal capacity to excrete calcium.
  - HHM is primarily due to the secretion of a parathyroid hormone-related protein (PThrP) by the primary tumour, which shares many characteristics with parathyroid hormone.
  - Ectopic parathyroid hormone and 1,25-dihydroxy vitamin D secretion have also been described as causative factors.

Tumour associations
- Squamous cell carcinomas.
- Myeloma.
- Gynaecological malignancy.
- SCLC.
- Breast cancer.
- Hodgkin's lymphoma.

Investigations
- Exclude underlying bone metastases first by bone scan or MRI.

Myasthenia Gravis
(See ▢ The patient with myasthenia gravis, p. 258).

Limbic Encephalitis (LE)

Features
- Inflammatory disorder involving the limbic structures.
- LE can be paraneoplastic or non-paraneoplastic (idiopathic).
- When paraneoplastic, the presentation of LE precedes the diagnosis of malignancy in 60% of cases (with median interval between diagnosis of LE and underlying cancer of 3.5 months).

Presentation
- Onset ranging from days to 3 months of any number of the following:
  - Short-term memory impairment.
  - Seizures.
  - Confusion.
  - Irritability.
  - Hypothalamic dysfunction.
  - Psychiatric disturbance.
- Improvement in neurological symptoms may be seen following treatment of the underlying tumour.

Investigations
- **MRI**
  - High signal on T2-weighted and FLAIR (Fluid Attenuated Inversion Recovery) sequences.
  - Typically involving the limbic structures, and sometimes brainstem.
  - Diagnosis requires exclusion of viral causes, such as herpes simplex.
- **Blood onconeural antibodies:**
  - Anti-Hu, anti-TA, Anti-Ma.

Tumour associations
- Bronchial carcinoma (50–59%), most commonly SCLC.
- Testicular tumours (6–20%).
- Breast cancer (3–8%).
- Hodgkin's lymphoma (3–4%).
- Thymoma (2–5%).
- Although a proportion of patients presenting with LE may turn out to have a non-paraneoplastic syndrome, the association between LE and malignancy is strong enough to warrant thorough investigation for malignancy.

Paraneoplastic cerebellar degeneration (PCD)

Features
- Severe pancerebellar dysfunction.
- Progresses over weeks to months.
- Usually stabilizes by 6 months.
- Precedes a diagnosis of cancer in approximately 60% cases.

Investigations
- Other causes of cerebellar degeneration, e.g. metastatic disease, infection, nutritional deficits, or treatment effects should be considered before a diagnosis of PCD is made.

- **FDG PET/CT**
  - Recommended if conventional imaging (chest/abdominal CT, mammography) does not reveal an underlying malignancy.
  - A thorough search for malignancy is advocated in patients with PCD.
- **MRI**
  - Often normal
  - Cerebellar oedema can be seen in early stages progressing to cerebellar atrophy in the late stages.
- **Blood onconeural antibodies**
  - Positive anti-Yo antibodies occur in post-menopausal women with gynaecological and breast malignancies.
  - Anti-Hu antibodies are associated with SCLC.

Tumour associations
- Lung (28%).
- Gynaecological (20%).
- Hodgkin's disease (16%).
- Breast (12%).
- Others—thymoma and testicular tumours.

Table 4.22 Paraneoplastic syndromes and associated tumours relevant to thoracic anaesthesia

System	Syndrome	Associated tumour
Dermatological	Seborrhoeic keratoses (Leser-Tralat syndrome)	NHL, gastrointestinal tumours
	Icthyosis	Lymphoma
	Acanthosis nigricans	Gastric cancer, other intra-abdominal tumours
	Paraneoplastic pemphigus	Lymphoma, epithelial tumours
	Sweet's syndrome	Lymphoma
	Erythema gyratum repens	Lung, oesophageal
Endocrine	SIADH	Lung cancer
	Ectopic ACTH secretion	Small cell lung cancer
	Cushing's syndrome	Lung cancer, neuroendocrine tumours
	Hypercalcaemia	Variety of epithelial tumours, lymphomas
	Hypoglycaemia	Mesothelioma, sarcoma

(Contd.)

Table 4.22 (Contd.)

System	Syndrome	Associated tumour
Haematological	Normocytic anaemia	Wide variety of neoplasms
	Disseminated intravascular coagulation	Epithelial tumours, lymphoma
	Idiopathic thrombocytopenic purpura	Lung cancer, lymphomas, sarcoma
	Thrombocytosis	Carcinomas, Hodgkin's lymphoma
	Cryoglobulinaemia	
	Leukaemoid reaction	Lymphoma, lung cancer
	Thrombotic thrombocytopenic purpura	Lymphoma, gastric and breast cancer
	Microangiopathic haemolytic anaemia	Oesophageal cancer
	Marantic endocarditis	Mucinous adenocarcinomas
	Autoimmune haemolytic anaemia	Mucinous adenocarcinomas
		Lymphoma, epithelial tumours
Neurological	Limbic Encephalitis	Lung, lymphoma
	Paraneoplastic cerebellar degeneration	Lung
	Opsoclonus-myoclonus	SCLC
	Subacute sensory neuropathy	SCLC, sarcomas
	Myasthenis Gravis	Thymoma
	Lambert-Eaton myasthenic syndromes (LEMS)	SCLC, lymphoma
Musculoskeletal	Hypertrophic osteoarthropathy	Lung cancer, mesothelioma, diaphragmatic neurilemmoma
	Dermatomyositis	Wide variety of malignancies

Further reading

Vedeler CA, Antoine JC, Giometto B, *et al.* Management of paraneoplastic neurological syndromes: report of an EFNS Task Force. *European Journal of Neurology* 2006; 13:682–90.

Rutherford GC, Dineen RA, O'Connor A. Imaging in the investigation of paraneoplastic syndromes. *Clinical Radiology.* 2007 Nov; 92(11):1021–35.

The patient with lung cancer

Involve the multi-disciplinary care team early to ensure patient optimization prior to surgery. This involves physiotherapy, occupational therapy, nursing, dieticians, psychologists and physicians.

All patients with known or suspected lung cancer should undergo a thorough history, physical examination, and standard laboratory tests as a screen for metastatic disease. This is based on level-B evidence and benefit is reported in the literature to be substantial.

A rough guide to assessment of fitness for surgery (after the BTS and Society of Cardiothoracic Surgeons of Great Britain and Ireland)

(See 📖 BTS Guidelines, p. 158).

- Age >80 years:
  - Independent predictor of mortality in pneumonectomy, but not lobectomy.
- Respiratory function:
  - Spirometry (FVC and FEV_1), estimation of transfer factor, post-operative lung function prediction using anatomical equations and if necessary quantitative isotope perfusions scans.
  - Pre-operative FEV_1 >1.5 L for lobectomy and >2 L for pneumonectomy generally indicates suitability. Lesser values should prompt a respiratory referral and further investigation (MDT approach).
- Cardiovascular fitness:
  - All patients should have an ECG.
  - Echocardiogram if murmur audible.
  - Refer to cardiology if previous MI or high risk (unstable angina)
- Nutrition, weight loss and performance status:
  - Patients with pre-operative weight loss of >10% are at increased risk of post-operative morbidity and mortality.
  - Review the serum albumin result.

Background

- Lung cancer is the most prevalent cancer worldwide and accounts for 1:3 cancer deaths in men and 1:6.5 cancer deaths in women.
- Lung cancer is recognized late; the 5-year survival rate is 10–13% and 80% will be inoperable at presentation.
- Mortality is 80–90% with a poor prognosis and a mean survival <6 months. In particular, female mortality from lung cancer now exceeds that from breast cancer.

Classification

- Two main types of lung carcinoma:
  - Non-small cell (80.4%).
  - Small-cell (16.8%).
- This histological classification has important implications for clinical management and prognosis of the disease (See Table 4.23).

Table 4.23 Types of lung malignancy

Histology	Location and behaviour
Adenocarcinoma	Accounts for 45% of all cases
	75% cases are peripheral
	Lymph node metastases are common
Squamous cell carcinoma	Accounts for 30% of all cases
	70% are centrally located near the hilum or major bronchi
	Often locally invasive
Large cell tumours	Account for 5–10% of tumours
	Usually peripherally located
	Poorly differentiated tumours may cavitate
	Early spread to distant sites
Small cell tumours (also known as 'Oat cell carcinoma')	Accounts for 20% of tumours
	80% centrally located
	Can produce neuroendocrine hormones
	May result in paraneoplastic syndromes
	Tendency to disseminate early

Risk factors

Smoking

- 20% of smokers will develop lung cancer.
- Over 90% of lung cancers occur in current or ex-smokers.

Atmospheric Pollution

- Persistently higher lung cancer rates in urban populations.
- Passive smoking.

Industrial exposure

- Asbestos fibre, aluminium industry, arsenic compounds, benzyl chloride, beryllium.

Signs and symptoms
- May not produce symptoms until the disease is well advanced.
- Early recognition of symptoms may be beneficial to outcome (See Table 4.24 for symptom list).
- When first diagnosed:
  - 20% have localized disease.
  - 25% have regional metastases.
  - 55% have distant metastases.
  - 10–20% of patients may present with symptoms/signs indicating a paraneoplastic syndrome.

Table 4.24 Tumour locations and associated symptoms/signs

Tumour location	Presenting feature
Pleural	Chest pain (27–49%)
	Dyspnoea (37–58%)
	Cough (45–75%)
Endobronchial	Cough (45–75%)
	Haemoptysis (57%)
	Bronchial obstruction
	Post-obstructive complications, e.g., pneumonitis, pneumonia, effusion
Mediastinal	Dyspnoea
	Postprandial coughing (oesophageal)
	Wheezing
	Stridor (upper airway obstruction, 2–18%)
	Hoarseness (left vocal cord paralysis due to recurrent laryngeal nerve impingement)
	Chylothorax (thoracic duct)
	Palpitations (pericardial)
Neurological spread	Arm weakness and paraesthesia (brachial plexus impingement)
	Miosis, ptosis and anhidrosis (cervical sympathetic chain, Horner syndrome)
	Dyspnoea (phrenic nerve)

(Contd.)

Table 4.24 (Contd.)

Tumour location	Presenting feature
Central nervous system involvement	Headache
	Altered mental status
	Seizure
	Meningism
	Ataxia
	Nausea and/or vomiting
Metastatic	Weight loss (8–68%)
	Cachexia
Vascular	Phlebitis, thromboembolism (Trousseau syndrome)
Musculoskeletal	Bone pain
	Spinal cord impingement

Paraneoplastic syndromes

(See 📖 The patient with a paraneoplastic syndrome, p. 268).
- Do not result from local tumour presence.
- Possibly an abnormal neuro-humoral response to neoplastic tissue (mediated by hormones or cytokines), or as a result of a compound produced by the tumour.
- Lung cancer commonly presents with a paraneoplastic syndrome and its presence does not preclude potentially curative therapy.
- Affects those of middle age or later.
- (See Table 4.25 for paraneoplastic syndromes relating to lung malignancy).

Table 4.25 Paraneoplastic manifestations of lung malignancy

Syndrome	Causal mechanism	Signs/symptoms
Cushing syndrome	Ectopic ACTH	Weight gain, central obesity, 'moon face', striae, polyuria, hyperglycaemia, hypertension
SIADH	Antidiuretic hormone	Hyponatraemia and concentrated urine without peripheral oedema or hypertension. Cerebral oedema causing seizures and coma
Hypercalcaemia	PTHrP, TGF-α, TNF, IL-1	Groans (constipation), moans (psychotic noise), bones (bone pain, especially if PTH is elevated), stones (kidney stones), and psychiatric overtones (e.g. depression & confusion)

(Contd.)

Table 4.25 (Contd.)

Syndrome	Causal mechanism	Signs/symptoms
Carcinoid syndrome	Serotonin, bradykinin	Flushing, diarrhoea, bronchospasm
Lambert-Eaton Myasthenic Syndrome	Immunologic	Progressive muscle weakness that does not usually involve the face or respiratory muscles
Paraneoplastic Cerebellar Degeneration	Immunologic	Subacute progressive cerebellar ataxia
Acanthosis Nigricans	Immunologic	Brown/black, poorly defined velvety hyperpigmentation of the skin. Usually found in body folds

Investigation of lung cancer

The aims of evaluating a patient with a lung tumour are to determine:
- Tumour histology:
  - Indicates potential responsiveness to chemo/radiotherapy.
  - Prognosis and time course.
- Anatomical extent of the disease:
  - Indicates surgical resectability.
- Functional status of the patient:
  - To assess need for further multi-disciplinary involvement.
  - To assess need for pre-operative optimization.

Investigations

Bloods
- **FBC.**
  - Anaemia, intercurrent infection, platelet count.
- **U+E.**
  - Electrolyte imbalance, e.g. paraneoplastic syndromes, renal failure due to metastatic involvement, tumour lysis and hyperkalaemia.
- **Calcium.**
- **LFTs**
  - Particularly if metastases known.
- **Clotting.**
- **ABG.**
  - To assess functionality, particularly in those with co-existent COPD.
  - (Refer to Chapter 4, BTS Guidelines).

Radiology
- **Chest X-ray.**
  - Lung cancer usually presents radiographically as a solitary pulmonary nodule or mass, pulmonary collapse, mediastinal lymphadenopathy, pleural effusion or as an area of persistent consolidation.
  - Adenocarcinoma and large cell carcinoma are more frequently seen peripherally.
  - Squamous and small cell carcinomas typically arise in the central bronchi and commonly extend into the hilum and mediastinum
  - Squamous cell carcinoma may also occur in the lung parenchyma and cavitate.
- **CT chest.**
  - To identify metastatic disease and/or evidence of local tumour invasion for staging purposes.
  - To guide further investigation, e.g. bronchoscopy.
- **CT Brain.**
  - If there are personality changes or neurological symptoms.
- **PET.**
  - Allows functional information of cells to be collected.
  - Not commonly used as not widely available.
- **Radionuclide bone scan.**
  - Extent of metastatic involvement.

Other
- **Bronchoscopy.**
  - Gold standard for histological diagnosis.
- **CT-guided percutaneous needle biopsy.**
- **Mediastinoscopy.**
  - As a means of staging cancers.
- Thoracoscopy.
  - A useful means to obtain a diagnosis of indeterminate solitary pulmonary nodules without the need for thoracotomy, when less invasive methods have failed to identify the lesion.

Surgical management
- Only 25% patients have resectable disease at presentation.
- Lung resection is best treatment for Stage 1 and 2 disease.
- 5-year survival decreases with extent of disease.
- Only surgery can cure non-small cell lung cancer. However, most are unsuitable for surgery.
- Aims of surgery are complete resection of the tumour with wide margins and clearance of involved intrapulmonary lymphatics. This can be achieved by:
  - Pulmonary lobectomy, pneumonectomy, sublobar resections or bronchoplastic resections depending upon the site, size and extent of disease.
- Mortality from lobectomy is 2–4%.
- Mortality from pneumonectomy is 6–8%.

Special considerations

- Pulmonary complications are the commonest cause of post-operative morbidity and mortality:
  - Acute lung injury occurs in 4–5% of resections.
- Arrhythmias, especially atrial fibrillation, are common after pneumonectomy. Many advocate prophylactic digitalization during surgery and post-operatively.
- Remember that patients with bronchial carcinoma may have 'non-metastatic' manifestations such as Lambert-Eaton Myasthenic syndrome that require adjustments to a usual thoracic anaesthetic technique.

Further reading

http://guidance.nice.org.uk/CG24/Guidance/pdf/Englishl NICE Guidelines for Lung Cancer (accessed 2/9/09)

Gould G, Pearce A. Assessment of suitability for Lung Resection. Continuing Education in Anaesthesia, *Critical Care & Pain* 2006; 6(3):97–100.

Armstrong P. Congleton J, Fountain S, *et al*. BTS Guidelines: Guidelines on the selection of patients with lung cancer for surgery. *Thorax* 2001; 56:89–108.

Chapter 5

Diagnostic and therapeutic procedures in thoracic anaesthesia

Bronchoscopy

PROCEDURE BASICS: inspection of tracheobronchial anatomy via a rigid or flexible scope. Biopsy/debulking stenting. (See Table 5.1 for indications).

TIME: 5–30 mins.

PAIN RATING: 1/5.

ANALGESIA: simple oral analgesia/IV Paracetamol.

BLOOD LOSS: usually minimal unless debulking.

HOSPITAL STAY: suitable for day case.

PREPARATION AND EQUIPMENT: standard monitoring. TIVA (propofol and remifentanil). Pre-medication. Sanders injector. Full oxygen or air cylinder. Range of ETT tubes small to standard. Separate suction for rigid and flexible bronchoscope.

Table 5.1 Indications for bronchoscopy

Classification	Indication
Diagnostic	Airway obstruction
	Persistent pneumonia
	Tracheo-oesophageal fistula
	Brushings for cytology
	Biopsy
	Failure to wean from ventilator
	Haemoptysis
	Staging
Therapeutic	Removal foreign body
	Suction mucus plugs
	Facilitate endobronchial intubation for OLV
	Debulking therapy
	Balloon dilatation
	Stenting

See Table 5.2 for a comparison of rigid and fibreoptic bronchoscopy.

Table 5.2 Rigid vs. fibreoptic bronchoscopy

Rigid	Fibreoptic
More suitable for foreign body removal	Better yield for biopsy in suspected bronchogenic carcinoma
Better control of moderate to massive haemoptysis	More detailed resolution
Enables packing of airway if bleeding	
If obstruction of airway, may be only scope passable	
Enables larger biopsies	
Preferred for visualization of carina, assessment of mobility and sharpness	More detailed assessment of tracheobronchial tree
Restricted to larger airways	Can be guided into 5th generation bronchi
	Improved patient comfort
	Can be performed in sitting position in those with poor ventilation
Needs heavy medication	Needs far less medication
	Suitable for patients with C-spine problems, atlanto-axial instability and vertebral artery insufficiency
	Allows better cooperation between anaesthetist and surgeon

Pre-operative assessment and preparation
Examine previous anaesthetic charts
- Could the larynx be visualized?
- Was there airway obstruction in any particular position at induction?
- Size of endotracheal tube and bronchoscope used?
- Any difficulty oxygenating during bronchoscopy?
- Did the patient suffer post-operative stridor?

History
- Discussion with the patient will help elucidate the underlying diagnosis.
- How do symptoms vary in relation to position?
- Inspiratory stridor suggests extrathoracic obstruction.
- Expiratory stridor suggests intrathoracic cause.
- Past medical history of lung disease may predispose the patient to barotrauma.
- Warn about post-op coughing, haemoptysis, sore throat and suxamethonium induced myalgia.

Examination
- Focus on airway and respiratory system.
- Anatomical abnormalities may dictate type of bronchoscopy (e.g. deformities of the cervical spine or possible spinal instability may warrant a fibreoptic scope).
- Examine range of movement of neck.

Investigations

Specific investigations may be required:
Radiology
- **CXR**.
  - To localize an inhaled foreign body.
- **CT chest**.
  - To evaluate a possible cause and location of an obstruction, tracheal tumour.

Anaesthesia for bronchoscopy

Pre-medication

Anxiolytic:
- Midazolam.
  - 0.03–0.05 mg/kg IV.
  - Give once cannula sited 2–3 mins prior to induction.

❶ Extreme caution if there is obvious airway obstruction or respiratory embarrassment.

Anticholinergic:
- Atropine.
  - 400–600 mcg IV-/IM.
  - Give IV at induction or can be given IM 30 mins prior to anaesthesia.
  - Vagolytic, antisialogogue, bronchodilator.

Steroid:
- Dexamethasone.
  - 8–16 mg IV.
  - Give slow IV injection prior to induction (can cause groin tingling and mild tachycardia).
  - Decreases swelling/oedema of airway.

Rigid bronchoscopy as sole procedure

Induction
- Pre-oxygenate with 100% O_2.
- Gas induction with 8% sevoflurane in 100% O_2 if anticipated difficulty.
- TIVA with propofol and remifentanil provides good airway reflex suppression, rapid emergence and decreased pollution, ± suxamethonium boluses.

Position
- Surgeon's preference, normally supine with a rolled towel across the back between the scapulae to extend the neck and push the upper trachea forward.

Ventilation
- Once rigid scope is passed through the cords, use side port of the bronchoscope, attach oxygen/air supply and connect to Sanders injector.
- Observe chest at all times to prevent over/under expansion.
- Hypercarbia will develop after only a short time, as expiratory phase is poor.
- Aim for maximal expiration, i.e. 5–10 s.

The end of the procedure
- Ask surgeon to administer suction at end.
- Once finished, allow spontaneous breathing to return. Can use facemask or pass LMA if relaxant has worn off.
- Patient should be awake with full airway reflexes BEFORE they are left in recovery.

Rigid bronchoscopy and follow-on procedure

As above and:
- Usually performed in anaesthetic room prior to passage and placement of DLT.
- If surgeon struggled, be prepared for a potential difficult intubation.
- Aim is to obtund stimulation during rigid scope, then pass, secure and check DLT once main scope removed.

The end of the procedure
- Turn patient biopsied side down to avoid aspiration/passage of blood into the good lung.
- Sit up as soon as full airway reflexes return.

⚠ **Special considerations**

- Seemingly benign procedure:
  - Complications are legion, be warned!
- Very stimulating:
  - Anticipate and obtund haemodynamic response.
- Arrhythmias:
  - Minor arrhythmias 70%, major 8%.
- Profound relaxation:
  - Rapid return of spontaneous breathing/airway reflexes once procedure is terminated.
- LA to cords:
  - 4% Lidocaine/(max 5–7mg/kg) will NOT obtund CVS response and can impair post-op cough.
  - Local anaesthetic toxicity is a well-recognized phenomenon. Be vigilant.
- Airway bleeding:
  - Can be catastrophic as a result of biopsy of vascular tumours.
- Airway complications:
  - Laryngospasm and bronchospasm are frequent. Be ready to intubate if necessary.
- Surgeon struggles to obtain view:
  - If bronchoscopy is difficult for the surgeon. It will most likely be difficult for you to intubate!
- Atropine:
  - A useful pre-medicant … but it may exacerbate tachycardia.
- Capnography:
  - Only possible intermittently with rigid scopes.
- Suction!
  - Don't forget to suction airway before de-instrumentation/extubation.

Further reading

Kaplan JA, Slinger PD. *Thoracic Anaesthesia*, 3rd ed. Philadelphia: Churchill Livingstone; 2003.

Broncho-alveolar lavage

PROCEDURE BASICS: alveolar protein is removed from one lung by repeated instillation and drainage of saline (10–20 L) via a double lumen endobronchial tube.

TIME: 2–4hrs.

PAIN RATING: 0–1/5.

ANALGESIA: not usually required.

BLOOD LOSS: N/A.

HOSPITAL STAY: at least one day. May require ICU/HDU.

PREPARATION AND EQUIPMENT: standard monitoring + arterial line. DLT/warming mattress/sterile warmed saline.

N.B. Ensure there is a physiotherapist available.

Therapeutic

Pulmonary alveolar proteinosis

- A rare respiratory disease in which there is an accumulation of surfactant derived protein in the lungs.
- May be acquired, characterized by a cough and dyspnoea that progresses to respiratory failure.
- The presence of anti-granulocyte colony stimulating factor (GM-CSF) antibodies helps establish the diagnosis.
- Secondary PAP can rarely occur with malignancies, immunodeficiency disorder, haemopoietic disorders and with acute inhalational syndromes.

Pre-operative assessment and preparation

History and optimization

- Marked dyspnoea worsening with exercise.
- Further detailed respiratory history to ascertain any cardiac and other respiratory causes for breachlessness.

Specific investigations

Bloods
- **U&E**
  - Lung lavage will lower K^+
- **LFT**
  - Proteinosis long-standing, may have lead to a low albumin state.

Other
- **PFT**
  - Restrictive picture.
- **DLCO**
  - Often markedly reduced.

Basics of the procedure
- Instill 500ml aliquots of warmed saline. After a few minutes allow fluid to drain into a container below the patient. The effluent fluid is milky in appearance.
- This is repeated 10–20 times until the effluent clears.
- Physiotherapist can administer percussion, vibration and pressure to increase efficacy of lavage.
- After the initial filling of the FRC, the volume returned should approximate the volume instilled.
- After the last exchange, suction the lavaged lung to aid removal of residual fluid.
- Further management then depends on the patient. Options include waking and extubating or a further period of ventilation.

Anaesthesia
Equipment
- Check equipment:
  - Fibreoptic bronchoscope, DLT.
  - Tubing, Y piece and connectors to attach warmed saline to DLT and enable effluent to drain into a receptacle where volume of fluid can be measured.
  - Line clamps (to direct flow of saline).
  - Large volume (20L) of saline warmed to body temperature.
- Physiotherapist present.

Induction and maintenance
- Light or no premedication.
- Site arterial line awake.
- Nasal temperature probe.
- 100% O_2 pre-oxygenation.
- Suitable induction and NMB:
  - Maintain anaesthesia with volatile agent or TIVA arterial oxygenation usually worse with TIVA.
- Intubating the non-lavaged lung (fluid pressure in treated lung may force DLT out). L DLT is normally suitable. Using a larger DLT may limit tube movement.
- Confirm optimal placement with a FOB:
  - Ensure the tube is well fix; consider a rigid collar to reduce/prevent tube movement during repositioning. Loss of DLT position can be disastrous and result in both lungs being flooded = drowning!
- Ensure good airway seal.
- Take baseline recordings of airway mechanics before and after the procedure (both lungs, then each individually). This allows gauge of effectiveness of the procedure.

Position
- Position the patient so the treated lung is dependent (lowermost).

Ventilation
- Ventilation with 100% O_2 allows de-nitrogenation to occur.
- Establish OLV to non-lavaged (independent \ uppermost)lung.
- Relatively high P_{AW} (40 cmH$_2$O) may be required.
- Replace the FRC of the dependent lung with saline SLOWLY (limits gas trapping).

Cautions

- ⚠ Only one lung should be done at a time; the most severely affected first, to minimize hypoxic time.
- ⚠ Maintain the lavaged lung in the dependent position to limit contamination of the other lung with fluid.
- Fluid balance:
  - Maintain strict in and out balance. 15L can be instilled; >90% should be recovered.
- Desaturation:
  - Blood flow increases to the non-ventilated side during drainage. Shunt therefore increases so may manifest as a desaturation.
  - Usage of PA catheter balloon inflation to this side has been performed with success, as has hyperbaric ventilation.
  - ECMO has been used to facilitate bilateral simultaneous whole-lung lavage.
- Airway pressure rises with filling of the lung and may limit size of fluid aliquots.
- Watch patient and fluid temperature! Patients can easily become cold.
- Watch for fluid leakage into the contra-lateral lung.
  - Avoid large aliquots. If leakage occurs drain both lungs and reposition DLT. May need to abandon procedure. Post-operative ventilation may be needed.

Completion and post-operative

- Patients should receive supplementary O_2 (or ventilation with suitable FiO_2).
- The patient should be observed on a HDU for ±24 hr.
- If performed CXR will show unilateral pulmonary oedema.
- May require K^+ supplements.
- Before the next lung is lavaged, allow baseline mechanics and gas exchange to return to normal. The freshly lavaged lung should now support gas exchange.
- Most patients report a vast symptomatic improvement.
- Some may require lavage every month; some can go for years without a repeat.

Diagnostic

- Adjunct to diagnostic bronchoscopy (See 📖 Bronchoscopy, p. 282).
- Commonly performed on patients on the ICU.
- Offers ability to remove airway debris and obtain material for culture of organisms, and biochemistry and cytology.
- Carried out under direct vision with fibreoptic bronchoscopy, enabling focused assessments of smaller lung areas.
- Whilst frequently performed under local anaesthesia alone it is more common for anaesthetists to perform this in the theatre or ICU environment under general anaesthesia/sedation.
- Its role in the diagnosis of ventilator acquired pneumonia is currently controversial.

Indications

- Diagnosis of ventilator acquired pneumonia.
- Diagnosis of atypical pulmonary infection (TB, PCP).
- Diagnosis of other pulmonary conditions including tumours.

Contraindications

- Severe refractory hypoxaemia (unless as part of therapeutic manoeuvre).
- Severe coagulopathy.

Procedure

- Thorough pre-oxygenation and aseptic technique.
- Adequate analgesia, sedation ± paralysis.
- Scope advanced under direct vision through tracheal tube/tracheostomy.
- Enter 'clean' side/lobe first to minimize risk of cross infection.
- Avoid suction prior to diagnostic sample.
- Enter segmental bronchus and instill 20 ml saline under direct vision then gentle suction to remove saline (only 40–60% return expected).
- Repeat in suspicious areas until adequate samples obtained (up to 100 ml instilled).

> NB: Samples may be sent for urgent microscopy to enable focused anti-microbial agent use in the context of pulmonary infection. This may be particularly important in immunocompromised individuals.

Complications

- Hypoxaemia:
  - May be improved with subsequent recruitment maneuvers and increasing PEEP (may need to abandon procedure).
- Bronchospasm:
  - May be minimized with β-agonist pre-medication.
- Hypercapnoea:
  - Occurs if minute volume falls due to tube obstruction.
- Cardiac arrhythmias
- Bleeding:
  - Usually minor but can be torrential.
- Death:
  - Has been reported and is usually due to one of the above mechanisms.

Further reading

Martin WJ, Smith TF, Sanderson DR, *et al.* Role of bronchoalveolar lavage in the assessment of opportunistic pulmonary infections: utility and complications. *Mayo Clinic Proceedings* 1987; 62:549–557.

Pue CA, Pacht ER. Complications of fibreoptic bronchoscopy at a university hospital. *Chest* 1995; 107(2):430–2.

Upper GI endoscopy, dilatation, and stent insertion

PROCEDURE BASICS: inspection of oesophagus via a rigid or flexible fibr-eoptic scope ± biopsy, dilatation, or stent insertion. (See Table 5.3 for indications).

TIME: 5–30 mins.

PAIN RATING: 1–2/5.

ANALGESIA: simple oral analgesia/IV paracetamol. May need opiates if oesophagus stented or dilated.

BLOOD LOSS: usually minimal, be prepared if dealing with varices which can bleed torrentially.

HOSPITAL STAY: generally suitable for day case, but may have multiple co-morbidities.

PREPARATION AND EQUIPMENT: pre-operative IV fluid rehydration + PPI/H_2 antagonist. Standard monitoring. Rapid sequence induction. SLT placed to the L of the mouth to allow access.

Table 5.3 Indications for oesophagoscopy

Classification	Indication
Diagnostic	Inspection ± biopsy, e.g. oesophagitis/Barrett's oesophagus
	Suspected TOF
	To assess motility disorders
	Staging of oesophageal malignancy
	To evaluate oesophageal anastomosis
	To evaluate response to therapy, e.g. ulcer healing
Therapeutic	Removal foreign body
	Insertion of feeding tube
	Insertion of brachytherapy catheter
	Treatment of oesophageal and gastric varices
	Stenting of oesophageal stricture/extrinsic compression/TOF
	Resection of small tumours

Pre-operative assessment and preparation

History

- Establish the indication for oesophagoscopy.
- Does the patient complain of heartburn, regurgitation or coughing on lying flat?
- Focused assessment of cardio-respiratory reserve. Many of these patients have multiple co-morbidities.
- Known or anticipated difficult laryngoscopy? The majority of these patients require a rapid sequence induction.
- Look for evidence of dehydration and malnutrition associated with dysphagia.
- Observe for drooling associated with obstruction by foreign body.
- Warn about post-operative coughing, nausea, sore throat and suxamethonium myalgia.

Anaesthesia

- Flexible oesphagoscopy may be performed under IV sedation; balance this with the potential risk of reflux.

Pre-medication

Proton pump inhibitor or H_2 blocker

- Ranitidine.
  - 150 mg PO,
- Omeprazole.
  - 20 mg IV/PO.
- Sodium citrate.
  - Consider 0.3M 30 ml PO immediately pre-operative.

Rapid sequence induction

- Suction nasogastric tube if present.
- Head up 45° to decrease the possibility of reflux.
- Adequately pre-oxygenate with 100% O_2.
- Intubate trachea with SLT; consider using an armoured tube.
- Secure tube at the left side of the mouth.

Top tip

- Oesophagoscopy can be an extremely quick procedure requiring relaxation; therefore, long-acting relaxants are not first choice.
- Suxamethonium is used as part of the R.S.I, and can also be used to maintain relaxation.

Maintenance relaxant suggestion

- Suxamethonium and atropine.
  - Mix 100 mg of suxamethonium with 300 mcg atropine.
  - Dilute to 5 ml with saline.
  - Give 1 ml increments as necessary if maintained relaxation is needed.
- Remifentanil TCI.
  - Can be used to provide apnoea, relaxation and to act as an anti-tussive.
  - Use with care to avoid bradycardia!

Position

- Patient may be supine or in lateral position.

Maintenance

- Watch for airway obstruction and tracheal tube displacement during the procedure.
- Complete muscle relaxation is required to allow safe passage of the oesophagoscope through the cricopharyngeal sphincter.
- May need to deflate tracheal tube cuff to aid passage of scope.
- A nasogastric tube is likely to be required in most cases.
- Cardiac arrhythmia can occur.
  - Most resolve spontaneously and are benign, but some can cause reduced cardiac output and hypotension.
- Oesophageal rupture and bleeding can occur during the procedure; consider cross-match in cases of oesophageal varices.
- Stent insertion may be guided by fluoroscopy.

The end of the procedure

- Awake extubation in left lateral position.
- Ensure adequate reversal of neuromuscular blockade.
  - If repeated suxamethonium has been used, be aware of phase II blockade.
- Suction nasogastric tube prior to extubation.
- Patients should be awake with full airway reflexes present before being left in recovery.
- Sit patient up as soon as full airway reflexes return.

Post-operative and analgesia

- Oesophageal stent insertion and dilatation are associated with increased pain.
  - Patients may require small doses of opioid in the immediate post-operative period.
- Risk of oesophageal rupture is low (< 0.5%). Liaise with surgical colleagues if suspected; most are treated conservatively.

Further reading

Low DE (2004). Complications of oesophageal instrumentation. In Little AG (Ed.), *Complications in Cardiothoracic Surgery*, 1st ed. Ch 13. Blackwell Futura.

Tracheal stenting procedures

PROCEDURE BASICS: often a palliative procedure used when airway resection and reconstruction are not possible or appropriate.

TIME: varies depending on the extent of the obstruction and pathology.

PAIN RATING: 1–3/5.

ANALGESIA: simple oral analgesia. Opioids are often required but take care not to render the patient apnoeic.

BLOOD LOSS: can be massive if there is tumour debulking involved.

HOSPITAL STAY: can be a day case if benign pathology, but more likely palliative in-patient.

PREPARATION AND EQUIPMENT: standard monitoring. Arterial line may be a good idea to monitor haemodynamics. Sander's injector with supply of air/difficult intubation equipment.

Introduction
- Patients with central airway obstruction may be within hours of death.
- Palliative debulking may not be an option.
- Developments in other specialities have been utilized to make stenting an increasingly used treatment option.

Mechanisms of obstruction
- Benign causes:
  - Tracheal stenosis (eg post intubation).
  - Tracheomalacia.
  - Granulomatous disease.
  - Amyloid.
  - Relapsing polychondritis.
- Malignant lesions may primarily be treated with "core out" procedures, laser therapy, electrocautery, brachy therapy or cryotherapy.
- Stenting of malignant disease is often reserved for recurrence or external compression.
- Stents are not licensed for non-malignant lesions.

Basics on stenting

- Early stents were cylindrical tubes composed of silicone.
- Progression to the "Montgomery T-Tube", inserted via a tracheostomy. Contains a limb allowing suction and anchoring of the stent giving it the "T" shape.
- Studded silicone allows a degree of anchoring, as does the addition of proximal and distal phlanges.
- Bifurcation of the stent assists positioning at the carina.
- Recent stents, self or balloon expanded, make use of advances in vascular surgery technology.
- Metal mesh may provide better anchoring.

Problems with stents

- Displacement (major complication).
  - Can cause airway obstruction.
  - It may be extremely difficult to reposition an established stent.
  - Many stents (eg metal) should be considered permanent.
- Imperforate walled stents (polyurethane, silicone).
  - Cause loss of cilia action.
  - Cause sputum retention.
- Meshed wall.
  - Ability to cross bronchi without obstructing distal airway.
  - Epithelization may occur, leading to cilia recovery, with time.
  - Tumour may grow through the spaces, leading to airway obstruction.
  - Balloon re-expansion may be possible.

Stents placed with X-ray guidance

- Becoming more common.
- During the procedure a guidewire is placed with fluoroscopic screening.
- The stent is aligned with the obstruction and a balloon is used to open the stent.
- ❶ There will be episodes of complete airway obstruction (balloon inflation).
- ❶ Anaesthetic back-up is often not present/immediately available.
- ❶ Staff may not be competent to deal with acute airway problems.

Bronchoscopic placement

- May be preceded by debulking of airway tumour.

Pre-operative assessment and preparation

- Patients may be very frail with advanced malignancy.
- Look for manifestations of paraneoplasia.

Investigations

Radiology
- **CXR** and **CT**
  - Review scans to determine site and severity of stenosis or obstruction.

Bloods
- **FBC, U&E, LFT** and **Clotting**
  - If end–stage malignancy, routine bloods may reveal results detrimental to anaesthesia without further optimization.
  - If liver function is deranged, clotting may also be deranged. Catastrophic airway bleeding is undesirable (particularly in a patient undergoing a palliative procedure)!

Anaesthesia for VATS

Induction
- Talk with the surgeon regarding the time and complexity involved in the procedure.
  - Allows tailoring of NMB.
  - You may want to induce the patient in theatre to minimize any hypoxia on ntransfer.
- BIS should be considered due to inability to monitor ET volatile level.
  - Minimum monitoring as recommended by the RCOA ± arterial line, dependent upon the pre-morbid condition of the patient.
- Pre-oxygenate.
  - May take a longer time than with a "non-obstructed" patient.
  - Avoid coughing as may result in complete airway obstruction.
  - Airway obstruction in this case may result in a "can intubate, can't ventilate" scenario.
- Gas induction with sevoflurane.
- Ensure that patient can be manually ventilated.
- Then consider neuromuscular blockade with suxamethonium or short acting non-depolarizing agent eg mivacurium.
- Await neuromuscular blockade, with gentle hand ventilation.
- Air trapping is the main issue with IPPV at this stage.
- When neuromuscular blockade complete, the surgeon can insert the rigid bronchoscope.

Position
- Usually sitting up.
  - Helps to maximize FRC and prevent atelectasis.

Maintenance and intra-operative
- TIVA maintenance anaesthesia (titrate to HR, BP and BIS score).
- Repeat neuromuscular blockade as necessary.
- Manual jet ventilation (via Sanders injector) can be utilized by attaching to the ventilating port of the rigid scope.

Caution

- ❶ Be aware of air-trapping behind obstructed airways (risk of pneumothorax).
- Do not ventilate whilst laser is active. Risk of airway fire.
- Attention to BP and HR.
- Maintenance of neuromuscular blockade, during stent insertion.

⚠ *The end of the procedure*
- A critical point in the anaesthetic.
- Ensure adequate haemostasis and meticulous airway toilet with the surgeons.
- Stop infusions.
- Maintain gentle jet ventilation until return of spontaneous ventilation
- Rigid bronchoscope may remain in situ until the cough reflex begins to return.
- ❶ Post-operatively, the patient should only be returned to the recovery room when adequate spontaneous ventilation and cough reflex are present.

Complications

Airway obstruction
- The most common complication.
- Recognition:
  - Inadequate ventilation ± cough reflex.
  - Loss of consciousness (inability to clear CO_2).
  - See-saw abdominal movements and respiratory effort (common indicators of respiratory obstruction) may be obtunded.
  - → pallor, desaturation, hypotension, dysrhythmias and death.
- Intubation and ventilation may be lifesaving. Airway toilet via rigid bronchoscopy may be required urgently.
- Suction of a stent is often all that is required. Foreign material may be present at the carina, trachea or stent.
- Rarely, stent displacement may be the cause of obstruction, but is usually a late complication.
- Airway perforation, airway laceration, erosion of local structures and tension pneumothorax are all recognized complications.

Tracheo-oesophageal foreign body removal

Anaesthetic management can be challenging!

Trachea or oesophagus?

Tracheal obstruction

⚠️⚠️ Urgent and can be acutely life threatening!
- Airway foreign bodies tend to fall down the right side.
- If the patient is breathing, with acceptable saturation and appears comfortable, they ARE NOT CRITICALLY OBSTRUCTED.
- The potential is for circumstances to worsen by dislodging the foreign body/worsen the obstruction with your intervention.

Oesophageal obstruction

⚠️ Urgent but usually not life threatening, however due to the proximity of the oesophagus to the trachea, even slight swelling may impact upon the airway!
- Points of oesophageal narrowing:
  - Normal anatomical points: Cricopharyngeus, aortic arch, GOJ
  - Any pathological narrowing.
- 70% of impactions occur in the cervical oesophagus, 20% in the upper thoracic oesophagus and 10% in the lower oesophagus.
- Adults
  - Food boluses > bones (particularly fish bones) > coins, fruit pips, pins and dentures.
  - >60 years consider oesophageal disease.
  - Incarcerated individuals and psychiatric patients.

Pre-operative assessment and preparation

- ❗❗ History of intoxication (alcohol or CNS depressants), stroke patients or those with parkinsonism should raise suspicion of aspiration.
- ❗ Surgical emphysema implies perforation.
- General anaesthetic assessment.
  - Thoracotomy may be required; ask surgeon.
- See Table 5.4 for presentation.

Table 5.4 Presentation of oesophageal and tracheal obstruction

Oesophageal	Tracheal
Dysphagia	Choking
Pain	Cough
Foreign body sensation	Stridor ❶❶
Regurgitation	Respiratory distress
Salivation	Pneumonia
Gagging	Wheeze
Cough	Pulmonary oedema
Choking	
Fever	

Examination
- Usually nil to find.
- Examination of the pharynx, neck, trachea, lungs and abdomen should be performed.
- If there are chest signs, be highly suspicious of aspiration.

Investigations

Bloods
- **FBC, U&E.**
- **ABG.**
  - Particularly if signs of respiratory distress.

Radiology
- **CXR/Cervical X-ray.**
  - AP and lateral.
  - Look for soft tissue swelling and air (aids location of foreign body).
  - Denture plates and other objects are sometimes radiolucent.
  - Because of the cartilaginous support of the trachea, tracheal foreign bodies tend to locate anteroposteriorly, while oesophageal foreign bodies are usually found in the frontal plane.
- **Contrast CT.**
  - Allows more information if suspecting perforation.
- **Swallowing studies.**
  - If object is radiolucent.

Other
- **Endoscopy.**
  - Beware; this can push the object further away.
  - Have equipment ready to grasp object.

Immediate emergency anaesthetic management

Acute life-threatening airway obstruction

- 100% O_2, ECG monitoring, pulse oximetry, IV access.
- In stridulous patients, epinephrine via a nebulizer may be a temporising measure until bronchoscopy can be performed.
- If the patient is coughing, wheezing, or is stridulous but maintaining an airway, DO NOT attempt to intervene; transport to the nearest facility where definitive treatment can be provided.
- If severe airway compromise or total obstruction occurs, attempt chest compressions, back blows, abdominal thrusts, or the Heimlich manoeuvre.
- If unstable, rapid sequence intubation may be needed. In these cases, be prepared with suction and Magill forceps.
- In emergency situations with tracheal foreign bodies below the level of the vocal cords, intubation may be required.
- The ET tube may be advanced to the hilt, thus moving the object from above the carina (total obstruction) down a mainstem bronchus.
- ET tube is then withdrawn to the normal position and the patient is ventilated after ensuring the tip of the tube is not occluded with the foreign body.
- Although only ventilating one lung, this will provide bide time to perform formal, more controlled bronchoscopy.

Pharmacological therapy in non-life threatening obstruction

- Glucagon:
  - 0.5 to 2.0 mg IV after a small test dose.
  - Can be repeated after 10 mins.
  - For distal oesophageal impaction.
  - Effective in 30 to 50%.
  - Relaxes smooth muscle, but is ineffective in the cervical oesophagus.
  - Followed by several sips of water.
- Other agents are out of favour now (Papain/bicarbonate therapy).

Equipment

- General anaesthesia.
- Operating table with variable head position.
- Rigid and flexible bronchoscopes and oesophagoscopes.
- Selection of grasping forceps.
- x2 rigid suction.
- Good light source.

- Venturi ventilator with sufficient gas.
- Thoracotomy set available if irretrievable by endoscopic route.
- Selection of ET tubes: may need DLT for thoracotomy.

Surgical procedure-airway retrieval

- Careful intubation of airway with rigid bronchoscope.
- Exploration of the entire bronchial tree.
- Grasp foreign body with rigid forceps, suction, Dormier basket.
- Flexible scope may be used prior to rigid.

Surgical procedure-oesophageal retrieval

Flexible scope

- Careful endobronchial intubation, secured to the LEFT side of mouth.
- Gentle inspection with flexible scope.
- Assess potential for removal with flexible scope with biopsy forceps, crocodile teeth forceps or Dormier basket.
- Impacted food bolus can be pushed into stomach rather than removed.
- Perforation rate 0.25%.
- Less potential for your tube to be dislodged.
- May not need GA for this.

Rigid scope

- Will need GA for this.
- Removal can be hazardous as may be hooked into the wall.
- Greater endotracheal tube movement.
- Allows larger instruments to be used.
- Breaking up of foreign body can facilitate removal.

Anaesthetic management of the stable patient

- Provide an adequate plane of anaesthesia.
- Prevent patient movement, and decrease the chance of laryngospasm.
- Ensure normoxia, normocarbia and rapid emergence with preservation of airway reflexes as far as is possible.
- Management options are divided according to the modality of ventilation chosen. Each has its advantages and disadvantages:

Controlled ventilation

- (−)Neuromuscular blockade needed.
  - Use short acting agent i.e. suxamethonium.
- (−)Risk of intra-operative laryngospasm.
- (−)Need for positive pressure ventilation and ensuing risk of critical airway obstruction due to dislodging foreign body; thus making retrieval more difficult or creating a "ball-valve" obstruction with clinical deterioration.
- (+)Lower risk of laryngospasm.
- (+)Ventilation can be stopped at critical retrieval moment
- (+)Easier to maintain normoxia and normocarbia.
- (+) Less cardiovascular compromise.
- (+)Lower risk of atelectasis.

Assisted ventilation

- (−)May require neuromuscular blockade.
- (−)Risk of intra-operative laryngospasm remains.
- (−)Use of positive pressure, even intermittently may cause acute obstruction with the foreign body.
- (+)Maintains SOME of the normal ventilatory physiology and therefore lower risk of dislodging foreign body into distal airway.

Spontaneous ventilation

- (−)Cardiovascular compromise is common due to the need for greater depth of anaesthesia to keep the patient still and attempt obtund laryngospasm.
- (−)Greater risk of atelectasis.
- (−)Movement and coughing may make retrieval of the foreign body extremely difficult.
- (+)Preservation of normal negative pressure generated ventilation.
- (+)Lower risk of dislodging foreign body with positive pressure causing life threatening acute obstruction.
- (+)Lack of a disruption to ventilation when the surgeon is attempting to retrieve the foreign body with the bronchoscope's eye piece open.

IV Vs. Inhalational anaesthesia

- Jury is still out!
- IV may offer a better plane of anaesthesia as inhalational agents may not enter the lungs as effectively due to obstructed ventilation.
- Short acting opiodes such as Remifentanil can provide excellent obtundation of airway reflexes, but care is needed not to overdo dosage as apnoea in a patient with hypercarbia and hypoxia will obviate the requirement to assist ventilation.

> **❶ Pitfalls**
>
> - Desaturation.
>   - Commonly into the low 90's due to atelectasis and impaired O_2 delivery secondary to obstruction.
> - Hypercapnia.
>   - Common to see $PaCO_2$ >8 kPa due to impaired ventilation.
> - Bradycardia
>   - Due to deep anaesthesia particularly with spontaneous breathing and vagal response to airway stimulation.
> - Coughing and laryngospasm.
>   - Common and difficult to manage.
>   - May need paralysis with its accompanying disadvantages.
> - Dislodgement of foreign body and distal critical airway obstruction.

Further reading

Limper AH, Prakash UB. Tracheobronchial foreign bodies in adults. *Annals of Internal Medicine.* 1990; 112(8):604–9.

Henderson CT, Engel J, Schlesinger P. Foreign body ingestion: review and suggested guidelines for management. *Endoscopy* 1987; 19:68–71.

Mediastinoscopy and mediastinotomy

PROCEDURE BASICS: mediastinoscopy is the introduction of an endoscope into the mediastinum from above the sternal notch.

Mediastinotomy is the surgical access of the mediastinum from a limited anterior thoracotomy.

The two procedures are complimentary but should not be confused as the positioning and anaesthetic requirements differ.

TIME: 30 minutes to 1 hour.

PAIN RATING: 2–3/5.

ANALGESIA: routine simple analgesia post-operatively.

BLOOD LOSS: minimal but potential for massive haemorrhage.

HOSPITAL STAY: short stay or day case.

PREPARATION AND EQUIPMENT: standard intubation. Large bore IV access. Consider invasive pressure monitoring if patient co-morbidities exist. DLT may be needed for mediastinotomy.

Brief anatomy of the mediastinium
- The mediastinium is the region between the two pleural sacs extending from thoracic inlet superiorly to diaphragm inferiorly.
- The sternum forms the anterior boundary and thoracic vertebrae form the posterior boundary.
- It is divided, somewhat arbitrarily, into a superior and inferior part by a plane that extends from the sternal angle to the lower border of the fourth thoracic vertebra.
- The inferior mediastinum is subdivided into the anterior mediastinum in front of the pericardium, the middle mediastinum containing the pericardium, and the posterior mediastinum behind the pericardium.

Mediastinoscopy or cervical mediastinoscopy
- A diagnostic procedure first described by Carlens in 1959.
- Although possible under local anaesthetic it is usually performed under a general anaesthetic.
- May be performed as a day case procedure. However, due to the potential complications, it should not be undertaken in a stand-alone day case centre.
- A 3 cm incision is made at the level of the suprasternal notch.
- Blunt dissection then continues between the trachea and aortic arch

A mediastinoscope is then inserted into the space and used to assess sample lymph nodes or a mass.

Indications
- Evaluate and biopsy mediastinal lymph nodes and masses.
- Staging of carcinoma of the lung (involvement of mediastinal lymph nodes may confer inoperability).

Contraindications
- Previous recent mediastinoscopy.
- Aortic arch aneurysm.
- Previous thoracic radiotherapy.
- Previous recurrent laryngeal nerve damage.
- Severe tracheal deviation.
- Limited neck extension

Pre-operative assessment and preparation
History and examination
- Many mediastinal masses are asymptomatic.
- In addition to the usual pre-operative assessment ask for symptoms suggestive of cerebral metastasis or an Lambert-Eaton myasthenic syndrome.
- Look for signs of upper airway distortion or superior vena caval obstruction.

Investigations

Bloods
- **FBC, U&E** and **Clotting**.

Radiology
- **CXR**.
  - PA view routine, lateral and thoracic inlet views as indicated.
- **Thoracic CT scan**.

Other
- **PFT**.
- **ECG**.
- **Erect and supine flow-volume loop**.

Anaesthesia
Premedication
- Consider short-acting benzodiazepine for anxiolysis; avoid if any suggestion of airway obstruction.
- Avoid if any suggestion of airway obstruction.

Induction
- At least one large bore cannula.
  - Consider placing in lower limb, especially if superior vena caval obstruction (SVCO) present.
- Monitoring as per AAGBI guidelines consider invasive arterial blood pressure.
  - If used, place on right side to allow early identification of compression of brachiocephalic artery by surgeon.
- Peripheral nerve stimulator mandatory in patients with myasthenia gravis or Lambert-Eaton myasthenic syndrome.
- ❶ Care with or avoidance of muscle relaxants in patients with or suspected myasthenia gravis or Eaton-Lambert syndrome.
- *No airway obstruction*
  - Consider IV induction, tracheal intubation with single lumen endotracheal tube and intermittent positive pressure ventilation.
- *Intrathoracic airway obstruction*
  - Muscle relaxation and positive pressure ventilation may worsen obstruction consider spontaneously ventilating technique.

Position
- 20° head up, sand bag under shoulders, head ring.

The end of the procedure
- Extubate awake.
- Simple and opiod analgesia usually sufficient.
- Post-operative CXR.

⚠ **Special considerations**

Be aware of the potential complications:
- Haemorrhage (particularly if SVCO), possibly torrential.
- Pneumothorax.
- Recurrent laryngeal nerve injury.
- Arterial compression.
- Tracheal compression.
- Dysrhythmia.
- Tumour implantation
- Phrenic nerve injury
- Oesophageal injury
- Air embolism
- Chylothorax
- Stroke.

Mediastinotomy or anterior mediastinotomy
- A limited anterior thoracotomy made in the second intercostal space, lateral to the sternal border.
- Usually performed on the left side.
  - A left anterior mediastinotomy is also known as a Chamberlains procedure.
- This approach allows biopsy of central lymph nodes particularly aortopulmonary nodes and mediastinal masses.

Pre-operative assessment and preparation
History, examination and investigations
- As for mediastinoscopy.

Premedication
- Consider short-acting benzodiazepine for anxiolysis.

Anaesthesia
- Position patient supine; consider a "sand bag" under shoulder on operative side.
- Insert large bore cannulae and consider invasive blood pressure monitoring.
- DLT and one lung ventilation is usually used to facilitate the surgery.
- Complications are less frequent (structures are more visible).
- Post-operative pain is more severe; an IV-PCA system is usually used.

> **Future developments**
>
> - The emergence of PET scanning has led to a reduction in the frequency of mediastinoscopy.
> - The use of endobronchial ultrasound guided lymph node biopsies (EBUS) has similarly reduced the need for mediastinoscopy.
> - Video-assisted mediastinal lymphadenectomy and lobectomy (VAMLA and VATS-lobectomy) are new minimally invasive techniques.

Further reading

Searl CP, Ahmed ST (2009). *Core Topics in Thoracic Anaesthesia*. Cambridge. Cambridge University Press.

Kaplan JA, Slinger PD (2003). *Thoracic Anaesthesia*. Elsevier Science (USA).

Ahmed-Nusrath A, Swaneveleder J. Continuing Education in Anaesthesia, *Critical Care & Pain* 2007; 7:6–9.

Staging laparoscopy

PROCEDURE BASICS: laparoscopic examination and lymph node biopsy to exclude local spread or metastases prior to curative surgery (usually oesophagectomy).

TIME: 15–45 mins.

PAIN RATING: 2/5.

ANALGESIA: simple analgesics +/– systemic opioids. Local anaesthetic infiltration.

BLOOD LOSS: minimal.

HOSPITAL STAY: may be performed as day case.

PREPARATION AND EQUIPMENT: basic anaesthetic equipment/basic monitoring/single lumen tube.

Background
- Most patients with upper GI cancer present at an advanced stage.
- 'Occult' deposits are often missed by conventional imaging techniques:
  - Sensitivity of detecting peritoneal metastasis; ultrasound 14%, CT 14% and laparoscopy 71%.
- Usually performed prior to major curative surgery for carcinoma of the oesophagus and stomach to exclude incurable oesophageal and gastric cancer and avoid unnecessary further surgery.
- Indications for staging laparoscopy in upper GI cancer is still evolving.
- Laparoscopy is usually intended to replace laparotomy in patients with 'resectable' tumour as judged by conventional imaging techniques to assess distant spread before curative surgery.
- Intra-vascular and gut access lines can be placed during laparoscopy.
- Re-staging is needed following neo-adjuvant chemotherapy and before surgery.
- Staging entails laparoscopic examination of:
  - The liver.
  - Peritoneum and lymph nodes.
  - Biopsies and cytology.
- Endoscopic ultrasound is useful to assess liver metastasis.
- ♥ Cellular and humoral immune response following laparoscopy is said to be significant and no different from that following laparotomy and concerns have been raised about adverse impact later on incurable cancer
- See Table 5.5 for staging of oesophageal cancer.

Table 5.5 Tumour- Node- Metastasis classification (TNM)

Stage	Tumour	Node	Metastasis	5-yr survival%
0	Tis	N0	M0	>95
I	T1	N0	M0	50–80
IIA	T2–3	N0	M0	30–40
IIB	T1–2	N1	M0	10–30
III	T3	N1	M0	10–15
IVA	AnyT	AnyN	M1a	<5
IVB	AnyT	AnyN	M1b	<1

Tumour invasion: Tis = in situ, T1= lamina propria, T2 = muscularis propria, T3 = adventitia, T4 = adjacent tissue.

Lymph node metastasis: T0 = no spread, N1 = regional

Metastasis (distant): M0 = no metastasis, M1a = cervical nodes in upper oesophagus and coeliac nodes in lower oesophagus, M1b = other distant nodes.

Pre-operative assessment and preparation

- Often pre-operative work up is as for oesophagectomy since definitive surgery may quickly (days) follow staging laparoscopy. (See 📖 Oesophagectomy, p. 444).
- Pre-operative co-morbidities contraindicating oesophagectomy (e.g. severe ischaemic heart disease) may contraindicate staging laparoscopy.
- Discussion of analgesic techniques (e.g. epidural or paravertebral), invasive monitoring and critical care stay after oesophagectomy can also be started at this time.

History
(See 📖 Oesophagectomy, p. 444).

Examination
(See 📖 Oesophagectomy, p. 444).

Investigations
(See 📖 Oesophagectomy, p. 444).

Discuss with patient
- Rapid sequence induction (gastro-oesophageal sphincter may be inadequate; food may be lodged above tumour).
- Day surgery advice (analgesia, driving, supervision at home etc).

Anaesthesia
- Rapid sequence induction.
- Tracheal intubation and controlled ventilation.
- Volatile or TIVA maintenance.
- Intra-operative analgesia.
  - Remifentanil infusion or longer acting opioids e.g. fentanyl or morphine.

Position
- Supine.

The end of the procedure
- Extubate on side or sitting (to minimize risk of aspiration).

Post-operative

Analgesia
- Paracetamol combined with medium to longer acting opioids.
- Ask surgeon to infiltrate incision sites with local anaesthetic solution.

Further reading

Enzinger PC, Mayer RJ. Gastrointestinal cancer in older patients. *New England Journal of Medicine*. 2003; 349: 2241–52.

Surgery to the lung and upper airway

Video-assisted thoracoscopic surgery (VATS)

PROCEDURE BASICS: minimally invasive surgery using a thoracoscope and two or more ports to perform diagnostic or therapeutic thoracic surgery. Increasingly used for lobectomy and has proven lower peri-operative morbidity and similar long term outcomes compared to thoracotomy.

TIME: varies depending on the intended surgery (See Table 6.1 for indications). Upwards of 45 mins dependent on surgery.

PAIN RATING: 3–5/5. Even though the procedure is minimally invasive, it can still be very painful.

ANALGESIA: simple analgesics, NSAID, PCA opioid ± single-shot paravertebral block. Thoracic epidural/paravertebral catheter recommended for "utility" thoracotomy, bilateral procedures, and for conversion to open thoracotomy.

BLOOD LOSS: minimal; potential for significant haemorrhage from pulmonary vessels during lung resection.

HOSPITAL STAY: dependent on indication ± subsequent surgery.

PREPARATION AND EQUIPMENT: standard monitoring. Majority require a DLT (speak to surgeon). Arterial line required in most cases except very minor. CVP line may only be needed if patient co-morbidities exist.

Introduction
- Video-assisted thoracoscopic surgery (VATS) procedures range from excision or biopsy of pleural/lung/mediastinal lesions to lung resection.
- VATS has opened the door to patients who otherwise would be considered inoperable due to severe respiratory disease.
- The physiological impact of VATS and the associated complexity of anaesthesia are no different to that for open thoracotomy. The approach to both should be of an equally high standard.

Table 6.1 Indications for VATS

Diagnostic	Therapeutic
Staging	*Parenchymal disease*
Lung cancer	Wedge resection
Mesothelioma	Lobectomy
Oesohogeal cancer	Pneumonectomy
	Lung volume reduction
Pleural disease	*Pleural disease*
Tuberculosis	Pleurodesis
Thoracocentesis	Decortication
Parenchymal disease	*Pericardial disease*
Interstitial fibrosis	Effusions, window
Solitary nodules	*Mediastinal disease*
	Thymectomy
	Chylothorax
	Other
	Sympathectomy
	Vagotomy

Basics on surgical technique (lobectomy)

- Three or four 10 mm incisions plus one 4–6 cm incision for specimen retrieval in endobag.
- Camera at 8th ICS, anterior axillary line, port at 9th ICS mid scapular line and a 5 mm accessory port at the tip of the scapula.
- Positive pressure insufflation (as in laparoscopy) is not used. The lung collapses when the bronchus is obstructed.
- Rib resection or spreading may be used (which can cause significant pain).
- Surgical approach for lobectomy:
  - Isolation of the lobar vasculature and bronchial structures in an anterior to posterior approach (similar to thoracotomy).
  - Complete mediastinal lymph node dissection is preferable to mediastinal lymph node sampling. This has better outcomes and requires high surgical skill.

Anaesthesia for VATS

Pre-operative assessment and optimization

- Pre-operative assessment and optimization as per thoracotomy.
- Discussion of PCA analgesia ± regional anaesthetic techniques.

Induction
- Epidural analgesia or paravertebral blockade (requires "utility" thoracotomy/conversion to thoracotomy).
- OLV is usually required. Ask surgeon.
- Standard IV induction or TIVA.
- The use of DLT or BB is acceptable.
- Pre-oxygenation not only has the obvious safety advantage but causes quicker lung collapse as oxygen will be absorbed faster than remaining nitrogen.
- Standard maintenance technique using volatile/TIVA plus relaxant.

Position
- Lateral decubitus position, operative side up (non-dependent).

Maintenance and intra-operative
- Peak airway pressure monitoring is essential.
  - Do not exceed 35 cmH$_2$O.
  - Drop in airway pressure may be first sign of bronchial cuff displacement and TLV.
  - Note airway pressure may be higher with BB than DLT for same tidal volume as lumen is smaller.
- Cuff pressure change can also indicate displacement.

Maintenance of normoxia
- Pressure controlled and volume controlled ventilation have similar effects on oxygenation.
- Maintain 6–8 ml/kg tidal volume during OLV.
- Peak airway pressure should not exceed 35 cmH$_2$O. Methods to treat hypoxaemia during OLV for VATS (See 📖 Postpneumonectomy pulmonary oedena (PPO) and OLV, p. 622).

The end of the procedure
- Apply suction catheter to collapsed lung.
- Slow manual inflation to 30–40 cmH$_2$O for re-expansion and testing of bronchial sutures.
- Apical and basal chest drains will be inserted (painful).
- Extubation at end of operation is the norm to allow spontaneous ventilation, cough and expansion of atelectatic lung.
- Most centres have a dedicated thoracic HDU.

Post-operative and analgesia
- Although less severe than thoracotomy, the pain post VATS is still significant and may lead to respiratory complications and inability to comply with physiotherapy.
- Thoracic epidural analgesia is 'gold standard'.

- Paravertebral block with LA, as a catheter infusion, provides equal analgesia to epidural but reduced hypotension, urinary retention and nausea.
  - Often a single-shot paravertebral block suffices to provide intra-post-operative analgesia. Typically, this is combined with regular simple analgesics, NSAID (if not contra-indicated), and PCA opioid. Consider thoracic epidural for bilateral procedures
- Intercostal blocks (single injection) are of inadequate duration and inferior analgesia compared to epidural.
  - Can be a rescue plan if epidural not possible.
- Interpleural anaesthetic not recommended as absorption of LA is high and analgesia is inferior to epidural.

> - Evidence comparing paravertebral blockade to epidural analgesia is equivocal. Different centres will consistently achieve greater success with one or other technique.

Complications and outcome

Intra-operative
- Conversion to thoracotomy 5–11%.
- Similar operative time to thoracotomy (~150mins lobectomy).
- Similar blood loss to thoracotomy.

Peri-operative
(See Table 6.2 for complication comparison).
- Chest drain days and length of hospital stay.
  - Each reduced by → 1 day vs. thoracotomy
- Improved FEV_1, SpO_2 and PaO_2 post-operatively vs. thoracotomy.

Table 6.2 Complications of VATS Vs. thoracotomy

Complication	VATS lobectomy	Open lobectomy
Death	1%	3–5%
Prolonged air leak	13%	19%
Atelectasis	5%	12%
Atrial fibrillation	13%	21%
Need for transfusion	4%	13%
Pneumonia	5%	10%
Acute renal failure	1.4%	5%
Post-operative pain	Less severe	More severe

> **Long-term outcome/advantages of VATS**
>
> - There is a growing evidence-base to support the use of VATS, but the data tends to be heterogeneous and originates from specialized centres.
> - Overall incidence of complications following VATS is 10%–15% with a mortality of 1–2%, compared with 1–12% for open lung resection.
> - Approximately 10% cases are converted to open thoracotomy.
> - Reduced post-operative mortality and morbidity (See Table 6.1).
> - Hospital stay reduced by 2–3 days compared to thoracotomy.
> - Improved access to post-operative adjunctive chemotherapy.
> - VATS 5-year survival for lung cancer is comparable to thoracotomy.
> - There is concern that VATS is not as oncologically safe as thoracotomy because the surgeon does not have tactile perception and lymphadeonectomy is more difficult.
> - Although only a few randomized controlled trials compare VATS and thoracotomy for long term outcome there is strong level 2 evidence (comparing cohorts with historic controls) that 5-year survival is similar (See Table 6.3).

Table 6.3 Long term survival between VATS and thoracotomy lobectomy (n=147)

Survival at year	VATS (%)	Thoracotomy (%)
1 year	96	91
2	82	83
3	78	77
4	72	66
5	71	64

Further reading

Fischer G, Cohen E. An update on anesthesia for thoracoscopic surgery. *Current opinion in anesthesiology.* 2010; 23:7–11.

Whitson B, Andrade R, Boettcher A. Video-assisted Thoracoscopic surgery is more favourable for resection of clinical stage I Non-small cell lung cancer. *Annals of Thoracic Surgery* 2007; 83:19–65.

Brodsky J. Lung separatiojn and the difficult airway. *British Journal of Anaesthesia* 2009; 103 (suppl 1):i66–75.

Tracheostomy

PROCEDURE BASICS: formation of an airway directly into the trachea via an incision made in the neck. This can be done surgically or percutaneously.

TIME: 10–30 minutes.

PAIN RATING: 1–2/5.

ANALGESIA: local infiltration by the surgeon is normally adequate.

BLOOD LOSS: minimal, however potential for significant haemorrhage from the thyroid vessels.

HOSPITAL STAY: dependent on indication ± subsequent surgery.

PREPARATION AND EQUIPMENT: may be performed under LA in emergencies. Otherwise use SLT/LMA as initial airway while anaesthetized. Use fibreoptic scope to guide percutaneous placement. If anticipated difficult airway, do not anaesthetize until the surgeon is scrubbed and ready.

Indications

Elective
- Long term ventilation of ITU patients (See also percutaneous tracheostomy below).
- Protection of the tracheobronchial tree from soiling, e.g. patients with absent laryngeal/pharyngeal reflexes.
- Pulmonary toilet.
- Temporary or permanent airway as part of another surgical procedure, e.g. laryngectomy, maxillofacial surgery involving the airway.

Emergency
- Relief from airway obstruction.

Complications

Early
- Malposition (false track) or dislodgment of the tube.
- Bleeding.
- Oesophageal perforation.
- Blockage of the tube.
- Pneumothorax.

Late
- Infection.
- Subcutaneous emphysema.
- Tracheal stenosis.
- Tracheal ulceration.
- Dislodgement of the tube.

Anaesthesia for surgical tracheostomy (performed in the operating theatre)

Pre-operative
- Airway assessment.
  - Consider how the airway can be managed if the procedure is for airway obstruction.
  - If in any doubt, awake tracheostomy under local anaesthetic may be indicated.
- Equipment should be available in case an emergency airway is required e.g. cricothyroidotomy kit.
- In patients with the potential for total airway obstruction, the surgeon should be in theatre, scrubbed and ready to perform emergency tracheostomy before induction of anaesthesia.
  - Consider prophylactic needle cricothyroidotomy in these patients.
- Ensure the patient is starved and any NG tubes aspirated.
- The type of tracheostomy tube should be decided on, and be available in a range of sizes (above and below).

Investigations

Bloods
- **FBC.**
  - Platelet count must be more than 50,000/μL.
- **Clotting.**
  - Prothrombin time or activated partial thromboplastin time must be less than 1.5 times the reference range.

Induction
- Standard volatile/IV induction.
- Secure the ETT so it is easy to loosen and withdraw. Ensure easy access to the pilot balloon.
- Patient must be draped to allow access to the head and ETT as this is a shared airway procedure.

Intra-operative
- Switch to 100% O_2 for 5 minutes prior to the tracheal incision, and ensure that the patient is paralysed (avoids coughing).
- Good communication with the surgeon is paramount for this procedure.
- When the surgeon is ready to insert the tracheostomy tube, withdraw the ETT so its tip lies just proximal to the tracheostomy incision.
  - This can be done with the aid of a fibreoscope if available.
- Once the tracheostomy tube is in situ, connect to ventilation tubing and confirm that ventilation of the lungs is possible, there is a viable CO_2 trace and the chest is moving adequately.
  - The ETT should only be removed only once these 3 factors are satisfied.

The end of the procedure and post-operative
- Ensure the tracheostomy tube is firmly secured as can be difficult to re-insert if dislodged during the first 72 hours.
- CXR in recovery to exclude:
  - Mal- position of tracheostomy tube.
  - Pneumothorax.
  - Significant pneumo-mediastinum.
  - Surgical emphysema.
- Humidify supplemental oxygen to preserve muco-ciliary function.
- Suctioning equipment should be on hand for all patients with a tracheostomy tube.

Percutaneous tracheostomy performed on the intensive care unit

- Percutaneous tracheostomy is often performed on ITU by a senior intensivist and is now considered a critical care skill.
- The peri-operative considerations and complications are similar to those for a surgical tracheostomy. Ensure that:
  - Clotting is normal.
  - NG feed has been stopped.
  - They have been ventilated on 100% O_2 for 10 minutes prior to the procedure.

Indications

- Percutaneous tracheostomies are normally performed on the unit in order to:
  - Facilitate weaning from mechanical ventilation (lower work of breathing than COETT)
  - Allow tracheal toileting and suction
  - Prevent complications that arise from prolonged endotracheal intubation, such as laryngeal and tracheal injury, vocal cord paralysis, and infection.

Advantages of PCT over surgical tracheostomy
- Avoids transfer of a critically ill patient from ITU to theatre
  - Avoids accidental extubation and intravascular catheter decannulation.
- Can be quicker than a surgical tracheostomy.
- If performed correctly causes less trauma to the trachea and may lead to a lower incidence of tracheal stenosis.
- Fewer instruments needed, technically easier, smaller operative scar, less bleeding and tracheal erosion, reduced likelihood of infection.

Comparison of PCT and ST

- Intra-procedural complications are similar for PCT and ST
- Post-procedural complications are less likely with the percutaneous procedure.
  - One study found a lower incidence of accidental tracheal decannulation, bleeding, and wound infection after PCT than after ST 13% compared to 41% respectively.

Contraindications

- Difficult neck anatomy, e.g. short neck, difficult palpation of the trachea.
- Coagulopathy.
- Large thyroid artery on initial neck ultrasound, large aberrant thyroid vessels on ultrasound.
- Neck tumours, oedema, burns over the area.
- Reliance on high PEEP for adequate oxygenation (e.g. severe ARDS).
- Maximal FiO_2 requirements.
- Obesity (BMI of 30 or higher).
- Severe haemodynamic instability.
- Would a surgical tracheostomy be more applicable?

Technique for ITU percutaneous tracheostomy

It is strongly recommended that a skilled bronchoscopist aids in the insertion process. This allows visualization of the wire/needle as it enters the trachea, minimizing false passage creation and allowing better centralization of the tracheostomy passage. Techniques vary but are all modifications of the Seldinger technique:
- Ultrasound scan of the area chosen in order to exclude:
  - Unusual anatomy.
  - Enlarged thyroid gland.
  - Superficial blood vessels which could be cut causing uncontrolled bleeding or bleeding into the airway.
- Infiltration of the area to be incised with xylocaine 1% + 1:200,000 epinephrine.
- Palpate for the angle of Louis; palpable rings above this correspond to 2nd/3rd tracheal rings.
- Bronchoscopist should now deflate the tracheal tube cuff and under fibreoscopic guidance, pull the tube back so that it is JUST ABOVE THE VOCAL CORDS.

- The aim is to withdraw the COETT far enough to allow the needle into the trachea, without passing it into the cuff of onto the bronchoscope (damaging it).
- The cuff can now be re-inflated above the cords, which will allow for better ventilation.
- An assistant can adjust ventilator settings to account for leakage.
- Make a 1–1.5 cm skin incision over the desired tracheal rings (correlates with 1st and 4th tracheal rings). The incision can be horizontal or vertical.
- Blunt dissection down to tracheal tissue.
- Pass the needle down until the trachea is cannulated (aiming needle in a caudad direction) and confirm aspiration of air.
  - The bronchoscopist should see the needle in direct view.
- Pass the wire through the needle into the trachea.
  - The bronchoscopist should see the wire passing down into the trachea.
- Remove the needle and pass the small introducer over the wire first.
- Remove the small introducer and then pass dilator of choice over the wire. There are 2 techniques used:
  - Progressive dilatation (Ciaglia technique). Rhinodilator is pushed gently in and out of the trachea over the wire, creating a circumferential hole.
  - Blunt dissection and passage of dilation forceps over the wire (Griggs technique). The forceps are opened, making a passage into the trachea.
- Tracheostomy tube is inserted over wire into trachea.
  - It is well worth a bronchoscopic check to ensure that the tracheostomy tube is patent, free of secretions and is placed high enough above the carina.

Complications are as per surgical tracheostomy.

Post-tracheostomy checks
- Check for bilateral, equal air entry by auscultation.
- Apply suction to clear excess secretions/blood.
- A tracheostomy tube with an inner cannula facilitates care and hygiene and ensures added safety (due to easy removal) if obstruction from secretions occurs.
- If decannulation occurs accidentally within 5–7 days, the patient may need to be re-intubated orally if the tracheostomy tube cannot be immediately reinserted, because the tracheostomy tract is still relatively immature.

Types of tracheostomy tube

A standard tracheostomy tube will consist of the following components:
- Outer tube.
- Removable inner tube to allow cleaning.
- 15 mm connector to fit all ventilator attachments.
- Obturator to assist tube insertion.

Cuffed or uncuffed tube
- High volume, low pressure cuff. The cuff is used to:
  - Facilitate CPAP or positive pressure ventilation.
  - Protect the airway.

Fenestrated or non-fenestrated tube:
- Fenestrated tubes incorporate holes (fenestrations) in the outer cannula. These fenestrations allow air to be exhaled via the larynx and mouth.
- A fenestrated tube allows:
  - Normal breathing.
  - Expectoration of secretions via the mouth.
  - Talking.

Bronchial lasering

Background

- When a gaseous medium, such as argon (Ar) or carbon dioxide (CO_2), is stimulated by an energy source, it emits energy in the form of light.
- Through a series of reflections this light becomes monophasic and monochromatic which are properties common to all lasers.
- The effect of the laser on tissues is dependent on wavelength.
- The most commonly used lasing media for bronchial surgery are CO_2 and Nd-YAG.
- The CO_2 laser emits a long wavelength (10,600 nm) and has less tissue penetrance than the Nd-YAG laser with a wavelength of 1.064 nm.
- CO_2 lasers are therefore commonly used for precise cutting of tissue and Nd-YAG lasers for tumour debulking.

Indications

- Resection of airway tumors, laryngeal papillomata, subglotic stenosis and vascular malformations.

Associated hazards

- Perforation of blood vessel or other structure.
- Gas embolism.
- Ocular damage to patient and staff.
- Airway fire.
- Other burns.
- Atmospheric contamination (smoke produced may be teratogenic and/or a vector for viral infection).

Anaesthetic technique

- Laser therapy may be administered with the aid of a flexible or rigid bronchoscope.
- General anaesthetic is required for rigid bronchoscopy and is recommended for fibreoptic bronchoscopy.
- Standard monitoring, as per AAGBI guidelines should be employed for laser surgery, with invasive monitoring as indicated.
- Options for airway management include intubating and non-intubating methods (see Table 6.4).
  - All techniques are aimed at reducing the risks of complications, especially airway fire.
- The final choice of technique should be based upon the experience of the clinician and the requirements of the individual patient.
- FiO_2 should be kept to a minimum, ideally less than 0.4.

- Avoid nitrous oxide and consider using helium, which has a high thermal conductivity and low density).
- If an intubating technique is used, the tube cuff should be inflated with saline water soaked swabs can be placed around the tube
  - Dyes have been placed into tube cuffs to indicate puncture.
- Laser power density should be limited to the lowest acceptable level.
- Surgical drapes should have a matt surface.
- The scrub practitioner should have a container of water at their immediate disposal.
- All theatre staff should wear appropriate protective equipment including eye protection.
- Entrances and exits to theatre should be locked and clearly marked "laser surgery in progress".
- Consider total intravenous anaesthesia (TIVA) as common volatile agents undergo pyrolysis producing potentially toxic compounds.

Management of airway fires

- Communication with surgical team is paramount.
- STOP surgery immediately, or finish as quickly as possible if at a vital stage.
- Remove oxygen source and extubate trachea.
  - This alone may be enough to allow fire to extinguish spontaneously.
- Have another team member extinguish the fire:
  - Remove cuff-protective devices and any segments of burned tube that may remain smoldering in the airway.
- Once fire is extinguished, re-establish the airway and resume ventilating with air until certain that nothing is left burning in the airway; then switch to 100% oxygen.
- Evaluate tissue damage and remove any debris with rigid bronchoscope.
- Consider re-intubation or low tracheostomy and transfer to intensive care unit.
- An extended period of ventilation may be required.
- Airway lavage and bronchoscopy may be required.
- Steroids may help to reduce inflammation.

Table 6.4 Intubating vs. non-intubating approaches to bronchial lasering

Intubating techniques	Non-intubating techniques
Conventional PVC endotraceal tube wrapped with metallic tape	Spontaneous ventilation
Specific laser resistant tube	Apnoeic technique
Conventional PVC endotraceal tube	Jet ventilation
Metal tracheal tubes	

Further reading

Kaplan JA, Slinger PD (2003). *Thoracic Anaesthesia*. Elsevier Science (USA) .

Ibrahim E. Bronchial Stents. *Annals of Thoracic medicine*. 2006; 1(2):92–7.

Tracheal resection and reconstruction

PROCEDURE BASICS: surgical resection of a segment of the trachea/carina and re-construction of trachea. May undergo segmental resection with primary anastamosis or prosthetic re-construction, otherwise T-tube insertion takes place.

TIME: 1–6h (Airway management and surgical procedure is very challenging and prolonged).

PAIN RATING: 3–4/5.

ANALGESIA: short acting opioids. Simple analgesia and oral opiates/PCA post-operatively. Epidural infusion in case of thoracotomy.

BLOOD LOSS: minimal/moderate.

HOSPITAL STAY: 7–10 days.

PREPARATION AND EQUIPMENT: standard equipment for fibreoptic bronchoscopy, ± high frequency jet ventilation (HFJV). Arterial pressure monitoring (left sided arterial line in right thoracotomy, to avoid damping of trace in case of compression of right innominate artery), OLV, precautions for laser surgery.

Introduction

- Uncommon surgery, which presents major challenges to both surgeon and anaesthetist; should ideally involve senior input.
- Can present as emergency with central airway obstruction and a critically narrowed airway.
- Usually cervicotomy (for high tracheal lesions), thoracotomy & midline sternotomy (for low tracheal or carinal lesions).

Indications

- Primary tracheal tumours (mainly cancers).
- Tracheal stenosis from prolonged invasive ventilation.
- Acquired tracheo-oesophageal fistula.
- Congenital anomalies.
- Vascular lesions

Pre-operative assessment and preparation

General considerations

- Technically challenging as major surgery involving shared airway.
- Aim to maintain ventilation with good gas exchange, whilst allowing optimal surgical access.
- Intra-operative; ventilation strategy should be ascertained pre-operatively between surgeon and anaesthetist. Good communication is paramount throughout the procedure.
- Post-operatively; fragile airway with awkward positioning.
- A need for elective post-operative ventilation is a relative contra-indication for the surgery.

History, examination and optimization

- Symptoms of airway obstruction.
  - Positional dyspnoea, altered sleeping position
- Able to lie supine?
- Able to cough and clear secretions?
- Airway evaluation.
- Respiratory examination.
- Assessment and optimization of other co-morbidities (IHD, COPD, PVD etc.).
- Cessation of smoking pre-operatively.
- Chest physiotherapy.
- Some lesions are non-resectable and may require palliative therapy with dilatation and stenting.

Investigations

Bloods

- **FBC, U&E, Clotting, ABG**

Radiology

- **CXR, CT chest, MRI chest**
  - Delineation of site of lesion
- **Barium swallow, Angiography**
  - Imaging of adjacent structures

Other

- **Bronchoscopy and biopsy**
- **PFT**
- **Spirometry**
  - Flow volume loop measurement helps confirm the location of the obstruction and severity of the lesion.

Anaesthesia

Pre-induction
- Sedative pre-medication may worsen repiratory function.
- Aspiration prophylaxis and anti-sialogogue to reduce secretions.

Induction
- Avoid airway irritation and coughing, which may worsen an already critically narrowed airway.
- Inhalational Vs Intra-venous.
- Maintaining spontaneous ventilation initially allows assessment of the adequacy of assisted ventilation under anaesthesia.
- In patients with severe respiratory distress who are unable to lie supine, the use of neuromuscular blocking agents may eliminate the only muscular tone which is keeping the airway patent.
  - However, the application of IPPV and PEEP may stent the airway open and actually improve tidal volume.

Position
- Initially, neck extended and roll between scapulae.
- Re-positioning required for tracheal re-construction and anastamosis with neck flexed and rolls deflated or removed.
- Right thoracotomy.
  - Neck flexed; approach to low or carinal lesions.
- Slight head down tilt helps to minimize aspiration of blood and secretions.

Maintenance
- TIVA is the optimal technique ± relaxant; volatile anaesthesia can also be used.
- Airway maintenance differs for high/low tracheal and carinal lesions:
  - Sequential change of means of ventilating the lungs during the surgery.
  - After the lesion is exposed ventilation of one or both lungs is achieved by a tracheal tube placed distal to the lesion via the tracheal incision. This allows resection of the lesion and repair of posterior wall of trachea.
  - A narrow tracheal tube or endobronchial tube is subsequently passed beyond the anastomotic site to aid the repair of the anterior wall of trachea.

- Ventilation strategies during tracheal resection include:
  - *For high tracheal lesions:* jet ventilator catheter passed through ETT (which is above resection) for manual or high-frequency jet ventilation. IPPV through sterile ETT inserted by surgeon into trachea below resection.
  - *For low lesions:* bronchial intubation by the surgeon and IPPV to one lung or both separately. Spontaneous ventilation (complicated by hypercarbia, coughing and possible airway soiling).
- Cardiopulmonary bypass (complications of systemic anticoagulation)
- After anastamosis, airway pressures must be minimized:
  - Use spontaneous ventilation or low tidal volume IPPV.
- **❶❶** Be vigilant to intraoperative soiling of the airway with blood → severe hypoxia.
- Aim for extubation at end of surgery to minimize exposure of anastamosis to positive airway pressure.

Post-operative management and complications

Management

- Beware fragile airway with awkward positioning.
- **▶▶** Keep the neck flexed after surgery to avoid tension to the tracheal repair. This is achieved by suturing the chin to the skin over the sternum and maintained until the trachea heals.
- HDU advised post-operatively.
- Analgesia:
  - PCA, epidural/paravertabral infusion in case of thoracotomy.

Complications

- Anastomotic dehiscence
  - Associated with poor outcome
  - Greater risk of dehiscence with post-operative ventilation, steroids, infection, extensive tracheal disease.
  - Reduced risk of dehiscence with use of vascularized flap covering anastomosis and application of fibrin glue sealant.
- Hemorrhage.

- Prolonged neck flexion may cause cervical spinal cord compression.
- Pulmonary infections.
- Re-stenosis.
- Tracheomalacia

Further reading

Ernst A, Central Airway Obstruction. *American Journal of Respiratory and Critical Care Medicine.* 2004; 169:1278–97.

Hermes C. Grillo. Development of tracheal surgery: a historical review. Part 1: techniques of tracheal surgery. *Annals of Thoracic Surgery.* 2003; 75:610–19.

Conacher ID, Feller-Kopman D, Becker HD, *et al.* Anaesthesia and tracheobronchial stenting for central airway obstruction in adults. *British Journal of Anaesthesia,* 2003; 90:367–74.

Pancoast tumour and resection

PROCEDURE BASICS: anterior transcervical or posterior thoracotomy. May involve resection of chest wall, vertebrae and subclavian artery.

TIME: 2–5 hours.

PAIN RATING: 5/5.

ANALGESIA: multimodal. Regional block + systemic opioids.

BLOOD LOSS: variable. May be extensive.

HOSPITAL STAY: days to weeks. ITU/step-down to HDU care

PREPARATION AND EQUIPMENT: standard equipment, range of DLT/CVP/ arterial line.

Pathology
- Originally described by radiologist, Henry Pancoast, in 1932. He described this apical tumor as being associated with:
  - Rib destruction.
  - Horner syndrome.
  - Atrophy of the hand muscles.
- 1–3% of all lung cancers.
- Apical bronchogenic (non-small cell) carcinoma arising in or near the superior sulcus and invading the adjacent extrathoracic structures by direct extension.
- Generally invades adjacent vital structures, including the brachial plexus, subclavian vessels, sympathetic chain, stellate ganglion, ribs, spine and chest wall.

Treatment options
- Surgery alone is not the prevalent course of treatment.
  - Indicated in patients who have very localized early disease; 5-year survival around 40%.
- Contraindications to surgery include:
  - Extension of the tumor into the neck or vertebrae.
  - Presence of substantial mediastinal lymph nodes.
  - Peripheral tumor dissemination.
- Peripheral metastases signal a poor prognosis, and surgery is contraindicated in such cases.
- Selected patients will receive pre-operative irradiation with 30 Gy of radiation over 2 weeks.
- Surgery is often performed within 2–4 weeks following irradiation therapy.

- Surgical options include:
  - Lung resection/lobectomy
  - Chest wall resection.
  - Resection of part of subclavian artery and grafting.
  - Vertebral body resections and resections of parts of the brachial plexus (particularly C8 and T1).
- Newer protocols that use combinations of irradiation, chemotherapy, and surgery are currently being studied to determine the best therapy.

Basics on the surgical technique

Anterior approach
Patient position
- Supine ± neck hyper-extension; head turned away from affected side.

Incision
- Cervical and upper thorax, may involve median sternotomy or removal of medial half of clavicle.
  - Affected part of the subclavian artery may be removed and a graft inserted.
  - May be completed with a posterolateral thoracotomy and upper lobectomy.

Posterior approach
Patient position
- Lateral decubitus, rotated slightly anteriorly.

Incision
- Posterolateral thoracotomy.
- Can involve division of T1 nerve root (weakness of intrinsic muscles of hand), or removal of C8 nerve root or lower trunk of brachial plexus (permanent paralysis of hand intrinsic muscles).

Vertebral body and epidural tumour
- Vertebral body infiltration only.
  - Posterolateral thoracotomy with chest wall resection, vertebral body resection and anterior stabilization.
- Vertebral body + posterior elements + epidural lesions.
  - Posterior cervico-thoracic stabilization (prone) followed by posterolateral thoracotomy and anterior resection and reconstruction (lateral).

Pre-operative assessment and preparation

History, examination, and optimization

- Pain (frequently relentless and un-remitting).
  - Shoulder and vertebral border of the scapula.
  - Along ulnar nerve distribution of the arm to the elbow and, ultimately, to the ulnar surface of the forearm and to the little and ring fingers of the hand (C8).
  - Patient usually supports the elbow of the affected arm with the opposite hand to ease the tension on the shoulder and upper arm.
- Sympathetic chain involvement
  - Ipsilateral Horner's syndrome (ptosis, meiosis, anhidrosis and nasal stuffiness).
- Weakness
  - Atrophic hand with absent triceps reflex.
- Paraneoplastic syndrome
  - Cushing syndrome, excessive antidiuretic hormone secretion, hypercalcaemia, myopathies, haematological problems, and hypertrophic osteoarthropathy (See 🕮 The patient with a paraneoplastic syndrome, p. 268).
  - The presence of paraneoplastic syndromes does not imply un-resectability, but most of these are associated with small cell cancer.

Investigations

Bloods

- **FBC, Clotting, U&Es**
- **LFT.**
  - Suspected metastases only.
- **X-Cross match.**
  - At least 2 units of blood (may need much more).
- **ABG.**

Radiology

- **CXR.**
  - May see lesion and or other pulmonary involvement.
- **CT chest/upper abdomen.**
  - To assess local extent of disease. Also facilitates percutaneous needle biopsy.
- **MRI of thoracic inlet.**
  - Including brachial plexus, subclavian vessels, spine and neural foramina.

- **MRI brain**
  - Metastases here are relatively common at diagnosis.
- **Whole Body PET**
- **Arteriogram or venogram**
  - If large vessel involvement.

Other

- **Sputum cytology**
- **ECG**
- **Mediastinoscopy**
  - Used for staging to delineate the metastases to mediastinal lymph nodes.
- **Flexible bronchoscopy**
  - Allows for targeted biopsy.
- **Physiological performance status:**
  - Renal and neurological function (to tolerate chemotherapy)
  - Pulmonary function and cardiac stress testing (to tolerate lung resection).

Anaesthesia for pancoast resection

Induction

- 2 x large bore IV access.
- IV induction, paralyses with non-depolarising muscle relaxant.
- Pre-procedure bronchoscopy often performed (as per pneumonectomy).
- DLT or bronchial blocker as OLV required.
- Place arterial line on opposite side to the surgery. Consider femoral central venous access.
- Temperature probe and urinary catheter.
- Patient warming devices (hot air blower, fluid warmers).
- DVT prophylaxis.

Maintenance and intra-operative

- Remifentanil TCI infusion
  - Useful because of variable length of procedure, often being very long with periods of intense surgical stimulation.
  - (See 📖 Thoracic epidurals, p. 686, regarding intra-operative epidural infusion)

Position

(Described above)

Post-operative and analgesia

Analgesia

- Epidural or paravertebral analgesia may be indicated for thoracotomy.
  - Epidural and paravertebral catheters are contraindicated if vertebral resection is anticipated because of the potential infection risk.

- Systemic opioids via PCA (morphine, diamorphine) plus simple analgesics are more frequently indicated.
- Regional blocks may be used
  - Continuous brachial plexus block should be considered in patients with severe pre-operative neuropathic cancer pain in the arm and shoulder.
  - A catheter can be placed via the posterior approach to the plexus (supraclavicular placement, under ultrasound guidance)
  - This technique may be better than the interscalene approach, as it is easier to secure for longer-term use and is less likely to work-loose.

Post-operative care

- Critical care environment
- Mortality rates are 2–5%.
- May require a period of post-operative ventilation if very extensive surgery or large blood loss. Aim to extubate as soon as possible.

Further reading

Rusch VW. Management of Pancoast tumours. *The Lancet Oncology*. 2006; 7:12:997–1005.

Empyema drainage (decortication)

PROCEDURE: surgical removal of pus—either video-assisted thorascopic surgery (VATS), open thoracic drainage, or thoracotomy and decortication.

TIME: drainage 20–40mins.

PAIN RATING: 3/5.

ANALGESIA: balanced analgesia, including opioids. Intercostal/paravertebral blocks useful for drainage procedures. Epidural if thoracotomy.

BLOOD LOSS: minimal if just simple drainage.

HOSPITAL STAY: 2–3 days following simple drainage; a week following thoracotomy.

PREPARATION AND EQUIPMENT: as for thoracotomy, or VATS. Intensive care bed may be required if complications arise.

Introduction
- Most present for operative drainage after failed catheter/drain eradication.
- 20% of patients with empyema die.

Pathophysiology
- Empyema.
  - Collection of pus within the lung pleura.
- Abscess.
  - Collection of pus in a newly formed cavity within the lung parenchyma.
- Both are slow to manifest and usually occur in a dependent section of the lung (R lung > L).
- Most commonly seen 1–2 weeks after aspiration of oropharyngeal secretions.
- Usually a secondary complication of pneumonia.
- Can also arise from penetrating chest trauma, oesophageal rupture, as a complication of lung surgery, or after thoracocentesis/chest tube placement.

3 progressive phases

Exudative

- Can be treated by thoracostomy tube and antibiotics.
- Fluid sample:
  - pH <7.2.
  - Glucose <40 mg/dL.
  - LDH >1000 IU/dL.
  - WBC >500/μL.
  - Specific gravity >1.018.
  - Thin serous or cloudy fluid, generally sterile.

Fibrinopurulent

- Can also be treated as with exudative, however more difficult as can be thicker pus and multiple loculations.
  - Thicker, opaque fluid or fluid with positive cultures.

Organizing phase

- Surgical intervention is indicated at this stage to adequately evacuate the infected material and to create a unified space for drainage.
- Organizing peel with entrapment of the lung.
  - Pleural fluid marker currently being studied is TNF-α.
  - In patients who have pleural effusions, a TNF-α level >80 pg/mL is suggestive of an empyema or complicated para-pneumonic effusion.

Risk factors

- Oral cavity disease.
- Altered consciousness.
  - Alcoholism.
  - Coma.
  - Drug abuse.
  - Anaesthesia.
  - Seizures.
- Immuno-compromised host.
  - Steroid therapy.
  - Chemotherapy.
  - Malnutrition.
- Multiple trauma.
- Oesophageal disease.
  - Achalasia.
  - Reflux disease.
  - Depressed cough and gag reflex.
  - Oesophageal obstruction.
- Bronchial obstruction.
  - Tumour.
  - Foreign body.
  - Stricture.

- Generalized sepsis, including a complication of severe or incompletely. treated pneumonia (particularly Staphylococci or Klebsiellae).
- Tricuspid endocarditis leading to septic pulmonary embolus.
- Extension of hepatic abscess.

Clinical features

Symptoms

- Often insidious (more acute if follows pneumonia).
- Spiking temperature with rigors and night sweats.
- Cough ± sputum production (often foul-tasting, foul-smelling and often blood-stained).
- Pleuritic chest pain.
- Breathlessness.

Signs

- Tachypnoea.
- Tachycardia.
- Finger clubbing in chronic cases.
- Dehydration.
- Pyrexia.
- Localized dullness to percussion (if consolidation also present or effusion).
- Bronchial breathing and/or crepitations (if consolidation present); look for signs of severe periodontal disease and infective endocarditis.

Management

This involves 3 core principles:

- Prompt initiation of appropriate antibiotics.
- Complete evacuation of suppurative pleural fluid.
- Preservation or restoration of lung expansion.

Medical vs. surgical management

A large literature review was undertaken in 2000 by the American College of Chest Physicians. They issued a statement regarding the treatment of parapneumonic effusions:

- The following findings suggest a moderate or high risk for a poor outcome:
  - Large, free-flowing effusion (at least half of a hemithorax).
  - Loculated effusion or effusion with thickened parietal pleura.
  - Positive cultures or Gram stains.
  - Pleural pus.
  - pH <7.20.
- When these findings are present, interventional drainage is recommended.

Exudative stage
- Thoracocentesis and antibiotics alone have been successful in 6–20% patients.

Fibrinopurulent stage
- Large-tube thoracostomy with or without the adjunctive use of fibrinolytics has been the traditional management with reported success rates of 24–78%.

Organizing phase
- Requires direct removal with open or thoracoscopic techniques.

Anaesthesia issues: thoracotomy vs. VATS

- Thoracoscopy and more recently, VATS present less invasive approaches to the management of empyema by minimizing access trauma.
  - Essentially, the same operation can be performed with VATS as in open surgery.
- VATS has been found to be particularly effective for treating the fibrinopurulent phase of empyema, in which multiple loculations can be easily disrupted to allow adequate drainage.
  - Comparitive studies between VATS and thoracotomy shows similar rates of success, but the former offers a substantial advantage in terms of disease resolution hospital stay, pain and cosmesis.

Anaesthetic management of empyema decortication
- In general, these patients have three major problems:
  - ❶ The remaining healthy lung can be soiled by the overflow of pus or infected fluid, resulting in a lung with decreased gas exchange capacity.
  - ❶ The remaining lung may also have the compromised function as a result of underlying pulmonary disease.
  - ❶ The patient's pulmonary function may be compromised because of a loss in tidal volume via a bronchopleural connection, which is a complication of empyema.

Pre-operative assessment and optimization
- Routine assessment for thoracic surgery.
  - ❶ Patient may be septic.
- O_2, IV fluids, antibiotics.
- Pre-operative physiotherapy to reduce secretions and improve oxygenation.
- Chest drain under LA—to drain any pus or fluid within the chest cavity and prevent spillage into the bronchial tree.

▶ By preventing the development of a positive pressure within the chest cavity, the chest drain can help to minimize mediastinal shift, compression of the remaining lung and haemodynamic instability.

Investigations

Bloods
- **FBC.**
  - Normocytic anaemia or neutrophilia.
- **Blood/sputum cultures**
  - Including AAFB.
- **ESR/CRP.**
- **ABG.**

Radiology
- **CXR.**
  - Walled cavity ±fluid level.
- **CT chest**
  - Multiple small abscesses.

Other
- **Fibre optic bronchoscopy**
  - Can exclude obstruction and provide samples for culture.
- **Trans-thoracic biopsy/aspiration**
  - Usually with ultrasound guidance or trans-tracheal biopsy.
  - Fluid/empyema sent for microscopy, culture and sensitivity.
- **Spirometry**.

Induction
- Objectives
  - Maintain oxygenation and ventilation.
  - Avoid soiling good lung.
- Induce in a semi-sitting position with the disease side dependent.
- Large bore IV cannula placed and drip run through a warmer.
- Arterial line.
  - Pre-induction insertion mandatory for haemodynamic monitoring and repetitive blood gas sampling.
- CVP.
  - May be needed, particularly if the patient is septic/needs longer-term antibiotic therapy.
- Spirometry:
  - Helpful to establish and quantify magnitude of air leak.

▶ The induction agent is irrelevant. However, it is important to ensure spontaneous respiration is maintained until the lung is isolated.

▶ Elective rigid bronchoscopy before double-lumen tube placement allows both surgical assessment of bronchial pathology and anatomy, and the efficient removal of airway secretions or pus.

Maintenance and intra-operative
- Intra-operative isolation of lung is mandatory and therefore the use of a double lumen tube is necessary, bronchial lumen to good side.
- While the lung containing the abscess is not being ventilated, there are both theoretical and practical benefits in connecting this lung to an oxygen reservoir at ambient pressure.
- Suction should be available at all times.

The end of the procedure
- Suction via the DLT lumen on operative side before re-expansion of the residual lobe will remove any purulent material that has drained from the abscess in the course of surgery.

Post-operative
- HDU/ITU may be indicated if the patient is septic, as they may require inotropic, vasopressor or even continued ventilator support.
- Analgesia.
  - The aim is to avoid deterioration of respiratory function, particularly if the patient is already compromised.
  - Epidural if thoracoscopic/thoracotomy drainage took place
  - However, controversy still exists as to whether this is a good idea in a septic/unstable patient.

• Consider simple analgesics as per WHO ladder, then step-up to more invasive measures to aid optimal respiratory function in the un-intubated patient (paravertebral blocks/intercostal blocks/ epidural).

Further reading

Davies C, Gleeson F, Davies R. BTS Guidelines for the management of pleural infection. *Thorax* 2003; 58:18–28.

American Thoracic Society. *An international scientific society which focuses on respiratory and critical care medicine.* www.thoracic.org (accessed 3/11/09).

Porcel JM, Vives M, Esquerda A. Tumour necrosis factor-alpha in pleural fluid: a marker of complicated parapneumonic effusions. *Chest* 2004; 125(1):160–4.

Broncho-pleural fistula repair

PROCEDURE BASICS: repair of tracheobronchial tree using glue, sutures or an allogenic tissue flap.

TIME: 2–4 hours.

PAIN RATING: 5/5.

ANALGESIA: epidural, paravertebral block, or opioid infusion.

BLOOD LOSS: usually minimal, can be torrential, XM 2–6 units.

HOSPITAL STAY: 7–14 days.

PREPARATION AND EQUIPMENT: invasive monitoring, large bore IV access, DLT, small ET tubes, bronchial blocker, airway exchange catheter, fibreoptic bronchoscope, suction catheters, forced air blower, fluid warmer.

Introduction
- A broncho-pleural fistula (BPF) is an abnormal communication between the conducting airways and pleural cavity → air leak.
- Post-operatively, BPF occurs more frequently on the right side.
- Small fistulae may be repaired endobronchially using tissue glue, while larger fistulae require surgical repair via a lateral thoracotomy (usually through a previous incision).
- BPF may be complicated by ipsilateral empyema which can potentially contaminate the unaffected lung.

Aetiology
- Typically occurs as a post-operative complication of pneumonectomy/lobectomy. Its development in this instance (particularly if early) is an independent predictor of mortality.
- Chest trauma; many victims do not reach hospital alive.
- Ruptured lung bullae.
- Necrotizing pneumonia.
- Lung abscess.
- Invasive neoplastic lesions; particularly if treated with chemo/radiotherapy.

Presenting features

Patients may present with:
- Cough ± haemoptysis.
- Sepsis 2° pneumonia/empyema.
- Respiratory distress, which is proportional to the size of fistula.
- Continuous bubbling of a chest drain or a falling fluid level in the hemithorax after pneumonectomy.
- Large air leaks may cause subcutaneous emphysema and tension pneumothorax.
  - These cases have high peri-operative morbidity and mortality and present a number of anaesthetic challenges that should not be underestimated.

Anaesthetic management

- The goals of anaesthetic management are:
  - Prevent spillage of empyema into the normal bronchus and contamination of the un-affected lung.
  - Control distribution of ventilation. An increase in the air leak from a non-isolated fistula reduces alveolar ventilation, increases pulmonary shunt, and could cause a tension pneumothorax, e.g. during IPPV.
- These can be achieved by:
  - Appropriate patient position, i.e. semi-sitting ± lateral tilt (affected side lowermost).
  - Endobronchial intubation of the main bronchus contra-lateral to the BPF using DLT/SLT, or by placement of a bronchial blocker in the main bronchus of the affected side.

Pre-operative assessment and optimization

- Patients may be increasingly debilitated for various reasons:
  - Co-existent medical co-morbidities.
  - Concurrent sepsis.
  - Recent major surgery.
- Patients may present in extremis with overt sepsis and severe respiratory failure.
- Review previous anaesthetic charts paying particular attention to ease of airway instrumentation, lung isolation and the patient's physiological behaviour during the case.
- Intercostal drains required to control air leak and drain any associated empyema.

Investigations

Bloods
- **FBC, U&E, LFT, ABG**.

Radiology
- CXR/CT chest:
  - CT useful to assess size and location of air leak
  - Look for any lower airway distortion caused by recent surgery as this can affect the placement of a DLT, endobronchial tube or bronchial blocker.

Other
- **ECG**.

Induction
- Choice of technique will depend on size of fistula, condition of patient and local expertise.
- Establish invasive arterial pressure monitoring awake.
- Thorough pre-oxygenation is essential as patients may desaturate rapidly.
- ▶ Fibreoptic guidance of endobronchial intubation is always recommended.
- ❶ Blind insertion of an endobronchial tube may enlarge the fistula.

Deep inhalational anaesthesia
- This is not especially cardio-stable.
- It can be difficult to achieve the depth of anaesthesia required for DLT insertion with sevoflurane.
- Delivery and uptake of volatile agents may be unreliable and induction of anaesthesia can be slow, especially with large air leaks.
- Passage of DLT can result in coughing and contamination of unaffected lung.

Rapid sequence induction
- Consider if no anticipated difficulty with upper airway anatomy.
- Position as above.
- Use suxamethonium.

Awake fibreoptic intubation (AFOI)
- Difficult to anaesthetize the upper airway sufficiently to allow passage of a DLT. Coughing will increase the risk of contamination.
- ❶ Deep sedation during AFOI is likely to cause significant cardio-respiratory depression and is best avoided. However, low dose remifentanil infusion may be a useful adjunct in this setting.
- Endobronchial anaesthesia is often poor. Consider induction of anaesthesia when the trachea is intubated, but prior to endobronchial intubation to avoid coughing.

Options for lung isolation

Intubation and subsequent lung isolation with an appropriately sized DLT is the method of choice. However, an adequate position may not be achievable. Alternative techniques include:
- Jet ventilation
  - Cautious jet ventilation via a rigid bronchoscope placed in the normal bronchus.
- Small standard ETT
  - A size 6 mm ID endotracheal tube may be inserted into the normal bronchus, either railroaded over a fibreoptic scope, or over a bougie placed by the surgeon via a rigid bronchoscope.
- COOK™ airway exchange catheter
  - Can be similarly placed via a rigid bronchoscope into the normal bronchus allowing temporary oxygenation.
- Bronchial blocker
  - Insert into the diseased bronchus as a temporary measure. Surgical handling may limit the effectiveness of this technique.

Post-operative
- Patients are best managed in a critical care environment with standard post-thoracotomy care.
- Extubate as soon as possible; ideally in theatre after gentle suction to the affected bronchus.
- Minimize airway pressure and PEEP if post-operative ventilation is required.
- If persistent air leak, consider independent lung ventilation or HFOV.
- ECMO has been used as a temporary bridge to recovery in refractory hypoxaemia.

Further reading

Ricci ZJ, Haramati LB, Rosenbaum AT, et al. Role of computed tomography in guiding management of peripheral bronchopleural fistula. *Journal of Thoracic Imaging* 2002; 17(3):214–8.

Hollaus PJ, Lax F, el-Nashef BB, et al. Natural history of bronchopleural fistula after pneumonectomy: a review of 96 cases. *Annals of Thoracic Surgery* 1997; 63:1391–6.

Khan NU, Al-Aloul M, Khasati N, et al. Extracorporeal membrane oxygenator as a bridge to successful surgical repair of bronchopleural fistula following bilateral sequential lung transplantation: a case report and review of literature. *Journal of Cardiothoracic Surgery* 2007; 2(28):Open Access.

Acquired tracheo-oesophageal fistula

PROCEDURE BASICS: repair of tracheo-oesophageal fistula using a muscle flap or reconstruction ± resection of the trachea.

TIME: 2–3 hours.

PAIN RATING: 3–4/5.

ANALGESIA: thoracic epidural/paravertebral depending on patient status as often manifesting sepsis.

BLOOD LOSS: usually minimal.

HOSPITAL STAY: depends on associated sequalae relating to the TOF.

PREPARATION AND EQUIPMENT: invasive monitoring advised, large bore IV access. Talk to surgeon regarding SLT and use fibreoscope to guide cuff past TOF.

Introduction

- Tracheo-oesophageal fistula (TOF) is an abnormal communication between the trachea and oesophagus.
- TOF develops as a result of apposing oesophageal and tracheal wall necrosis.
- TOF allows passage of food, saliva, and gastric contents into the lower respiratory tract. This results in atelectasis, pneumonia and respiratory distress.
- This chapter will not discuss congenital TOF.

Aetiology

Iatrogenic

- Tracheal intubation is the most common non-malignant cause of acquired TOF.
  - 75% injuries relate to prolonged, excessive ETT cuff pressure, i.e. >30 mmHg.
- Percutaneous tracheostomy.
- Previous oesophageal/tracheal surgery.
  - 4% post-oesophagectomy.
- Oesophageal instrumentation, e.g. stenting, endoscopy, echocardiography.

Blunt/penetrating trauma
- Antero-posterior crush injury to chest caused by steering wheel impact is most commonly implicated.

Malignancy
- 50% all cases secondary to mediastinal malignancy.
- 77% oesophageal cancer.

Granulomatous infection
- Tuberculosis.
- Mediastinitis.
- HIV.

Ingestion of caustic material/foreign body

Presentation
Spontaneously breathing patient
- Coughing after swallowing (Ohno's sign) ± haemoptysis.
- Chest pain.
- Breathlessness.
- Dysphagia ± hoarseness.
- Recurrent chest infection.

Ventilated
- Recurrent chest infection.
- Failure to wean.
- ↑ airway pressures, i.e. positive pressure ventilation forces gas into the stomach via the fistula, causing gastric distension and diaphragmatic splinting.
- Unexplained weight loss.

Pre-operative assessment and preparation
- The goal is to optimize cardio-respiratory function prior to surgery by:
    - Isolation of defect to prevent further tracheal soiling.
    - Identification and treatment of pneumonia.
    - Attention to nutritional status.

Specific investigations

Accurate localization is the key to management.
Radiology
- **CXR.**
  - Look for consolidation and atelectasis.
- **Barium swallow**
  - Identifies the lesion and the extent of the fistula.

Other
- **Oesophagoscopy**
- **Flexible/rigid bronchoscopy**
  - Identifies the lesion and allows broncho-alveolar lavage; thus targeted antibiotic therapy.

Initial management strategy
- Nurse head-up.
- Suppress gastric acid production, e.g. omeprazole.
- Replace existing ETT/tracheostomy tube.
  - Ensure cuff is positioned below TOF.
- Remove naso-gastric tube.
  - Insert drainage gastrostomy and feeding jejunostomy tube.
- Targeted antibiotic therapy & chest physiotherapy/pulmonary toilet.
- Aim to wean if ventilated, i.e. post-operative ventilation associated with anastomotic breakdown/stenosis and poor outcome.

Subsequent management

Inoperable
- Typically occurs in TOF caused by malignancy.
- Options to minimize further airway soiling include oesophageal stent insertion (under sedation) or tracheal stent insertion.

Surgery
- Majority have lesions in the upper two thirds of the trachea.
  - Proximal lesions require anterior/low cervical approach.
- Most TOF repairs in the adult are undertaken through a thoracotomy or an open transcervical approach.
- Large TOF may require tracheal resection/reconstruction (See 📖 Tracheal reconstruction and resection, p. 332).
- Placement of a pleural or muscle flap is used for the repair.
- Thoracoscopic approach is also possible.

Anaesthesia for repair of TOF

- The goals of anaesthetic management are to:
  - Avoid tracheal soiling.
  - Isolate TOF rapidly.
- These can be achieved by:
  - Pre-operative suppression of gastric acid production.
  - Induction of anaesthesia in semi-sitting position.
  - Knowledge of site and extent of TOF.

Induction

- Standard monitoring.
- Arterial line inserted awake.
  - Consider central venous line when patient is anaesthetized.
- Insert naso-gastric tube.
  - Leave on free drainage to mitigate/reduce gastric dilatation.
- Pre-oxygenate well.
- RSI as further aspiration will merely amplify the existing issue of tracheal/lung soiling.
- IV induction.
  - Use rocuronium or suxamthonium to facilitate intubation.
  - Pre-curarise if using suxamethonium as fasciculation can precipitate tracheal soiling.
- Use a SLT in most cases.
- Placement of the ETT cuff below the level of the TOF must be guided by fibreoptic observation.
  - Carinal TOF may necessitate endobronchial intubation with SLT; consider DLT in this instance.

Pitfalls during induction

- Positive pressure ventilation causes passage of gas via the TOF into the stomach resulting in gastric dilatation.
  - Minimize IPPV until TOF is isolated.
- The ETT cuff must lie below the level of the TOF to ensure adequate ventilation and avoidance of gastric dilatation.
- Failure to ventilate following tracheal intubation can occur when the ETT has traversed the TOF.

Maintenance and intra-operative

- IV or volatile maintenance of anaesthesia.
- Leak test, i.e. ETT cuff withdrawn to lie above repaired TOF.
- Maintain neuromuscular paralysis.
- Avoid high airway pressures at this stage.
- Analgesia dependent on surgical approach.
- Aim to extubate at end of surgery; avoid stressing suture line with high airway pressures caused by coughing.

Post-operative
- Avoid positive pressure ventilation
- Manage on HDU/ITU.

Further reading

Grebenik C. Anaesthetic management of malignant trachea-oesophageal fistula. *British Journal of Anaesthesia*, 1989; 63(4):492–6.

Diddee R, Shaw I. Acquired trachea-oesophageal fistula in adults. *Continuing Education in Anaesthesia, Critical Care & Pain* 2006; 6(3):105–8.

Radioactive pellet implantation (brachytherapy)

PROCEDURE BASICS: insertion of radioactive seeds or pellets directly into, or adjacent to an endobronchial or interstitial lung tumour. Allows delivery of targeted high dose rate radiation therapy. Usually administered in the outpatient setting using bronchscopy or CT guidance under local anaesthesia. May be inserted at the time of primary lung resection in selected cases.

TIME: variable, depending on method of insertion.

PAIN RATING: minimal if administered in outpatient setting.

ANALGESIA: post thoracotomy analgesia (Thoracic epidural/paravertebral) if inserted at time of lung resection. Basic analgesia sufficient if inserted as an outpatient.

BLOOD LOSS: minimal.

HOSPITAL STAY: home if procedure done as outpatient.

PREPARATION AND EQUIPMENT: standard equipment.

Anaesthesia for brachytherapy
- Patients may have been deemed unfit for surgery or be terminally ill with intractable symptoms.
- Most radioactive seed implantations will occur in the outpatient setting.
- Patients will have undergone the usual diagnostic and staging procedures, including lung function testing.

High dose rate brachytherapy (palliation of endobronchial symptoms)
- Treatment option in patients with endobronchial symptoms. It may be utilized for inoperable primary endobronchial lung tumours, recurrent or metastatic tumours.
  - Current NICE guidelines in the UK advise its use for palliation where other treatment options have failed.
- Catheter is inserted via a bronchoscope into the diseased bronchus through which brachytherapy treatment is given.
  - The catheter may stay in place for as little as 45 minutes and then be removed. This will usually occur in the outpatient setting under local anaesthesia.

Brachytherapy for interstitial tumours (pre-resection)
- Performed under CT-fluoroscopy guidance with local anaesthesia. Seeds or pellets can be placed directly into the tumour, and then the tumour treated under computer control.
- Radioactive pellets (containing 125I) can be implanted at the time of primary lung resection when gross or microscopic positive surgical margins are discovered.
- Gel foam radioactive plaques may also be inserted along the tumour beds at the time of resection.

Post-operative
- Those patients undergoing the procedure in the outpatient setting under local anaesthesia will require a minimal hospital stay.
- Low dose radiation will be emitted from the seeds, so patients are advised to avoid contact with pregnant women and young children for a few weeks after the procedure.
- Patients who have undergone thoracotomy and lung resection will require the usual post-operative care and analgesia in an appropriate facility.

Special considerations
- Currently, radioactive seed implantation is undergoing further evaluation as a treatment modality for lung tumours, including rare tumours such as mediastinal carcinoid tumours.
- Advantages of this treatment include the ability to direct high dose radiation direct to the tumour whilst reducing radiation injury to nearby structures.
- It may be particularly useful in patients with recurrent tumours where external beam radiation offers limited success.
- Other indications for radioactive pellet implantation in the future may include bleeding from an endobronchial lesion, and in the treatment of in situ lung cancer.

Further reading
Kennedy MP, Jimenez CA, Chang J, et al. Optimization of bronchial brachytherapy catheter placement with a modified airway stent. *European Respiratory Journal.* 2008; 31:902–3.

Mutoa P, Ravoa V, Panellia G, et al. High-Dose Rate Brachytherapy of Bronchial Cancer: Treatment Optimization Using Three Schemes of Therapy. *The Oncologist.* 2000; 5(3):209–14.

Anaesthesia for lung transplantation

Introduction

- 1963 first lung transplant (LT)—patient survived just 18 days.
- Between 1963 and 1974 136 lung transplants were done worldwide—only two patients survived for >2 months.
- Introduction of Cyclosporin A in 1981 and other steroid sparing immunosuppressants have improved the outcome.
- Survival after single lung transplant (SLTX).
  - 90% for 3 months.
  - 80% for 1 year.
  - 60% for 3 years.
  - 45% for 5 years.
- Survival outcome is slightly better after Double Lung Transplant (DLTX).
- Living lobar transplants (LLT) are performed in special units.
  - Right and left lower lobes are harvested from two living donors and transplanted sequentially preceded by pneumonectomy on the corresponding side.

Indications

- Indications for surgery depend on pulmonary ± cardiac disease and local guidelines (See Table 6.5).
- ☞ Lung allocation score (LAS) was introduced in 2005 based on predicted survival with and without transplant.

Table 6.5 Indications for lung transplantation

SLTX	DLTX	Heart & Lung
End stage pulmonary disease, limited life expectancy (<1 yr)	End stage pulmonary disease, limited life expectancy (<1 yr)	End stage cardiac and Pulmonary disease
<65 yrs	<60 yrs	<55 yrs
Emphysema (FEV$_1$ <25%, PaCO$_2$ >7.3 kPa, pulmonary hypertension).	Cystic fibrosis (FEV$_1$ <30%, rapid worsening, PaCO$_2$ >6.7 kPa, PaO$_2$ <7.3 kPa)	Eisenmengers with uncorrectable cardiac defect
Idiopathic pulmonary fibrosis (hypoxia at rest, FVC <70%, DLCO <50%)	Bronchiectasis (same as above)	NYHA class III or IV
α- 1 antitrypsin deficiency	α -1 antitrypsin deficiency	
Primary pulmonary hypertension (NYHA class III or IV, CI <2 L/min/m^2, RAP >15 mmHg, mean PAP >55 mmHg)	Emphysema	

Donor criteria
Criteria vary between institutions and are influenced by demand and experience.
- 👉 Donor characteristics:
  - Age <55 yrs.
  - Smoking <20 pack years.
  - Clear chest x-ray.
  - PaO_2 >40 kPa on 100% FiO_2 and PEEP 5 cmH_2O.
  - Absence of previous chest trauma and surgery, and current infection.
- 👉 Lung characteristics:
  - Ischaemia time <6 hours.
  - Total lung capacity matched using height and sex.
  - ABO and HLA compatibility matching.

> 25% of mortality from transplant failure is attributed to poor quality of donor lung; importance of rigorous screening of donors and maintenance of good organ function in the donor after brain stem death.

Pre-operative assessment and preparation
Except in LLT, surgery is done as an emergency, with <6 hrs to prepare patient.

Transplant program entry
- If BMI <17 kg/m^2 feeding via enteral route.
- Steroids should be weaned to <20 mg prednisolone/day.
- Repeated courses of antibiotics—cystic fibrosis (CF).

Assess the need for Cardio-Pulmonary-Bypass (CPB)
- COPD and interstitial lung disease—no need for CPB.
- CPB is routinely used during LLT to avoid entire CO going through the first transplanted lobe and when pulmonary hypertension is severe.
- ECMO—preferable when no cardiac support is needed, only need partial anti-coagulation.

- There is emergent use of partial CPB or ECMO as a last resort in cases of:
  - Reperfusion injury of 1st transplant lung during sequential DLTX—severe and intractable hypoxia.
  - Unexpected right heart failure—CI <2.0 L/min/m^2, SvO$_2$ <60%, MPAP >45 mmHg when clamped.
  - Severe hypoxia due to troublesome thick secretions eg. Cystic fibrosis.

Immunosuppressant therapy

- Cyclosporin A (10 mg/kg) or tacrolimus is best given orally 5–7 hrs pre-operatively to avoid interaction with anaesthetic agents if given IV at induction.
- Azothioprine (2 mg/kg) or mycophenolate mofetil, prednisolone and prophylactic antibiotics should be administered 60 mins before GA.

Anaesthesia for lung transplant

Induction

- Gentle and slick anaesthetic technique.
- Use drugs with minimal cardio-depressant and histamine releasing properties.
- Close monitoring and aggressive management of physiological derangement is essential.
- Invasive monitoring should be instituted before induction.
  - Arterial line, CVP line, PAFC, trans-oesophageal-echocardiogram (TOE, after induction), non-invasive cardiac output monitoring.
- Fluid restriction to minimize pulmonary oedema.
- Exemplary asepsis is mandatory.

⚠ Epidural blockade is invaluable but its placement must be delayed if full or partial CPB is indicated or anticipated → use remifentanil IVI per-operatively.

⚠ Special considerations and difficulties

See also Table 6.6

- The recipient, by normal criteria for thoracotomy, will be very high risk for surgery.
- There are 5 main problem areas:

Induction

- Poor pulmonary reserve → serious and precipitous hypoxia at induction.
  - If severe consider femoral vessel cannulation for ECMO.
- Poor cardiac reserve → acute drop in cardiac output (CO) and BP.
  - If severe acidosis → consider femoral vessel cannulation for CPB before induction.

Airway options

- Segmental lavage via an ETT is useful before lung isolation in cystic fibrosis (CF).
- OLV is achieved with DLT (usually L) in CF & bronchiectasis to enable suction of secretions.
- ETT with a bronchial blocker located on the side of pneumonectomy is adequate in other cases.
- ETT alone if CPB is used.

Initiation of one lung ventilation (OLV)

- Emphysema → dynamic hyper-inflation → hypoxia and hypotension.
  - Disconnect from ventilator, allow deflation and reconnect. Exclude pneumothorax if patient fails to improve.
  - Use smaller tidal volume, no PEEP and prolonged expiratory time at a slower rate → permissive hypercapnia.
  - Use a ventilator with flow and pressure measurements.
- Interstitial lung disease → poor compliance.
  - Use protective ventilation strategy (low V_T, higher frequency or pressure limited).

Pulmonary artery clamping

- Pre-existing pulmonary hypertension and clamping of PA → severe PH, RV failure, hypoxia and systemic hypotension.
  - ∴ do not use N_2O → may worsen pulmonary hypertension. Norepinephrine and inhaled NO are shown to help.
  - If severe PH use CPB electively.

Pulmonary artery un-clamping

- Give 2nd dose of prednisolone prior to un-clamping.
- Washout of pneumoplegic solution along with PGE_1 and products of ischaemia → short period of hypotension.
- If hypotension is persistent or severe, exclude the following using TOE:
  - Pulmonary artery stenosis or kinking → hypotension.
  - Pulmonary vein stenosis or thrombosis → hypotension.

- RVF due to R coronary artery occlusion → hypotension
- ☛ Aprotinin may reduce graft dysfunction but may risk renal impairment.

▶ Laparotomy to harvest omentum for wrapping around the bronchial suture line is no longer done. Current telescopic surgical technique to anastomose the bronchus is adequate.

Post-operative

2 main approaches:
- Extubation in theatre is possible and has advantages:
  - No need to exchange SLT for DLT.
  - Optimization of cough and sputum clearance.
  - Avoid IPPV → anastamotic leak and barotrauma.
  - Early awakening and mobilization.
- IPPV on ICU and early extubation (within 6 hours).
  - 90% will have reperfusion injury ∴ protective ventilation.
  - Restrictive fluid regim.

Early post-operative mortality caused by

- Infection.
- Rejection.
- Hypoxic ischaemic encephalopathy.
- Ischaemic reperfusion injury.
- Others.
  - Neurological injury, drug toxicity, excess bleeding, acute RVF and muscle weakness.

Key post-operatively care points

Good analgesia

- Multi-modal—opioid sparing agents (tramadol and paracetamol) and regional anaesthesia.
- Allows effective coughing and ventilation.
- Avoid NSAID's to minimize renal failure (already at risk from cyclosporine induced nephrotoxicity).

CXR infiltrates

- Almost universal after transplant.
- Caused by ischaemic re-perfusion injury associated with alveolar and endothelial leakage and poor interstitial fluid clearance due to absent lymphatics.
- Also caused by rejection and infection.

COPD patients with SLTX

- Native lung at risk of hyper-inflation due to its high compliance
- Leads to mediastinal shift and haemodynamic compromise
- May consider differential lung ventilation to minimize pressures.

- Post-operative oxygen therapy.
  - Allograft lacks stretch receptors.
  - Makes recipient prone to CO_2 retention.
  - If used to hypoxia-stimulated chemoreceptors for respiratory drive ... may only need pre-op O_2 saturation (87–92% sometimes suffices).
- Continue triple immunosuppressive therapy for life.
  - Co-trimoxazole for life, gancyclovir and itraconazole for 6 months.
- Monitor for and treat rejection.

Table 6.6 Intra-operative problems and their management

Event	Problem	Management
Onset of one lung ventilation	↓ SpO$_2$	↑ FiO$_2$, clamp pulmonary artery early, correct low CO; CPB if severe and intractable
	↑ PaCO$_2$	↑ minute ventilation, permissive hypercapnia if CVS stable, CPB if unstable
Clamping pulmonary artery	↑ Pulmonary Artery Pressure	Norepinephrine, inhaled nitric oxide; if severe RVF then CPB
Donor lung perfused	↓ SpO$_2$	Clamp PA if being ventilated
		Low volume ventilation with 100% O$_2$ via tube inserted into bronchus by surgeon
		CPB if hypoxia during sequential DLTX

Further reading

Orens JB, Estenne M, *et al.* International Guidelines for the selection of Lung Transplant Candidates: 2006 Update—A consensus Report from the Pulmonary Scientific Council of the International Society for Heart .and Lung Transplantation. *Journal of Heart Lung Transplant* 2006; 25:745–55.

De Perrot M, Bonser RS, *et al.* Report of the ISHLT Working Group on Primary Lung Graft Dysfunction Part III: Donor-related Risk Factors and Markers. *Journal of Heart Lung Transplant* 2005; 24:1460–7.

Chapman S, Robinson G, Stradling J, *et al* 2005. Lung Transplantation. In: *Oxford Handbook of Respiratory Medicine*. Oxford University Press, pp. 380–9.

Pulmonary embolectomy

Surgical and percutaneous embolectomy are treatment options for massive PE. However the quoted mortality is high.

Why is embolectomy being tried?

- Massive PE is life-threatening, with a high mortality rate despite standard medical treatment.
- In massive PE recommended practice is to use thrombolysis. However this may be contraindicated or be ineffective.
- Some case series report as high as 86% 1 year survival after surgical embolectomy, suggesting improvement in outcome with invasive techniques. However, currently there is insufficient evidence to establish definitive guidelines for its use.

Indication for embolectomy

- BTS suggest invasive approaches should be considered in massive PE where facilities and expertise are readily available.
- Where thrombolysis is contraindicated, or has failed, and the patient is critically ill, large emboli can be successfully fragmented using mechanical techniques via a right heart catheter, or removed with surgical embolectomy.
- Some evidence suggests embolectomy can facilitate reduction of pulmonary hypertension, and recovery of right ventricular function.

Open surgical embolectomy

- CTPA or echocardiography will reliably diagnose clinically massive PE:
  - CTPA reliably demonstrates both proximal thrombus and acute right ventricular dilatation.
  - Transthoracic echocardiography will demonstrate a massive PE, but TOE is more reliable for demonstrating intrapulmonary and intracardiac thrombus. However, availability is limited.
- If considering embolectomy after failed thrombolysis, re-image if feasible, to ensure surgically accessible clot remains—i.e. proximal to the first pulmonary artery branches.
- Surgical approach is commonly via median sternotomy.
- Cardiopulmonary bypass (CPB) is frequently used, and may give the best chance of stabilizing the circulation in the patient with severe haemodynamic compromise.

Conduct of anaesthesia

- Challenging as a result of the hemodynamic instability.
- Compromised cardiac function results in systemic blood pressure becoming predominantly dependent on compensatory increases in systemic vascular resistance and heart rate.

- Consequently, haemodynamic deterioration during induction is common, as the ability to compensate for any myocardial depression or systemic vasodilatation is limited.
- Haemodynamic collapse after induction, with hypotension refractory to inotropes or fluid administration, will require cardiopulmonary resuscitation followed by urgent institution of CPB.
- Patients should be prepared and draped before induction, and a cardiac surgical team should be immediately available for emergency institution of CPB.
- Consideration should be given to using femoro-femoral CPB prior to inducing anesthesia in patients with severe right ventricular dysfunction. The risk of venous thromboembolism associated with instrumentation of the femoral vein has to be weighed against the risk of hemodynamic collapse on induction.

Percutaneous embolectomy
- Minimally invasive option when thrombolysis fails/contraindicated, as an alternative to surgical embolectomy.
- Three catheter interventional techniques are currently available:
  - aspiration thrombectomy.
  - fragmentation thrombectomy.
  - rheolytic thrombectomy.
- A recent review suggests all these devices may be useful, with clinical success over 70%, and low rates of serious complications.
- Devices remove, fragment, macerate or aspirate embolic mass, aiming to relieve central obstruction to improve haemodynamics.
- Complications include perforation or dissection of cardiovascular structures, pericardial tamponade, pulmonary haemorrhage, distal thrombus embolization.

The future?
- The transfer of patients, who do not respond to thrombolysis, to a cardiothoracic centre that can offer embolectomy could be considered.
- Extracorporeal life support has also been used for massive pulmonary embolism, as a supportive measure to enable embolectomy or emboli resolution with anticoagulation. A case series reported an overall survival rate of 62%. This may represent an improvement in prognosis in an otherwise near fatal condition.

Surgical embolectomy—Key points
- High risk invasive procedure performed on patients who are likely to have profound haemodynamic instability.
- No established evidence for its use, but recent literature suggests improved outcomes with surgical and catheter embolectomy in massive PE.
- RCTs are required to confirm the validity of these claims.
- Availability limited to specialist centres.

Further reading

British Thoracic Society Guidelines for the management of suspected acute pulmonary embolism, 2003. The British Thoracic Society Standards of Care Committee, Pulmonary Embolism Guideline Development Group. *Thorax*. 2003; 58:470–84.

Kucher N, Rossi E, De Rossa M, *et al.* Massive Pulmonary Embolism. *Circulation* 2006; 113(4):577–82.

Rosenberger P, Shernan SK, Shekar PS, *et al.* Acute hemodynamic collapse after induction of general anesthesia for emergent pulmonary embolectomy. *Anesthesia and Analgesia* 2006; 102:1311–5.

Pneumonectomy

PROCEDURE BASICS: excision of entire lung. Right pneumonectomy presents more of a physiological insult than removal of the left.

TIME: 1–4 hrs.

PAIN RATING: 4–5/5.

ANALGESIA: thoracic epidural analgesia or paravertebral analgesia ± PCA advised.

BLOOD LOSS: mild/moderate.

HOSPITAL STAY: 4–7 days; ITU will be required with step-down to HDU after 24 hours or so.

PREPARATION AND EQUIPMENT: jet ventilation for initial bronchoscopy. Standard monitoring. R DLT for L pneumonectomy (speak to surgeon). Arterial line and CVP line required (particularly important for post-operative fluid monitoring).

Removal of one lung may represent a significant physiological challenge to the patient.

Indications
- Bronchial carcinoma that can not be adequately excised with a lesser resection.
- Traumatic lung injury.
- Inflammatory/Infective lung conditions.
- Congenital lung disorders.

Pre-operative assessment and preparation
History and optimization
- Patients should have a pre-operative assessment in line with the BTS guidelines regarding fitness for surgery and operability.
  - (See 📖 BTS Guidelines, p. 158).
- Potentially multiple medical co-morbidities.
- Illicit smoking history and inter-related problems.
- Pre-operative staging.
  - Underestimates extent of disease in up to 50%.
  - Patient MUST be free of pleural metastases or mediastinal extension.
  - Spinal, chest wall, diaphragmatic and mediastinal invasion should be excluded.

Pulmonary hypertension
- Constitutes a relative contraindication to pneumonectomy.
- Particularly important for right-sided surgery since the right lung receives the greater proportion of the cardiac output.

Nutrition
- An area frequently overlooked is the nutritional status, although in reality little can be done to normalize this in the time window available for cancer surgery.

Anaesthetic charts
- Patients may have had recent staging procedures such as bronchoscopy, mediastinoscopy and thoracoscopy and these anaesthetic charts may offer further valuable information.

Blood loss
- Usually minimal but potentially catastrophic. Therefore, patients should be cross-matched pre-operatively.

Anaesthesia for pneumonectomy

Induction
- More than 2 large bore IV cannulae.
- Invasive arterial monitoring and CVP monitoring.
- Urinary catheter.
- Insert mid-thoracic epidural (if used) prior to induction.
  - Consider paravertebral analgesia ± PCA.
- Propofol/remifentanil TIVA.
  - A useful technique to cover the rigid bronchoscopy prior to the main procedure.
  - Bronchoscopy immediately prior to surgery dictates that there is a minimum of 2 cm of main-stem bronchus free of tumour.
- Maintenance via TIVA or volatile/relaxant technique.
- Following this a double lumen endobronchial tube (DLT) is inserted and its position confirmed clinically and with fibreoptic bronchoscopy.

Right or left DLT?

- Consider a R DLT for a Left pneumonectomy.
- Ask the surgeon what they would prefer.
  - Special care must be taken to avoid obstruction of the right upper lobe bronchus during its placement.
  - Check and re-check!
  - If a left DLT is used for left pneumonetomy the tube must be pulled back prior to bronchial cross-clamping.

Position
- Left or right lateral decubitus with table break or bridge.
- DLT movement may occur during movement and its position should be re-checked with fibreoptic bronchoscopy.

Maintenance and intra-operative

- Institution of OLV should occur prior to thoracotomy.
- Once OLV is established either pressure limited or volume limited ventilation may be used.
  - The jury is out as to which mode is more appropriate regarding 30-day morbidity.
- Use a V_T of 6–8 ml ideal body weight and a PiP of <30 cmH$_2$O.
- Desaturation and problems with tube position are discussed. (See 🕮 Post-pneumonectomy pulmonary oedema (PPO) and OLV, p. 622).
- It is worth taking a blood gas sample at the mid-way point of the procedure in order to assess how well the patient is coping with the procedure physiologically.
- Normothermia should be maintained and forced air warming blankets are useful in this context.

The end of the procedure

- Take a final ABG to assess final physiological status of the patient.
- Ensure that the patient is physiologically as near normal as is possible.
  - Warm, haemodynamically stable, good effective analgesia.
  - Is there anything else that can be done to further optimize the patient with the insight of the ABG result?

Post-operative

ITU/HDU

- Initial 12–24 hours on ITU recommended.
- Step-down to a dedicated HDU/Thoracic HDU.

Intercostal chest drains

- Although some surgeons do not use a drain most patients have one basal drain.
  - The drain is largely to determine if the patient is bleeding.
  - Drain management protocols vary.
  - A common practice is to clamp the drain immediately after surgery and then to release the clamp for 5 min every hour to reveal any haemorrhage.
  - ❶ Applying suction to the chest drain after a pneumonectomy can be catastrophic and should be avoided!

Nutrition

- Early enteral nutrition is encouraged in most centres.

IV fluids

- Excessive intravenous fluid should be avoided and a careful fluid balance maintained.
  - (See section below).

Chest physiotherapy
- An important post-operative adjuvant, reducing atelectasis, sputum retention and subsequent respiratory infections.

Pain team and epidural analgesia
- Regular reviews of analgesia are appropriate and an input from the hospital pain team may be helpful.
- Thoracic epidural/paravertebral infusions should be weaned off after 24 hours or so and, replaced with the appropriate regimen (e.g. IV PCA with simple analgesia as adjuncts).
  - Early epidural fall-out is a huge problem in the UK.
  - If fall-out occurs early, there should be serious consideration of re-insertion to minimize morbidity.
  - Those that fail/fall-out within the required analgesia period should be reviewed as early as possible with a view to PCA/other forms of analgesia as later re-insertion may be associated with higher morbidity.

⚠ Special considerations and problems

Intravenous fluid therapy
- Controversial area.
  - Although hypovolaemia should be avoided, excessive fluid administration is associated with a worse outcome in patients who develop post-pneumonectomy pulmonary oedema (See 📖 Post-pneumonectomy pulmonary oedema (PPO) and OLV, p. 622).

❶ CVP rise on clamping of the pulmonary artery
- If a significant rise occurred on test clamping of the pulmonary artery, this suggests an un-compliant RV.
  - This should alert the clinician to post-operative complications including arrhythmias, ischaemia and RV infarction which carries a high mortality.

Intra-operative hypotension
- This often results from the vasodilatory effects of general anaesthesia and the thoracic epidural induced sympathectomy.
- Should be treated with vasoactive drugs, not excessive fluids.

Arrhythmias
- Particularly common during the surgical handling that takes place during an intra-pericardial pneumonectomy.
  - It may be prudent to ask the surgeon to stop temporarily.
  - Atrial fibrillation is a common complication of pneumonectomy.
  - The use of intra-operative drugs to reduce the incidence of AF remains controversial.

Other considerations
- *Tracheal stump* once the resection is complete the surgeon will usually ask for a valsalva manoeuver to check integrity of the bronchial stump. Gentle endobronchial suction is advisable, to remove blood and debris. An airway pressure of 20–30 cm H_2O is usually appropriate. This is usually done with hand ventilation.
- After a pneumonectomy there is a slow build up of serous fluid within the pleural cavity. Complete opacification of the cavity takes several months and in some patients an-air fluid level persists indefinitely.
- *Extubation* is possible in the vast majority of cases and is performed awake in a sitting position with established good-quality analgesia. Short acting volatile agents/remifentanil can be useful in achieving rapid extubation conditions.
- *Post-pneumonectomy pulmonary oedema* occurs in approximately 2–4% of cases and carries a high (>50%) mortality. The exact pathogenesis remains unclear but is unlikely to be simply due to increased hydrostatic forces seen in hypervolaemia. It appears to mimic ARDS, and lung injury from mechanical ventilation, circulating inflammatory mediators and oxidative stress may all be implicated in its development.
- *Post-pneumonectomy syndrome*—a late complication, usually seen in children and young adults after right sided surgery. Manifests as progressive exertional dyspnoea, stridor, recurrent infection and occasionally syncope. It results from mediastinal shift towards the side of surgery with the heart, great vessels and occasionally the remaining lung herniating to the contralateral hemithorax and may require surgical correction.

Other complications
- Operative mortality should not exceed 8% for pneumonectomy. Post-operative morbidity is relatively common (>50%) and includes:
  - Post-operative respiratory failure.
  - Arrhythmias.
  - Infection.
  - Cardiac herniation (on resumption of supine position).
  - Bronchopleural fistulae.
  - Haemorrhage.
  - Chylothorax.
  - Myocardial infarction (commonly right ventricular infarct).
  - Pulmonary embolism.

Further reading

British Thoracic Society Guidelines on the selection of patients for lung cancer surgery. *Thorax* 2001; 56:89–108.

Jordan S, Mitchell JA, Quinlan GJ, *et al.* The pathogenesis of lung injury following pulmonary resection. *European Respiratory Journal* 2000; 15(4):629–30.

Fernandez-Perez ER, Keegan MT, Brown DR, *et al.* Intra-operative tidal volume as a risk factor for respiratory failure after pneumonectomy. *Anesthesiology* 2006; 105(1):14–8.

Lobectomy (open & video-assisted)

PROCEDURE BASICS: as for thoracotomy, sternotomy or video-assisted thoracoscopy.

TIME: 2–4 hours.

PAIN RATING: 2–4/5, highest after thoracotomy.

ANALGESIA: thoracic epidural, paravertebral block, intercostal nerve block and PCA as appropriate.

BLOOD LOSS: minimal.

HOSPITAL STAY: 5–7 days following thoracotomy. HDU needed; ITU governed by patient co-morbidity and surgical outcome (complications etc.).

PREPARATION AND EQUIPMENT: as for thoracotomy, sternotomy or VATS. Arterial line, CVP line as per patient co-morbidity.

Introduction

- Lobectomy describes the surgical removal of an entire lobe ± associated lymph nodes.
- Cancer is the most common indication for lobectomy. Other indications include benign tumours, TB and bronchiectasis.
- ~45% of all lung carcinomas are limited to the chest. Surgical resection is an important therapeutic modality and is effective in disease control.
- Patients with T1N0 and T2N0 tumours have early lung cancer, and most are curable by resection.
- T1N0 status patients have 5-year survival rates in the range of 75–80%.
- Lobectomy is the "gold standard" surgery, regardless of tumour size at presentation.

Pre-operative assessment and preparation

- BTS guidelines state factors determining fitness for surgery:
  - Age.
  - Pre-operative pulmonary function.
  - Cardiovascular fitness.
  - Nutrition and performance status.

- Guidelines also state factors determining operability:
  - Diagnosis and staging.
  - Adjuvant therapy.
  - The available operations.
  - Locally advanced disease.
  - Small cell lung cancer.

Lung function tests—BTS guidelines

- FEV_1 >1.5 L is recommended by the BTS as this is associated with a <5% mortality.
- (See 📖 BTS Guidelines, p. 158).
- Higher value is placed upon the calculation of % predicted FEV_1 (ppoFEV_1) for lung resection surgery.
- Pre-operative DLCO (%predicted) is more closely correlated to post-operative mortality than %predicted FEV_1.

Exercise testing

(See 📖 Cardio-pulmonary exercise testing, p. 208).
- Should be performed if lung function testing provides unclear results.
- Inverse relationship between exercise tolerance and post-operative complications.
- CPEX is the 'gold standard'.
- ∴MWT or shuttle testing follow this if no CPEX available.
- Shuttle test is most comparable screening test to VO_2 max.
- Flights of stairs give a rough surrogate for FEV_1
  - → flight is 20 steps, each of 6 inches in height.
  - 3 flights=1.7 L
  - 5 flights= 2 L.

Anaesthesia for open lobectomy

Induction

- Awake thoracic epidural insertion.
- Awake one-shot paravertebral block.
- IV access; x2 large bore cannulae.
- Arterial line; consider insertion pre-induction in patients with significant cardiovascular disease.
- Lobectomy is usually preceded by bronchoscopy.
- Pre-oxygenate.

- TIVA or IV induction followed by volatile maintenance after bronchoscopy.
- Deep neuromuscular blockade required to prevent coughing during bronchoscopy.
- Consider central line (operative side) insertion.
  - Central venous access may not be needed if the patient is medically/physiologically fit.

Airway and lung isolation

- Left-sided double lumen tube most common technique.
  - Advantages of DLT include ease and speed of lung deflation and re-inflation.
- Check position clinically and with fibreoscope.
- Bronchial blocker may be used, although lung deflation may take longer.
- Remember that a left-sided lobectomy may be converted to a left pneumonectomy, i.e. a tube in the left main bronchus will hinder surgery.
- Use spirometry to assess the impact of one lung ventilation on respiratory mechanics.

Maintenance and intra-operative

- Avoid nitrous oxide.
- Ventilation:
  - Use an appropriate ventilation strategy, i.e. ~6–8 ml/kg during TLV or OLV.
  - PEEP on the dependent lung may be necessary for oxygenation, but the increased airway pressure may increase shunt through the non-ventilated lung and exacerbate VQ mismatch (See 🕮 Abnormalities of Q and V, the diffusion of gases and hypoxic pulmonary vasoconstriction, p. 2).
- Conservative fluid management is recommended to avoid post-operative pulmonary oedema.
- Maintain normothermia:
  - IV fluid warmers and forced air warmers are essential.
  - Hypothermia predisposes to shivering which increases O_2 demand and CO_2 production which may delay extubation.
- Suck out secretions thoroughly before gently re-inflating the lung.

The end of the procedure

- Ensure good quality analgesia prior to extubation.
- Aim to extubate immediately after surgery; sit patient up.
- Humidified oxygen.
- Appropriate maintenance fluids.

- CXR.
- Level 2 care in the immediate post-operative phase. Respiratory complications are common and may necessitate a step to level 3 care or return to theatre.
- Low threshold for vasopressor therapy (especially with concurrent epidural).
- Be aware of a tendency for the development of pulmonary oedema in the manipulated lung.

Post-operative and analgesia

Thoracic epidural

- Considered the gold the standard. This should be placed whilst awake, and an assessment of effectiveness made prior to induction.
- Level chosen should cover the thoracotomy scar (T8-T9).
  - Test doses of choice vary between clinicians, some favour lidocaine/bupivacaine mix.
  - The key is cautious awake test dosing to assess for subarachnoid placement.
  - Epidural opioid may also be used, e.g. fentanyl 50–100 mcg/diamorphine 2.5–5 mg stat.

Should you run an intra-operative epidural infusion?

- There is continued debate as to whether to run an epidural intra-operatively, or leave dosing up to full surgical anaesthesia until the end of the procedure.

Disadvantages

- Unwise to run an infusion in a haemo-dynamically unstable patient.
- Unwise to run an infusion during a procedure where there is anticipated heavy blood loss, as physiological compensatory responses are blunted.
- Tachycardia and hypotension could be your epidural, or continued blood loss; difficult to know?
- Vasodilatation creates an effectively hypovolaemic circulation.
  - Over-infusion of IV fluid to bring haemodynamic parameters back to normal levels may result in fluid overload, intra/post-op pulmonary oedema, un-necessary cardiac workload, and at worst an ischaemic cardiac event.
  - Use bolus dose vasopressors, and/or infusions.

Advantages
- Good intra-operative analgesia.
- More stable haemodynamic parameters.
  - Smoothing of BP and heart rate swings intra-operatively.
- A more comfortable, settled patient in recovery and immediately post-operatively.
- Possibly lower incidence of immediate post-operative nausea/vomiting.
- Lower incidence of opioid narcosis/respiratory depression; permits swifter extubation.

- One shot paravertebral block in the anaesthetic room pre-operatively, with surgically-placed catheter inserted towards the end of the procedure has been used with success.
- Simple analgesia should not be forgotten, i.e. paracetamol and NSAIDs (if no contraindication).

VATS assisted lobectomy
(See 📖 Video-assisted thoracoscopic surgery (VATS), p. 316).
- This procedure makes use of a smaller incision (5 cm) and there is no need for rib excision or spreading and extensive muscle dissection.
- This leads to a more comfortable and rapid recovery.
- Candidates include those with early disease, peripheral lesions (surrounded by normal parenchyma), and no previous chest wall surgery or radiotherapy/chemotherapy for lung cancer.

Analgesia
- Paravertebral block ± PCA.
- Endoscopic placement of paravertebral catheters is possible.
- If converted to thoracotomy epidural insertion should be considered prior to waking.
- Evidence suggests that there are similar survival rates compared to open lobectomy via thoracotomy.

Wedge resection/segmentectomy (open & video-assisted)

PROCEDURE BASICS: surgical resection of part of a pulmonary lobe (frequently for a tumour) by either an open thoracotomy or by a video-assisted thoracoscopic approach (VATS).

TIME: 1–4h (Segmentectomy can be challenging).

PAIN RATING: 2–5/5.

ANALGESIA: thoracic epidural or paravertebral block appropriate for open surgery. Paravertebral block and/or IV-PCA system appropriate for VATS procedure.

BLOOD LOSS: minimal/moderate.

HOSPITAL STAY: 3–5 days.

PREPARATION AND EQUIPMENT: DLT, arterial line, ± CVP line if patient co-morbidity necessitates.

Introduction
- Pulmonary resections of less than an anatomic lobectomy.
- Initially wedge resections were largely undertaken for diagnosis or resection of non-malignant conditions, but now metastatic tumours as well as primary cancers are removed via this approach.
- Segmental resections are the least common type of pulmonary resection performed and can be technically more challenging than either a lobectomy or pneumonectomy.

Two distinct categories
- Anatomic.
  - Resection demarcated by the lymphatic drainage and bronchial branches of the segments resected.
  - Otherwise known as segmentectomy.
  - Provides a theoretical, but unproven, advantage over non-anatomic wedge resection in the treatment of primary lung cancer.
- Non-anatomic
  - Commonly referred to as a wedge resection.

Indication
- Resection of pulmonary metastasis.
- Diagnosis of pulmonary nodules or diffuse pulmonary disease if needle biopsy inappropriate or unsuccessful.
- Resection of pulmonary primary in patients unable to tolerate a lobectomy.

- Research has demonstrated that segmentectomy and wedge resection are realistic and reasonable alternatives to complete lobectomy in cancer patients.
- In general, segmentectomy and wedge resection are reserved for those patients with small peripheral tumours, (<3 cm in diameter confined to the outer 1/3 of the lung parenchyma).
- Peripheral tumours at the lung apex, lung base or adjacent to a fissure are most amenable to wedge resection.

Pre-operative assessment and preparation

History and optimization

- A range of patients are scheduled for wedge resections. These include otherwise fit patients with for example lung metastasis and patients with primary lung cancer who are not considered to have sufficient pulmonary reserve to undergo more extensive resections.
- New guidelines suggest that patients who would previously have been considered unsuitable for resective lung surgery should now be considered for surgery.
- The poor pulmonary function of patients considered, 'not fit', for more extensive resection increases their risk of post-operative pulmonary complications.
- Radiotherapy/chemotherapy may be more risky for these patients than surgery.
- Moderate to severe COPD may need medical optimization with treatment of any underlying infections.
- Patients on steroids may require peri-operative corticosteroid replacement therapy (See 📖 Steroids, p. 68).

Investigations

Bloods
- **FBC, U&E, LFT, X-match, ABG.**

Radiology
- **CXR.**
  - Extent and location of lesion.
  - COPD and/or infective exacerbations.
  - Other pathology.
- **CT chest and PET.**
  - Particularly important in localizing/identifying lymph node involvement.
  - Sub-lobar resections are contraindicated in those with nodal disease.

Other
- **SPO$_2$** on air
- **ECG.**
- **Echocardiogram.**
  - If warranted by clinical history.
- **PFT.**
  - Assessment of COPD/operability.
- **Flow-volume loops**
  - Assessment of COPD/operability.

Anaesthesia for wedge resection/segmentectomy

- Bronchoscopy will frequently be performed at the time of the main procedure in order to identify:
  - Areas of extrinsic segmental compression.
  - Presence of endoluminal tumour.
  - Areas of abnormal segmental anatomy to aid surgical planning.

Induction

- For open surgery.
  - DLT, invasive monitoring and thoracic epidural or paravertebral.
- For VATS.
  - DLT, arterial pressure monitoring and paravertebral/PCA.
  - Consider thoracic epidural if poor pulmonary function.
- Maintenance with volatile or TIVA.

Position

- Lateral decubitus position.

Maintenance and intra-operative

- Minimize peak airway pressures:
  - Pressure limited ventilation (<25 cmH$_2$O).
  - Low tidal volume ventilation (≈6 ml/kg).

Post-operative, analgesia and complications

- Post-operative complications include:
  - Pulmonary infections.
  - Respiratory failure requiring ventilation.
  - Persistent air leaks.
- Patients may benefit from specialized physiotherapy.

- Good pain management is important particularly after open surgery.
  - A regional technique is recommended and the choice is between thoracic epidural analgesia and a continuous paravertebral block.
  - Systemic opioids and non-opioid analgesics should be added as appropriate.
- Pulmonary rehabilitation programmes may be available in some institutions.
- Mortality rate following wedge resection is related to the pre-operative status, overall mortality is less than 5%.

Further reading

Hoffmann TH and Ransdell HT. Comparison of lobectomy and wedge resection for carcinoma of the lung. *The Journal of Thoracic and Cardiovascular Surgery*. 1980; 79:211–17.

Lung Cancer Study Group (prepared by Ginsberg RJ, Rubinstein LV). Randomized trial of lobectomy versus limited resection for T1 N0 nonsmall cell lung cancer. *Annals of Thoracic Surgery*. 1995; 60:615.

Sleeve resection

PROCEDURE BASICS: resection of a cancerous lobe along with part of the bronchus supplying it. The remaining lobe(s) are then re-anastomosed to the remaining distal bronchus. May be performed in isolation with complete preservation of lung parenchyma, or with a lobectomy. More commonly performed as an open procedure, but successful VATS sleeve resections have been reported. Associated nodal resection is also performed.

TIME: 2–5hrs.

PAIN RATING: 4–5/5.

ANALGESIA: thoracic epidural or paravertebral ± PCA.

BLOOD LOSS: mild; may be considerably more if resection of pulmonary artery is required. X match 2–4 units.

HOSPITAL STAY: 3–5 days.

PREPARATION AND EQUIPMENT: standard monitoring. DLT. Arterial line. CVP line also advised.

Introduction and indication

- Most commonly performed for bronchogenic and non-bronchogenic tumours (benign or malignant) arising at the origin of a lobar bronchus.
  - Thus ruling out simple lobectomy, but not infiltrating enough as to require a pneumonectomy (parenchymal preservation).
- Utilized for 5–13% of resectable lung cancers.
- The mortality rate for sleeve lobectomy is slightly higher than for routine lobectomy (3%–5%).
- Good oncological outcomes if adequate resection margins free of tumour are achieved (<5% recurrence), and nodal involvement limited to N1 status.
- Also performed for:
  - Traumatic bronchial disruption.
  - TB.
  - Bronchial stenosis.
  - Congenital abnormalities.
  - Vascular lesions.
- Local invasion may necessitate pulmonary artery resection or patching, which may involve harvesting of pericardium.

Pre-operative assessment and preparation

General considerations

- As for all lung resections, in particular:
  - Careful assessment of cardio respiratory reserve.
  - An estimate of post resection lung function.
  - Assessment of the patient's airway with respect to DLT placement.
- Also ascertain:
  - Evidence of previous thoracic procedures?
  - Chest irradiation recently?
  - Use of high-dose steroids or systemic illnesses that might interfere with bronchial anastamotic healing?
- Decide with patient, a plan for post op analgesia.
- Mediastinoscopy may be performed in patients with malignant disease
- Patients who have mediastinal nodes of >1.0 cm on CT scan undergo mediastinoscopy before thoracotomy.
  - If the mediastinoscopy is negative → thoracotomy.
  - If the mediastinoscopy reveals ipsilateral N_2 disease → pre-operative chemo- or chemoradiation therapy and return later for resection.
  - Those patients with contralateral N_3 disease are referred for chemoradiation therapy and are not offered surgical resection.

Investigations

Bloods

- **FBC, U&E, glucose, clotting, X-match 2–4 units.**
- **ABG.**

Radiology

- **CXR**
  - Extent and location of lesion/other pathology.
- **CT chest and PET**
  - Particularly important in localizing/identifying lymph node involvement.

Other

- **SPO$_2$** on air.
- **ECG**
- **Echocardiogram**
  - If warranted by clinical history.
- **PFT**
  - Assessment of COPD/operability.
- **Flow-volume loops**
  - Assessment of COPD/operability.

Anaesthesia for sleeve resection

Induction
- Induction of choice.
- Rigid or flexible bronchoscopy will be performed.
  - Allows visualization of the lesion and planning of the resection.
- Prepare a means of maintaining ventilation, e.g. jet ventilation.
- Right-sided sleeve resection:
  - Left DLT.
- Left-sided sleeve resection:
  - Right DLT.
- For sleeve pneumonectomy/carinal sleeve resection:
  - Sterile anaesthesia circuit is required to allow direct ventilation from the surgical field.
- Wide bore intravenous access.
- Invasive arterial monitoring.
- CVP if indicated by patient co-morbidity or if likely to be needed post operatively.

Position
- Lateral decubitus position for unilateral surgery.

Maintenance and intra-operative
- Once anastomosis is complete, the surgeon will request a leak test under saline with manual ventilation (20–30 cm H_2O normally).
  - Confirm with the surgeon the maximum airway pressure to test at.
- Suction of the operative collapsed lung, prior to re-inflation will help reduce atelectasis, but if not done gently and with care, may damage the anastamosis. Discuss with the surgeon.
- Once two lung ventilation resumes, avoid high airway pressures so as not to place undue pressure on the anastomosis.

Post-operative
- Aim to extubate at the end of the case, if possible, thus avoiding prolonged positive pressure ventilation.
- A CXR will be required in recovery to assess lung inflation and intercostal drain placement.
- HDU environment with nursing staff trained in epidural management is ideal.
- Epidural normally remains in place until 12 hours after chest tubes are removed.

- Begin ambulation on post-operative day → 1 if possible.
- Monitor blood loss via the chest drain and Hb measurement, as transfusion may be necessary.

Complications

- Atelectasis is common but can be reduced by managing the basics well:
  - Ensure adequate analgesia.
  - Sit the patient up.
  - Supply humidified oxygen where possible.
  - Aggressive pulmonary toilet that may include frequent bronchoscopy, if necessary.
  - Incentive spirometry as soon as the patient is awake.
- Dehiscence of the anastamosis is rare, but will result in a bronchopleural fistula. Suspicion is aroused by:
  - Expectoration of thin bloody fluid.
  - Continued air leak via the chest drain.
- This is likely to require surgical exploration as it may be associated with infection/empyema.
  - May require completion pneumonectomy.
    (See 📖 Pneumonectomy, p. 374).
- If pulmonary artery resection has occurred, significant blood loss may occur during the post operative course.
  - The pulmonary artery is a low pressure vessel and slow leakage from the anastamosis may go unnoticed intra-operatively.

Special situations and problems

Difficulty achieving OLV

- Bronchial blockers are not ideal, as to facilitate OLV, as they are normally very near to or at the site of resection—thus hampering operative progress.
- If DLT placement fails, discuss the potential options with the surgeon.
  - If a bronchial blocker is not feasible viable, consider advancing an armoured single lumen tube over a FOS under direct vision into the non operative endobronchial lumen.
  - Again this is not ideal, but once the operative bronchial lumen is open, ventilation to the dependent lung would otherwise be impossible.
  - This however limits the ability to manage persistent hypoxia on OLV.

Persistesnt hypoxia on OLV during sleeve resection

❶ If hypoxia is persistent and not responding to other methods, then this must be communicated to the surgeon and a solution found.

❶ Once the bronchial tree is open, CPAP cannot be applied to operative side as it will be ineffective and may hamper the surgical view.
- Ventilation of the lung segments distal to the bronchial defect intra-operatively may be achieved by bridging the gap with and airway exchange catheter or bronchial blocker.
- Surgical assistance is likely to be required for correct and adequate placement.
- Ventilation is then achieved by available means.
- Care must be taken to prevent barotrauma in the distal lung segments.
- Although not universally available, HFJV is reported as successful with lower pleural pressures, better maintenance of venous return and cardiac output and a lower incidence of barotrauma.
- It may also be continued throughout resection with minimal inflation of the lung, therefore maintaining surgical access.

If the bronchial resection extends to the carina
- Occasionally surgery will extend as far as, or include the carina to achieve good resection margins around the pathology.
- In elective situations this should be known prior to surgery following bronchoscopy.
- Discuss with the surgeon the available intubation options:
  - If a DLT is not suitable, a single lumen armoured ETT advanced into the dependent bronchus bridging the defect created at the carina during resection may afford adequate surgical access
  - Alternatively Cardiopulmonary bypass may be required.

Further reading

Erino A Rendina. '*Bronchial and Pulmonary Arterial Sleeve resection*' The Cardiothoracic Surgery Network. www.ctsnet.org (accessed 10/3/10).

Mahtabifard A, Fuller CB, McKenna RJ Jr. 'Video-assisted thoracic surgery sleeve lobectomy: a case series'. *Annals of Thoracic Surgery*. 2008 Feb; 85(2):729–32.

Ju-Mei Ng. 'Hypoxemia During One-Lung Ventilation: Jet Ventilation of the Middle and Lower Lobes During Right Upper Lobe Sleeve Resection' *Anesthesia and Analgesia*. 2005; 101:1554–5.

Lung volume reduction surgery

PROCEDURE BASICS: as for thoracotomy, sternotomy or VATs.

TIME: 2–4 hours.

PAIN RATING: 2–4/5, highest after thoracotomy.

ANALGESIA: thoracic epidural; consider paravertebral block.

BLOOD LOSS: minimal.

HOSPITAL STAY: 7–10 days following thoracotomy. ITU needed as per complications of case/patient co-morbidities.

PREPARATION AND EQUIPMENT: as for thoracotomy, sternotomy or VATS.

Introduction
- Lung volume reduction surgery (LVRS) was tried for the management of end-stage emphysema in 1957. It was associated with high mortality (18%) and abandoned.
- LVRS reintroduced in 1990's.
- Improved surgical technique and case selection → ↑ functional capacity + ↓ mortality → widespread acceptance of LVRS.

Pathophysiology of emphysema
(See 📖 The patient with severe emphysema, p. 230).

Physiologic improvements associated with LVRS
- Resection of the most hyperexpanded (∴ least functional) lung tissue → re-expansion of more functional tissue. The aim of surgery is to see an immediate improvement in ventilatory mechanics and work of breathing via:
  - Improvement in elastic recoil.
  - ↓ expiratory flow limitation.
  - ↓ dynamic hyperinflation.
  - ↓ intrinsic PEEP.
- Reduced TLC → re-'doming' of diaphragm → ↑ –ve pressure generation.
- Improved cardiac output and venous return.

Surgical techniques for LVRS

Patients with the following will require lung transplant (See 📖 The patient with a lung transplant, p. 220).
- FEV$_1$ < 20% predicted.
- DLCO < 20% predicted.
- Homogeneous emphysema.

Anaesthesia issues

Unilateral vs. bilateral resection?
- Some evidence that the functional gain of unilateral LVRS is more durable than the results of bilateral LVRS.
  - ∴ staged unilateral LVRS advocated to provide longer periods of palliation.
- However, bilateral LVRS results in greater postoperative functional improvement with similar length of hospitalization, morbidity, and mortality as unilateral LRVS.

Thoracotomy vs. sternotomy vs. VATS resection?
- Thoracotomy divides ++ muscle and is ++ painful. ∴ not popular.
- Sternotomy and VATS approach to bilateral LVRS have similar:
- Early and late mortality.
  - Complication rates.
  - Improvements in spirometry.
  - Improvements in exercise capacity.
  - Improvements in quality of life.

VATS approach is superior to sternotomy in facilitating earlier recovery, reducing hospital LoS, and reducing health care costs.

Case selection for LVRS

Based on National Emphysema Treatment Trial Group Outcomes.
- RCT with 1218 patients, comparing LVRS to medical therapy.
- 90-day mortality following LVRS is 5.2%. LVRS is associated with increased short term mortality, but survival at 2½ years is identical.

- Exercise capacity and Health Related Quality of Life (QOL) showed:
  - Progressive decline from baseline in the medical therapy group.
  - Improvement in the LVRS group. A gradual decline was also noted, but the benefit remained above baseline at 24 months F/U.
- Subgroup analysis: LVRS in patients with *predominate upper lobe emphysema* and *low exercise capacity* → ↑ functional status + ↓ long-term mortality (mean F/U = 29 months).

Establish patient has emphysema

- History and signs.
  - Smoking.
  - FEV_1 >20% and <40% (spirometry).
  - TLC >100% (plethysmography).
  - RV >150% (plethysmography).
  - CT evidence of emphysema.

Establish patient will benefit from LVRS (Also NICE Recommendations)

- Upper lobe emphysema + low exercise capacity → best survival, ↓ symptoms and ↑ exercise.
- Upper lobe emphysema + high exercise capacity → ↓ symptoms and ↑ exercise only. There is no survival benefit.
  - ❶ Exercise limitation must be due to emphysema alone and not due to other respiratory or cardiac disease.
- Patients with solitary tumours can benefit from LVRS if the tumour is in the emphysematous site.

Specific investigations

- **Echocardiography**
  - To exclude pulmonary hypertension (MPAP <35 mmHg).
- **Myocardial perfusion scanning**
  - To exclude ischaemia.
- **Inspiration/expiration high res. chest CT**
  - To exclude bronchiectasis and establish presence of compressed normal parenchyma.

Exclude contraindications

- Asthma, non-emphysematous COPD, bronchiectasis are the main ones.
- Severe and advanced co-pathology.
  - ↓ predicted survival <2 years.
- HIGH RISK population identified in which LVRS was associated with 29% mortality at 90 days and no functional benefit, homogeneous emphysema.
- Summary of inclusion criteria (See Table 6.7) and mortality (See Table 6.8).

Table 6.7 Criteria for inclusion for LVRS

Inclusion	Exclusion
End-stage emphysema refractory to medical therapy	Active smoking (nicotine level)
	Prior thoracotomy
Compliance with pulmonary rehabilitation program	Other significant pulmonary disease (pulmonary hypertension, bronchiectasis, extensive lung cancer, pleural disease)
$PaO_2 \geq 6$ kPa	
$PaCO_2 \leq 7.3$ kPa	Significant co-morbidity
FEV_1 <45% predicted (post-bronchodilator)	Systemic steroid use ≥ 20 mg prednisone/day, e.g. COPD, Asthma
∴MWT >140 m with O_2 supplement ≤ 6 L to maintain $SpO_2 \geq 90\%$	FEV_1 <20% predicted (post-bronchodilator)
	DLCO <20% predicted
	Poor exercise tolerance due to heart or other lung disease
Radiographic evidence of heterogeneous emphysema, especially involving upper lobes.	Radiographic evidence of homogeneous emphysema.

Table 6.8 Mortality, exercise capacity and quality of life in patients undergoing LVRS (relative to conventional medical therapy)

	Mortality		Exercise capacity	QOL
	90 day	Total		
All Patients	↑	N/S	↑	↑
High Risk	↑	N/S	N/S	↑
Other	↑	N/S	↑	↑
Subgroups				
Upper lobe emphysema				
Low exercise capacity	N/S	↓	↑	↑
High exercise capacity	N/S	N/S	↑	↑
Non-upper lobe emphysema				
Low exercise capacity	↑	N/S	N/S	↑
High exercise capacity	↑	↑	N/S	N/S

↑ = Statistically significant increase; ↓ = Statistically significant decrease; NS = non-significant.

Pre-operative assessment and optimisaization
- Multi-disciplinary care team consists of physiotherapy, occupational therapy, nursing, dieticians, psychologists and physicians.
- Patients should be enrolled in pulmonary rehabilitation program to maximize exercise capacity.
- Medical optimization with long-acting bronchodilators and steroid dose reduced (inhaled ± systemic).
- ❶ Sedative pre-medication should be either avoided or sparingly used
  - If required, short acting agents are preferred to minimize the risk of respiratory depression at time of emergence.

Anaesthesia for LVRS
Induction
- Awake thoracic epidural as indicated.
  - LA ± opioid infusions can be used.
- Pre-oxygenation:
  - Patients with severe dyspnea and air trapping may require prolonged periods of O_2 in a semi-sitting position to achieve adequate pre-oxygenation.
- Drugs with short T1/2 such as propofol, atracurium and remifentanil are ideal for induction.
- 2x large bore IV cannulae.
- Standard monitoring.
- Invasive monitors:
  - Arterial line useful for repetitive ABG sampling.
- No evidence to support the routine use of PAFC or TOE.
- Flow volume loops are useful in order to quantify any air leaks.

Lung Isolation Techniques
- L DLT most commonly used. Advantages include:
  - Easy selective ventilation of either lung during bilateral LVRS.
  - Large lumina which facilitate collapse of the non-ventilated lung (especially given the decreased elastic recoil characteristic of severe emphysema).
  - DLT are useful to inflate the surgical lung during surgery for assessment of emphysema.
- Bronchial blockers may be required in patients who are difficult to intubate.

Maintenance and intra-operative
- An appropriate ventilation strategy is essential to minimize air trapping and avoid auto-PEEP complications.
  - Pressure control ventilation with low-moderate sized tidal volumes. (6–8 ml/kg during TLV, 4–6 ml/kg during OLV).
  - Adequate expiratory period (Inspiratory: Expiratory ratios ≤1:3)
  - Low respiratory rates (<12 breaths/min.).
  - Avoid the use of PEEP.
- Maintenance can be achieved using inhalational agents, eg desflurane.
- ❶ AVOID Nitrous Oxide.
- Conservative fluid management is recommended to facilitate early extubation.
- Maintain normothermia.
  - IV fluid warmers and forced air warmers are key.
  - Hypothermia predisposes to shivering which increases O_2 demand and CO_2 production which may delay extubation.
- Suck out secretions thoroughly before gently re-inflating the lung.

The end of the procedure
- Extubate immediately after surgery to minimize the development or worsening of air leaks.
- Optimization of lung function prior to extubation includes:
  - Reversal of neuromuscular blockade.
  - Tailoring the anaesthetic to ensure only minimal, and ideally, no sedation at the time of emergence.
  - Excellent pain control.
  - Use of bronchodilators to minimize the risk of bronchospasm.
  - Positioning the patient head-up.

Post-operative and analgesia
- Excellent pain management is essential to encourage maximal post-operative ventilatory effort. Common strategies include:
  - Thoracic epidural.
  - Adjuvant analgesia, NSAIDs (if not contraindicated) and Paracetamol.
- ❶ Adequate pain control is essential prior to extubation.
- ❶ Opioids should be used cautiously.
  - Somnolence and hypoventilation in this severely respiratory compromised group must be avoided!

Identifying and managing critical events during LVRS
For management of general intra-operative problems.

Table 6.9 Management of intra-operative problems during LVRS

Problem	Cause	Management
Hypotension	Dynamic hyperinflation (air trapping) → ↓↓↓ venous return. Commonly occurs during bag/mask ventilation and initiation of mechanical ventilation	Disconnect circuit from ETT
	Tension pneumothorax (see below)	AVOID aggressive fluid resuscitation. Treat with a vasoconstrictor
	Thoracic epidural sympathetic blockade	
	Myocardial Ischemia	
Tension Pneumothorax	Hyperinflation	
	Kinked or obstructed chest tube. Special care is required during bilateral VATS or thoracotomy LVRS when positioning the 1st operative lung in the lateral decubitus position	
Hypercapnoea	Hypercapnoea may result from strategies to minimize auto-PEEP and is generally well tolerated.	Enhance minute ventilation by increasing the RR

▶▶ Summary of LVRS anaesthetic goals

- Optimize peri-operative pulmonary function.
  - Use bronchodilators!
- Use short acting sedatives, induction agents, and maintenance drugs to minimize respiratory depression at the end of surgery.
- Ensure excellent pain control prior to extubation.
- Early tracheal extubation.
- Persistent air leak may require a Heimlich valve.

Alternatives to surgery

- One-way valves positioned in the bronchi of emphysematous segments allow air to leave alveoli → collapse and atelectasis. (Emphasys®).
- Biological LVR can be achieved by injecting substances from two syringes that mix in the bronchi and seal them off. (Aeris® therapeutics).
- Both techniques are performed bronchoscopically and in initial trials have achieved comparable results but at extremely reduced risk.

Further reading

Brister NW, Barnette RE, et al. Anesthetic Considerations in Candidates for Lung Volume Reduction Surgery. *Proceedings of the American Thoracic Society* 2008; 5:432–7.

Hillier J, Gillbe C. Anaesthesia for lung volume reduction surgery. *Anaesthesia* 2003;58: 1210–9.

National Emphysema Treatment Trial Research Group. A Randomized Trial Comparing Lung-Volume-Reduction Surgery with Medical Therapy for Severe Emphysema. *New England Journal of Medicine* 2003;348 (21):2059–73.

Bullectomy

PROCEDURE BASICS: surgical resection of bullae (thin walled, air filled spaces secondary to alveolar destruction) or cysts (sac-like structures that can be either gas or liquid filled) by either thoracotomy, midline sternotomy (for bilateral surgery) or thoracoscopic approach.

TIME: 2–4hrs.

PAIN RATING: 3–4/5.

ANALGESIA: thoracic epidural advised for open surgery. Paravertebral block can be useful.

BLOOD LOSS: minimal/moderate.

HOSPITAL STAY: 3–5 days.

PREPARATION AND EQUIPMENT: standard equipment ± provisions for ventilation in case of bronchopleural fistula. Arterial line and CVP line advised.

Introduction
- Bullae are air filled sacs that do not take part in effective ventilation. The walls can be formed from almost any part of the tissue within the lung.
- Causes.
  - Most commonly associated with emphysema (particularly in chronic smokers).
  - Genetic, e.g. α-1 antitrypsin deficiency.
  - Idiopathic.
  - Associated with connective tissue disorders.
- Tend to enlarge progressively over a period of months to years.
- May lead to pneumothorax.
  - Commonly occurs with small bulla affecting lung apices
  - May be difficult to differentiate large bulla from pneumothorax
  - Edge of a pneumothorax will usually parallel the chest wall curvature whereas edge of a bulla frequently curves inwards away from the chest wall
  - CT may help

- Infected bullae can be distinguished from abscesses
  - Bulla contains less fluid
  - Much thinner wall
  - No surrounding pneumonitis
  - Patients less sick with infected bulla

Types and locations
- Type 1
  - Originate in a sub-pleural location usually in upper part of lung.
  - Narrow neck.
  - Produce passive atelectasis of adjacent lung tissue.
- Type 2
  - Superficial in location.
  - Very broad neck.
  - Anterior edge of upper and middle lobes and along diaphragm.
  - Contain blood vessels and strands of partially destroyed lung.
  - Spontaneous pneumothorax common with these bullae.
- Type 3
  - Lie deep within lung substance.
  - Like type 2, contain residual strands of lung tissue.
  - Affect upper and lower lobes with same frequency.

Indications for surgery
- Bullae occupying >30% of the hemi-thorax.
- Normal lung parenchyma elsewhere.
- Moderate to severe dyspnoea.
- Recurrent pneumothoraces.
- Pain.
- Recurrent infection/haemoptysis.

Pre-operative assessment and preparation
History and optimization
- Patients are likely to have significant co-morbidities.
- Moderate to severe COPD will need medical optimization as well as treatment of any underlying infections.
- Patients on steroids will require peri-operative corticosteroid replacement therapy (See 📖 Steroids, p. 68).
- Thorough cardiac assessment is necessary as patients are high risk for IHD, pulmonary hypertension and right heart failure.

Investigations

Bloods
- **Routine bloods** and **ABG.**

Radiology
- **CXR**
  - Extent and location of bullae/other pathology.
- **CT chest.**

Other
- **ECG.**
- **Echocardiogram.**
  - RHF/LVF.
- **PFT's.**
  - Assessment of COPD/operability.

Anaesthesia for bullectomy

Induction
- (See 📖 Lung volume reduction surgery—LVRS, p. 396.)
- For open surgery—a DLT, invasive monitoring and thoracic epidural are essential.

Position
- Lateral decubitus position for unilateral surgery
- Supine, both arms by sides for midline sternotomy if bilateral surgery.

Maintenance and intra-operative
- Similar to LVRS (See 📖 Lung volume reduction surgery, p. 396).
- Minimize peak airway pressures:
  - Pressure limited ventilation (<25 cmH$_2$O).
  - Low tidal volume ventilation (4–6 ml/kg).
  - Prolonged I:E ratio (1:4).
  - Intermittent disconnection from ventilator if gas trapping suspected.

Post-operative

- Patients may require periods of post-operative ventilation during which all precautions to prevent high airway pressures and 'gas trapping' should be taken.
- Common post-operative complications include:
  - Pulmonary infections.
  - Respiratory failure requiring ventilation.
  - Persistent air leak.
- These patients will require specialized physiotherapy.

- Good pain management is essential with the gold standard for open surgery being a thoracic epidural infusion.
- Pulmonary rehabilitation programmes may be available in some institutions.
- Overall mortality rate following bullectomy surgery is 2.3%.

⚠ Special considerations

- Avoid nitrous oxide to prevent expansion and possible rupture of poorly ventilated bullae.
- Aim to minimize rupture of bullae and subsequent pneumothorax.
- High index of suspicion of intra-operative simple/tension pneumothorax if:
  - Increasing airway pressures.
  - Desaturation.
  - Cardiovascular collapse.
  - Unilateral hyperexpansion.
  - Tracheal shift.

Further reading

Conacher ID. Anaesthesia for the surgery of emphysema. *British Journal of Anaesthesia* 1997; 79:530–8.

Surgery to the chest wall and pleura

Chest wall tumours

PROCEDURE BASICS: resection of benign/malignant tumour, ± bony stabilization, ± reconstruction with muscle flap.

TIME: dependent on degree of resection and reconstruction.

PAIN RATING: 5/5.

ANALGESIA: many patients on pre-operative opioids; thoracic epidural/paravertebral advisable.

BLOOD LOSS: dependent on extent of surgery; XM 6 units.

HOSPITAL STAY: 5–7 days following thoracotomy. HDU/ITU may be needed according to patient co-morbidity and procedure difficulty/complications.

PREPARATION AND EQUIPMENT: can be a long procedure as patient may require thoracotomy and free flap surgery; invasive monitoring, large bore IV access, ± DLT, urinary catheter, forced air warmer, fluid warmer, careful positioning to avoid decubitus ulceration.

Classification of chest wall tumours
(See Table 7.1)
- Primary tumours are rare, with 50–80% being malignant.
- Metastatic.
  - Sarcoma.
  - Carcinoma.
- Adjacent neoplasm with local invasion.
  - e.g. lung, breast, pleura.
- Non-neoplastic disease.
  - e.g. cyst, inflammation.

Table 7.1 Examples of chest wall tumours

Benign	Malignant
Osteochondroma	Myeloma
Chondroma	Malignant fibrous histiocytoma
Desmoid	Chondrosarcoma
Fibrous dysplasia	Rhabdomyosarcoma
Lipoma	Ewing's sarcoma
Fibroma	Liposarcoma
	Lymphoma
	Leiomyosarcoma
	Haemangiosarcoma

Clinical features

- Slow growing.
- May be asymptomatic initially.
- Pain is a feature of nearly all malignant and 2/3 of benign tumours.
- Fever, leucocytosis and raised inflammatory markers may also be present.

Pre-operative assessment and preparation

- Chest wall resection requires careful pre-operative planning with respect to:
  - Extent of resection.
  - Options for bony stabilization.
  - Method of tissue coverage (often a muscle flap).

Investigations

Bloods
- **FBC, U&E** and **Clotting** profiles.
- **X match** 6 units.

Radiology
- **CXR**.
  - PA and Lateral.
- **CT chest.**

Other
- PFT's.
- ECG.

Anaesthesia for chest wall tumour resection

(See other procedures requiring thoracotomy)
- X2 wide bore IV access.
- Invasive monitoring desirable.
  - Arterial line/CVP line.
- Careful positioning to prevent pressure ulcers.
- Analgesia difficult to manage post-operatively, particularly as many will have been on high dose opioids pre-operatively.
- Consider thoracic epidural.
- Manage post-operatively in HDU/ITU setting.
- Consider period of post-operative ventilation to allow for re-warming and optimization of analgesia and any deranged physiology.

Complications

- Respiratory distress/failure due to altered pulmonary mechanics.
- Pneumonia secondary to sputum retention if pain not well controlled.
- Bleeding.
- Pneumothorax and abdominal wall hernia; dependent on muscle group harvested for muscle flap.
- Wound infection.
- Muscle flap necrosis.

Further reading

Searl CP. *Anaesthesia for pleural and chest wall surgery*. In Searl CP, Ahmed ST (Eds.), Core Topics in Thoracic Anaesthesia. Cambridge University Press 2009.

Warwick J. *Free flap surgery*. In Allman K, Wilson I (Eds.), Oxford Handbook of Anaesthesia. Oxford University Press, 2006.

Pectus correction surgery

PROCEDURE BASICS: open or thoracoscopic assisted procedure where a bar is inserted into the chest to correct the deformity.

TIME: 2–3 hours.

PAIN RATING: 3–4/5.

ANALGESIA: thoracic epidural advised; paravertabral usually unsuitable as involves both sides of the chest.

BLOOD LOSS: usually minimal.

HOSPITAL STAY: 2–3 days. Ward-based recovery usually suffices.

PREPARATION AND EQUIPMENT: standard monitoring. Arterial line not usually required. DLT for Nuss/SLT for Ravitch procedure.

There are two main types of deformities of the sternum, pectus carinatum (pigeon chest) and pectus excavatum (funnel chest). Surgery is undertaken for cosmetic reasons. Currently two surgical procedures are used to treat patients in the UK, the Ravitch and the Nuss procedures.

Pathophysiology

- Abnormal growth of bone and cartilage in the anterior chest wall.
- Typically affecting 4–5 ribs on each side of the sternum.
- No known genetic defect is directly responsible.
- Male: Female ratio 3:1.
- 20% may have other musculoskeletal conditions (Marfan's, Ehlers-Danlos and Poland's Syndromes).
- Familial occurrence of pectus deformity is reported in 35% of cases.

Indications for surgery

- Nearly always for cosmetic reasons.
- Psychosocial factors.

The Ravitch procedure

- In addition to being used for the standard pectus excavatum patient it is used to correct patients with pectus carinatum and complex pectus excavatum.
- An open procedure.
- Horizontal chest incision.
- Ribs are detached from sternum.
- A metal bar (temporary or permanent) may be used to maintain the position during healing.

The Nuss procedure

- Also called MIRPE (minimally invasive repair of pectus excavatum).
- A thoracoscopic procedure during which one or two curved steel bars are placed behind the sternum and used to force it back into position.
- Increasingly used for the treatment of children.
- The bar is then removed usually between 2–5 years later.
  - Pre-operative assessment and preparation

History

- Young patient usually fit and well.
- May be a history of chest pain, shortness of breath and poor exercise tolerance for their age.

Examination

- CVS
  - May hear a 'click' after 1st heart sound signifying mitral valve prolapse (Marfans).
  - Listen for other heart murmurs.
- RS
  - Auscultate lung fields to exclude other causes of shortness of breath.
- Examine thoracic spine with a view to thoracic epidural placement as many have scoliosis.

Investigations

No specific laboratory studies are necessary as most patients are young and otherwise fit.

Bloods:

- **FBC, U+E, G+S.**

Radiology:

- **CXR**; 2 views (antero-posterior and lateral views) in all patients. This provides information about:
  - Possible associated intrathoracic pathology.
  - Severity of the lung compression, and mediastinal displacement.
  - Degree of posterior displacement of the sternum, particularly in relation to the spine.
  - Assessment of the spine and possible associated scoliosis, a common finding in many patients with pectus excavatum.
- **CT chest** to determines the Haller index:
  - Transverse chest diameter ÷ antero-posterior diameter.
  - Index > 3.2 has been correlated with a severe deformity that requires surgery.
  - CT used only in selected cases of asymmetric pectus excavatum or if significant cardiac displacement and rotation is suspected.

Other:
- **Echocardiogram**
  - Un-necessary unless symptomatic due to cardiac compression or suspected mitral valve prolapse.
- **ECG**
  - If mitral valve prolapse murmur, other heart murmurs or to detect any A-V conduction delay.
- **PFT**
  - Normally un-necessary unless overt breathlessness on minimal exertion.

Anaesthesia for pectus correction

Induction
- If planned place awake mid-thoracic epidural
- Standard IV induction, paralysis and maintenance using volatile or TIVA
- Intubation
  - For the Nuss procedure OLV is required and a DLT is recommended. (Bronchial blockers are not advised, as sequential lung deflation requires repositioning of the bronchial blockers with associated time delays).
  - For the Ravitch procedure a single lumen tube is suitable.

Position
- Supine position
- For the Nuss procedure the patient's arms are abducted 90° to the body and fixed to arm supports (crucifix position).

Ventilation
- Sequential collapse of the lungs is required for the Nuss procedure.
- OLV not required for the Ravitch procedure.

Post-operative and analgesia
- Pain can be considerable and a suitable analgesic technique should be used.
- A major risk to the patients undergoing the Nuss procedure is the dislodgment of the steel bar.
- This can result in acute severe compression of the mediastinum and heart → cardiac standstill and cardiopulmonary arrest.
- In this situation, CPR is ineffective and the chest may have to be opened in order to relieve the compression.

Pleurectomy

PROCEDURE BASICS: partial removal of parietal pleura frequently combined with removal of ruptured bullae. May be performed by VATS or open thoracotomy.

TIME: 1–2 hours.

PAIN RATING: 3–4/5.

ANALGESIA: morphine IV-PCA, paravertebral catheter and non opioid analgesics. Consider thoracic epidural.

BLOOD LOSS: minimal loss with VATS; up to 500 ml with thoracotomy.

HOSPITAL STAY: 2–3 days. Ward-based recovery usually suffices However, if there is significant patient co-morbidity HDU may be required.

PREPARATION AND EQUIPMENT: as per VATS or thoracotomy.

Introduction
- Partial removal of parietal layer of pleura.
- Several indictions but most commonly for recurrent pneumothorax.
- Most commonly performed as VATS procedure, but may require thoracotomy.
- Patients may have underlying conditions requiring pre-optimization, e.g. asthma, COPD or cystic fibrosis.
- An alternative to pleurodesis.
- If the patient has a connective tissue disorder, acquire more information regarding its other associated morbidities.

Indications
- Recurrent pneumothorax.
- Recurrent pleural effusion, especially malignant.

Pre-operative assessment and preparation
- Patients usually either fit and young or older with COPD.
- Discuss operative plan with surgeon.
- Inspect recent CXR to assess for pneumothorax or extent of effusion.
- Consider placing an intercostal chest drain prior to anaesthesia if pneumothorax is present.

Anaesthesia for pleurectomy

Induction

- Chest drain, if present, should be left in situ and unclamped until OLV on contra-lateral lung established to prevent development of a tension pneumothorax.
- Can be a painful procedure and analgesia should reflect this. Consider thoracic epidural or paravertebral block.
- One-lung anaesthesia is required to assist surgical access.

Maintenance

- Minimize peak airway pressure and avoid nitrous oxide in patients with recent pneumothorax.

Position

- Patients typically positioned in lateral decubitus. Beware that large pleural effusions (half hemithorax on CXR) may cause cardiovascular compromise when positioned operative (effusion) side up. Consider pre-operative drainage.

The end of the procedure

- A chest drain is surgically placed at the end of the procedure to aid re-expansion of the lung and drainage of blood.
- Fully re-expand the lung at the end of the procedure to ensure apposition of parietal and visceral pleura.
- Consider carring for patients initially in an HDU setting to allow for optimization of analgesia and care of chest drain.

Post-operative problems

- Pain.
- Acute respiratory distress/failure.
- Prolonged air leak.
- Failure to correct the presenting complaint.
- Infection e.g. wound, pleura, systemic.

Pleurodesis

- Pleurodesis: (pleuro + Greek desis, binding together—from dein, to bind).
- Numerous benign, infectious, and malignant diseases can lead to recurrent pleural effusions.
- Approximately half of all patients with metastatic cancer will develop a pleural effusion, with lung and breast cancer accounting for 75% of cases.
- Development of a malignant pleural effusion, (MPE), significantly reduces the quality of life.
- Pleurodesis produces fibrosis between the visceral and parietal pleura, thereby obliterating the pleural space. If successful, it prevents the re-accumulation of pleural effusion with permanent relief of symptoms.

History

- Dyspnoea is the most common symptom associated with pleural effusion relating more to the distortion of the diaphragm and chest wall during respiration, than to hypoxaemia.

Examination

- Physical findings, which do not usually manifest until pleural effusion exceeds 300 ml include:
  - Decreased breath sounds.
  - Stony dullness to percussion.
  - Decreased tactile fremitus.
  - Pleural friction rub.
  - Mediastinal shift away from the effusion.

Anaesthetic considerations for thoracoscopic pleurodesis

- For malignant pleural effusion consider associated manifestations of the malignancy (eg malignant pericardial effusion).
- Determine the size of the pleural effusion (usually un-drained to facilitate thoracoscopy).
- In the lateral position a large effusion can cause mediastinal distortion and compromise the cardiac output.
  - May require supine repositioning.
- Remember re-expansion pulmonary oedema (pleural effusion is drained to allow thoracoscopy and to enable pleurodesis).
- Consider appropriate post-operative analgesia.
  - Some patients may be opioid tolerant.

Sclerosing agents

- Almost all sclerosing agents can produce fever, tachycardia, chest pain and nausea.
- As sclerosing agents may cause pain, the patient should be premedicated with pain medication prior to instillation of the sclerosing agent.
- Talc is the agent of choice for pleurodesis (level of evidence 1a to 1b; recommendation grade A).

- Both thoracoscopic pleurodesis (in the operating theatre) and bedside instillation of talc slurry were equivalent in effectiveness (level of evidence 1b; recommendation grade A).
- Rotation of the patient's body to enhance dispersal of the sclerosing agent is not recommended (level of evidence 1B; recommendation grade B).

Talc

- Considered to be one of the most successful sclerosing agents used to achieve pleurodesis.
- It is a soft anhydrous compound mainly composed of magnesium silicate and contains particles of varying size.
- Typically, a slurry of 5 g in a solution of 50 to 100 ml saline (with or without lignocaine) is instilled.
- Precise mechanism by which talc induces pleural sclerosis is unclear. However, there is evidence to suggest that basic fibroblast growth factor plays an important role in this process.

Bleomycin

- An anti-neoplastic antibiotic used to treat head and neck, cervical, and germ cell malignancies.
- Successfully utilized as a pleural sclerosing agent for many years.
- 60 units has been shown useful and may be of equivalent effectiveness to tetracycline.

Tetracycline (Doxycycline)

- Tetracycline is a broad spectrum antibiotic derived from *Sterptomyces*.
- Parenteral form of the drug is no longer commercially available in USA, thereby precluding its use as a sclerosing agent.
- Doxycycline, a close pharmacological relative, has been used as an alternative with similar efficacy.

Conclusions

- Talc is the sclerosing agent of choice for the treatment of symptomatic malignant pleural effusion (level of evidence 1; recommendation grade A).
- A patient with a malignant pleural effusion who is deemed a candidate for pleurodesis should be offered thoracoscopic insufflation of talc to optimize the likelihood of achieving durable symptomatic relief (level of evidence 1; recommendation grade A).

Further reading

Light RW. Management of pleural effusions. *Journal of Formosan Medical Association* 2000; 99:523–31.

American Thoracic Society. Management of malignant pleural effusions. *American Journal of Respiratory Critical Care Medicine* 2000; 162:1987–2001.

Schafers SJ, Dresler CM. Update on talc, bleomycin, and the tetracyclines in the treatment of malignant pleural effusions. *Pharmacotherapy* 1995; 15:228–35.

Upper gastrointestinal and mediastinal surgery

Thymectomy

PROCEDURE BASICS: excision of thymic tissue—complete or partial.

TIME: 2–4hrs.

PAIN RATING: 1/5 to 4–5/5.

ANALGESIA: Epidural analgesia is strongly advised (T8–10) for trans-sternal resection.

BLOOD LOSS: mild/moderate.

HOSPITAL STAY: 3–7 days. Ward-based recovery usually suffices; unless severe myasthenia associated.

PREPARATION AND EQUIPMENT: standard equipment, range of DLT/CVP/arterial line for trans-sternal approach.

Introduction

Tumours of the thymus are rare, with an incidence of 1–5 per million population, per year. Thymomas are the commonest mediastinal tumour in adults, followed by lymphomas.

- Due to the association of autoimmune disease with thymomas and thymic hyperplasia, the commonest indication for thymectomy is in the treatment of myasthenia gravis. (See 📖 The patient with myasthenia gravis, p. 258).
- Thymectomy is indicated in young patients with a short history of symptoms and poor response to medical treatment.
- Isolated ocular symptoms or good control on medical management → surgery not indicated.

Treatment options

Surgical

- Surgical options are still evolving
- For maximal thymectomy: trans-sternal (partial and median), trans-cervical or a combination (Clamshell approach if tumour is very large).
- For non-maximal thymectomy → video-assisted thoracoscopic thymectomy:
  - With one lung ventilation (OLV)
  - Without OLV → capnothorax.
- Invasive thymoma will require adjuvant radiotherapy and surgery.

✒ Controversy still exists if maximal thymectomy is absolutely necessary.

Pre-operative assessment and preparation
(See 📖 Pre-op assessment)

History and optimization

Thymectomy is an elective procedure; so there is time to optimize.

- Are bulbar symptoms present?
  - Ability to protect and maintain their airway may be compromised.
- Assess crude respiratory muscle strength:
  - Cough efficient enough to clear secretions?
- Chest infection is common and must be adequately treated
- Ensure MG is well controlled:
  - Perform plasmapheresis if bulbar weakness, respiratory failure or on large doses of steroids.
  - High dose steroids → muscle weakness ... taper dose ± azothioprine/cyclosporin.
  - Anticholinesterase dose must be optimized and continued until surgery.
  - If oral pyridostigmine not possible, convert to IV or IM neostigmine.

Dose of anticholinesterase

- Pyridostigmine
  - 30 mg PO OD.

Equivalents for conversion:
- Pyridostigmine 0.5–1 mg IV OD.
- Neostigmine 1.5–2 mg IV/IM OD.

Relevent investigations

- Assess formal respiratory muscle strength:
  - **FVC**
  - **Maximum inspiratory pressure**
  - **TOF**—sub-maximal?
- **Flow volume loops**—if CXR/CT/MRI imaging shows large anterior mediastinal mass (intrathoracic airway obstruction). Perform supine and erect to ascertain whether fixed or dynamic obstruction.

If dynamic obstruction, awake intubation is a safe option if needed.

Radiology

- **CT/MRI** scan to establish:
  - Large thymoma → sternotomy
  - Hyperplasia → less invasive surgery.

Pre-operative planning to avoid post-operative ventilation

Pre-operative predictors of post-operative ventilation, See 📖 p. 606.
- Reduce dose of steroids:
  - Adequate dose of pyridostigmine.
  - Add Cyclosporine and azothioprine.
- Plasmapheresis
- Plasmapheresis if severe generalized muscle weakness (dysphagia, dysphoria, respiratory failure) or high steroid dose.
- Less invasive surgical approach.
- Avoidance of neuromuscular blocking agents:
  - Depolarising & non-depolarising.
  - If non-depolarising used, allow spontaneous recovery (do not reverse).
  - Avoid aminoglycosides and polymyxin.
  - Avoid β blockers.
  - Optimize analgesia.
- Timing of surgery:
  - Optimal control of MG.
  - Control of chest infection.
- Re-start pyridostigmine within six hours.

Anaesthesia for thymectomy

Induction

- Avoid sedative pre-medication:
  - Respiratory depression risk.
- Awake thoracic epidural analgesia:
  - May help decrease the possible need for ventilation in post-operative period.
- Invasive arterial monitoring:

- Recommended in all patients.
- Trans-sternal resections for large thymic tumours/previous trans-cervical surgery all tend to involve more extensive surgery.
- CVP monitoring.
- Pre-oxygenation and intubation with SLT.
- Rapid sequence induction if reflux risk:
  - If using suxamethonium, a large dose is required (1.5–2.0 mg/kg).
  - Remifentanil 2 mcg/kg induction dose is preferable.
- Awake intubation:
  - If dynamic airway obstruction.
  - 4% lidocaine topical spray + careful remifentanil TCI sedation.

Maintenance
- Non-muscle relaxant based anaesthetic technique (See below):
  - TCI remifentanil useful as relaxant sparing/avoiding agent.
  - ± epidural usage intra-operatively.
- Temperature monitoring:
  - Essential, to avoid the deleterious effects of hypothermia upon neuromuscular function.
- Neuromuscular monitoring is essential.
- IV hydrocortisone:
  - For patients taking >10 mg prednisolone PO OD.

Neuromuscular blocking drugs and MG

Depolarising relaxants
- Suxamethonium block prolonged due to:
  - Inhibition of cholinesterase by pyridostigmine.
  - Depletion of cholinesterase by plasmapheresis.
- Risk of phase II block with single dose suxamethonium.

Non-depolarising relaxants
- Better if totally avoided by using volatile agents and remifentanil.
- If decision to use them:
  - <10% of normal dose; titrate dose using NM monitoring.
  - Allow spontaneous recovery as reversal with neostigmine → risk of phase II block and cholinergic crisis.
- Neuromuscular monitoring is essential.
  - May involve a peripheral nerve stimulator or more advanced methods such as EMG, MMG or acceleromyography.

❶ Avoid calcium channel blockers, β blockers and aminoglycosides, which will prolong NM blockade

The end of the procedure
- Ensure that the patient has adequate respiratory muscle strength and is fully conscious prior to extubation with:
  - Ability to maintain head lift for greater than 5 seconds.
  - Ability to generate an inspiratory force of >25cm H_2O.

- Sub-maximal TOF: if fade or T4:T1 <0.9 implies significant muscle weakness.
- Short term post-op ventilation (See Table 8.1) may be required if:
  - Surgery was extensive.
  - Poor NM recovery/weakness with or without prior usage of muscle relaxants.
  - Patient had pre-operative bulbar muscle involvement (may require extended period of airway protection).

Table 8.1 Management of post-operative ventilatory failure

Causation	Management suggestion
Muscle weakness	Sedate and ventilate
Phrenic nerve damage at surgery	Sedate and ventilate
Myasthenic crisis	Plasmapheresis or Ig therapy
Cholinergic crisis	Sedate and ventilate
Infection	Sedate and ventilate

Post-operative

- All patients require close monitoring of their respiratory function in the post-operative period, and should be cared for in a high dependency or intensive care setting.
- Serial PEFR or vital capacity measurement may be useful.
- Patients who had pre-operative plasmapheresis tend to bleed post-operatively.
- Type II respiratory failure may result from cholinergic crisis, myasthenia or phrenic nerve damage.
- Chest physiotherapy and incentive spirometery are of value in assisting the clearance of secretions.
- The dose of anticholinesterases may need to be reduced post thymectomy.

⚠ Special considerations

Cholinergic crisis

Excess anticholinesterase drug dosage → excess ACh acting at muscarinic and nicotinic receptors.

- Nicotinic symptoms—lack of muscle co-ordination.
  - Twitching.
  - Fasciculation.
  - Muscle weakness.
- Muscarinic symptoms.
  - Bradycardia.
  - Bronchospasm.
  - Nausea, vomiting and hyper-salivation.
  - Miosis—distinguishes from incomplete reversal.
- Nicotinic symptoms predominate if the crisis is induced by reversal of neuromuscular blockade.
  - Differentiation from inadequate neuromuscular transmission (myasthenic crisis) may require a Tensilon® test.
- Treatment consists of respiratory support and antimuscarinics.

Further reading

Leventhal SR, Orkin FK, Hirsh RA. Prediction of the need for postoperative mechanical ventilation in myasthenia gravis. *Anesthesiology* 1980; 53(1):26–30.

Naguib M, el Dawlatly AA, Ashour M, *et al.* Multivariate determinants of the need for postoperative ventilation in myasthenia gravis. *Canadian Journal of Anaesthesia* 1996; 43(10):1006–13.

Eisenkraft JB, Book WJ, Mann SM, *et al.* Resistance to Succinylcholine in Myasthenia Gravis: A Dose-response Study. *Anesthesiology* 1988; 69(5):760–2.

Hiatus hernia repair

PROCEDURE BASICS: surgical repair of abnormal diaphragmatic oesophageal hiatus (allows a portion of the stomach or other abdominal contents to herniate into the chest). Can be performed open, via the abdomen, open via the thorax, laparoscopically or endo-luminally via an endoscope. Aims to treat gastro-oesophageal reflux disease, dysphagia and prevent incarceration.

TIME: open: 2–4hrs/laparoscopic: 3–5hrs/endo-luminal 2–4hrs.

PAIN RATING: open 3/5/laparoscopic 2/5/endo-luminal 1–2/5.

ANALGESIA: thoracic epidural advised for open surgery/thoracotomy. Paravertebral block also possible. Simple analgesia for endo-luminal.

BLOOD LOSS: minimal/moderate especially if incarcerated.

HOSPITAL STAY: open 2–5 days/laparoscopic1–2 days/endo-luminal 1–2 days. HDU advised post thoracotomy or if obese.

PREPARATION AND EQUIPMENT: standard equipment. CVP, arterial line. SLT uaually suffices; discuss with the surgeon.

Causes
- Straining during labour, defecation, weight training.
- Obesity.
- Hereditary.
- Smoking.
- Old age and loss of tissue elasticity.
- Chronic oesophagitis.

Indications
- Para-oesophageal hernia (except the very frail).
- Severe reflux refractory to medical therapy.
- Complicated oesophagitis.
- Strictures, ulcers, and bleeding.
- Barrett's oesophagus with high grade dysplasia.
- Those with pulmonary complications, i.e. asthma, recurrent aspiration pneumonia, chronic cough, or hoarseness linked to reflux disease.

Treatment options
Thorough investigation MUST precede decision making on treatment.

Medical
Treatment aims to:
- Control existent reflux.
  - Lifestyle modifications.
- Improve oesophageal clearance.
  - Motility agents.
- Reduce acid production.
  - Proton pump inhibitors.
- Treat iron deficiency anaemia (2° to erosive gastritis/oesophagitis).

Surgical
- Advised for complicated oesophagitis despite medical therapy and para-oesophageal hernias.
- The goal of surgery is to remove the hernia sac and close the abnormally wide oesophageal hiatus.
- Involves a wrap of stomach fundus around the inferior part of the oesophagus, preventing herniation of the stomach through the hiatus in the diaphragm (fundoplication); 80–90% cure rate.

Laparoscopic approach
- Lower morbidity and mortality, shorter hospital stay and less painful compared to the open procedure.
- Relatively high incidence of post-operative complications, such as dysphagia and gas bloating.
- Dumping and achalasia also reported.

Open approach
- Stomach and lower esophagus are placed back into the abdominal cavity.
- Hiatus is tightened and the stomach is stitched in position within the abdominal cavity.
- Necessary to deal with compromised viscera or shortened oesophagus.

Pre-operative assessment and preparation
History and optimization
- Do not forget that all patients have refflux and are an aspiration risk!
- Pre-operative course of proton pump inhibitor is mandatory … at least a month's worth.

- Consider IV ranitidine 24 hours pre-operatively.
- If pulmonary symptoms are apparent, consider bronchodilator therapy and pre-operatively CXR to ensure no LRTI.
- Encourage weight loss prior to GA as many will be obese.
- Advise smoking cessation at least 1 month prior to surgery.
- Consider ferrous sulphate therapy to raise Hb level if patient has Fe deficiency anaemia 2° to Camerons ulcers; may need transfusion.

Investigations

Bloods
- **FBC, U+E, Clotting, X match** 2–4 units.
- **ABG.**
  - If significant SOB

Radiology
- **CXR**
  - Defines nature of HH and allows assessment of co-pathologies (COPD/heart size in obese patients).
- **Barium upper gastrointestinal series**
  - Out-pouching of barium at the lower end of the oesophagus, a wide hiatus through which gastric folds are seen in continuum with those in the stomach, and, occasionally, free reflux of barium.
  - Helps distinguish a sliding from a para-oesophageal hernia.

Other
- **ECG.**
  - Exclude cardiac cause of assumed reflux associated chest pains.
- **Endoscopy**
  - Diagnosis of a hiatus hernia is usually incidental.
  - Endoscopy is used to diagnose complications such as erosive oesophagitis, ulcers, Barrett oesophagus, or tumour.
  - Confirmed HH when the endoscope is about to enter the stomach or on retrograde view once inside the stomach.
  - Also permits biopsy of any abnormal or suspicious area.
- **Oesophageal manometry**
  - To document reflux and identify gastro-oesophageal junction, particularly when shortened.

Anaesthesia for hiatus hernia repair

Induction
- Standard monitoring.
- Speak to surgeon, if requires lung down (thoracotomy approach) use DLT/bronchial blocker.
- Invasive monitoring is advised for thoracotomy.

- NGT to decompress stomach.
- Urinary catheter.
- RSI as high risk for aspiration.
- Pre-oxygenate well, particularly obese patients.
- Maintenance via TIVA or volatile/relaxant technique.

Position
- Laparoscopic.
  - Modified lithotomy position with the head of the table tilted up 25 degrees.
- Open procedure.
  - Supine laparotomy or left lateral thoracotomy.

Maintenance
- Pressure controlled/limited ventilation advised. Patients are often obese.
- Increase ventilation to remove systemically absorbed CO_2 2° to pneumoperitoneum.

❶ Post-operative
- HDU advised post-operatively, particularly obese patients/those with pulmonary co-pathologies.
- Be wary of and treat shoulder tip pain (may have to increase opioid dose? Role of pre-emptive gabapentin).
- Diet of pureed foods for 1–2 weeks.
- Normal diet after 4–6 weeks.
- Light activity is encouraged and heavy lifting is avoided for 4 weeks.
- Analgesia is given in liquid form for the first two weeks and all pills are crushed.

⚠ Special considerations
- Overall complication rate is 1–2%.
- Conversion from laparoscopic to open procedure is <1–2%.
- Pneumothorax <1%, beware of pneumomediastinum, pneumopericardium.
- Oesophageal perforation or gastric perforation: <1–2%
- Peri-operative mortality <0.5%.
- Splenic injury or hepatic Injury is rare.
- If perforation occurs, mortality rate is high.
  - Many surgeons advise elective repair when the diagnosis is made.
- Don't forget systemic CO_2 absorption 2° to pneumoperitoneum.
- Ask surgeon to infiltrate phrenic nerve with LA to prevent shoulder tip pain (⚠ those with COPD).

Further reading

Hinder R.A, Filipi C.J. The technique of laparoscopic Nissen fundoplication. *Surgical laparoscopy and Endoscopy*. 1992; 2(3):265–72.

Anti-reflux surgery

(See also hiatus hernia repair).

PROCEDURE BASICS: also known as Nissen Fundoplication. The gastric fundus is wrapped around the lower end of the oesophagus. Usually performed laparoscopically, but has also been performed via laparotomy and left thoracotomy.

TIME: 2–3hrs.

PAIN RATING: laparoscopic 2/5.

ANALGESIA: simple analgesics, NSAID, + morphine. Consider thoracic epidural or paravertebral catheter + morphine PCA for thoracotomy.

BLOOD LOSS: minimal.

HOSPITAL STAY: 1–2 days (has been done in day surgery).

PREPARATION AND EQUIPMENT: standard, SLT normally; DLT if thoracotomy.

Open vs. laparoscopic

- Both techniques eliminate the need for acid suppression.
- Laparoscopy may not be appropriate for certain patients, dependent on the severity of co-morbidity or previous abdominal surgery.
- Laparoscopic approach offers the following advantages:
  - Reduced post-operative pain.
  - Shorter hospital stay.
  - A faster return to work.
  - Improved cosmetic result.
- Laparoscopic Nissen Fundoplication is relatively safe and effective:
  - Studies have shown that after 10 years, 90% of patients are still symptom free.

Pre-operative assessment and preparation

- Optimize lifestyle factors. Surgery is only performed once lifestyle changes/medical therapy have failed:
  - Encourage weight loss if obese.
  - ↓ alcohol intake.
  - Stop smoking.

- CXR & pulmonary function tests as indicated by history
- Advise patient to continue their anti-reflux medications up to and including the day of surgery. Consider IV ranitidine the night before surgery.

Patient selection

The following categories indicate groups of patients who may be considered for anti-reflux surgery:
- Persistent complications due to GORD, e.g. peptic stricture
- Barrett's oesophagus; these patients usually have severe GORD
- Respiratory complications refractory to medical therapy:
  - Recurrent pneumonia, asthma.
  - Hoarseness, chronic cough, laryngitis.
- Persistent regurgitation:
  - PPIs often neutralize the acid stopping the heartburn, but regurgitation persists.
- Patients < 40 years old with severe GORD, i.e. they are at high risk of progressive disease.
- Failure to respond to medical therapy:
  - ❶ Patients whose symptoms do not respond to PPIs should be treated with caution. Consider cardiac, pulmonary, musculoskeletal or other gastro-intestinal diagnosis.
  - Likely to have an inferior response to surgery as confounding diagnosis will not respond to stopping gastro-oesophageal reflux.

Anaesthesia for anti-reflux surgery

Induction
- All patients require rapid sequence induction; consider awake intubation in known or anticipated difficult laryngoscopy.
- Consider thoracic epidural for open surgical technique; DLT required for left thoracotomy.
- NGT to decompress stomach.

Position
- Position for laparoscopic technique:
  - Patient supine, legs apart with arms alongside body.
  - Patient then placed in reverse-trendelenburg to improve exposure.
  - May result in sudden hypotension.

Maintenance
- Increase minute volume to remove CO_2 absorbed from pneumoperitoneum.
- ⚠ Iatrogenic pneumothorax may occur intra-operatively, i.e. insufflated gas passes from the peritoneal to pleural space.
  - Application of PEEP has been found to resolve the pneumothorax with no need for a chest drain.

- Maintain muscle relaxation throughout surgery.
- Extubate awake.

Post-operative

- Routine post-operative care on the ward. HDU requirement dictated by underlying co-morbidities, e.g. limited cardio-respiratory reserve, obesity, obstructive sleep apnoea.
- Regular anti-emetics to control vomiting and retching for 24 hours.
- Simple analgesics, NSAID + S/C morphine PRN. Oral analgesics may need to be in liquid form for first week.
- Care of epidural/paravertebral catheters, PCA in thoracotomy patients.
- Clear fluids day one with light diet from day two.
- Avoid bread and fizzy drinks for 4–6 weeks.
- Anti-reflux medications should no longer be required.

Fundoplication complications

- Mortality < 1%.
- Dysphagia.
- Gas bloat syndrome:
  - 2–5% of patients.
  - Unable to belch.
  - Causes an accumulation of gas in the stomach or small intestine.
  - Commonly believed to be related to the tightness of the "wrap".
  - Usually self-limiting within 2 to 4 weeks, but in some it may persist.
- Dumping syndrome.
- The fundoplication can loosen over time in about 5–10% of cases, leading to recurrence of symptoms.
- Difficult to vomit.
- Achalasia (rare).

Further reading

Joris J, Chiche J, Lamy M. Pneumothorax during laparoscopic fundoplication: Diagnosis and treatment with positive end-expiratory pressure. *Anesthesia and Analgesia* 1995; 81:993–1000.

Dupont F. Anaesthesia for oesophageal surgery. *Seminars in Cardiothorac and Vascular Anesthesia* 2000; 4:2–17.

Ackroyd R, Watson D, Majeed A, *et al*. Randomized clinical trial of laparoscopic versus open fundoplication for gastro-oesophageal reflux disease. *British Journal of Surgery* 2004; 91:975–82.

Oesophageal tumours and their considerations

- Oesophageal tumours are mainly of 2 types:
  - Squamous cell carcinoma.
  - Adenocarcinoma.
- Less common types of oesophageal cancer include:
  - Leiomyosarcomas.
  - Metastatic cancers.
- These tumours may develop anywhere in the oesophagus and appear morphologically as:
  - Strictures.
  - Lumps.
  - Plaques.
  - Fistulae between the oesophagus and the airways.
- Oesophagogastric junctional tumours are classified as:
  - Type I (distal oesophageal).
  - Type II (cardia).
  - Type III (proximal stomach).

Risk factors

- Both squamous and adenocarcinoma are more common in men.
- Tobacco abuse predispose to both squamous and adenocarcinoma.
- There are various risk factors:
  - Alcohol abuse (predisposes to squamous carcinoma).
  - Certain human papillomavirus infections.
  - Previous radiation to the oesophagus as a result of treatment of nearby cancers.
- Existing disorders of the oesophagus may predispose:
  - Achalasia.
  - Oesophageal web (Plummer-Vinson syndrome).
  - Narrowing due to having once swallowed a corrosive substance (such as highly alkaline substances).
- Barrett's oesophagus:
  - A pre-malignant condition whereby specialized columnar epithelium replaces healthy squamous epithelium.
  - Cells are exposed to gastric acid repeatedly and undergo: metaplasia → low grade dysplasia → high grade dysplasia → adenocarcinoma.

Symptoms

- Symptoms are often minimal until the oesophagus is nearly occluded:
  - The first symptom is usually dysphagia to solid foods.
  - Later, dysphagia to liquids and saliva may develop.
  - Weight loss and anorexia.
- Atypical chest pain, often radiating to the back, with normal ECG during episodes.

- Compression/invasion of adjacent structures causing:
  - Hoarseness.
  - Horner's syndrome.
  - Spinal pain.
  - Hiccups.
- Signs of un-resectability include metastases:
  - To the lungs causing shortness of breath.
  - To the liver with ascites.
  - To the bones causing bony pain.
  - To the brain causing headache, confusion, and seizures.
- In late stages, the tumour may completely occlude the oesophagus. Swallowing becomes impossible leading to build up of secretions in the mouth, causing severe distress.
- Trapped food debris can become infected with bacteria as the food material is not exposed to gastric acid. Aspiration of this material in patients with poor laryngeal reflexes or during induction may result in pneumonia/lung abscess.

Investigations

Bloods
- **FBC, U&E.**
- **LFT.**
  - Nutritional status may be poor due to inability to swallow, cachexia. Check albumin level.
- **ABG's.**

Radiology
- **CXR.**
  - Look for gross metastases or collapse/consolidation.
- **Barium swallow.**
- **CT, MRI.**
  - Initial staging assessment should include spiral computed tomography (CT) of the thorax and abdomen to determine the presence or absence of metastatic disease.

Other
Staging needs to be thorough and accurate for all patients in order to plan optimal therapeutic options.
- **ECG.**
- **PFT.**
- **CPEX.**
- **Endoscopic biopsy** or brush cytology.
- **Bronchoscopy.**
- **Staging laparoscopy.**
- **Transabdominal ultrasound.**

Prognosis

- Because oesophageal cancer is usually not diagnosed until the disease has spread the mortality is high.
- Fewer than 5% of people survive more than 5 years.

Treatment

- A multidisciplinary team approach, with plans for treatment selection (radical and palliative), treatment provision and post-treatment care is recommended.
- Surgery remains the best potentially curative option for most patients. However, <40% of patients are operable at presentation.
- Pre-operative chemo radiation may improve long term survival.
- Chemo radiation is the definitive treatment of choice for localized squamous cell carcinoma of the proximal oesophagus.
- Radiotherapy is more effective for squamous cell carcinoma than adenocarcinoma. Complications of this treatment include pneumonitis, bleeding, myelitis and tracheo-oesophageal fistula.
- Neoadjuvant chemotherapy with cisplatin and 5-fluorouracil (5-FU) improves short term survival over surgery alone.

Pre-operative assessment and preparation

- Haematological and biochemical abnormalities should be corrected.

Cardio-respiratory

- Patients with known or symptomatic ischaemic heart disease need careful evaluation.
  - More detailed investigations such as exercise electrocardiography, echocardiography, thallium imaging, and V/Q scanning may be considered.
- Pharmacological treatment of angina, hypertension, asthma, and COPD should be optimized.
- Pulmonary complications are increased when FEV_1 is reduced by >20%.
  - Pre-operative chest physiotherapy may be beneficial.
- Patients should be encouraged to stop smoking.

Other measures

- Most patients should have anti-thrombotic and antibiotic prophylaxis instituted at an appropriate time.
- Quality of life at presentation should be assessed and taken into consideration in treatment planning.

Preparation for operation

- Four units of blood should be cross matched prior to surgery. However, transfusion should be avoided if possible as the immuno suppressant effect can adversely affect survival
- Chemotherapeutic agents can cause various side-effects relevant to anaesthesia:
  - Doxorubicin can cause myelosupression, dose-related cardiomyopathy, cardiac dysrhythmias & conduction defects.
  - Bleomycin also causes myelosuppression and pulmonary toxicity, worsened by a high inspired oxygen content.

Surgical techniques

These are discussed in detail (See 📖 Oesophagectomy, p. 444).

Oesophagectomy

PROCEDURE BASICS: usually laparotomy followed by thoracotomy. Sometimes a neck anastamosis is necessary.

TIME: 3–6 hours.

PAIN RATING: 4/5.

ANALGESIA: thoracic epidural/paravertebral +/- PCA.

BLOOD LOSS: minimal-moderate.

HOSPITAL STAY: up to 72 hours on ITU. HDU care is the minimal requirement. Further week to 10 days to establish enteral feeding.

PREPARATION AND EQUIPMENT: as for thoracotomy and laparotomy.. Intensive care provision should be available. DLT needed to permit any thoracotomy. Invasive monitoring with arterial line AND CVP line.

Introduction
- There are approximately 2000 oesophagectomies performed each year in the UK. With a national 30-day mortality reported to be 10% and a 5-year survival of 25%.
- Local reporting from centres performing regular oesophagectomies give lower 30 day mortality figures (often <5%).
- Post-operative morbidity is also common, reportedly up to 40%.

History
- The first (documented) successful transthoracic oesophagectomy was performed in 1913 by Dr Franz Torek.
- By 1933 Grey Turner had success with the transhiatal route and Ohsa reported successful transthoracic resection of lower oesophageal tumours.

Surgical procedure
- Involves excision of the oesophageal tumour, part of the oesophagus and usually part of the stomach. The gastric remnant is usually tubularized and used to re-establish continuity.
- There are several approaches to this, and choice of surgical technique is determined by location of tumour and surgeon's preference.

Ivor Lewis oesophagectomy

Described in 1946 By Ivor Lewis.

- Mid to distal third oesophageal tumours
- This involves a laparotomy to:
  - Mobilize the stomach.
  - Check for sub-diaphpagmatic spread that may have been missed.
  - Resect lymphatic spread to para-aortic, cardiac and lesser curve nodes.
- Followed by position change and a right sided thoracotomy to access, mobilize and excise the tumour.
  - This will involve a skin incision from the midpoint between spinous process of T3 and the medial border of scapula, extending in a curved fashion around, to below the right nipple.
  - The fifth rib is exposed and the posterior 2 cm excised to allow adequate retraction.
  - The oesophagus is mobilized and an appropriate excision margin is determined.
- The stomach is then passed into the thoracic cavity, via the oesophageal hiatus, taking care not to rotate the stomach on its longitudinal axis and disturb the vasculature.
- The specimen is then excised completely and the stomach anastamosed with the "clear" proximal oesophageal stump.

McKeown three stage oesophagecomy

Described in 1976 by KC McKeown. the three stages refer to:

- Laparotomy, as per Ivor Lewis.
- Right thoracotomy.
- Cervical incision and anastamosis of gastric tract.
  - This involves "thyroidectomy" positioning.
  - Incision from the posterior triangle (2 cm above clavicle) to the midline, just above the suprasternal notch.
  - The cervical oesophagus is located and then the thoracic oesophagus is gently pulled into the neck.
  - The cervical oesophagus is then anastamosed to the fundus.
  - The oesophagogastric anastamosis is then passed back into the upper thoracic cavity.

Left thoracotomy

- Favoured by many thoracic surgeons.
- Allows access to the thoracic oesophagus and stomach, via one skin incision, by dividing the left hemidiaphragm.

Transhiatal approach

- This involves laparotomy with no thoracotomy.
- The thoracic oesophagus is mobilized, via the oesophageal hiatus, with blunt dissection and a cervical oesophagogastric anastamosis is performed.

- This procedure has been suggested as appropriate for low oesophageal tumours only, as the clearance of thoracic nodes is not possible.
- There is no need for one lung anaesthesia. However, similar rates of respiratory complications and wound infections have been shown between Ivor Lewis and Transhiatal approaches.

Thoracoabdominal incision
- Combines a thoracotomy with a laparotomy, through one incision.

Minimally invasive oesophagectomy
- Various combinations of open and video-assisted thoracotomy and laparotomy are used, often with a neck incision.

Pre-operative assessment and preparation
- Malnutrition is common, as most patients will have dysphagia.
- >50% of patients are over 70 yr.
- Respiratory disease is common, and pulmonary function tests should be performed.
- Immunosuppression from chemotherapy.
- CVS problems are common and a functional status assessment should be performed.
  - Dukes activity status index.
  - Shuttle walk test.
  - CPEX testing.

Anaesthesia for oesophagectomy
Induction
- Establish good awake thoracic epidural.
- Insert invasive lines asleep.
  - Use a CVP line with 5 lumens if possible; TPN may be necessary post-operatively.
- Catheterize and insert an NG tube (this cannot be easily re-positioned later!).
- RSI/modified RSI should be performed and the airway secured with a (left) DLT.
- ❶ Fibreoptic checking of the DLT position is mandatory after initial intubation and after ANY re-positioning of the patient.

Position
Described above.

Maintenance and intra-operative
- Intra-operative warming with temperature monitoring.
- Pressure supported ventilation with the use of PEEP (bearing in mind that PEEP may increase shunt through the dependent lung, hence worsening hypoxaemia).

- Avoidance of hypoxaemia during one-lung anaesthesia.
- Care with intra-operative fluids as these patients are prone to post-operative ALI/ARDS. Fluid shifts secondary to extensive peri-operative inflammation increase risk of airway oedema.
- Surgeon may ask you to withdraw or advance the NG tube until it is in the optimal position.

- It is well worth taking an ABG early, in the middle and towards the end of the procedure
  - Together with this, the intra-operative haemodynamic and respiratory behaviour of the patient can inform the decision to extubate or not.

The end of the procedure
- Suction to non-dependent lung prior to re-establishment of TLV.
- Sling NG tube once surgeon is happy with the position as this will be needed for post-operative course.
- Decide as to whether the patient is suitable for extubation or whether they will be taken to ITU intubated (See below).

Post-operative course
- Thoracic epidural is gold standard at present, and should be able to cover thoracotomy, and to a certain extent the abdominal wound, but sometimes, a multimodal approach is necessary due to the large dermatomal spread of the wounds.
- For a left thoracotomy, paravertebral blocks (with surgical placement of catheter) have been employed. This offers no cover for the laparotomy in other approaches.
- For minimally invasive oesophagectomy, paravertebral infusion and PCA may be appropriate.

To ventilate or not to ventilate after the procedure?

- There are numerous studies demonstrating the safety of immediate post-operative extubation, assuming the intra-operative course has been unremarkable.
- Many centres will not embark on the procedure if there are no level three (ITU) care provisions available.

Immediate extubation
- The advantages of immediate extubation are both financial and practical, as the level 2 (HDU) patients are less staff intensive.
- Early extubation is only really feasible if there is good analgesia on-board for the immediate post-operative period (normally a thoracic epidural with established block).

Late extubation
- Elective post-operative ventilation allows further optimization of the patient prior to extubation:
  - Any hypothermia can be addressed.
  - Electrolytes and clotting can be corrected.

- Excessive intra-operative blood loss/transfusion sequalae can be dealt with.
- Analgesia can be optimized.
- Acid-base status can be normailzed.
- Haemodynamic status correction +/- vasopressor/inotropic support can be given.
- The anastomosis is theoretically protected in the immediate post-op period (lack of retching, patient immobility, correction of correctible adverse conditions whilst intubated).
- Adverse effects of the described fluid shifts can be controlled with a supported airway.
- Biliary reflux and aspiration is minimized.
- However, the incidence of ventilator-associated pneumonia increases at 48 hours.
- Patients who are extubated later, generally have a longer ITU stay than those who were extubated early.
- The bottom line is that it is down to the clinician and experience!

Feeding

- This is often controversial, some clinicians preferring not to feed at all.
  - However, these patients are sometimes malnourished and malnourishment has been linked to poor wound healing, difficulty weaning and adverse outcome.
- Oral feeding will usually commence following a satisfactory contrast swallow, usually at day 5.
- Many centres will commence parentral feeding immediately post-operatively.
- Often a feeding jejunostomy will be performed. If ileus is present or the jejunal tube becomes displaced, consideration of early parentral feeding should be made.

Complications

- Three conditions have been implicated in early post-operative death:
  - Pulmonary disorders.
  - Anastamotic leak.
  - Dysrhythmias.

Pulmonary complications (25%)

- Up to 25% of patients suffer pulmonary complications.
- Pain from extensive incisions can be a major contributor to decreased ventilation and atelectasis, leading to pneumonia and respiratory failure.
- Respiratory problems have also been linked with pre-operative respiratory issues, low FEV_1 and smoking.
- Incisions of the diaphragm may impair its movement and extensive lymphadenectomy can cause poor lymphatic drainage of the pulmonary alveoli, resulting in a form of acute pulmonary oedema.
- The use of thoracic epidural anaesthesia has been shown to significantly decrease the incidence of respiratory complications.
- There is a well established link between hypoxaemia during OLV and ALI/ARDS. ARDS in the post-operative oesophagectomy carries 50% mortality.
- There is a small step to be made between poor practice of one-lung anaesthesia and development of post-operative ALI/ARDS.
- Hypoxaemia during one-lung anaesthesia is often due to displacement of the double lumen tube, and failure to identify and reposition.

Anastomotic leak (10–15%)

- Early disruption (within the first 72 hours) usually reflects technical error.
  - Once confirmed, if the general condition of the patient is good, then re-exploration and repair is appropriate.
- The majority of disruptions occur later (up to two weeks) and probably reflect local ischaemia and/or tension in the anastomotic site.
- A high index of clinical suspicion is important.
  - Although water soluble contrast radiology should be used to establish that leakage has occurred, the technique is not completely accurate and may miss clinically significant leaks as well as demonstrate radiological leakages of no clinical significance.
  - The majority of anastomotic leakages, whether in the neck or the chest, can be managed conservatively with nasogastric suction, appropriate local drainage, antibiotics, and jejunal feeding.
- At worst, mediastinitis, systemic sepsis, ARDS and death can result.
- Improvement of O_2 delivery, by way of increasing cardiac output, has demonstrated a reduction in gastric ischaemia.
- It has been shown that O_2 delivery and consumption in survivors is higher than in non-survivors in the immediate 6-hour post-op period.
- Suggesting a role for optimization of O_2 delivery in HDU.

CVS complications (11%)
- Includes MI and dysrhythmia.
- It has been shown that myocardial ischaemia increases with thoracotomy and this is also linked to adverse outcome.

Recurrent laryngeal nerve injury
- More common during dissection of the upper third of the oesophagus.
- Recurrent laryngeal nerve injury impairs the patient's ability to cough in the early post-operative period and adequately protect the airway during swallowing, hence increases pulmonary morbidity.
- In most patients there is adequate compensation from the opposite cord.
- Tracheostomy should be considered to protect the airway and improve pulmonary toilet. Thyroplasty or vocal cord injections are rarely required.

Thoracic trauma, emergencies, and special cases

General approach to thoracic trauma

Thoracic trauma can be daunting to the assessing physician. Individual aetiologies will be discussed at length later. The following offers a brief overview.

Pathophysiology

- Thoracic trauma can result in global hypoxaemia and hypoperfusion. Ultimately, the Pasteur point is reached, aerobic switches to anaerobic metabolism and cellular hypoxia ensues with eventual cell death.
- Patients presenting with profound acidosis (pH <7.0 and lactate >6) as a result of thoracic trauma, are at significant risk of imminent death.
- Therefore, a thorough primary survey with immediate, rapid and effective resuscitation is the key to minimize associated morbidity and mortality.

Types of trauma

- Blunt.
  - >10% will require a definitive operation.
- Penetrating
  - 15–30% require operation.
- Majority.
  - Require simple resuscitation.

Life-threatening injuries

Immediate threat—ATOM FC

- **A**irway obstruction/laryngotracheal injury.
- **T**ension pneumothorax.
- **O**pen pneumothorax.
- **M**assive haemothorax.
- **F**lail chest & severe pulmonary contusion.
- **C**ardiac tamponade.

Potential threat

- Simple pneumothorax may tension during IPPV.
- Pulmonary contusion.
- Tracheobronchial injury.
- Haemothorax.
- Blunt cardiac injury.
- Great vessel injury.
- Blunt oesophageal rupture.
- Traumatic diaphragmatic rupture.

Rib fractures and associated injuries

Ribs 1–3

- High mortality.
- Severe force needed to produce injury.

- Associated injuries:
  - Great vessels.
  - Cardiac tamponade.
  - Tension pneumothorax.
  - Tracheobronchial/oesophageal injury.

Ribs 4–9
- Pulmonary contusion.
- Pneumothorax.

Ribs 10–12
- Likely abdominal injuries, e.g. hepatic, splenic.

Management of all trauma
Should follow suggested ATLS algorithms.

Airway maintenance with C-spine control
- Deliver high flow oxygen (15 L/min) via a trauma mask with reservoir.
- Basic airway manoeuvres if needed (chin lift, jaw thrust).
- Use basic airway adjuncts if needed.
  - Do not insert a nasal airway if there is a suspected base of skull fracture.
- Intubate if necessary:
  - Anticipate that laryngoscopy will be difficult, i.e. have a McCoy laryngoscope and bougie available.
  - Immobilize the head and neck with manual in-line stabilization (MILS).
  - Undo the hard collar and remove sandbags and tape. If not removed, the hard collar impedes/prevents mouth opening.
  - Maintain MILS until the hard collar, sandbags and tape are re-applied.
- Thoracic trauma may ultimately require a DLT to be placed in order to facilitate surgery.
  - This IS NOT AN IMMEDIATE PRIORITY. The aim is to secure the airway as best one can to prevent death from hypoxia.

Breathing
- Consider the need to assist ventilation.

Circulation
- Wide bore IV access and take blood samples.
  - **FBC, U&E, Glucose, Clotting and X-match, ABG.**
- Rapid IV fluid infusion; the colloid vs. crystalloid debate continues without definitive strong evidence in support of one or the other.
  - The key is to support the failing circulation, and improve O_2 flux.
  - There is evidence to support judicious intravascular volume replacement to obtain a goal systolic BP of NO HIGHER than around 90–110 mmHg. Any higher may increase active bleeding.
  - Never use 5% dextrose.
  - **There is an exception to the rule, whereby 'C' may need to be addressed prior to 'B' in the algorithm of the primary survey.

****❶** It may be prudent to consider wide bore IV access BEFORE draining a suspected haemothorax.
- The aim is to allow rapid infusion of fluid/blood products if catastrophic blood loss results after the intercostal drain is placed. In addition, the tamponade effect of a large haemothorax will be lost.

Definitive management
- The majority of thoracic trauma can be managed with oxygen, intercostal chest drainage, analgesia, and appropriate fluid management.
- However, some patients will require immediate/urgent thoracotomy/ median sternotomy and repair of intra-thoracic injuries.

When to intubate and ventilate

General
- If the patient has a GCS <8, whether due to head trauma or not, the airway may be un-supported. Therefore, consider intubation to secure their airway.
- If the patient is in shock, fractious, combative, acidotic and requires further investigation or theatre.
  - It may be prudent to intubate and ventilate the patient, as these signs are often the result of poor O_2 flux.
  - Provision of a definitive airway with 100% O_2 may improve the O_2 flux.
- Immediate surgery required:
  - Patient stable for brief transfer to theatre. ⚠ Transfer with full equipment and intubate in theatre with surgical standby.
  - Patient unstable; ⚠ consider securing their airway prior to transfer to theatre.

Pneumothorax
- Intubation and IPPV in the presence of a simple pneumothorax can convert it to a tension pneumothorax.
- Consider chest drain insertion PRIOR to intubation.

Cardiac tamponade
- Deciding the optimal time to intubate a patient for open evacuation of a cardiac tamponade is important.
  - IPPV will have deleterious haemodynamic effects as a result of the loss of the negative intrathoracic pressure. Physiological compensation may not be possible.
  - Intubation and IPPV can be considered early if there is a skilled surgeon on immediate standby to immediately decompress the tamponade once intubation is achieved.
  - If intubation cannot be delayed because of very low oxygen saturation or imminent cardiac arrest, high ventilatory pressures should be avoided and consideration given to percutaneous drainage of the pericardial sac before induction of anaesthesia.

When is an emergency department thoracotomy (EDT) warranted?

- The rationale for performing an EDT is to:
  - Attempt resuscitation in a patient with an agonal rhythm secondary to penetrating cardiothoracic injuries.
  - Release cardiac tamponade by evacuation of pericardial blood.
  - Immediately control haemorrhage and repair cardiac or pulmonary injury.
  - Enable open cardiac massage to be performed.
  - Place a descending thoracic aortic cross-clamp to improve the perfusion the brain and heart
  - Control massive air embolism.
- Following emergency thoracotomy, the overall survival rates for penetrating thoracic trauma are around 9–12% but have been reported to be as high as 38%.
- The decision to perform emergency thoracotomy involves careful evaluation of the scientific, ethical, social and economic issues.
- New agreed consensus is that EDT should be considered for:
  - Any penetrating thoracic injury and pulseless electrical activity arrest/refractory cardiovascular collapse.
  - Presence of an appropriately skilled cardio-thoracic surgeon.
  - THERE IS NO PLACE FOR EDT IN BLUNT TRAUMA.

Pitfalls

- Consider co-morbidities, medication, age and patient fitness when assessing initial haemodynamics and further resuscitation.
- Simple pneumothorax may become a tension pneumothorax with IPPV.
- Needle decompression of any pneumothorax MUST be followed by insertion of a definitive chest drain.
- Low threshold for insertion of an ICD, particularly when:
  - Moving the patient ANYWHERE.
  - Air transfer.
  - Positive pressure ventilation is required.

- Beware of the retained haemothorax.
- DO NOT USE N$_2$O during operative procedures.
- Diaphragmatic injuries may not be apparent until much later.

**Do not be fooled by a head injury!
- If the patient has a mechanism of injury and visible injuries/clinical signs of thoracic trauma; it is almost certain that the thoracic injuries are causing the shock, NOT the head injury.

Laryngo-tracheal trauma

Background

Direct trauma to the airway is fortunately rare, and is seen in <1% of patients presenting to emergency departments following trauma. The bony protection afforded to the airway by the sternum and mandible as well as death from asphyxia at the scene may account for the rare presentation of this type of injury.

- Typical victim is male and 30–40 years old.
- Penetrating laryngo-tracheal trauma is more common.
- Blunt trauma and the need for an emergency airway are independent predictors of mortality.
- Overall mortality for this spectrum of injury is up to 30%.

Classification

Blunt injury

- Typically, both the larynx and trachea are injured together.
- Mechanism of injury:
  - Direct impact, e.g. from steering wheel/dashboard.
  - Crush, e.g. strangulation
  - Flexion/extension, e.g. clothesline injury.
- 45% of injuries involve the cervical trachea:
  - Crico-tracheal junction is prone to transection. Oedema and/or air dissecting through the epiglottic submucosa may result in worsening airway obstruction.
- 35% of injuries are above the cricoid:
  - Result in supra/subglottic oedema, haematoma, thyroid and arytenoid cartilage fracture.
- 15% of injuries involve cricoid cartilage ± RLN damage.

Penetrating injury

- The trachea is more commonly injured.
- Mechanism of injury:
  - Gunshot.
  - Stab wound; most commonly in anterior triangle of neck (two thirds of these injuries involve the cervical trachea).
  - Iatrogenic, e.g. percutaneous tracheostomy, intubation.

Associated injuries

Blunt trauma

- Closed head injury.
- Maxillofacial injury.
- Cervical spine injury.
- Cervicothoracic vascular injury.
- Thoracic trauma.

Penetrating trauma
- Cervicothoracic vascular injury in 25–50% cases.
- Oesophageal injury (30%).
- Neurological (12%), especially RLN.
- Pulmonary injury (10%).

Presentation and assessment
* >25% patients with laryngo-tracheal injury have no symptoms and signs until 24–48 hours following injury.

Symptoms
- Respiratory distress/stridor.
- Hoarseness/dysphonia/dysphagia
- Cough.
- Neck pain.

Signs
- Haemoptysis.
- Subcutaneous emphysema, neck swelling/bruising.
- Sucking chest/neck wound.
- Patient prefers to sit forwards.

Immediate trauma management
- Manage as per ATLS guidelines, i.e. identify and treat immediate threats to life using an ABC approach.
- Do not delay definitive airway management for investigations.
- >50% patients require emergency airway intervention.
- Typically, these patients can be managed with an endotracheal tube.
- It is vital that the airway is secured distal to the injury.
- If necessary, the trachea can be intubated through an open neck wound.
- Remember, a partially obstructed airway can rapidly obstruct.

Emergency
Stridulous/obstructed with signs of laryngo-tracheal injury.
- Intubate:
  - IV vs. inhalational induction.
  - Endotracheal tube may not advance past a tracheal transection.
  - Consider rigid bronchoscopy.
- Perform needle cricothyroidotomy & jet ventilation.
  - May be futile in cases of cricoid disruption or distal tracheal injury.
- Perform tracheostomy.
  - LA vs. GA; likely to be technically difficult in a patient who is in extremis.

Urgent
- Administer humidified oxygen.
- Ensure that a surgeon is immediately available and able to create a surgical airway.
- Ensure that equipment for cricothyroidotomy is available.

- Airway management options are:
  - Awake fibreoptic inspection/intubation. Observe the patient in a critical care environment if fibreoptic examination demonstrates normal or minor findings.
  - General anaesthesia as above and intubate/tracheostomize.
- Consider IV steroids once all other life-/limb-threatening injuries excluded.

Investigations

Bloods
- **FBC, coagulation.**
- **X-match.**
- **U&E.**
- **ABG.**

Radiology
- **X-Ray.**
  - C-spine: inspect for fracture/dislocation.
  - Chest: inspect for pnuemomediastinum/subcutaneous emphysema/pneumothorax/haemothorax/scapula, upper rib, clavicle fractures.
  - Pelvis: inspect for pelvic disruption.
- **CT** chest
  - Airway calibre, cartilaginous and soft tissue injury, associated c-spine/chest/abdominal injury.

Other
- **Nasendoscopy.**
  - Inspect for oedema, haematoma, vocal cord paralysis, cartilage disruption, laryngeal inlet patency.
  - Oesophagoscopy/contrast swallow study to exclude oesophageal injury.

Pitfalls/difficult situations

- A high index of suspicion for cricoid/cervical spine/tracheal injury is vital.
- Cricoid pressure and paralysis in a patient with occult cricoid injury or laryngo-tracheal transection can be disastrous.
- Cricothyroidotomy may be impossible.
- Positive pressure ventilation can exacerbate air leaks and rapidly worsen pneumothoraces, pneumomediastinum and subcutaneous emphysema.
  - If possible, the patient should be allowed to spontaneously ventilate until the endotracheal tube has been placed distal to the tracheal injury.

Tracheo-bronchial trauma

- True incidence of tracheo-bronchial injury (TBI) is unknown; 30–80% of patients will die before arrival at hospital; estimated that up to 3% traumatic deaths may have an associated TBI.
- Reported incidence of up to 2% patients presenting to Emergency Department (ED) following blunt chest trauma.
- >80% injuries associated with blunt chest trauma are within 1 inch of the carina.
- The majority of penetrating TBI involves the cervical trachea.
- Patients who reach ED with a TBI may not require emergent airway intervention. Therefore, other life-threatening injuries may be appropriately addressed first.

Presentation and assessment

- Findings may be subtle.
  - Subcutaneous emphysema.
  - Tachypnoea.
  - Hoarseness.
  - Haemoptysis.
  - Reduced air entry/breath sounds.
  - Signs related to associated injuries.

Associated injuries

- Simple/tension/open pneumothorax; may fail to drain adequately with one chest drain in-situ due to large air leak.
- Haemothorax.
- Flail chest.
- Pulmonary contusion.

Specific investigations

- A high index of suspicion is required.
- CT can detect >90% of TBIs.
- Bronchoscopy is the gold standard diagnostic tool.

Management

- Assess and treat immediately life-threatening injuries as described above.
- Conservative management of TBI is an option.
- Rapid progression of subcutaneous/mediastinal emphysema, mediastinitis, or difficulty with ventilation to all indicate that urgent surgical repair of the injury is indicated.
- Endobronchial intubation with a single/double lumen tube may be required in order to isolate a distal TBI.

Surgery

Surgical approach is tailored to the specific injury. Typically, the following applies:

- A collar incision is used for cervical tracheal injury.
- A median sternotomy is used for injuries high in the mediastinal trachea or where great vessel injury is suspected.
- Right postero-lateral thoracotomy is used for lower mediastinal tracheal injuries.
- Ipsilateral postero-lateral thoracotomy is used where TBI is associated with pneumothorax or there is a diagnosed bronchial injury.
- Tracheal resection may be necessary if the injured tracheal segment is beyond repair. (See 📖 Tracheal reconstruction and resection, p. 332).

Further reading

Beed M, Sherman R, Majahan R (2007). *Emergencies in Critical Care*. Oxford University Press. p. 26.

Hurford W E, Peralta R. Management of tracheal trauma. *Canadian Journal of Anaesthesia* 2003; 50(6):1–6.

Bhojani R, Rosenbaum D, Dikmen E, *et al*. Contemporary assessment of laryngo-tracheal trauma. *Journal of Thoracic and Cardiovascular Surgery* 2005; 130:426–32.

Pneumothorax

Definition
Free gas in the pleural cavity. The gas is usually air but can be medically administered gas such as CO_2 or nitrous oxide.

Classification

Spontaneous pneumothorax
Primary
- No apparent underlying lung disease. Usually occurring due to a congenital pleural bleb or bulla (found in 80–90% of patients investigated with either a CT chest or thoracoscopy).

Secondary
- Underlying lung disease, e.g. TB, bullous emphysema, asthma, pulmonary fibrosis.

Traumatic pneumothorax
Closed
- Occurs due to damage of the visceral or parietal pleura, e.g. by fractured ribs.

Open
- Defect in the chest wall which exposes the pleural cavity to atmospheric pressure.

> - **Tension pneumothorax** can occur if there is a flap mechanism in either the visceral pleura or the chest wall.
> - The flap mechanism allows air to enter the pleural cavity on inspiration but closes on expiration. Thus, air becomes trapped in the pleural cavity and the pneumothorax expands with each breath.
> - Tension pneumothorax impedes venous return to the heart and if untreated, results in cardiac arrest, i.e. pulseless electrical activity.

Presentation

History
- Pleuritic chest pain and progressive dyspnoea.
- Patients with a tension pneumothorax are very distressed and, if able to talk, will describe the feeling of being unable to breathe.
- Patient risk factors for pneumothorax include:
  - Tall stature (Marfan's syndrome, other connective tissue diseases).
  - Male.
  - Smoker.
  - Previous pneumothorax.
  - History of underlying lung disease.
  - History of chest trauma.
  - Excessive coughing.

Clinical examination

(See Table 9.1)

- The clinical presentation can vary depending on the size of the pneumothorax and the patient's pre-morbid physiological condition.
- Clinical signs may be absent in small pneumothoraces in fit patients.
- Pneumothorax rarely occurs during mechanical ventilation and normally only if high airway pressures are used or if the patient has underlying lung disease, e.g. bullous emphysema.

Table 9.1 Clinical examination findings for pneumothorax

Examination	Clinical Findings
Inspection	Tachypnoea
	Evidence of chest trauma
	Cyanosis
	Distended neck veins (tension pneumothorax)
Palpation	Trachea deviated away from pneumothorax
	Reduced chest expansion of side with pneumothorax
	Subcutaneous emphysema
Percussion	Hyper-resonant on side of pneumothorax
Auscultation	Reduced or absent breath sounds on side of pneumothorax
CVS Exam	Tachycardia
	Hypotension
	Cardiac arrest can occur in tension pneumothorax
Ventilation	Increasing airway pressures
	Rising $PaCO_2$
	$EtCO_2$ may fall with reduction in cardiac output

Specific investigations

- BP, pulse oximetry, ECG.

Bloods
- **ABG.**

Radiology
- **Erect CXR.**
  - Lung edge with absent lung markings beyond the edge of the collapsed lung.

Radiological considerations

- CXR findings of a pneumothorax in supine patients (e.g. after trauma, unstable ITU patients) may not be obvious due to the air moving toward the anterior chest rather than the apex.
- Radiological signs to look for are:
  - Deep sulcus sign—abnormally prominent or deep costophrenic angle.
  - Etched diaphragm—diaphragm contrasted with air in pleural space.
  - Etched mediastinum—heart border outlined with air in pleural space.
- Ultrasound can be used in the diagnosis of a pneumothorax when the plain radiograph is unclear, e.g. the supine ventilated patient.

Immediate treatment priorities

- An ABC approach should be taken to all these patients.
- Administer 100% oxygen.
- IV access.

Tension pneumothorax
- ⚠ This is an immediately life-threatening emergency. It is a clinical diagnosis and treatment should not be delayed for radiological confirmation.
- Perform needle thoracocentesis with a 14G cannula in the 2nd intercostal space, mid-clavicular line. The patient should improve after decompression of the tension.
  - However, the cannula can become kinked and the patient deteriorates again. In this instance repeat decompression.
- Needle thoracocentesis is a temporising measure. An intercostal chest drain should be inserted as soon as possible.

Open pneumothorax
- Consider early intubation. This should not delay chest tube placement and closure of the wound with an occlusive dressing.
- Do not insert the intercostal drain through the chest wound.
- If an intercostal chest drain is not imminent then a dressing may be applied over the wound and taped on 3 SIDES ONLY.
  - This acts as a one-way valve allowing air to escape on expiration but becomes sucked closed on inspiration.

Simple pneumothorax

- Spontaneously breathing patients with a small pneumothorax (<2 cm rim between lung edge and chest wall on CXR) and not breathless may be managed conservatively by observation alone.
- Aspiration is the first line treatment for all symptomatic patients with a primary pneumothorax.
  - This is less likely to succeed. in patients with secondary pneumothorax and should be limited to those patients <50 years with a small pneumothorax (<2cm rim) and minimal dyspnoea.
- Intercostal drainage is reserved for those patients where aspiration has failed, or in those patients with secondary pneumothorax who are breathless, or where the pneumothorax is large (≥2cm rim); see 📖 Insertion of intercostal drains, p. 744 for a description of the procedure.
- All mechanically ventilated patients with a pneumothorax require an intercostal chest drain due to the risk of tension pneumothorax as a result of IPPV.

Transfer of patients to another hospital—considerations

If involved in transfer of a patient with a simple pneumothorax:
- Insert a chest drain BEFORE leaving origin hospital.
  - Placement of a chest drain in an ambulance is not easy!!
- If transferring by air:
  - ALWAYS insert a chest drain, as pressure changes/lack of space to work in an air ambulance will make conversion to tension likely/will leave little room to work in!

Anaesthetic procedures with risk of pneumothorax

Airway/Breathing

- Percutaneous tracheostomy.
- Mechanical/non-invasive ventilation.
- Valsalva manoeuvre.

Circulation

- Central venous puncture, i.e. internal jugular/subclavian vein.
- Rib fracture associated with chest compressions.

Regional Analgesia Techniques

- Paravertebral block.
- Intercostal nerve block.
- Interpleural block.
- Brachial plexus block, i.e. infra-, supra-clavicular, interscalene.
- Cervical plexus block.

Anaesthesia for a patient with a pneumothorax

- Ensure a chest drain is in-situ and is draining/bubbling before mechanical ventilation is commenced.
  - This may not always be immediately possible in the acute trauma setting, e.g. decompressed tension pneumothorax awaiting intercostal drainage after needle thoracocentesis.
- Avoid the use of nitrous oxide as this diffuses into air filled cavities and will expand the pneumothorax.
- Avoid using high ventilation pressures if visceral injury is suspected.

Surgical management of pneumothorax

Aims

- Suture any visceral perforation or resect any blebs which may be responsible for the pneumothorax.
- To create a pleural symphysis to prevent recurrence.

Indications for surgical intervention

- Second ipsilateral pneumothorax.
- First contralateral pneumothorax.
- Bilateral spontaneous pneumothorax.
- Persistent air leak (>5–7 days of tube drainage, air leak or failure to re-expand).
- Spontaneous haemothorax.
- Profession at risk, e.g. pilot, diver.

Surgical options

- Open thoracotomy and parietal pleurectomy.
- Video-assisted thoracoscopic surgery (VATS).
- Pleurectomy.
- Chemical pleurodesis.
- Trans-axillary mini-thoracotomy.

Further reading

Henry M, Arnold T, Harvey J. BTS guidelines for the management of spontaneous pneumothorax. *Thorax* 2003; **58**: 39–52.

Advanced Trauma Life Support Course Manual. 8th Edition. 2009.

Traumatic cardiac tamponade

Definition

A haemodynamically significant cardiac compression caused by pericardial fluid.

Acute traumatic cardiac tamponade may be caused by haemopericardium or pneumopericardium and represents an immediate threat to life. The chapter focuses on acute haemopericardium (HP).

Causes

Traumatic haemo pericardium (HP) is caused by:

- Blunt/penetrating chest and upper abdominal trauma.
- Iatrogenic.
  - Central venous catheter insertion.
  - Percutaneous coronary intervention.
  - Pacing wire insertion.
  - Endocardial biopsy.
  - Post cardiac surgery, valve surgery, ± abnormal coagulation.
- Haemorrhage may result from:
  - Coronary artery/vein laceration.
  - Cardiac chamber rupture.
  - Diffuse myocardial haemorrhage.
  - Intra-pericardial aortic root rupture.

Pathophysiology

▶ Filling pressure = intra-cardiac—intra-pericardial pressure

- Normal pericardial volume = 30–50 ml. Typically, rapid accumulation of 200–300 ml pericardial blood → fatal cardiac tamponade.
- During acute HP there is a rapid increase in pericardial volume. Initially, the pericardium accommodates the increased volume and there is only a slow rise in the intrapericardial pressure.
- Subsequently, the limit of pericardial stretch is reached and intrapericardial pressure increases rapidly and exponentially (cf Monroe-Kellie doctrine).

Thus:

- ↑ intrapericardial pressure → cardiac chamber compression.
- ↓ myocardial diastolic compliance → ↓ cardiac filling & ↓SV.
- ↑ sympathetic activity to maintain cardiac output.
  - ↑ HR.
  - ↑ contractility.
  - ↑ SVR—maintains coronary perfusion.

- Ultimately, intra pericardial pressure ≈ diastolic intra-cardiac pressure
  ∴ cardiac filling ceases and cardiac arrest occurs (pulseless electrical
  activity).
- The low-pressure right heart is affected first.

⚠ During the initial phase of aggressive fluid therapy in acute trauma
patients cardiac filling pressures will increase ∴ the effects of cardiac tamponade will be temporarily masked.

Presentation and assessment

- Signs of acute traumatic cardiac tamponade are subtle and non-specific
  - Therefore easily missed during the initial assessment and treatment
    of a trauma victim.

⚠ High index of suspicion is required, especially in cases of blunt chest
trauma.

Signs

- ↑ HR.
- ↓ BP.
  - Disproportionate to estimated blood loss ± unresponsive to fluid
    therapy.
- ↑ RR.
- Signs of hypoperfusion despite high CVP.
  - Cool and cyanosed periphery.
  - Prolonged CRT.
  - Rising lactate.
- Chest/upper abdominal wounds.
  - Cardiac tamponade has been associated with wounds anywhere
    between the umbilicus and root of neck.
- Beck's triad (10% of trauma patients with cardiac tamponade).
  - ↓ BP.
  - Muffled heart sounds.
  - Distended neck veins.
- Exaggerated jugular venous pulsation.
- Pulsus paradoxus is diagnostic.
  - ↓ systolic pressure 10 mmHg during inspiration
  - Clinically undetectable in extreme hypovolaemia.

▶▶ Presence of a praecordial entrance wound, ↓BP, ↑ HR and distended
neck veins is pathognomonic of cardiac tamponade 2° acute haemopericardium. Look for arrhythmias on ECG.

Immediate life threatening differential diagnoses

Tension pneumothorax
- ⚠ immediate threat to life
  - Exclude clinically: hyperresonant percussion note and absent breath sounds.
  - Immediate decompression by needle thoracocentesis with subsequent intercostal drain insertion.

Severe heart failure/myocardial contusion.
PE and acute heart failure
- Possible, however they may have been responsible for the accident.

Investigations

- **FAST scan** (Focused assessment sonography in trauma).
  - Visualization of haemopericardium.
  - 89% sensitivity & 99% specificity for cardiac tamponade.
  - Permits immediate diagnosis in the hypovolaemic patient.
  - Non-invasive.
  - Improved patient outcomes 2° to rapid diagnosis and ∴ access to definitive treatment.
- **Echocardiogram**
  - Usually right ventricle and atrium collapse during early and late diastole respectively.
  - Right atrial collapse is also seen in hypovolaemic patients.
  - Left atrial collapse is highly specific for cardiac tamponade (25% patients with tamponade).

Immedite trauma management

☞ Needle pericardiocentesis
Merely a temporary manoeuvre prior to urgent sternotomy/thoracotomy, affording a short-lived reduction in intrapericardial pressure.
- Ideally, echocardiographic guidance should be used to facilitate needle pericardiocentesis.
- ECG chest lead may be attached to needle hub. Needle tip contact with the myocardium is identified by a current of injury = ST elevation ± ectopics.
- Using a cannula-over-needle (16 - 18G) technique, advance slowly and continually aspirate.
- Leave the cannula in the pericardial sac to permit further drainage as required prior to definitive treatment.
- May not be helpful in acute haemopericardium with clotted blood.
- ⚠ Complications of needle pericardiocentesis:
  - Coronary artery/vein laceration.
  - Puncture/laceration of cardiac chamber.
  - Ectopic beats.

- Arrhythmia.
- Pneumothorax.
- Liver laceration

Ultrasound
- Recent opinion states that needle pericardiocentesis has been superceded by ultrasound guided drainage.

Definitive thoracotomy
- Ultimately, nearly all trauma patients with cardiac tamponade will require thoracotomy or median sternotomy.
  - Left antero-lateral thoracotomy/median sternotomy.
  - Allows evacuation of pericardial blood/clot and exploration/repair of thoracic contents.
- Many trauma centres proceed to immediate thoracotomy in the operating theatre and do not attempt needle pericardiocentesis/ sub-xiphoid pericardiotomy; see Table 9.2.

Anaesthesia for traumatic acute cardiac tamponade
- The anaesthetic management of a patient with acute traumatic cardiac tamponade and any associated blunt trauma injuries is challenging.
- The cardio-depressant effects of anaesthetic agents and positive pressure ventilation conspire against the patient with acute haemopericardium.
  - Discuss with the surgeon regarding whether to intubate or not.
  - You may have no choice but to intubate—do not allow the patient to die as a result of acute hypoxia!!

- 🔴🔴 Maintenance of compensatory cardiovascular mechanisms is paramount during induction of anaesthesia, and before drainage of acute haemopericardium. Drugs and anaesthetic technique should be chosen with the following in mind:
  - Avoid bradycardia.
  - Ensure adequate volume replacement and cardiac filling.
  - Optimize inotropy—need for CVP line.
  - Minimize vasodilatation.

Useful strategies
- Pre-operative ultrasound guided percutaneous drainage of acute tamponade; catheter left in-situ.
- Ketamine may be the induction agent of choice as it has minimal cardiovascular depressant effects.
- Minimize intra-thoracic pressure.
- Low V_t/pressure limited ventilation.

- CVP, invasive arterial pressure monitoring.
- Inotropic support.
- Local anaesthesia/analgesia.

Table 9.2 Approaches to emergency needle pericardiocentesis

Approach	Puncture site	Angulation	Direction
Paraxyphoid	Between xiphoid & left costal margin	15° to skin to pass deep to costal margin	Left shoulder
Sub-xiphoid	1–2cm inferior to left xiphocondral junction	45° to skin	Tip of left scapula

Further reading

Rozycki G, Feliciano DV, Ochsner M, *et al.* The role of ultrasound in patients with possible penetrating cardiac wounds: prospective multicentre study. *The Journal of Trauma: Injury, Infection, and Critical Care* 1999; **46**(**4**):543–52.

Flail chest

Definition

Fracture of 2 or more consecutive ribs in 2 or more places. The resultant flail segment is not in bony continuity with the thoracic cage. This leads to paradoxical movement of the flail segment during spontaneous breathing.

- Flail chest may be classified according to anatomical position:
  - Sternal.
  - Anterior.
  - Lateral.
  - Posterior.

Causes

Direct high-energy impact, typically occurring after road traffic collisions and falls. Diagnosis at presentation is missed in up to 20% of patients.

Pathophysiology

Flail chest results in acute respiratory failure 2° to:

- Inefficient chest wall mechanics, i.e. paradoxical chest wall movement
- Severe pain
  - → shallow breathing due to pain and mechanical inefficiency.
    ⚠ pooling of secretions.
  - → infection.
- Pulmonary contusion (46% flail chests).
  - → hypoxaemia 2° to ↑ pulmonary shunt fraction and hypoventilation.
- Constant movement of the flail segment may puncture the pleura and lung.
  - disruption of intercostal vessels leading to pneumo and haemo thorax.

Presentation and assessment

Symptoms

- Severe pain.
- Fatigue.

Signs

- ↓ SpO$_2$ ↑ RR ↑ HR.
- Un-coordinated, asymmetrical chest wall movement.
- Chest wall bruising, tenderness & crepitus.
- Flail segment better appreciated on palpation.
- ❶ May not be obvious due to chest wall splinting.

Investigations

Bloods
- **Routine trauma blood series** (See 📖 General approach to thoracic trauma, p. 452).
- **ABG.**
  - ↓ PaO_2 ± ↑ $PaCO_2$

Radiology
- **CXR.**
  - Multiple rib fractures as per definition.
  - Lateral and anterior fractures are often missed.
  - Pulmonary contusion; may only become apparent 4–6 hours after injury.
- **CT chest**
  - More likely to demonstrate rib fractures and pulmonary contusion compared to routine chest radiography.
  - Perform on all intubated patients.

- **⊕⊕ Blunt trauma ± lung contusion ± pneumothorax ± haemothorax = high probability of rib fractures**

Diagnosis
- Essentially a clinical one, based on observation of paradoxical movement of the flail segment and often crepitations by palpation.
- A history of blunt trauma involving high energy impact.
- X-Ray evidence of lung contusion, haemothorax or pneumothorax.
  - Rib fractures may are not always seen—special views and CT are not indicated in an otherwise uncomplicated case.

Associated injuries
- Pneumothorax, haemothorax or haemo-pneumothorax (70–80% patients).
- 1st and 2nd rib fractures imply significant force and are associated with head, neck, abdominal and cardiac injuries.
- 9th–12th rib fractures associated with hepatic (↑ × 1.4), renal and splenic injuries (↑ × 1.7).

Immediate trauma management

- Immediate assessment and treatment of flail chest should follow Advanced Trauma Life Support guidelines (See 📖 General approach to thoracic trauma, p. 452). Lung contusion—mangaement goals:
  - Adequate oxygenation.
  - Adequate ventilation.
  - Airway toilet.
  - Prevention of secondary pneumonia.
- Flail segment—mangaement goals:
  - IPPV to correct hypoxia from contusion will provide stabilization.
  - Surgery is rarely indicated.
  - Prophylactic chest drains if undergoing prolonged non-thoracic surgery.

Prevention of hypoxaemia

- High-flow, humidified O_2.
- Incentive spirometry.
- Coughing and deep breathing exercises.
- Ventilatory support required in up to 60% of patients with an isolated flail chest.
- In the presence of pulmonary contusion, 50–75% of patients require ventilation dependent on the severity of the lung injury.
- Consider ventilation in the following circumstances:
  - Progressive fatigue
  - RR   >35 bpm or <8 bpm
  - PaO_2 <8 kPa at $FiO_2 \geq 0.5$
  - $PaCO_2$ >8 kPa at $FiO_2 \geq 0.5$
  - FEV_1 ≤10 ml/kg
  - A-a DO_2 >60 kPa at FiO_2 of 1.0
  - PaO_2/FiO_2 ≤200.
- Non-invasive ventilation can be used in appropriately selected patients as a first line treatment.
- Patients with flail chest treated with CPAP demonstrate lower rates of hospital-acquired pneumonia and mortality compared to matched patients treated with IPPV.
  - Length of ICU stay remains the same.
- Judicious fluid management to avoid exacerbation of acute lung injury.

Acute pain management

(See table 9.3)
- Adequate analgesia → ↓ chest wall splinting.
- ∴ pulmonary gas exchange improves 2° to re-expansion of collapsed lung and clearance of pulmonary secretions.

Table 9.3 Strategies for pain management of flail chest

Technique	Advantages	Disadvantages/ complications
Systemic opioids	Simple	Cough, respiratory & CNS depression
Oral analgesics/ NSAIDs	Simple	Peptic ulceration
	Lack of CNS/CVS side effects	Renal dysfunction
		Platelet dysfunction
		Inadequate analgesia
TENS	Safe	Inadequate analgesia
	Simple	
	More effective than NSAID	
Intercostal LA	No CNS effects	Pneumothorax, multiple & frequent injections
		LA toxicity
Intrapleural LA	No CNS depression	↓ efficacy with adhesions
	Single injection	Chest tube clamped
		LA toxicity
Paravertebral LA	Stable haemodynamics	Pneumothorax
	No CNS depression	LA toxicity
		Unpredictable block
Epidural opioids	Low dose required	Urinary retention
	No sensory/motor block	Respiratory depression
	Stable haemodynamics	Breakthrough pain
Epidural LA	No CNS depression	↓ BP
	Superior pain control	Urinary retention
Epidural LA + opioids	Improved analgesia	As per epidural LA/opioids

There is a lack of class 1 evidence to support the efficacy of epidural analgesia in the context of flail chest. Anecdotally however, a correctly managed epidural is invaluable.

Purported advantages of epidural analgesia for flail chest:
- ↓ mortality in patients >65 years. (10% vs. 16%).
- ↓ pulmonary complications.
- ↓ respiratory depression.
- ↑ subjective pain control.

Operative management
- Uncommon
- Indications:
  - Existing need for thoracotomy.
  - Chest wall instability hindering ventilatory wean.
- Benefits:
  - ↓ ventilator days, ↓ pneumonia & ↑ return to work when surgical stabilisaization combined with epidural analgesia and aggressive pulmonary toilet.
- Benefits confined to patients with minimal or no underlying pulmonary contusion.

Outcome
- The impact of rib fractures and thus, flail chest, is greatest in the elderly $2°$ to co-morbidities and physiological reserve.
- Mortality (See Table 9.4).
  - ↑ by 132% for every 10 years after the 2nd decade.
  - ↑ by 30% with each unit increase of the injury severity score.
  - ↓ by 23% for each day survived in hospital.
- ARDS (up to 30% patients).
- Patients >65 years have significantly worse outcome measures:
  - ↑ Number of ventilator days
  - ↑ Length of ICU stay
  - ↑ Length of hospital stay
  - ↑ incidence of ARDS. There is a linear increase with each rib fracture. The incidence plateaus for younger patients after 3 rib fractures.

Table 9.4 Injury related mortality and risk of pneumonia

Injury	Pneumonia	Mortality
Isolated flail chest		16%
Isolated pulmonary contusion		16%
Flail chest & pulmonary contusion		42%
3–4 rib fractures*	31%	19%
>6 rib fractures*	51%	33%
Each additional rib fracture*	+16%	+19%

*isolated rib fractures in patients >65 years.

Long-term sequelae
Two thirds of patients with a flail chest will suffer from long-term disability:
- Chronic dyspnoea (66% patients).
- Chronic chest wall pain (50% patients).
- Chest tightness (25% patients).

Further reading

Gunduz M, Unlugenc H, Ozalevli M, , et al. A comparative study of continuous positive airway pressure (CPAP) and intermittent positive pressure ventilation (IPPV) in patients with flail chest. *Journal of Emergency Medicine* 2005; 22:325–9.

Karmakar HK, Ho AM. Acute pain management of patients with multiple fractured ribs. *Journal of Trauma* 2003; 54:615–25.

Massive haemothorax

Definition
- The accumulation of a large volume of blood within the pleural cavity.
- Most result from lacerations to the lung, pulmonary vasculature or chest wall as a result of either blunt or penetrating trauma.
- A massive haemothorax is a life threatening emergency resulting from the rapid accumulation of >1500 ml (or >1/3 total blood volume) into the chest cavity.
- It should be suspected when hypovolaemic shock and hypoxia coexist.

Pathophysiology
- Blood within the pleural cavity can produce both respiratory and haemodynamic compromise.
  - Dyspnoea and tachypnoea result as the haemothorax interferes with normal respiratory mechanics by compressing the lung.
  - The haemodymamic response varies depending on the rate and volume of blood lost.
  - Sufficient blood volume can be contained within the pleural cavity (>4 L in an average male) for hypovolaemic shock to occur, without external signs of bleeding.

Presentation
- Varies according to the rate and volume of blood loss, age and pre-morbid state of the patient, and presence/mechanism of associated injuries.

Symptoms
- Dyspnoea.
- Anxiety.
- Pain from associated injuries e.g. rib fractures.

Signs
- Bruising, crepitus, deformity, flail segments associated with rib fractures following blunt trauma.
- Tachycardia, hypotension, hypovolaemic shock, oliguria, delayed capillary refill.
- Flattened neck veins (but may be distended if haemopneumothorax present).
- Trachea deviated to opposite side.
- Tachypnoea, cyanosis and hypoxia.
- Stony dull percussion note with absent/reduced breath sounds on ipsilateral side (best assessed in sitting, rather than supine, position).
- Increased airway pressure in the volume control ventilated patient; decreased tidal volume in the pressure control ventilated patient.

Investigations

Bloods
- General trauma series of bloods. (See 📖 General approach to thoracic trauma, p. 452).
- **ABG.**
- **X-match 6 units.**
- **FBC, U&E, clotting.**

Radiology
- **CXR.**
  - Obliteration of costophrenic angle (if >400 ml blood).
  - Associated injury (pneumothorax, rib fractures, widened mediastinum).
  - Tracheal shift.
- **Ultrasound.**
  - Useful for determining size of haemothorax, but not for visualizing associated bony injuries.
- **CT chest.**
  - Although very accurate, not appropriate in the acute setting unless patient stable.

Other
- **Echocardiogram.**
  - Particularly if arrhythmias are present.
  - May exclude cardiac tamponade.

Immediate trauma management
- 100% O_2 ABC approach.
  - May need to intubate in extreme situations.
- Needle decompression of chest if associated pneumothorax.
- Insert large bore IV cannulae BEFORE insertion of ICD as torrential blood loss can occur.
- Insert large bore ICD.
- Restore circulating volume with colloid, crystalloid and ultimately blood.

Further management
- Consider thoracotomy if blood loss persists at >200 ml/hr.
- CXR to confirm position of ICD and to assess radiological change.
- Invasive monitoring.

Massive pulmonary haemorrhage

Massive pulmonary haemorrhage is a life-threatening complication of a wide range of pulmonary disorders. Initial management involves airway protection, aggressive resuscitation, and correction of coagulopathy. The site and cause of bleeding must be established, to enable bleeding to be controlled.

Definition

There is no consensus on the definition of massive haemorrhage, which has been defined as:
- >150 ml per hour of blood loss, or >600 ml in 24 hours.
- Loss of 50% circulating blood volume in 3 hours.
- Loss of whole blood volume within 24 hours.
- Alternatively, it can be considered as a volume loss that is life threatening due to airway obstruction or blood loss.

Presentation

- Massive haemoptysis:
  - 90% of cases from bronchial circulation; bronchial artery bleeding is more likely to cause massive haemorrhage as it is a high pressure (systemic) circulation.
  - 5% from pulmonary circulation.
- Respiratory failure.
- Cardiovascular compromise secondary to hypovolaemia and anaemia.

Aetiology

Common

- Chronic pulmonary inflammatory diseases e.g. bronchiectasis, TB.
- Lung neoplasm.

Less common

- Blunt or penetrating thoracic trauma usually results in massive haemothorax (See 📖 Massive haemothorax, p. 482). rather than massive haemoptysis.
- Other infection, e.g. lung abscess, fungal or parasitic infection, necrotizing pneumonia.
- Congenital heart disease.
- Cystic fibrosis.
- Peri-operative haemorrhage.
- Iatrogenic, e.g. Swan-Ganz catheterization, bronchial biopsy.
- Vascular.
  - Pulmonary infarct/embolism
  - AV malformation.
  - Arterio-bronchial fistula.
  - Haemorrhagic telangiectasis.
  - LVF.

- Coagulopathy.
- Vasculitis, e.g. Wegener's granulomatosis, Behcet's disease.
- Autoimmune, e.g. SLE, Goodpasture's Syndrome.
- Parasitic, e.g. Hydatid cyst.

Investigations

Bloods
- **General trauma series bloods** (See 📖 General approach to thoracic trauma, p. 452).
- **X-match** 6–8 units.
- **ABG**.

Radiology
- **CXR**.
  - Alveolar shadowing may indicate pulmonary haemorrhage.
- **CT Chest**.
  - Should be performed before bronchoscopy in stable patients.

Other
- **Pulmonary angiography**.
  - Will identify whether bleeding is from bronchial or pulmonary circulation, and determine if embolization is possible.
- **Microbiology and cytology of sputum**.
  - Chronic infection and tumours are common causes of haemoptysis. Early diagnosis will help determine definitive management once the patient is stabilized.

Medical management

Aim to manage these patients in a critical care environment, so that invasive airway, respiratory and cardiovascular support can be provided as necessary. Supportive measures alone may be effective at controlling the haemorrhage in some conditions, e.g. coagulopathy.

- High flow humidified oxygen.
- Avoid soiling of the non-bleeding lung by positioning the patient with bleeding side (if known) down to prevent aspiration into the non-bleeding lung.
- Consider invasive ventilation early. Use a large bore ETT +/– bronchial blocker or DLT to isolate the non-bleeding lung.
  - Endobronchial intubation may help to protect against aspiration and enable suctioning and bronchoscopy of the bleeding lung.
- ⚠ The administration of large volumes of crystalloid before haemorrhage control can:
  - Reverse vasoconstriction and displace early clot.
  - ↓ oxygen carriage.
  - Cause a dilutional coagulopathy.
  - Contribute to hypothermia.

- Contact the Blood bank staff:
  - Activate local massive haemorrhage protocol if applicable.
  - Patient may require blood component therapy.
- Establish invasive cardiovascular monitoring as soon as practicable; inotropic support may be required despite adequate fluid resuscitation.
- Involve the physicians, surgeons, radiologists and intensivists early.
- Massive transfusion and coagulopathy:
  - In order to successfully treat the coagulopathy associated with massive haemorrhage/transfusion, control of haemorrhage must be achieved first.
  - (See Table 9.5).

Table 9.5 Blood component therapy for massive haemorrhage

Component	When?	Initial dose	Target
FFP (contains all clotting factors & fibrinogen 2–5 g/dl)	After 50% BV loss, or earlier if indicated	15–20 ml/kg	PT & PTT < x1.5 control
Cryoprecipitate (VIIIc, won Willebrand factor, fibrinogen 3–6 g per 10 units)	After 150% BV loss, or earlier if indicated	10 units	Fibrinogen >1.0 g/l
Platelets	After 200% BV loss, or earlier if indicated	1–2 adult doses	>50 x 10^9/l (Consider >75 x 10^9/l)

- Drug therapy to optimize haemostatic capacity:
  - Anti-fibrinolytics e.g. tranexamic acid 1 g bolus with maintenance dose of 0.25 mg/kg/hr delivered over time periods of one to twelve hours.
  - Ca^{2+}.

Activated factor VIIa
The use of factor VIIa in massive haemorrhage is an "off-label" use of a licensed drug. Therefore, the clinician takes ultimate responsibility for any adverse events related to it administration.

Suggested criteria for administration of activated factor VIIa in the absence of a local protocol:
- Consultant/senior trainee decision.
- Liaise with senior haematological staff.
- Bleeding cannot be controlled. surgically.
- >8 units RBC transfusion.
- PT & PTT < ×1.5 control.
- Fibrinogen >0.5 g/l.
- pH >7.2.
- Temperature >36°C.

Non-surgical control of bleeding
Bronchoscopic haemorrhage control
- Local tamponade with balloon tipped catheter placed into a bleeding bronchus.
  - Temporising measure to gain control until a specific treatment is possible.
  - Not suitable for tracheal bleeding, or patient who would not tolerate temporary occlusion of the affected airway.
- Instillation of adrenaline solutions may reduce bleeding and aid visualization of bleeding point.
- Insertion of cellulose mesh, sealants/glues or use of laser coagulation. These are newer, unproven techniques, but with good results reported so far in the literature.

Bronchial artery embolization
- May be preferable in conditions unsuitable for surgery, e.g. multiple bleeding sites, inoperable tumours, or for patients with major co-morbidities where surgery is inappropriate.
- Success rates of 64–100% for immediate haemorrhage control.
- May avoid the higher mortality and morbidity associated with emergency surgical intervention, or allow stabilization and resuscitation of the patient prior to surgery.
- Failure particularly associated with bleeding from non-bronchial arterial sources. Recurrent bleeding and serious complications can also occur.

Surgical control of bleeding

- Preferred definitive treatment for those with localized bleeding that is amenable to surgery where bronchial artery embolization is either unavailable, unsuitable or has failed.
- Surgery is likely to be the treatment of choice in:
  - Thoracic vascular injury/trauma.
  - Arterio-venous malformation.
  - Leaking thoracic aneurysm with bronchial communication.
  - Bleeding from the pulmonary rather than the bronchial circulation
- Emergency thoracotomy and pulmonary surgery can be life-saving.

Key points

- Airway protection and oxygenation is the immediate priority.
- Aggressive resuscitation, correction of hypovolaemia and coagulopathy, invasive cardiovascular and respiratory support.
- Establish site and aetiology of bleeding.
- Consider non-surgical and surgical treatment options to rapidly control the bleeding.
- A multi-disciplinary approach is required, with co-ordination between critical care, respiratory physicians, thoracic surgeons and interventional radiologists.

Further reading

Lordan Jl, Gascoigne A, Corris PA. Assessment and management of massive haemoptysis. *Thorax* 2003; 58:814–19.

Reisz, G. Topical Hemostatic Tamponade—another tool in the treatment of massive hemoptysis (editorial). *Chest* 2005; 127:1888–9.

Jean-Baptiste, E. Clinical assessment and management of massive hemoptysis. *Critical Care Medicine* 2000; 28:1642–7.

Haemorrhagic shock

Thoracic trauma may present with haemorrhagic shock. Assessment and management should involve a rapid, systematic approach with good communication throughout.

Medical triage should move from initial contact with accident and emergency physicians, through to anaesthesia/ITU personnel and the thoracic surgical team. Individual life threatening conditions are dealt with separately in this chapter.

Thoracic trauma and haemorrhage

Haemorrhagic shock
- Haemorrhage is the major cause of shock after thoracic trauma.
- Haemorrhage can be a consequence of either blunt or penetrating trauma to the chest wall, lung, heart or great vessels.
- As a result, the extent of blood loss is often not obvious to the assessing physician.
- It is important to follow the basic principles of trauma management (See 📖 General approach to thoracic trauma, p. 452).
- Primary survey evaluation and detection and treatment of any immediate life threatening conditions should be the first steps.
- DO NOT ADVANCE to secondary survey until the primary survey allows.

Non-haemorrhagic causes of shock
These should always be considered:
- Tension pneumothorax.
- Cardiac tamponade.
- Cardiac contusion.
- Great vessel injury.
- Cardiogenic shock.
- Neurogenic shock.

Monitoring needed
- ECG.
- BP.
- Pulse oximetry.
- Arterial line.
- CVP line when safe to do so.

Diagnosis of acute haemorrhage
- Signs of hypovolaemic shock (See Table 9.6)
  - Do not forget to look for visible blood loss (chest drains, gaping wounds, visible tracheal/oral blood loss).

- Perform clinical examination looking for signs of immediately life threatening conditions.
- Use appropriate urgent investigations.
  - Bloods.
  - Necessary ultrasound scanning.
  - Trauma series of films: CXR, pelvic X-Ray.
- Involve other teams EARLY.

Table 9.6 The classical 'tennis score' approach to shock classification

Clinical Sign	15% (750ml)	15–30% (750–1500ml)	30–40% (1500–2000ml)	>40% (>2000ml)
Conscious level	Normal	Anxious	Confused	Lethargic
BP	Normal	Normal	Decreased	Hypotension
Heart Rate	<100	>100	>120	>140
Pulse pressure	Normal	Decreased	Decreased	Decreased
Respiratory Rate	14–20	20–30	30–40	>35
Urine Output	>30 ml/hr	20–30 ml/hr	5–15 ml/hr	Negligible

Investigations

Bloods

Trauma series of blood tests.
- **FBC.**
- **Clotting.**
- **U&E.**
- **X-match.**
- **ABG.**

Radiology
- **CXR.**
- **Pelvic X-ray.**
- **US chest:**
  - Can be done in Emergency Department (FAST scan).
- **CT chest:**
  - Only when the patient is stable!

Immediate trauma management via ATLS protocol
(See 📖 General approach to thoracic trauma, p. 452.)

The key is to perform a detailed rapid primary survey looking for acute life threatening injuries, then to consider whether the patient needs theatre immediately, or whether they are stable enough to undergo further investigation with further resuscitation. The clinician MUST RE-EVALUATE regularly.

Airway and cervical spine control
Breathing and ventilation
- Most cases of massive haemorrhage will need immediate surgical intervention.
- Securing the airway rapidly is a priority and can usually be done safely using a single lumen tube.
  - Passage of a DLT may be difficult and hazardous in the acute situation.
  - If required OLV can usually be achieved with a bronchial blocker inserted later via the SLT.
- On occasions initial insertion of a DLT, or change to a DLT, may be necessary for example to:
  - Ventilate the patient in the presence of a disruption of a major bronchus.
  - Isolate, protect and ventilate of one lung in the presence of major intra-bronchial haemorrhage in the contralateral lung.
- Bronchoscopy and suction of airways may be required to maintain adequate oxygenation in patients with ongoing bleeding into the tracheobronchial tree.

Circulation
- Large bore IV cannulae.
- Fluid resuscitation as appropriate.
- Blood transfusion, starting with O⁻ blood, followed by type specific blood and ultimately fully cross matched blood.
- Insertion of two large bore chest drains in massive haemothorax.
- Monitoring of blood loss from the chest drains. If the loss is more than 200 ml per hour for four hours or immediate blood loss >1L, immediate thoracotomy should be considered.
- Assess the response to fluid resuscitation:

Responder
- BP↑ and pulse rate↓.

Transient responder
- BP↑ and pulse rate↓ but reversion to hypotension and tachycardia within a short time of fluid challenge.

Non-responder with continuing severe blood loss
- No change in shock haemodynamics after fluid bolus.

> **❶❶** IV access should be secured BEFORE large bore chest drains are inserted in cases of massive haemothorax, as ensuing rapid blood loss into the drains may lead to complete circulatory collapse and cardiac arrest.

Further management

If the patient is stable

- CT scan of thorax should be considered.
  - If the bleeding is focal, localization of the bleeding may enable angiographic embolization or if a thoracotomy is required, inform the surgeon as to the site of bleeding.

If the patient is unstable

- If the bleeding can be localized bronchoscopically, endobronchial tamponade should be considered.
  - If bronchoscopy does not determined the site of bleeding an angiogram should be considered to ascertain the bleeding site.

- Emergency thoracotomy should be considered if the bleeding is massive and is originating from a focal lesion. This may necessitate pneumonectomy and is associated with a high mortality.

Blunt thoracic trauma

Thoracic trauma is common and ranks third behind head and extremity trauma. The aetiology of thoracic trauma in Europe is summarizsed (See Table 9.7). Ultimately, injury occurs as a result of rapid deceleration and crushing forces.

Table 9.7 Major causes of thoracic injury in Europe

Mechanism	% cases
Road traffic accident	60
Industrial accident	15
Domestic accident	10
Sports injury	10
Assault/Suicide	5

Pathophysiology
- Considerable mechanical force is required to produce significant blunt thoracic trauma.
- Consequently, blunt thoracic trauma seldom presents in isolation.
- Typically, there may be associated injuries to the abdomen, head, neck and extremities (See Table 9.8 for injury summary).

Table 9.8 Blunt thoracic injuries

Immediate threat to life	Potential threat to life
Airway obstruction	Blunt aortic injury
Tension pneumothorax	Tracheobronchial tree disruption
Open pneumothorax	Pulmonary contusion
Massive haemothorax	Diaphragmatic rupture
Flail chest	Myocardial contusion
Cardiac tamponade	

- The most common intrathoracic injuries secondary to blunt trauma are haemothorax, pulmonary contusion and great vessel disruption.
- Thus, the pathophysiological sequelae of blunt thoracic trauma are:
  - Hypoxia.
  - Hypercarbia.
  - Hypovolaemia.
  - Hypoperfusion.
  - Mixed acidosis.

Injury prediction

(See table 9.9)

- Blunt thoracic trauma is predominantly due to road traffic accidents.
- The severity of injury in this context may be predicted from knowledge of the type and speed of impact, and whether the individual was wearing a seat-belt.
- Ultimately, restrained passengers fair better than their unrestrained companions in head-on collisions and rollovers. However, restraint does not confer any benefit in a side-on collision.

- Significant injury occurs at an impact velocity of 10–20 mph in unrestrained passengers compared to at least 30 mph in restrained passengers.
- Significant intra-thoracic injury occurs in the absence of bony thoracic injury in up to 25% of cases.

Table 9.9 Prediction of chest wall & intrathoracic injuries

Mechanism of injury	Chest wall injury	Intrathoracic injury	Associated injury
High velocity	Often intact	Aortic rupture	Head
	± sternal fracture	Myocardial contusion	Maxillo-facial
	± bilateral rib fractures with anterior flail	Tracheo-bronchial disruption	Cervical spine
		Diaphragmatic rupture	Hepatic/splenic
			Long bone fracture
Low velocity	Lateral impact: unilateral rib fracture	Pulmonary contusion	Hepatic/splenic
		Myocardial contusion	Maxillo-facial
	Anterior impact:		
	sternal fracture		
Crush	Antero-posterior: bilateral rib fractures	Bronchial rupture	Thoracic spine fracture
		Myocardial contusion	
	± anterior flail	Pulmonary contusion	Hepatic/splenic
	Lateral: ipsilateral rib fracture		
	± flail segment		
	± contralateral rib fractures		

Management
- Initial assessment and management of blunt thoracic trauma aims to rapidly identify and treat immediately life-threatening injuries.
- Ultimately, the majority of injuries may be treated with humidified oxygen, adequate analgesia, intercostal chest drainage, ventilatory support and judicious fluid therapy.
  - Only 10–15% of blunt thoracic injuries require operative intervention.

Trauma management of immediately life-threatening injuries

- The management of open/tension pneumothorax, massive haemothorax, flail chest, and cardiac tamponade is discussed in the relevant sections of this chapter.

Partial/complete airway obstruction
Can occur secondary to:

Haemorrhage
- Results in distortion and compression of trachea
  - Airway must be secured rapidly
  - Options include endotracheal intubation, surgical cricothyroidotomy, and surgical tracheostomy.

Laryngeal fracture
- May be supraglottic, glottic, sub-glottic, hyoid, crico-arytenoid, or crico-thyroid.
- Presents with hoarseness, surgical emphysema, palpable fracture, respiratory distress, stridor.
  - These rare injuries may be missed initially and their management requires the input of an experienced ENT surgeon.
- Minor injuries may be managed conservatively with humidified oxygen and close observation.
- Severe injuries require surgical tracheostomy, direct laryngoscopy, oesophagoscopy, exploration and repair, ± stent insertion.
  - Standard endo-tracheal intubation under general anaesthesia may be impossible.
  - In cases of cricotracheal separation, induction of anaesthesia results in a loss of tone of the strap muscles splinting the injured larynx.
  - Consequently, the trachea and larynx distract and sublux.
  - Fibre-optic intubation is a possibility where time, skill and resources permit.

❶ Potentially life-threatening injuries

The management of injuries of the great vessels, tracheo-bronchial tree, and the diaphragm is discussed in the relevant sections of this chapter.

Pulmonary contusion

- CT appearances represent a pulmonary laceration surrounded by intra-alveolar blood.
- Commonly found in association with rib fracture/flail chest.

Myocardial contusion

- Common in blunt thoracic trauma, but may be subtle.
- Suspicion raised by tenderness, bruising, and/or crepitus of the anterior chest.
- May result in impaired contractility.
- As yet, there are no firm diagnostic criteria ∴ reported incidence variable.
  - Arrhythmia—85% of patients with an abnormal ECG on admission develop complications of blunt cardiac injury.
  - Haemodynamically stable patients with a normal ECG on admission do not develop arrhythmias or cardiac failure. Therefore, this group does not require further investigation of myocardial contusion.
- Patients with an abnormal ECG on admission should be monitored for 24–48 hours post-injury.
- ↑ Troponin I/T—these patients should also be monitored for 24–48 hours post-injury.
  - Routine echocardiographic examination should be avoided as there is no evidence to support its use as a screening tool in blunt thoracic trauma.
  - However, it may be used in patients suspected of having a complication of blunt cardiac injury.
- Management of cardiac contusion is supportive.

☛ Emergency thoracotomy in blunt trauma

- The survival rate of blunt thoracic trauma victims following emergency thoracotomy has been reported as 1–2%.
- In contrast, victims of penetrating trauma have an overall survival rate of 9–12%.
  - Emergency thoracotomy is inappropriate in blunt trauma patients presenting to the Emergency Department without signs of life.

Further reading

Karmy-Jones R, Jurkovich GJ. Blunt chest trauma. *Current Problems in Surgery* 2004; 41(3): 211–311.

Hunt PA, Greaves I, Owens WA. Emergency thoracotomy in thoracic trauma—a review. Injury, *International Journal of Care of the Injured* 2006; 37:1–19.

Gunshot, stabbing, and impaling injuries

Introduction

- Penetrating chest trauma is the result of an object piercing and entering the thoracic cavity. Causes include: gunshot, stabbing and impaling injuries.
- Not commonly seen in the UK.
- Rapid diagnosis, treatment and recognition of potential sequelae are paramount to the prevention of mortality.
- Severity of the injury depends upon:
  - Tissues involved.
  - Type of penetrating object.
  - Amount of kinetic energy transferred to the tissues.
- Approximately 15–30% of patients with penetrating chest injury will require thoracotomy as opposed to blunt chest trauma where 10%–15% will require this intervention.

Mechanism of injury

- Low velocity; only the structures penetrated are damaged—e.g.
  - Impaling.
  - Stabbing injuries.
- Medium velocity; may include other structures—e.g.
  - Bullets fired from handguns, shot guns and air-powered pellet guns.
- High velocity; cause the most primary tissue destruction e.g.
  - High-powered rifles and military weapons.

The amount tissue damage caused is directly related to the kinetic energy transmitted and can be calculated by the following equation:

$$KE = \frac{1}{2}mv^2$$

KE = kinetic energy
M = mass
V = Velocity

Indications for thoracotomy

Emergency (resuscitative) thoracotomy

- Release of pericardial tamponade in patients unresponsive to CPR.
- Direct control of intra-thoracic exsanguination.
- Massive blood loss originating from below the diaphragm requiring cross clamping of descending thoracic aorta.
- Patients requiring internal cardiac massage.

Urgent thoracotomy
- Blood loss from chest drain of >1500 ml total or >200 ml/hr.
- Massive air leak.
- Proven great vessel injury.
- Proven oesophageal or diaphragmatic injury.
- Cardiac tamponade.
- Penetration of mediastinum.

Immediate trauma management

- ❶ All trauma patients should undergo a primary survey to rapidly assess for life threatening injuries according to Advanced Trauma Life Support guidelines; 100% O_2/ABCDE approach with cervical spine immobilization (See ▢ General approach to thoracic trauma, p. 452).
- ❶ BEFORE ADVANCING TO THE SECONDARY SURVEY, the patient's primary survey must be re-assessed after any critical clinical intervention.
- ❶❶ **Penetrating objects should not be removed if present**. Await surgical opinion.

Life threatening injuries found on primary survey
ATOM FC
- **A**cute airway obstruction.
- **T**ension pneumothorax.
- **O**pen pneumothorax.
- **M**assive haemothorax.
- **F**lail chest.
- **C**ardiac tamponade.

Life threatening Injuries detected on secondary survey
- Simple pneumothorax.
- Haemothorax.
- Tracheobronchial tree injury.
- Mediastinal traversing wounds.
- Diaphragmatic injuries.

Diagnosis and management of specific injuries
Most of these are discussed individually in other areas within this section.

Acute airway obstruction
- Basic airway maneuvers, followed by advanced; endo-tracheal intubation, surgical cricothyroidotomy, and surgical tracheostomy. Followed by continued treatment/removal of cause.

Tension pneumothorax
(See 📖 Pneumothorax, p. 464).

Open pneumothorax
(See 📖 Pneumothorax, p. 464).
Caused by a large defect in chest wall, resulting in a continuous, 'sucking' chest wound.
- Treatment:
  - Closure of the wound using sterile occlusive dressing secured on three sides creating a 'flutter-valve' effect.
  - An intercostal drain with under water-seal should also be inserted.
  - A thoracotomy may be considered when the patient is stable.

Massive Haemothorax
(See 📖 Massive haemothorax, p. 482).
The pleural cavity can hold up to three litres of blood.
- Treatment:
  - ❶ Insertion of wide bore access BEFORE insertion of ICD. Massive rapid blood loss can ensue leading to cardiovascular collapse. (Due to 'C' being high priority, this is one situation where ABC approach becomes A**C**B.
  - Emergency thoracotomy may be indicated if continued blood loss. (See above).

Cardiac tamponade
(See 📖 Traumatic cardiac tamponade, p. 470).
- Tension pneumothorax can manifest in a similar manner (distended neck veins, muffled heart sounds, tachycardia.
  - However, with tension pneumothorax there will be no air entry, hyper-resonant percussion note and tracheal shift.

Tracheo-bronchial tree injury
(See 📖 Blunt thoracic trauma, p. 494).
These injuries can be associated with both blunt and penetrating trauma.
- Treatment:
  - Prompt intubation and ventilation may be required in the unstable patient.
  - One lung ventilation via a DLT may be necessary to provide adequate oxygenation.
  - For tracheal injuries a single lumen tube may be passed with bronchoscopic guidance past the injury to enable ventilation.
  - Surgical treatment options include repair, lobectomy or pneumonectomy depending on the injury.

Mediastinal traversing wounds
- There may be damage to the tracheobronchial tree, oesophagus, spinal cord, heart or great vessels.
  - Surgical opinion should be sought immediately.

❶ In the unstable patient, tension pneumothorax, cardiac tamponade or severe intra-thoracic haemorrhage should be identified and rapidly treated.

Diaphragmatic injuries
(See 📖 Blunt thoracic trauma, p. 494).
Can result from blunt thoraco-abdominal trauma or penetrating injuries. These injuries can be easily missed and a high index of suspicion should be maintained.
- Presentation:
  - Decreased breath sounds on side of injury.
  - Chest pain.
  - Respiratory distress.
- Investigations:
  - **CXR**—raised hemi-diaphragm, bowel or stomach in the chest.
- Treatment:
  - After the patient has been stabilized, the defect can be repaired either by a thoracotomy, thoraco-abdominal incision or laparotomy.

Further reading
Advanced Trauma Life Support Course Manual. 8th Edition: American College of Surgeons Committee on Trauma.

Great vessel injury

- Injuries to the great vessels in the chest can be considered in two groups:
  - Injuries likely to occur following blunt chest trauma.
  - Injuries likely to occur following penetrating chest trauma.
- Although immediate treatment to all chest traumas should follow an ATLS approach, the underlying pathology differs as do the surgical and anaesthetic requirements.
- Fluid replacement has important implications for re-bleeding, clotting and lung injury as well as organ perfusion.

Blunt chest trauma

Aortic injury

- Blunt aortic dissection is nearly always associated with other injuries.
- It is either contained or open to the hemithorax.
- The majority of patients with open wounds will die at the scene but a small proportion reach hospital.
- These patients are often haemodynamically stable due to intact pleura and adventitial layers.
- Although the thoracic aorta may be ruptured at any point, the most common site is at the isthmus just distal to the left Subclavian artery.
- The aorta is relatively fixed at this point, therefore shearing or pinching forces above or below this point may cause rupture.

 ❶ The presentation of aortic disruption with ongoing bleeding is an indication for immediate surgery but is a rare occurrence (<10%).

Presentation of aortic injury

History and mechanism of injury

- High speed road traffic accident.
- No seat belt worn.
- Broken steering wheel.
- Ejection from vehicle.
- Pedestrian hit by car.
- Falls greater than 3 m.
- Crush injuries.

Symptoms and signs

- Fracture of sternum, 1st rib, clavicle, scapula or multiple ribs.
- Steering wheel imprint on chest.
- Disparity in limb blood pressures.
- Dyspnoea.
- Hoarse voice.
- Back Pain.
- Haemothorax.
- Paraplegia or paraparesis.
- Haemodynamic shock with all other causes excluded.

Investigations

Bloods
- **Trauma series of bloods.**
- **Cross match**.
  - At least 6 units of blood (may need much more).
- **ABG**.

Radiology
- **CXR**:
  - Widened mediastinum on the CXR (may be easily missed if there is an associated Haemothorax); however, this alone is not sensitive enough to guide intervention.
  - Rightward tracheal shift.
  - Blurred aortic contour.
  - Loss of aortic knob.
  - Depression of left main bronchus.
  - Presence of significant chest trauma; multiple rib #, thoracic spine #, pulmonary contusion.
- **CT scan**:
In a trauma setting, if time is available, CT chest is advantageous:
  - Allows rapid assessment.
  - Does not rely too heavily on highly trained interpretation.
  - Is readily available.
  - Not too costly.
  - Maintains good standards of sensitivity and specificity.
  - CT angiography is also an option in some centres.
- **MRI/Aortography**:
  - If diagnostic doubt on CT.
  - If patient is stable with no other immediately life threatening injuries.

Others:
- **ECG**.
- **TOE**:
  - May aid in the diagnosis if suspicion is high, but urgency of other surgical interventions such as a craniotomy or laparotomy may take clinical priority.
  - May be more prudent to perform TOE once the patient is anaesthetized and ongoing treatment of other pathologies is occurring.

Immediate trauma management

Resuscitation

100% O_2, ATLS approach.

- **A**
  - With C-spine control.
- **B**
  - Examine for signs of tension pneumothorax/massive haemothorax.
- **C**
  - With identification and control of other life threatening haemorrhage.
  - Prevent further exsanguination if obvious, i.e. stabilize long bone #.
  - Fluid and blood resuscitation as indicated via large bore IV access.
  - ❶ Careful blood transfusion or fluid replacement is required so as not to precipitate fatal bleeding.
- **D**
  - Consider airway protection (intubate) if head injury present with rapid deterioration in conscious level or GCS <8.

If haemodynamically unstable

- Or transient responder, proceed to surgical intervention as indicated i.e. laparotomy, thorocotomy, pelvic stabilization/embolization.

If haemodynamically stable

- If there is an intracranial lesion, craniotomy takes priority.
- If there are other injuries requiring no immediate intervention, proceed to CT of chest.
- If there is evidence of head injury and history of significant trauma, but a normal GCS, then it is prudent to obtain a head CT at the same visit as this will help guide surgical and anaesthetic management.

Anaesthetic management

Pre-operative assessment and optimization

- Rapid anaesthetic assessment:
  - With AMPLE history.

Induction
- RSI probably safest, minimize cardiovascular collapse.
- DLT or use of bronchial blocker as lung isolation is ideally required to aid surgical access and reduce operating time.
- Insert invasive arterial monitoring as soon as possible:
  - This is ideally required in both the upper and lower limbs.
  - Check with the surgeon regarding their preferred site of femoral cannulation, if required, and place arterial line in opposite vessel. Usually the left femoral vessels are chosen by the surgeon.

Position
- The patient will be positioned in the right lateral decubitus position with hips slightly flexed to allow access to femoral vessels.
- Left Thoracotomy.
  - May require median sternotomy if disruption in proximal aorta.

Maintenance and intra-operative
- Avoid hypertension:
  - Increases the shear stress across the aortic walls.
  - Analgesia may be effective if it is pain related.
  - Alternatively, an infusion of a short acting β blocker or GTN can be used.
  - Aim for systolic BP <130 mmHg.
- Cell savage:
  - Should be available and can be started using blood drained from a haemothorax if present.
- Cardiopulmonary bypass:
  - If used then deep hypothermic circulatory arrest, cardioplegia and full heparinization will be required.
  - This is more likely with proximal dissections (i.e. the aortic arch) or if repair cannot occur with the cross clamp on.

❶ If it is likely that full cardiopulmonary bypass (CPB) is needed, a qualified technician will be required.
- Heparin:
  - Decisions regarding heparinization should ideally be discussed prior to surgery.
  - This will be governed by possible bypass/shunt maneuvers.
  - The surgeon may prefer to maintain lower limb perfusion, but this may be contraindicated by the presence of head injury.

Special points
- Axillary vessels may also be prepped and accessed as may the legs for saphenous vein grafts.
- ?Anti-fibrinolytics.
- If the surgeon chooses just to 'clamp and go' with no form of lower limb perfusion, it is reasonable to tolerate mild hypothermia (no lower than 34°C), as this may confer some spinal protection.
  - Care must be taken to rewarm as soon as possible to avoid coagulopathy.

Penetrating chest trauma

- 85–90% of traumatic injuries to the great vessels are due to a penetrating mechanism.
- Unlike blunt trauma there is no distinct pattern of injury.
- There are many factors governing the degree of injury, most important of which relates the velocity of penetrating object and therefore its energy transfer:
- Low velocity.
  - Knife wound; extent of injury will depend upon the length or distance of penetration into the thorax.
- Medium velocity.
  - Air rifles.
- High velocity.
  - Military guns or shrapnel.
- The site of entry and the trajectory of the penetrating object will predict the likely structures damaged within the thorax.
- If the patient sustains other significant injuries e.g. during an explosion or blast, then these injuries must be borne in mind when prioritizing treatment.

Investigation

(As for blunt great vessel injury)

Immediate trauma management

Resuscitation

ATLS approach (as for blunt vessel injury).
- Also:
  - Chest drain for therapeutic and diagnostic purposes; place as early as possible.
  - ❶ Do not wait for signs of shock to develop.
  - ❶ >1500 ml blood is an indication for urgent thoracotomy within investigation.
  - If persistently hypotensive or shocked consider tension pneumothorax and cardiac tamponade as potential causes and manage appropriately.
  - If a patient remains stable after initial resuscitation then it is appropriate to undertake further investigation.

Anaesthetic management
(As for blunt great vessel injury) also:

Induction
- DLT
  - Ideal for thoracotomy.
  - Placement can be difficult in the emergency setting when a rapid sequence induction is utilized.
  - The surgeon may proceed without lung isolation, or a bronchial. blocker can be placed once manual control of haemorrhage is achieved.
- Invasive monitoring.
  - Should be considered and placed as soon as possible.
  - CVP and arterial lines.
  - Placement of invasive lines should not delay operation and can be done after incision if needs be.

Position
- Choice of incision is based on the most likely site in injury if there was no time for imaging.
- Medium sternotomy allows access to most mediastinal vessels and can be extended into the neck. It will be required for any injury with an entry point within the area bounded by the mid-clavicular lines, xiphisternum and thoracic inlet, regardless of haemodynamic stability.
- Thoracotomy is performed for injuries to the descending aorta.

❶ Significant blood loss can occur from injury to the internal mammary or intercostal vessels without concomitant injury to a major vessel.
- Cell savage:
  - Of chest drain loss if available.
- CPB:
  - Lacerations of the proximal aorta and larger more complex injuries to the pulmonary vessels or the vena cava may require CPB.
- Have blood ready:
  - Be prepared for significant drops in blood pressure once a contained haematoma is released. Have blood products and fluid resuscitation ready.

Special points
- Antifibrinolytics? Discuss this with surgeon.
- Warming devices:
  - For fluid and blood; helps prevent worsening acidosis and coagulopathy.

- Clamps:
  - Most simple penetrating vessel injuries are amenable to repair with relatively short clamp times; even if grafting is required without the use of bypass or shunting measures.
- Air embolus:
  - Consider air embolus if there is sudden decompensation during repair to the vena cava or pulmonary veins.
  - Some surgeons prefer CPD when repairing the pulmonary veins to reduce the risk of air embolus to the brain.
- Once control of bleeding is achieved other organs can be explored
- Due the proximity of the great vessels, penetrating trauma results in a high incidence of associated bronchial and oesophageal injuries.

Endovascular stenting of aortic dissection

- At the time of writing there are currently no randomized controlled trials comparing endovascular with open for traumatic aortic transection.
- There are however a significant number citations describing successful endovascular stent grafting (EVSG) in this setting.
- EVSG may be chosen due to:
  - The presence of other significant injuries or co-morbidity.
  - Advanced age resulting in an unacceptable level of risk if open repair were attempted.
- Further studies are required to define a patient subgroup for which it may become a first line treatment.
- Can be performed under local anaesthesia, but can be prolonged procedure and may be performed in an isolated angio. suite rather than a familiar theatre environment.
- The patient is also likely to have other significant injuries and may need to be transferred from ITU.
  - General anaesthesia may be the only feasible option, as a rupture during EVSG will require an open procedure.

❶ Timing of such intervention must be considered balancing the risks of the need to intervene with a stable aortic rupture and leaving the relatively safe environment of the ITU.

Non-aortic vessel injury following blunt thoracic trauma

Isolated non-aortic vessel injury secondary to blunt chest trauma is rare. Incidence is unknown and one can find a scattering of case reports.

Brachiocephalic, left carotid or left subclavian artery laceration.

- Median Sternotomy incision.
- May require CPB depending upon extent or aortic damage.
- Isolated injury to one of the branches is unlikely to need CPB and the left Subclavian may be accessed from a left posterolateral thoracotomy.

Pulmonary artery/venous rupture

- Likely to present with cardiac tamponade due to pericardial extension.
- Massive haemothorax or tamponade may cause decompensation prior to surgical intervention.
- Median sternotomy provides access and CPB may required.

Extension of rupture into neck vessels

- In addition to thoracic injuries.
- Median sternotomy can be extended and graft repair undertaken.

Further reading

Maloney JT, Fowler SJ, Chang W. Anaesthetic Management of Thoracic Trauma. *Current Opinion in Anaesthesiology*. 2008; 21:41–6.

Gleason T GI, Bavaria J El. Trauma to Great Vessels. In: Cohn LH, Edmunds LH Jr, eds. *Cardiac Surgery in the Adult*. New York: McGraw-Hill. 2003: 1229–50.

Pulmonary artery rupture

Pulmonary artery rupture (PAR) is rare but the outcome may be fatal. It represents a less common cause of haemoptysis; bleeding from systemic vessels being the commonest. Depending on the cause and site of rupture the clinical presentation can range from mild to life threatening.

Causes

PAR occurs as a result of direct trauma, following the development of an aneurysm or pseudoaneurysm and with AV malformation of the pulmonary artery.

- Aneurysms are caused by:
  - Trauma (blunt or penetrating).
  - Iatrogenic (Pulmonary artery floatation catheter—PAFC).
  - Infection (TB, syphilis, aspergillus).
  - Behcet's syndrome.
  - Rare—chronic pulmonary hypertension, congenital heart disease, connective tissue disease (Marfan's), neoplasm and Hughes Stovin syndrome.
- AV malformations are seen in:
  - Rendu–Osler–Weber (ROW).

PAFC

The wide availability of non-invasive CO monitoring has resulted in reduced PAFC use. PAFC induced rupture (due to tip perforation or balloon rupturing vessel) can be immediate after manipulation of the catheter or delayed up to seven months following the formation of an aneurysm.

- Risk is 0.1% to 1.5% and influenced by:
  - Hypothermia (catheter more rigid and less compliant).
  - Coagulopathy.
  - Female gender.
  - Pulmonary hypertension.
  - Age—lower distending pressures tolerated as age advances >50 yrs.

Rules to minimize PA rupture when using a PA catheter

- Always inflate the balloon slowly while constantly monitoring the waveform and the resistance to inflation.
- Never inflate the balloon with a wedge pattern.
- Never fast flush the catheter with a wedge pattern.
- Never leave the balloon inflated for more than 20 s.
- Never use liquids to inflate the balloon.
- Where possible use a pilot balloon to minimize accidental overpressure.

Always leave the tip of the catheter in a central artery ie volume of air needed to wedge should be >0.8 ml.

Presentation
- Bleeding—haemoptysis and/or haemothorax.
- Pressure effect from large aneurysm—symptoms of airway compression, radiological changes.
- Pseudo-aneurysm—93% in right lower and middle lobes.

Diagnosis
Identification of side and site of rupture is fundamental to the management.
- PAFC related rupture.
  - New infiltrate on CXR at the tip of catheter.
  - Haemothorax.
  - Shock.
- Aneurysms and pseudo-aneurysms related rupture.

Management

Mild haemoptysis
- Lung isolation.
- Positive pressure ventilation with PEEP.
- Correction of any coagulation abnormalities.

▶ Pseudoaneurysms should be looked for and treated, as these can be inherently unstable. They involve the parenchyma of the lung, which provides vital structural support.

Massive haemoptysis or large haemothorax
- Mortality of 33–80%.

⚠ **Immediate management**

- **100% O$_2$/ABC/Get help.**
- **Resuscitate** with blood or fluids.
- **Position** the patient with the side of the tip of PA catheter down to protect the normal lung from blood soiling and reverse the position after isolation of the lung to reduce PA pressure at the site of bleeding.
- **Immediate lung isolation** is important to maintain gas exchange—may prove difficult if there is continuing blood loss into the airway.
  - Endobronchial blockers can be advanced into the side of rupture to provide endobronchial tamponade. (Blind placement described in chapter 12 p. ***).
  - A long ETT rotated through 180 with the head rotated to the right has a 92% chance of entering the left main bronchus.
  - If the rupture happens in a radiology department or access to it is rapid, then a standard radio-opaque bronchoscope can be directed into the bronchus under fluoroscopic control. An endobronchial tube can then be advanced over it.

- If the degree of shock is out of proportion to the evident blood loss, exclude cardiac tamponade.
- **Interventional radiology and or surgery.**

Specific investigations
Bloods
- Routine trauma blood series.

Radiology
- **Contrast enhanced spiral CT scan.**
  - Investigation of 1st choice.
  - Aneurysm—confirmed if the main diameter >29 mm or right PA diameter >17 mm.
- **Pulmonary angiography.**
  - May be done via PA catheter but special catheters produce better images and offer therapeutic advantage.

Interventional radiology or surgery

Pulmonary artery angiography and embolization
- Management of choice when PA catheter has caused the rupture or the patient is high risk for surgery.

Surgery
- Can include:
  - Thoracotomy and lobectomy.
  - Pneumonectomy.
  - Vessel repair.
  - In extreme dissections → heart/lung transplant.

⚠ Balloon tamponade using PA catheter is not recommended.

Indication for surgery

- Persistent hypotension despite adequate transfusion.
- Excessive blood loss ie haemoptysis +/− drain loss >300 ml/hr for >4hrs.
- On-going haemorrhage >2 l.
- Left haemothorax with widened mediastinum.
- Bleeding from bronchial vessels as opposed to from pulmonary artery (high pressure system).
- Continuing hypoxia despite successful embolization eg large AV malformations ROW syndrome.
- Extreme forms of dissection of PA may require Heart-Lung transplant.

Further reading

Nguyen ET, Silva CIS *et al*. Pulmonary artery aneurysms and pseudoaneurysms in adults: Findings at CT and radiography. *American Journal of Radiology* 2007; 188:126–34.

Chapman S, Robinson G, Stradling J, *et al*. (2005). Haemoptysis. In: *Oxford Handbook of Respiratory Medicine*. Oxford University Press, pp. 22–5.

Ruptured diaphragm

PROCEDURE BASICS: usually laparotomy, may be as part of polytrauma. Thoracotomy for right side or late diagnosis. Laparoscopic and thoracoscopic approaches are becoming popular.

TIME: 2–4 hours.

PAIN RATING: 3–5/5 dependent on approach.

ANALGESIA: multimodal. Morphine PCA/epidural/regional analgesia.

BLOOD LOSS: depends on associated trauma.

HOSPITAL STAY: HDU/ITU dependent on associated trauma and patient status.

PREPARATION AND EQUIPMENT: COETT (unlikely to need DLT—discuss with the surgeon, particularly if thoracotomy). Arterial and CVP lines advised. NG tube, ± chest drain, active warming, blood products must be available if emergency, deep muscle relaxation and neuromuscular monitoring.

Introduction

- Diaphragmatic injury is relatively uncommon, comprising only 3% of all traumatic injuries.
- 80–90% result from blunt thoraco-abdominal trauma, i.e. motor vehicle crashes. The remainder occur as a result of penetrating trauma, e.g. gunshot wound, stabbing.
- Rupture is more common on the left side (protective effect of the liver on the right). Bilateral injury occurs in approximately 2% of patients with diaphragmatic trauma.
- Up to 15% of diaphragmatic lacerations can be missed, especially injuries on the right and very posterior on the left.

Pathophysiology

- Blunt thoraco-abdominal trauma creates a sudden, high pressure gradient between the pleural and abdominal cavities, which can result in disruption of the diaphragm, e.g. acceleration-deceleration injury.
- Right-sided tear results from a higher force of injury (expect other associated injuries) and has more cardiovascular instability (most die before hospital).
- The most common injury from blunt trauma is a 10–15 cm radial tear posterolaterally (the embryological weak point of the diaphragm). Penetrating injury causes 2–3cm tears.
- Herniation of abdominal contents into the hemithorax occurs causing:
  - Atelectasis with associated hypoxaemia ± hypercapnia.
  - ↓ venous return and impaired ventricular filling can mimic tension pneumothorax.

Early diagnosis

- Can be occult; consider mechanism of injury and maintain a high index of suspicion.
- Incidental finding at laparotomy for associated injuries.
- Laparoscopy/thoracoscopy can be used to confirm the diagnosis. where there is a high index of suspicion, laparotomy is not indicated, and there are equivocal radiological findings.
- Physical signs include tachypnoea, shifted trachea, decreased chest expansion, dull or resonant percussion (nonspecific), and auscultation of bowel sounds in chest.
- Associated injuries:
  - Pelvic fractures in 40%.
  - Splenic rupture in 25%.
  - Liver laceration in 25%.
  - Thoracic aortic tear in 10%.

Late diagnosis

- May be years after initial trauma.
  - An asymptomatic phase is followed by visceral herniation, obstruction, ischaemia and possible rupture.
  - Eventual lung compression and respiratory distress.
  - Cardiac tamponade or tension viscerothorax in severe cases.

Investigations

Bloods
- **Trauma series of bloods.**

Radiology
- **CXR**.
  - Initial CXR non-diagnostic in up to 40% of ruptures.
  - Pneumothorax/haemothorax in up to 50% ruptures.
  - Elevation of hemidiaphragm, +/− bowel pattern in chest.
  - NG tube may descend into stomach then ascend into chest (pathognomonic).
  - Intubation and IPPV may reduce herniation, masking diagnosis.
  - Contrast studies (via NG tube or enema) for delayed diagnosis.
- **CT chest**.
  - May detect a large tear even without herniation.
  - Unable to consistently identify diaphragmatic laceration.
- **MRI**
  - May be used in equivocal diagnosis to avoid unnecessary laparotomy.

Initial trauma management
- ABC approach to resuscitation.
- NG tube can decompress abdominal herniation.
- Associated pneumothorax or haemothorax requires a chest drain.
  - This should be placed superiorly and with extreme caution.

Surgery
- Repair is necessary because the defect does not heal, and any herniated abdominal contents must be returned to the peritoneal cavity.
- The usual approach is laparotomy.
- The timing of surgery and the haemodynamic state of the patient depends on associated injuries.
- Thoracotomy may be necessary for right-sided injuries or in patients with a delayed diagnosis as the hernia is more difficult to reduce.
- Thoracoscopic and laparoscopic approaches are becoming more popular. Multiple ports will be used.

Laparoscopic surgery
- Reverse Trendelenburg position is used which causes venous pooling and decreased cardiac output.
- CO_2 insufflation:
  - Pneumothorax can develop from pneumoperitoneum at initial insufflation or on reduction of hernia.
  - Increased peak airway pressure will be first sign.
  - Deflate the abdomen and insert a chest drain.

Anaesthesia for repair of ruptured diaphragm

Pre-operative preparation and assessment
- Haemothorax or pneumothorax requires intercostal drain.
- IPPV can turn simple pneumothorax into tension pneumothorax.
- Resuscitate with crystalloid/blood products as necessary.

Induction
- Aspirate NG tube if in-situ.
- Rapid sequence induction in acute trauma or if there is bowel obstruction in patients who present late.
- Otherwise, routine induction but minimize/optimize facemask ventilation as this can cause gastric distension.
- Muscle relaxant, endotracheal tube, and IPPV.

Maintenance and intra-operative
- Avoid N_2O.
- Avoid increases in intra-abdominal pressure:
  - Coughing/straining at intubation and extubation.
  - Ensure deep muscle relaxation.
- TIVA or volatile suitable.
- Low threshold for invasive cardiovascular monitoring.
- Beware, CVP reading may be falsely high if large diaphragmatic hernia.

Analgesia

- Epidural may be considered in patients who present late where the surgical approach necessitates laparotomy/thoracotomy.
- Epidural is seldom appropriate in the acute trauma setting. Parenteral opioid is used in this instance.

Post-operative

- Extubate if ABG satisfactory and other injuries stable.
- Send to HDU/ITU.

Complications

- Mortality is related to associated injuries.
- Good prognosis with early repair.
- Re-expansion pulmonary oedema:
  - More likely if lung has been compressed for >24hr.
  - Treatment; sit up, oxygen, CPAP or IPPV+PEEP, furosemide.
  - Usually resolves well.
- Paralysis or incoordination of the diaphragm usually resolves
- Reccurence is decreased with mesh repair.

Further reading

Power M, McCoy D, Cunningham AJ. Laparoscopic assisted repair of a traumatic ruptured hemidiaphragm. *Anesthesia and Analgesia*. 1994; 78:1187–9.

Rashid F, Chakrabarty M, Singh R, *et al*. A review on delayed presentation of diaphragmatic rupture. *World Journal of Emergency Surgery* 2009; 4:32.

Superior vena cava obstruction

Pathophysiology

- Superior vena cava (SVC) obstruction usually results from progressive mechanical compression of this thin walled low-pressure vessel by its relatively rigid surrounding structures.
- Venous return is maintained by collaterals and flow through the azygous, internal mammary and long thoracic venous systems.
- Patients typically present with a gradual worsening of symptoms.
- May present with life-threatening manifestations.
- Historically, the syndrome was most commonly caused by syphilitic aortic aneurysms and tuberculous mediastinitis; with the advent of antimicrobial agents, thoracic malignancy is now the leading cause.

Causes

- Bronchogenic carcinoma (80%).
- Lymphoma (15%).
- Mediastinal fibrosis.
- Vascular diseases.
  - Aortic aneurysm, vasculitis, and arterial-venous fistulas.
- Benign mediastinal tumors.
  - Teratoma, cystic hygroma, thymoma, and dermoid cyst.
- Infections.
  - Histoplasmosis, tuberculosis, syphilis, and actinomycosis.
- Cardiac causes.
  - Pericarditis and atrial myxoma.
- SVC thrombosis (may be intra-vascular device related).

Presentation and assessment

Early in the disease there may be no symptoms. If compression develops slowly there is time for collateral venous vessels to dilate and symptoms may develop late in the disease process.

Symptoms

- Dyspnoea 63%—often relieved by sitting forwards.
- Orthopnoea.
- Headache + visual disturbance.
- Cough, and hoarseness and nasal congestion.
- Hoarseness.
- Dysphagia
- Chest pain.

Signs

- Facial swelling
- Papilloedema.
- Upper limb swelling.
- Horners syndrome (ptosis, meiosis, anhidrosis and nasal stuffiness).

- Stridor (life threatening).
- Venous distension of neck and chest wall.
- Plethoric facies with obvious demarcation.

Immediate emergency management

- ❶ SVC obstruction may be associated with significant tracheal compression.
  - Patient may present as an emergency with impending complete lower airway obstruction or respiratory failure.
- ❶ Patients who are asymptomatic awake, may develop complete airway obstruction once anaesthetized.
- ❶ If the obstruction is caused by a large mediastinal mass there may also be compression of the heart and pulmonary vessels in the supine position, compromising cardiac output.
- ❶ If cerebral oedema or acute thrombosis is present these may warrant appropriate emergency treatment.

Management options

Goals of the management of SVC obstruction are: obtain a diagnosis, relieve symptoms and if possible cure of the primary disease process.

Conservative

- Supplemental oxygen, humidified if possible.
- Raising the patients head, steroids and diuretics are used to alleviate symptoms (care with steroids if lymphoma suspected as this may result in rapid shrinkage of lymph nodes and make tissue sampling difficult).
- Radiotherapy.
  - Has been advocated as a standard treatment for most patients with SVC obstruction.
  - It is used as the initial treatment if a histologic diagnosis cannot be established and the clinical status of the patient is deteriorating; however, recent reviews suggest that SVC obstruction alone rarely represents an absolute emergency that requires treatment without a specific diagnosis.
  - If the tumour is sensitive a response may be seen in several days.
- Chemotherapy.
  - May be indicated in chemo-sensitive tumours (e.g. small-cell lung cancer, lymphoma).
- Anticoagulation
  - If SVC obstruction is due to thrombus around a central venous catheter, patients may be treated with a fibrinolytic agent (eg, streptokinase, urokinase, recombinant tissue-type plasminogen activator) and/or an anticoagulant.
  - Removal of the catheter should if possible be combined with anticoagulation to reduce embolization.

Surgical
- Many patients have advanced intrathoracic disease amenable only to palliative therapy (i.e. after failure of radiation therapy and chemotherapy).
- Stenting and angioplasty.
  - Can provide rapid symptomatic relief within few days in most patients with SVC obstruction as well as allowing for long-term access (TPN, haemodialysis).
- Surgical bypass.
  - Technically difficult (done via median sternotomy) but may be indicated.
  - No trial evidence to compare this to stenting in benign disease.

Pre-operative assessment and preparation
- Majority of cases presenting to the anaesthetist will be scheduled to undergo a procedure to acquire a tissue diagnosis or possibly stenting of a compressed trachea.
- It is likely that some of the following tests have been performed and the results should be reviewed before proceeding with anaesthesia.
- A specific diagnosis is usually suspected but as treatment is varied depending upon the cause, further investigation may be necessary.

Rapid general anaesthetic assessment.
- May be needed in the emergency situation.

Bloods
- **FBC, U&E, Glucose, X match** (6 units may be appropriate as blood loss can be massive).
- **ABG.**

Radiology
- **CXR.**
  - Abnormal in 80%; however it is not particularly helpful as the diagnosis is largely clinical.
  - Widened mediastinum or mediastinal mass.
  - Pleural effusions.
  - Lobar collapse.
  - Cardiomegaly.

- **CT.**
  - Most useful test.
  - Identification of the level of compressing structure.
  - Assess the extent of involvement of other structures/ lymphadenopathy.
  - It may also guide the technique for gaining tissue samples (via CT guidance itself or bronchoscopy/mediastinoscopy).
- **MRI.**
  - Provides images in multiple planes with differing signal and allows for the direct observation of blood flow.
  - Does not require iodinated contrast.
  - But study times are longer than CT and may not be tolerated in severe cases. Monitoring will be an issue (requires MRI compatible equipment)
- **Venography with contrast.**
  - Contrast media injected within the vascular system can elucidate the exact level of the obstruction and assess the blood flow and run off via collateral vessels.
  - This is helpful is surgical intervention is planned. Care needed in renal failure patients.
- **Cytology.**
  - If lung cancer is suspected sputum and pleural fluid may have been sent already.
- **Histology.**
  - Biopsy of lymph nodes or mass may have occurred previously during brochoscopy, under radiological guidance or surgically from superficial nodes.

Others
- **ECG.**
- **Flow volume loops.**
  - Upright and supine position if dynamic airway obstruction is suspected.
- **Echocardiography**
  - If related to cardiac cause, or there is suspicion of heart and pulmonary vessel compression by a large mediastinal mass.

Anaesthetic management
- General anaesthesia in patients with SVC obstruction may be challenging.
- Patients may be scheduled for bronchoscopy, mediastinoscopy or sternotomy.
- Severe symptoms or radiological evidence of significant airway compression should prompt consideration of pre-operative radiotherapy.

When general anaesthesia is required the following principles and precautions should be taken.

SVC obstruction associated with tracheal compression

Induction and maintenance

- Give Supplemental O_2, humidified if possible.
- The aim is to avoid coughing (worsens obstruction) and induction must be smooth.
- Keep the patient head up.
- Consider using an anti-sialogogue.
- Obtain large bore IV access in a leg or other vein draining into the inferior vena cava.
- Invasive blood pressure monitoring.
- Classic guidance is to maintain a spontaneously breathing patient.
  - This may be achieved by an awake fibreoptic Intubation (where dynamic collapse may be seen) or by inhalational induction.
- If presenting for stenting of the trachea however, many units use TIVA (± muscle relaxation) and insertion of rigid bronchoscope with jet ventilation for the deployment of the stent.
- The technique chosen should be based upon operator skill and experience, and in line with locally accepted practice.
- ❶ Caution should be exercised with muscle relaxation as complete airway collapse may occur.
- Have a small ETT ready that is likely to pass through sub-glottic narrowing (note degree of narrowing on pre op CT).
- ❶ Be prepared to change the patient's position quickly as obstruction may be less severe in the lateral or prone positions.
- Note IPPV will worsen SVC obstruction.
  - Consider high frequency jet ventilation.
- ❶ Positive pressure ventilation in the presence of a partially obstructed airway may result in air trapping which if undetected can result in a tension pneumothorax or barotrauma.
- In the emergency situation, heliox may be considered as a temporising measure while equipment and personnel are organized.
- A rigid bronchoscope and a skilled operator should be present to bypass obstruction if airway is lost.
- Cardiopulmonary bypass may be required and should be available.

SVC Obstruction associated with heart and pulmonary vessel compression

- Invasive blood pressure monitoring is recommended.
- Be prepared to alter patients position.
- Maintain preload with judicious fluids.
  - Too much worsens obstruction, however, too little augments hypotension associated with an already obstructed venous system.
- Avoid negative inotropes.
- Cardiopulmonary bypass should be available.

Post-operative

- Increased risk of respiratory failure due to:
  - Acute laryngospasm.
  - Acute bronchospasm.
  - Impairment of the muscles of respiration.
  - Residual tumour causing compression.
- The patient should be care for on the ITU.
  - If any of the above conditions exist, it may be prudent to maintain intubation in the immediate post-op period in the ITU.

Further reading

Abner A. Approach to the patient who presents with superior vena cava obstruction. *Chest* 1993; 103(4S):394–7.

Rowell NP, Gleeson FV. Steroids, radiotherapy, chemotherapy and stents for superior vena caval obstruction in carcinoma of the bronchus: a systematic review. *Clinical Oncology* 2002; 14(5):338–51.

Conacher ID. Anaesthesia and tracheobronchial stenting for central airway obstruction in adults. *British Journal of Anaesthesia.* 2003; 90(3):367–74.

Extra corporeal life support (ECLS)

Introduction

- Since the advent of membrane oxygenators, cardiopulmonary bypass (CPB) for more than a few hours has been feasible.
- The role of extracorporeal membrane oxygenation (ECMO) support widened to encompass patients with respiratory failure.
- ECMO was first successfully utilized in neonatal respiratory failure in 1975 and has since become a potential treatment option for patients with respiratory and/or cardiac failure, who fail to respond to maximal conventional therapy.
- Currently systems using the principles of extracorporeal circuits (CPB) are increasingly called extra corporeal life support (ECLS) to emphasize CO_2 removal as well as oxygenation.
- The aim of ECLS is to provide cardiopulmonary support to enable the FiO_2 and ventilatory pressures to be greatly reduced, allowing the respiratory system to recover.
- It DOES NOT treat the underlying pathology.

Indications

(See Table 9.9) for conditions amenable to ECMO therapy.

Adult respiratory failure & CESAR

- Whilst the use of ECLS in neonatal practice is established, the same is not true for adult respiratory failure.
  - Even with best management, mortality is still 30–40%.
  - Numerous studies have failed to show an advantage of ECLS over conventional treatment in adults with ARDS.
- The recent CESAR trial conducted in the UK in adults with severe respiratory failure compared ECMO and conventional treatment.
  - It concluded a relative risk in favour of ECMO of 0.69 (95% CI 0.05–0.97; p = 0.03).
- Adult patients who may benefit from ECLS include those with an A-a gradient of >600 mmHg on days 2 to 4 following intubation, and who have been ventilated for less than 5 days.
  - Mortality risk is 80%, but recovery with ECLS is approximately 70%.

Adult Cardiac Failure

- Patients considered for ECLS will usually be inadequately supported on inotropes and intra-aortic balloon pumping.
- ECLS may be instituted in patients who are candidates for ventricular assist devices or transplant.

- If the prognosis is unclear, some centres will institute ECLS to stabilize cardiopulmonary function and assess other organ failure, thereby enabling more informed decisions about further treatment.
  - Mortality with ECLS for these patients is 50–60%.

Cardiopulmonary resuscitation & ECLS

- For this to be successfully used, an ECLS system needs to be available within minutes of resuscitation.
  - Consequently, this is infrequently instituted after cardiac arrest in the UK.

Inclusion criteria

Suitability for ECMO closely follows the entry criteria for the CESAR trial:

- Adult patients aged 18–65.
- Severe, but potentially reversible respiratory failure
  - Severe respiratory failure defined as a Murray Score* >/= 3.0 or
  - Uncompensated hypercapnoea with a pH <7.20.
- No contraindication to anticoagulation.
- IPPV with high pressure or high FiO_2 <7 days.
- Optimum conventional treatment tried.

Exclusion

- Patients who have received high pressure (>30 cmH$_2$O) and/or high FiO_2 (>0.8) ventilation for more than 7 days.
- Single organ failure only is not a necessary criterion.
- Contra-indication to limited heparinization.
- Advanced malignancy.

---

*The Murray score

- PaO_2/FiO_2 ratio (mmHg) on 100% O_2 for at least 20 mins.
  - 300 = 0
  - 225–299 = 1
  - 175–224 = 2
  - 100–174 = 3
  - <100 = 4
- PEEP level (cmH$_2$O)
  - ≤5 = 0
  - 6–8 = 1
  - 9–11 = 2
  - 12–14 = 3
  - ≤15 = 4

- Lung compliance (ml/cmH$_2$O)
  - 80 = 0
  - 60–79 = 1
  - 40–59 = 2
  - 20–39 = 3
  - >19 = 4
- Number of quadrants with infiltration on the CXR
  - Normal = 0
  - ⚠ point per quadrant infiltrated

▶ Total score/4

❶ Murray Score of >2.5 = significant lung injury

Table 9.10 Conditions where ECMO may be considered for thoracic surgical patients

Condition
Aspiration pneumonia
ARDS post thoracic trauma
ARDS sepsis
Pneumonia
viral
bacterial
atypical
Pulmonary embolus
Post CPB failure to wean

Practicalities of ECLS

Veno-venous (V.V)

- For respiratory support only.
- Cannulation relatively easy; jugular and/or femoral veins.
- Venous blood is oxygenated and/or CO$_2$ is removed; it is warmed and then returned to the patient.
- Low risk of distal emboli.
- V.V has few haemodynamic consequences except reducing PAP due to improved oxygenation.
  - Patients who are unstable requiring vasopressor support prior to ECLS often tolerate V.V well once hypoxia and acidosis are treated.

Veno-arterial (V.A)

- For respiratory and cardiac support.
- Cannulation more difficult via IJV and carotid artery or femoral vessels.
- V.A ECLS should be used with specific indications, not as a panacea for severe circulatory collapse.
  - Poor outcomes have been seen when using ECLS for failure to wean from CPB.

- Arterial return from the circuit increases LV afterload.
  - Ischaemia and papillary muscle rupture have been reported, but the effects of ECLS and the pre ECLS status cannot be easily differentiated.
- Reduction in preload and increase in afterload during VA ECLS can lead to a marked reduction of the intrinsic cardiac output i.e. total bypass.
  - Coronary arteries are perfused with oxygenated blood, but flow is unspecified.
- Risk if arterial emboli.

Ventilation

- Once on ECLS, patients usually rapidly stabilize.
  - Only minimal ventilatory support is provided in order to rest the lungs and allow recovery to occur.
  - Pump flow is adjusted to maintain a mixed venous SO_2 of 65–70%.
- Patients are usually protectively ventilated with a low FiO_2, low tidal volumes, low respiratory rates (<6 ml/kg/min) and PEEP 10–15 cmH_2O to prevent atelectasis.
- Simplistically, to increase oxygen delivery, blood flow to the oxygenator is increased.
- $PaCO_2$ is inversely proportional to the gas flow across the membrane. To increase CO_2 clearance, increase the gas flow.

Anticoagulation

- ACT is usually kept 180–200s using heparin to avoid clot formation in the oxygenators.
  - Along with platelet dysfunction, clotting activation and fibrinolysis, haemorrhage is a common and potentially fatal problem.
- Use in polytrauma victims must be carefully considered. Newer systems of centrifugal pumps and heparin bonded circuits may reduce the requirement for heparin.

Circuit

- 3 main components:
  - Pump, oxygenator, heater.
- There are a number of safety mechanisms including pressure monitors to indicate blockages and leaks.

Fluid balance
- Total body water is increased and aggressive diuresis is instituted after the first 24 hours. Renal dysfunction is common; a haemofilter can be placed in the circuit.

Weaning off ECLS
- As the patient's condition improves, the ECLS flow rate is weaned. A trial off ECLS is performed. It is usually apparent within 30 minutes if ECLS can be withdrawn.
- Percutaneously placed lines may be removed with attention to clotting profile and direct pressure compression. Surgically placed V.A lines may require operative closure.

Common Problems
- Haemmorhage secondary to heparin.
- Mechanical/technical failure
- Organ failure:
  - Renal, hepatic, neurological.
- Neurological insult secondary to hypoxia/haemodynamic instability prior to ECLS.

Extracorporeal CO_2 removal [$ECCO_2R$]
Main Points
- An emerging technology is $ECCO_2R$ where primarily, CO_2 removal is required.
- New devices [e.g. Novalung iLA®] may be utilized using primarily Arterio-Venous [A.V], but also V.V or V.A configurations, preferentially via femoral vessels.
- With adequate blood pressure pumpless A.V can be used. 1–2L/min CO is diverted though the exchange membrane. CO_2 removal is dependent on O_2 gas flow rate.
- Oxygenation depends on shunt and SaO_2. Additional oxygenation although limited, may be potentially lifesaving. In the low CO states of hypoxic respiratory failure, a pumped V.V or V.A configuration should ideally be used to increase the blood flow through the membrane.
- Conventional ventilation using a protective strategy should be implemented.
- The portability, avoidance of pump-related complications, reduced requirement of heparinization and reduced extracorporeal circuit volume are leading to an increasing popularity, particularly in non-cardiac ICUs, as an alternative to ECLS.

Further reading

Lewandowski K. Extracorporeal membrane oxygenation for severe acute respiratory failure. *Critical Care* 2000; 4:156–68.

National Institute for Clinical Excellence (NICE). *Extracorporeal membrane oxygenation (ECMO) in adults.* Interventional Procedure Guidance 39. London, UK: NICE; January 2004. http://www.nice.org.uk/Guidance/IPG39.

Bein T, Weber F, Philipp A et al. A new pumpless extracorporeal interventional lung assist in critical hypoxaemia/hypercapnia. *Crit Care Med* 2006; 34:1372–7.

Bronchial carcinoid tumours

Introduction
- Rare neuroendocrine tumour arising from neural crest amine precursor uptake decarboxylation (APUD) cells.
- Majority are benign.
- Approximately 90% are located in the gastrointestinal system (enterochromaffin cell origin or Kulchitsky cells) of which the most common sites are the appendix (35%) and terminal ileum (20%).
- Remaining 10% arise from the endobronchial mucosa; account for <2% all of pulmonary neoplasms:
  - 90% confined to the bronchus.
  - 10% have regional lymph node involvement.
- M:F = 3:1 (40–60 years).

Classification
- World Health Organization (WHO)/International Association for the Study of Lung Cancer (IASLC) classify these tumours as part of the neuroendocrine tumour spectrum:
  - Typical carcinoid.
  - Atypical carcinoid.
  - Large cell neuroendocrine carcinoma.
  - Small cell carcinoma.
- Typical and atypical carcinoid tumours manifest in similar ways clinically and biochemically; hence are grouped together.

Presentation
- Incidental radiological finding in 25–40% patients who are asymptomatic.
- Clinical presentation is dependent on the presence of the following features (see Table 9.11):
  - Bronchial obstruction.
  - Tumour secretion of pharmacologically active peptides/amines causing cardiovascular, respiratory, electrolyte, endocrine disturbance.

Diagnosis
- 24 hour urine collection:
  - ↑ urinary 5-Hydroxyindoleacetic acid (5-HIAA); a breakdown product of serotonin metabolism.
  - Normal urinary 5-HIAA is <10 mg/24h (<52µmol/24h); in bronchial carcinoid, excretion usually >50 mg/24h (>260 µmol/24h).
- Plasma chromogranin A is the most sensitive tumour marker.

Carcinoid syndrome (Crisis)

- 10% of tumours give rise to the carcinoid syndrome.
- Pharmacologically active mediators secreted by tumour include serotonin, histamine, and bradykinin.
- Serotonin causes hypertension, bronchospasm, sedation and diarrhoea.
- Bradykinin causes flushing, hypotension and bronchospasm.
- Mediators undergo hepatic metabolism.
  - ∴ only tumours with hepatic metastases and bronchial carcinoid tumours (non-portal venous drainage) will give rise to carcinoid syndrome.

Table 9.11 Clinical presentation of bronchial carcinoid tumour

Site	Effect	Signs
Local	Direct bronchial obstruction	Persistent cough
		Haemoptysis –vascular tumours
		Wheeze
		Chest pain
		Dyspnoea
		Recurrent pneumonia
Systemic (i.e. Paraneoplastic syndrome)	↑ serotonin production → Carcinoid syndrome— 2–12% patients	Tachycardia, hypertension, flushing, bronchoconstriction, haemodynamic instability, diarrhoea and acidosis
	Syndrome of inappropriate ADH secretion	More commonly associated with small cell lung carcinoma
		Causes ↓Na 2° to water retention.
		Weight gain, weakness, lethargy, and mental confusion
		In severe cases, can → convulsions and coma
	Inappropriate melanocyte stimulating hormone secretion	↑ skin pigmentation
	Cushing's syndrome	Classic features often absent

Pre-operative assessment and preparation

- Many patients have simple carcinoid disease in which case there are no additional anaesthetic concerns.
- Patients with carcinoid syndrome require symptomatic therapy and optimization.

- Pre-operative investigation guided by history. Specifically, consider/review the following:
  - CXR/CT chest to assess tumour location, bronchial obstruction. There may be atelectasis, consolidation, compensatory hyperinflation, or bronchiectatic changes.
  - PFTs.
  - Bronchoscopic findings.
  - Echocardiogram (TOE may be most sensitive versus TTE).
- Discuss surgical plan with surgeon. Options include:
  - Thoracotomy with sleeve/segmental/wedge resection or lobectomy/pneumonectomy.
  - Endoscopic laser ablation of tumour via a bronchoscope; reserved for alleviating bronchial obstruction or tumour debulking before complete surgical resection.
- Consider pre-operative benzodiazepine.

Carcinoid syndrome

Symptomatic treatment of carcinoid syndrome
- Bronchodilators may be effective in reducing wheeze
- Ranitidine is associated with reduced plasma serotonin levels and is useful for treatment of severe itching, flushing, and urticaria
- Correction of dehydration/electrolyte imbalance.

Optimization of carcinoid syndrome
Prevent the release of mediators
- Octreotide
  - 100 µg SC TDS for 2 weeks prior to surgery.
  - 100 µg IV slowly at induction (diluted to 10 µg/ml).
  - 50–100µg subcutaneously 1 hr preoperatively.
- Ketanserin ($5HT_2$ antagonist).
  - 10mg given over 3 mins followed by an infusion of 3mg/hr can also counter vasoactive mediator effects.
- Clonidine useful to treat hypertension and tachycardia
- Investigate and treat heart failure.

Anaesthesia for the patient with carcinoid
Induction
- Awake arterial line insertion is essential. Induction and surgery may cause large BP swings due to vasoactive amine release.
- Thoracic epidural for thoracotomy.
- CVP monitoring; consider cardiac output monitoring in selected patients.

- Careful intra-operative fluid management is important as inadvertent fluid overload and pulmonary oedema are common.
- Propofol and etomidate used successfully; avoid thiopentone
- Prevent pressor response to intubation:
  - Magnesium/β blockade/IV lidocaine (all tried with varying success).
  - Consider careful administration of remifantanil.
- Avoid rigid bronchoscopy in order to minimize airway irritation. Consider flexible bronchoscopy via a single lumen tube if necessary.
- Double lumen tube to isolate the lung.

Maintenance and intra-operative
- Anaesthesia:
  - TIVA (remifentanil/propofol/vecuronium).
  - Volatile + relaxant (vecuronium/pancuronium).
- Analgesia:
  - IV opiate (fentanyl/remifentanil) intra-operatively.
  - Thoracic epidural; establish block slowly and carefully so as to minimize haemodynamic swings.
  - Consider paravertebral catheter or intercostal blocks (limited duration of analgesia) combined with PCA fentanyl.
- Avoid factors which may trigger a carcinoid crisis:
  - Catecholamines.
  - Anxiety.
  - Drugs which release histamine, e.g. morphine, atracurium.
- Major problems include severe hypo/hypertension, bronchospasm, and electrolyte/fluid shifts.
- Be prepared to manage a carcinoid crisis:
  - ↓ BP. Octreotide 10–20 µg IV ± phenylephrine or metaraminol. (the vasopressors of choice in carcinoid surgery since they are not catecholamines. Norepinephrine infusion has also been used uneventfully).
  - ↑ BP. Labetolol or esmolol may be used. Consider Ketanserin 10 mg IV bolus.
- Regular arterial blood gas analysis and blood glucose (carcinoid tumours may secrete insulin or glucagon).

> **❶❶ Critical point**
>
> - When the surgeon handles/manipulates the tumour there can be release of vasoactive amines into the circulation.
>   - At worst, this can lead to cardiac arrest!
>   - (See Fig. 9.1); data of a real-time cardiac arrest during bronchial carcinoid resection.
> - There must be good communication as to when this is going to take place.
> - 'Fore-warned is fore-armed'; the anaesthetist can then be prepared to deal with such events in a controlled fashion.
> - Even when any afferent and efferent vessels supplying the tumour are clamped, these physiological insults are still common.

Postoperative
- ICU or HDU is required.
- Patients may awaken very slowly, i.e. serotonergic sedation.
- Treat hypotensive episodes with octreotide 10–20 µg IV. Wean regular octreotide over 7–10 days.

Top tips

- Have epinephrine to hand as there are reported cases of complete cardiac standstill following tumour manipulation.
- Consider ondansetron (anti-5HT$_3$).
- Consider chlorpheniramine (anti-H$_1$), ranitidine (anti-H$_2$) and aprotinin (anti kallikrein).
- ❶ Severe haemorrhage has been reported in association with biopsy of a bronchial carcinoid tumour during bronchoscopy.

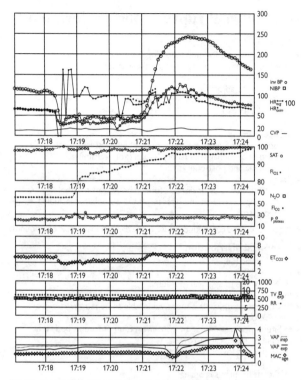

Fig. 9.1 Real-time recording of heart rate, invasive blood pressure, ETCO₂ and plateau airway pressure with internal cardiac massage; cardiac standstill.

The systolic pressure overshoot can be seen as a result of I.V adrenaline. This was a consequence of manipulation of the tumour. (Datex AS/3 monitor—data points at 5 second intervals; BP mmHg, CVP mmHg, P$_{plateau}$ cm H₂O, TV ml, SAT%, FiO₂%, ETCO₂, MAC$_{age}$, VAP%).

Further reading

McMullan DM, Wood DE. Pulmonary carcinoid tumors. *Seminars in Thoracic and Cardiovascular Surgery* 2003; 15(3):289–300.

Chinniah S, French J, Levy D. Serotonin and anaesthesia. *CEACCP* 2008; 8(2):43–5.

Wilkinson JN, Nickalls RWD. *Anaesthesia for bronchial carcinoid resection: a case report with multiple peri-arrests and real-time trend data.* 2010 (In press).

Oesophageal rupture and perforation

Causes
- 65% iatrogenic perforation following:
  - Rigid endoscopy at sites of natural narrowing.
  - Endoscopic sclerotherapy.
  - Surgery to adjoining tissue.
  - Percutaneous tracheostomy accidents.
  - Misplaced ETT.
  - TOE.
- 16% post emesis.
  - Boerhaave's Syndrome (transmural at left postero-lateral lower third of oesophagus), Mallory-Weiss (non-transmural).
- 18% trauma and post-operative.
- 1% other.
  - Caustic, peptic ulcer disease, foreign body, aortic pathology, straining, child birth and diseases of the oesophagus including neoplasm.

▶ Ingested alkaline compounds cause more damage than acidic compounds!

Anatomical distribution
- Intrathoracic (54%).
- Cervical (27%).
  - Mainly due to aggravated trauma.
- Intra-abdominal (19%).
- ▶ Cervical oesophagus is more vulnerable to penetrative trauma; thoracic oesophagus to blunt trauma.
- ▶ Site of perforation due to instrumentation or foreign body is at points of anatomical narrowing:
  - Upper and lower sphincters.
  - At aortic arch crossing.
  - At left bronchus crossing.

Pathophysiology
- The oesophagus has no serosal layer, therefore it is vulnerable to rupture or perforation.
- Gastric contents, saliva, bile, and other substances may enter the mediastinum, resulting in mediastinitis.
- If not dealt with rapidly, sepsis and eventually, death may result.
- 90% are left sided, around 2cm from the GOJ.
- Sympathetic pleural effusion often occurs secondary to mediastinal pleural rupture.

Mortality

Delay in treatment increases mortality:
- Treatment within 24h mortality = 25%.
- Treatment >24h mortality = 56%.
- Treatment >48h mortality = 75–89%.

Mortality is further influenced by complications of perforation, management strategy and other associated injuries.

Presentation and assessment

History
- Classically in Boerhaave's; middle-aged, male, dietary overindulgence and overconsumption of alcohol.
- Others include history of instrumentation, trauma, choking, swallowing caustic substances etc.

Symptoms and signs
▶ Symptoms and signs depend on the cause, site, duration, size, contamination and other injuries.

Early signs
- Non-specific and vague.
- Cervical lesions produce mild symptoms eg neck pain.
- Intrathoracic perforation produces the following:
  - Pain of variable location, commonly in the lower anterior chest or upper abdomen. Can present as back pain.
  - Fever.
  - Dyspnoea.
  - Crepitus.
  - Chest pain, subcutaneous emphysema and vomiting = Mackler triad (seen in 50%).

Within hours
- Seepage of gastric fluid will produce intense mediastinitis, sepsis and shock:
  - Fever and diaphoresis.
  - Cyanosis.
  - Tachycardia.
  - Hypotension.
  - Dyspnoea.
  - Tachypnoea.
- Vomiting, haematemesis, melaena.
- Dysphagia.
- Atypical symptoms.
  - Shoulder pain, facial swelling, hoarseness, and dysphonia.
- Upper abdominal rigidity.
- Local tenderness.

▶ Cervical perforation can be silent ∴ always exclude after high energy trauma to neck and torso.

Investigations

- General anaesthetic assessment.

Bloods
- **FBC.**
  - Leucocytosis.
- **Clotting screen and fibrinogen**.
- **U&E's, LFT's and glucose**.
- **Full septic screen**.
  - If febrile.
- **CRP** and **ESR**.
- **ABG's and lactate**.
  - If pH <7.2 or lactate >2, high likelihood of intra-thoracic penetrance.

Radiology
- **CXR**.
  - PA and lateral films looking for: hydrothorax, hydro-pneumothorax, pneumothorax, pneumomediastinum ("V sign"), pleural effusions (90% on left side).
  - Subcutaneous emphysema, mediastinal widening, sub diaphragmatic air.
  - Pneumomediastinum will be apparent within an hour.
  - Effusions and wide mediastinum will take several hours.
- **Lateral c-spine film**.
  - ► Lateral neck x-ray will show air in pre-vertebral fascia long before any chest x-ray changes in cervical injury.
- **CT scan with oral contrast**.
  - Investigation of choice.
  - Helps to identify pleural collections and co-morbidity.
  - Very useful for surgical planning.

Look for:
  - Air in soft tissue of mediastinum surrounding the oesophagus.
  - Abscess cavities in pleural space/mediastinum.
  - Communication of oesophagus with mediastinal fluid collections.
  - Check for metasteses if patient suspected of cancer.
- **Oesophagogram**
  - Gastrograffin (water-soluble contrast). 20% false negative rate.
  - Barium oesophagram. More specific.

Other
- **Thoracocentesis**
  - May reveal acidic pH, elevated salivary amylase, purulent malodorous fluid, or the presence of undigested food in pleural aspirate, which help confirm the diagnosis.
  - OGD under general anaesthetic is an essential part of surgical. management.
- **ECG**
  - To exclude cardiac cause of chest pain.

Management options (see Fig. 9.2)

Surgical

- To control leak, eradicate sepsis, re-expand lung, prevent gastric reflux.
- Procedures:
  - Endoscopic examination.
  - Primary closure with buttress or patch of small iatrogenic performations in only very early presentation i.e. before sepsis.
  - Diversion and exclusion.
  - Resection of damaged, necrotic tissues/T-tubes.
  - Stent.
  - Drainage gastrostomy and feeding jejunostomy.
  - Thoracic drainage and irrigation (Open/Thoracoscopic).
- Features supporting surgical therapy include the following:
  - Clinical instability with sepsis.
  - Recent postemetic perforation.
  - Intra-abdominal perforation.
  - Lack of medical contraindications to surgery (eg, severe emphysema, severe coronary artery disease).
  - Leak outside the mediastinum (ie, extravasation of contrast into adjacent body cavities).
  - Malignancy, obstruction, or stricture in the region of the perforation.

Medical/conservative

- Usually involves admission to medical/surgical HDU, nil by mouth, IVI, TPN, NG suction, broad-spectrum antibiotics and opiate based analgesia.
- Features supporting conservative therapy include the following:
  - Minimal symptoms.
  - Absence of sepsis.
  - Contained perforation in the mediastinum.
  - Recent iatrogenic or late iatrogenic perforation.
  - Perforation draining back into the esophagus.
  - Medical contraindications to surgery (e.g., severe emphysema, severe coronary artery disease).
  - No malignancy, obstruction, or stricture in the region of the perforation.

- ▶ Some authors believe that if treatment is instituted more than 24 hours after the perforation, the mode of treatment does not influence the outcome and can be conservative.
- Minimalistic approaches may be the preferred option tube thoracostomy or repair/diversion/drainage via VATS approach.

Anaesthetic management
- The unstable patient will need brisk resuscitation prior to surgery.
- Invasive monitoring and inotropic/vasoactive support may need to be initiated before induction.
- Post-op care will include ICU, IPPV, inotropes etc.
- Overall mortality following perforation is 18%:
  - 1° repair 12%.
  - Oesophagectomy 17%.
  - Exclusion and drainage 24%.
  - Drainage alone 37%.

Further reading
Smock ED, Andrew A. A case of traumatic rupture of the distal oesophagus: the importance of early diagnosis. *European Journal of Emergency Medicine*. 2008; 15:95–6.

Mamun M. Spontaneous oesophageal perforation: long known but still not easy to diagnoses. *Hospital Medicine* 1998; 58:968–9.

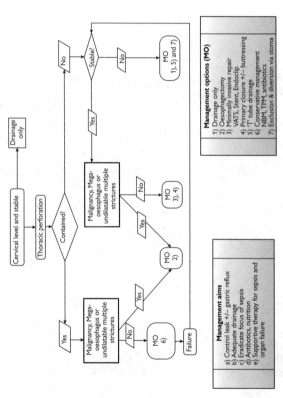

Fig. 9.2 Management of oesophageal perforation.

Management of intra-operative problems

Double lumen tube misplacement/ movement

Introduction

Double lumen tube (DLT) or bronchial blocker (BB) misplacement or movement has an incidence of 12%. Failure to recognize it can lead to saturation, difficulty with lung isolation, post-operative atelectasis and increased morbidity.

Causes

- Unrecognized incorrect placement after initial intubation of the trachea with the DLT or BB.
- Use of an inappropriately sized DLT.
- DLT or BB migration during patient positioning.
- DLT or BB migration during surgical manipulation of the airways, mediastinum or lung parenchyma.
- Inadequate muscle relaxation leading to coughing.

Prevention

- A pre-operative assessment and review of prior bronchoscopy reports, chest x-rays and CT scans will provide information on the anatomy of the airways and aid in the selection of an appropriate method and size of device for lung isolation.
- The DLT should be securely tied in and the tube length at incisors noted.

- ❶ DLT or BB placement must be confirmed clinically and with a fibreoptic bronchoscope:
  - After initial placement.
  - Before the knife-to-skin.
  - After ANY re-positioning of the patient.
- Clinician vigilance and access to a fibreoptic bronchoscope is mandatory throughout the entire procedure.

Effects of misplacement or movement of the DLT

- Proximal movement of a DLT can lead to obstruction of the lower trachea by the bronchial cuff and impaired ventilation of the contra-lateral lung.
- Distal movement of a DLT beyond the secondary carina can lead to single lobe ventilation.
- Minimal movement of a right sided DLT can result in mal-alignment of the opening to the right upper lobe.

Recognition of DLT migration intra-operatively

- Early desaturation following attempts at lung isolation.
- Failure to adequately deflate the operative lung.
- Appearance of leaks, increases in airway pressure, decrease in lung compliance or flattening of the flow volume loop.
- A sudden drop in end-tidal CO_2.

> ⚠ Always save a 2-lung initial flow volume loop at the start of the procedure. Once lung isolation is achieved, this may be used as a reference point for change.

Management

Address hypoxaemia first

- Hypoxaemia must be managed rapidly.
- Deflation of the bronchial cuff should allow for 2 lung ventilation, which can be observed directly.
- If this remains inadequate, the DLT should be withdrawn so that the tip of the bronchial lumen is above the carina and both lungs are ventilated.

Repositioning the DLT

- Fibreoptic bronchoscopy should be used to reposition and confirm correct placement of the DLT_1 as clinical confirmation will be difficult once the patient has been positioned and draped.
- The correct main bronchus can be identified with the fibreoscope, and the DLT railroaded over it straight into the desired position, all under direct vision.
- Another option is for the surgeon to actually palpate the main bronchi and confirm tube position.
- Resuming one lung ventilation and direct visual observation of collapse of the operative lung will further confirm correct placement.

Solutions for problematic lung isolation intra-operatively

- Alternative methods for lung isolation such as a single lumen tube passed into the appropriate main bronchus, a BB, or a different sided DLT can be tried.
- At worst, you may have to continue surgery with two lung ventilation?

Further reading

Slinger PD. One Lung Ventilation. In: Atlee JL, editor. *Complications in Anaesthesia.* 2nd ed. Philadelphia: Saunders; 2007. pp. 365–371.

Karzai W, Schwarzkopf K. Hypoxaemia during one-lung ventilation. *Prediction, prevention, and treatment. Anesthesiology* 2009; 110:1402–11.

Intra-operative pulmonary oedema

Introduction

Intra-operative pulmonary oedema is an uncommon problem in thoracic anaesthesia, but can have devastating clinical consequences. Pulmonary oedema can be multi-factorial and is most commonly cardiovascular in origin.

This topic will focus on re-expansion pulmonary oedema.

Causes

- Fluid overload.
- Cardiac failure secondary to arrhythmias, ischaemia or myocardial infarction.
- Aspiration.
- Negative pressure pulmonary oedema secondary to an obstructed airway in a spontaneously breathing patient.
- Re-expansion pulmonary oedema.
- Post pneumonectomy pulmonary oedema.
  - This is usually seen in the 2nd or 3rd post-operative day (See 📖 Post-pneumonectomy Pulmonary Oedema (PPO) and OLV, p. 622).

Re-expansion pulmonary oedema (RPE)

- Commonly occurs in lungs that have been collapsed for a prolonged period of time by pleural effusions or pneumothorax.
- Rapid re-expansion of a collapsed lung can lead to the development of pulmonary oedema.
- Typically seen in lungs collapsed for more than 3 days.
- Associated with pleural fluid drainage volumes exceeding 2 litres.
- RPE has also been described following one-lung anaesthesia with durations as short as 60–90 minutes.
- Re-expansion of the dependent lung, if done too rapidly and with high inflation pressures can lead to pulmonary oedema.

Pathophysiology

- Changes to pulmonary capillaries causing increased fragility.
- Destruction of capillaries due to stretching caused by re-expansion.
- Decrease in surfactant activity and amount.
- Increased permeability across capillaries due to reduced capillary-alveolar pressure gradient.
- Abnormalities of lymphatic drainage.

Clinical features

- SpO_2.
- Reduced cardiac output and hypotension in myocardial ischaemia or infarction.
  - ST segment elevation or depression.
- Pink frothy secretions from endo-tracheal tube.
- Decreased lung compliance.
- Acute elevation of airway pressures.
- Onset of pulmonary oedema occurs within 60 minutes in cases of RPE.

Management

- Management should be directed towards the underlying cause
- Increase FiO_2.
- Rapid correction of arrhythmias and attention to myocardial ischaemia.
- Positive pressure ventilation and addition of PEEP.
- CPAP or NIV is useful in extubated patients.
- Diuretics.
- Fluid restriction to 8 ml/kg/hr for the first hour intra-operatively and no more than 1.5 litres in the first 24hrs post-op.
- Avoid rapid re-expansion of lungs
- Avoid inflation pressures in excess of 30 cmH$_2$O.
- Avoid excessive and rapid drainage of pleural effusions or pneumothorax.
- HDU or ITU care post-operatively.

Further reading

Sohara Y. Re-expansion pulmonary edema. *Annals of Thoracic and Cardiovascular Surgery* 2008; 14(4):205–9.

Barotrauma

Patients undergoing thoracic surgery have an increased risk of developing barotrauma intra-operatively due to the pre-existing lung pathology, as well as the surgery itself. Anaesthetists must be familiar with the clinical manifestations of barotrauma to enable early detection and rapid management of this potentially fatal complication of mechanical ventilation.

Definition

- A type of ventilator-induce lung injury, caused by raised airway pressure/volume, resulting in an air leak and the accumulation of extra-alveolar air.

Manifestations

- Pneumomediastinum.
- Subcutaneous emphysema.
- Pneumothorax—simple or tension.
- Pneumopericardium.
- Pneumoretroperitoneum.
- Pulmonary interstitial emphysema.
- Sub-pleural air cysts.
- Systemic air embolism.

Physiological concepts

Barotrauma

- The concept that high airway pressures during positive pressure ventilation can cause injury manifesting as air leak is well known.
- Current evidence gives no clarity as to which pressure (peak, mean, positive end-expiratory pressure) is of most importance and what values cause injury.
- If the pressure gradient between the alveoli and bronchovascular sheath is transiently increased, air can gain access into the interstitial tissues.
- Gas then dissects within this sheath towards the mediastinum from where it decompresses through other fascial planes producing the manifestations of barotrauma listed above.

Volutrauma

- Refers to the concept that the critical variable causing injury is not airway pressure per se, but rather volume.
- Some authors suggest that the volume of regional lung distension, rather than the absolute pressure reached, is the critical feature of this type of lung injury.

Strategy to reduce barotrauma

- The use of ventilatory strategies such as pressure targeted ventilation with permissive hypercapnia, which may limit overdistension, may prevent or limit alveolar rupture and subsequent air leak.
- Expert opinion currently recommends:
  - Ventilation to low tidal volumes (e.g. ~5ml/kg).
  - Traditional teaching of large tidal volumes (10–12 ml/kg) in OLV to prevent atelectasis in the dependent lung has now been identified as being associated with ventilator-induced lung injury and an increased risk of barotrauma.
  - Adding PEEP with caution, as many patients will develop auto-PEEP
  - Limiting plateau inspiratory pressures to <30 cm H_2O.
  - High I: E ratios (1:3 to 1:5) recommended to prevent hyperinflation.
  - Avoidance of nitrous oxide as gas filled spaces such as bullae or pneumothoraces may expand due to the increased absorption of nitrous oxide.
- Early extubation at the end of surgery and restoration of spontaneous ventilation is a primary goal to prevent post-operative air leak secondary to disruption of suture lines or adjoining lung tissue.
- To enable the above, short acting anaesthetic agents and excellent post-operative analgesia are required.

Pathophysiology and barotrauma risk

- Patients undergoing thoracic surgery, particularly those with emphysema and severe airflow obstruction, are more susceptible to:
  - Intra or post-operative air leaks.
  - Development of gas trapping or dynamic hyperinflation (auto-PEEP) during ventilation, which can cause hypotension even without a pneumothorax.
- Tension pneumothorax in the contralateral lung can develop from a ruptured bulla where the contralateral pleura is still intact (See chapter on pneumothorax on the dependent side).

Other causes of air leak

- Tracheo-bronchial disruption after DLT placement.
- Lung injury after central venous line placement or epidural placement.
- Mediastinoscopy causing pneumothorax.
- High Frequency Jet Ventilation (HFJV) or techniques of jet insufflation with obstruction to expiration causing increased airway pressure resulting in alveolar rupture.

Clinical presentation
- Barotrauma in mechanically ventilated patients may present as acute, life-threatening respiratory and cardiovascular compromise.

Signs of air leak
- Increased airway pressure.
- Decreasing tidal volume.
- Hypoxaemia from impaired gas exchange.
- Decreased cardiac output.
  - Increasing intra-thoracic pressure exceeds venous and cardiac end-diastolic pressures, limiting cardiac filling, stroke volume and blood pressure.

Management

Action in the event of suspected air leak
- Inform surgeon and resume two-lung ventilation if possible.
- Increase oxygen delivery to 100%.
- Check breathing circuit and ensure there are no occlusions.
- If hyperinflation is the cause of hypotension disconnection of the ventilator circuit from the ETT should release the pressure and lead to a rapid resolution of hypotension.
- Fibreoptic check of tube position/blockage from secretions or blood through both lumens if DLT.
  - Possible to see circumferential compression and inward bulging of the bronchial mucosa if tensioning.
- Vasopressor bolus to support CO (e.g. metaraminol, phenylephrine)
- Ask surgeon to inspect for signs of pneumothorax of the dependent lung (e.g. mediastinal herniation into non-dependent hemi thorax, elevation of mainstem bronchus).
- Intra-operative chest x-ray.
- Surgical release of pressure and placement of chest drain.

Helpful tips

- Barotrauma from excessive tidal volume and high airway pressure may occur if a DLT is positioned too distally such that the entire tidal volume is directed to only one lobe.
- High tidal volumes and airway pressure can be delivered especially during re-expansion of the previously collapsed surgical lung, so vigilance is required at this time.
- Flow volume monitoring may be helpful in detecting the presence of air-trapping or auto-PEEP.
- If using HFJV, it is important to use a device with airway pressure monitoring, and alarm limits set which, if activated, cuts off the gas supply, to reduce the risk of barotrauma (See 📖 Jet ventilation, p. 728).
- If a large air leak develops, HFJV may be better than conventional ventilation in achieving adequate oxygenation and CVS stability.

Further reading

Marcy TW. Barotrauma: detection, recognition, and management. *Chest.* 1993; 104:578–84

Slutsky AS. Lung Injury Caused by Mechanical Ventilation. *Chest.* 1999; 116:9S–15S.

Slinger PD. Acute Lung Injury After Pulmonary Resection: More Pieces of the Puzzle. *Anesthesia & Analgesia* 2003; 97:1555–7.

Minimizing acute lung injury

- Respiratory complications account for almost half of all post-operative morbidity in thoracic surgical patients.
- ALI is the most common cause of mortality following lung resection.
- Recognition of factors that predispose patients to ALI, or which increase the severity of ALI, is vital to limit associated morbidity and mortality.
- A perioperative strategy to avoid exacerbation of risks can have a significant survival benefit.

The critical care implications and management of ALI/ARDS are discussed elsewhere in this book.

ALI

- ALI is defined as a syndrome of inflammation and $\uparrow$ in permeability which cannot be explained by, but may coexist with, left atrial or pulmonary hypertension.
- It can be caused by either a direct insult to the lung or by a cytokine mediated systemic inflammatory process.
- Clinically and histologically, ALI and ARDS represent a continuum of the same pathology.

Susceptibility

- Predisposition is multi-factorial
  - A complex interaction between genetic susceptibility and exposure to conditions that stress the alveolar-vascular interface determine the severity along a spectrum of normal to ALI to ARDS.

Factors which increase susceptibility to ALI

- Pneumonectomy R > L.
- Sub-lobar resection.
- Pre-operative excessive alcohol consumption.
- Return thoracotomy.
- Long duration of surgery.
  - Prolonged volutrauma to dependent lung.
  - Prolonged hypoxia of non-ventilated lung.
  - Increased cytokine release from tissue trauma.
- Genetic factors.
- Neo-adjuvant chemotherapy may be a contributory factor for ALI.
  - True incidence of interstitial pneumonitis and reduced DLCO following chemotherapy may be as high as 15%, as opposed to the commonly quoted figure of 5%
  - Neo-adjuvant chemo. by precipitating conduction blocks and cardiomyopathy may indirectly worsen ALI.
- Remaining lung perfusion <55%.

Factors not associated with a higher incidence of ALI

- Age.
- Pre-operative lung function.
- Staging of cancer.
- Pre-operative radiotherapy treatment.
- Sex.

Exacerbating factors

- Peri-operative management may determine the development of ALI.
- The following conditions contribute to the development of the lung injury.

Direct

- ↑ intra-operative pressure index
  - Volutrauma—Vt >7 ml/kg.
  - Barotrauma—PAwP >35cmH$_2$O.
- Hyperoxia
  - FiO$_2$ >0.8 (reactive O$_2$ species).
- Inadequate lung isolation
  - Soiling.
  - Micro-aspiration.
- Post-operative hyperinflation.
  - Mediastinal shift.
- Increased PVR.
- Pneumonia.
- Reperfusion injury.
  - Pulmonary capillary stress failure.

Indirect

- Excessive fluid administration.
  - Increased hydrostatic pressure → LVF.
  - Increased capillary pressure.
  - Increased RAP.
  - Increased PVR → RV dysfunction.
- Transfusion of blood or blood products.
- Neutrophil activation.
- Sepsis.
- PE.

Preventative strategies

- The aim is to maintain the lowest ventricular filling pressure consistent with adequate tissue perfusion, and to minimize sheer stresses within the lung whilst providing adequate tissue oxygen delivery.

Anaesthetic considerations

- Targeted fluid management
  - Avoid large volume loads and replace only physiological and surgical losses.
  - The chest has no third space!
- Pristine lung isolation
  - Avoid micro-aspiration.
- Optimize LV function as far as possible.
- Use lowest Vt that will provide SpO_2 >92%.
- Minimize peak airway pressure <35 cmH_2O.
- PEEP to ventilated lung.
  - Maintain alveolar patency.
  - Decrease intra-pulmonary shunt.
- O_2 to unventilated lung.
  - Avoid alveolar hypoxia.
- ❶ Propofol TCI as opposed to a volatile technique may potentiate ALI.

Surgical considerations

- Haemostatic surgery.
  - Avoid blood or blood product transfusion.
- Total positive balance in first 48 hours <20 ml/kg/day.
- Balanced drainage system to avoid mediastinal shift.

Management

- The principle of ALI management is to maintain adequate gas exchange until cellular damage resolves without incurring ventilator association lung injury.
- Good supportive ICU care with judicious exclusion of concurrent pathophysiology e.g. pneumonia, LV dysfunction, pulmonary embolus (See 📖 Acute lung injury and ARDS (ALI/ARDS), p. 616).
- The following therapies have been used without conclusive evidence of benefit:
  - Steroids.
  - Pulmonary vasodilators.
  - Elective re-intubation.
  - Colloid avoidance.
  - ECMO.

Prognosis
- Up to 58% hospital mortality at the ARDS end of the spectrum.

Further reading
Slinger PD. ALI after pulmonary resection: more pieces of the puzzle. *Anaesthesia and Analgesia.* 2003; 97:1555–7.

Mackay A, Al-Haddad M. ALI and ARDS. *CEACCP* 2009; 9(5):152–6.

Pneumothorax on the dependent side

A pneumothorax developing intra-operatively in the dependent hemithorax is an unusual but potentially life-threatening complication of thoracic surgery. During IPPV the pneumothorax may rapidly tension. The main challenge facing the anaesthetist is to be vigilant, detect it and deal with it rapidly.

Predisposing factors
- Bullous lung disease.
- Asthma/COPD.
- Previous pneumothorax.
- Cigarette smoking.
- Pneumonia.
- Recent CPR.
- Previous pleural breach (thoracotomy, needle biopsy, central line insertion).
- Airway trauma (rigid bronchoscopy, intubation, jet ventilation).
- Penetrating/blunt chest trauma.
- Baro-/volutrauma (can be caused by malpositioned DLT).
- Use of nitrous oxide.

Presenting features

These may develop before, or even during the onset of one-lung ventilation. Particular attention must be paid to any changing physiological signs.
- May be undetected initially.
  - May only be discovered on post-op CXR.
- Refractory hypoxaemia.
- Increased airway pressures.
- Reduced cardiac output/blood pressure.
- Tachycardia & dysrhythmias.
- Reduction in ECG amplitude.
- Progressive increase in CVP.
- Reduction in $ETCO_2$.

Differential diagnosis
Other things to exclude:

A
- Acute upper airway obstruction.
  - Laryngospasm.
  - Anaphylaxis.
  - ETT blocked with secretions.
  - Cuff herniation.
  - ETT malposition.
  - ETT kinking.
  - Surgical obstruction.

B

- Bronchospasm.
- Anaphylaxis.
- Aspiration of gastric contents.
- Severe pulmonary oedema.
  - Intra-op MI → acute pulmonary oedema.
  - Fluid overload.
  - Handling of the lung.
- Machine fault.
- Blockage of circuit.
- Stuck inspiratory/expiratory valves.

Diagnosis confirmation

- Access to examine the chest is almost impossible; aseptic surgical field, patient position and an open chest on the opposite side.
- Therefore, detection is extremely difficult.
- Signs may be very different to the situation of a large/tension pneumothorax in an awake patient/single ETT anaesthetized patient.
- It comes down to a high index of clinical suspicion; however:
  - Surgeons may notice mediastinum rising.
  - Fibreoptic bronchoscopy should be performed to exclude ETT malposition/cuff herniation.

Immediate management

Urgency will depend on severity!
- Ask surgeons to STOP.
- 100% O_2.
- Re-institute two-lung ventilation and consider ceasing ventilation to the dependent lung once operative lung is re-expanded.
- If a VATS is being performed, may be able to turn patient supine for assessment and needle thoracocentesis/ICD insertion.
- If open procedure, surgeons can open contralateral pleura and allow gas to escape into the operative field.
  - Large air leaks will still require the presence of a contralateral ICD.
- If after identification and treatment, it may be that the operation has to be postponed until the situation is stabilized.

Further reading

Akindipe O, Fernandez-Bussy S, Baz M, Staples ED. Intraoperative contralateral pneumothorax during single-lung transplantation. *General Thoracic Cardiovascular Surgery* 2008; 56(6):302–5.

Finlayson GN, Chiang AB, Brodsky JB, Cannon WB. Intraoperative contralateral tension pneumothorax during pneumonectomy. *Anesthesia and Analgesia* 2008; 106(1):58–60.

Malik S, Shapiro WA, Jablons D, Katz JA. Contralateral tension pneumothorax during one-lung ventilation for lobectomy: diagnosis aided by fibreoptic bronchoscopy. *Anesthesia and Analgesia* 2002; 95(3):570–2.

Hypotension

- Hypotension in the peri-operative phase of thoracic anaesthesia is common and usually multifactorial in origin.
- A systematic assessment combined with good communication skills is essential in establishing early and accurate diagnosis.

Pre-operative causes

Massive haemoptysis

(See 📖 Massive pulmonary haemorrhage, p. 484).

- Expectoration of >600 ml of blood/24 hr or 600 ml in 16 hours.
- Commonly due to erosion of bronchial arteries within the low-pressure pulmonary arterial system.
- The patient should be monitored within a HDU/ITU setting in the first instance whereby they can be stabilized along with invasive monitoring.
  - Arterial line, CVP, cardiac output monitoring (LiDCO/TOD).
  - This will permit close haemodynamic monitoring and allow guided intra-vascular volume replacement.

Intra-operative causes

Individual entities are discussed below.

Respiratory system

- Dynamic pulmonary hyperinflation (DPH)
  - (See below).
- Excessive IPPV at induction of Anaesthesia.
- Extrinsic Positive End Expiratory Pressure (E'PEEP).
- Pnuemothorax in the ventilated closed chest.
  - All of the above lead to increased RV afterload and eventual increased LV afterload.
  - This in turn leads to decreased cardiac output (all other variables remaining unchanged).

Cardiovascular system

- Vasodilatation following induction of anaesthesia.
  - Counteract with the appropriate vasopressor agent/decrease volatile MAC where possible.
- Sympathetic blockade secondary to thoracic epidural blockade.
  - Counteract with the appropriate vasopressor agent.
  - Delay the next epidural dosing or decrease the infusion rate if running.

- Hypovolaemia resulting from per-operative bleeding, particularly from pulmonary vasculature.
  - Again, this requires good communication with the surgeon; ask them what is going on and are there any continuing concerns.
- Air embolism.
- Cardiac manipulation during surgery.

DPH

- DPH manifests as a result of incomplete expiration of ventilated gases resulting in breath stacking.
- Accumulation of gases in the lung causes progressive increase in end expiratory pressure and volume.
- This hyper-inflated lung causes a tamponade like effect on the right atrium and ventricle.
- Hyperinflation also increases intra-alveolar pressure and compresses alveolar blood vessels.

⚠ The above changes results in right ventricular dysfunction followed by left ventricular dysfunction and electro-mechanical disassociation.

Aggravating causes of DPH
- Inadequate expiratory time during IPPV.
- High resistance endo-tracheal tube (DLT).
  - If there was difficulty in passing the desired size tube, a smaller one may have been inserted
  - In a patient prone to the effects of auto-PEEP (asthmatics), this increased resistance may have a deleterious effect.
- Application of E'PEEP during OLV.
- Moderate to severe Emphysema.

Diagnosis
- High index of suspicion coupled with monitoring peek and mean airway pressure (as a surrogate measure of pulmonary air trapping) and flow volume loops are helpful in recognising DPH.
- Flow volume loop monitoring should always be considered during thoracic anaesthesia.
- Commencement of inspiration before the expired volume reaches baseline along with increasing peak and mean airway pressure and hypotension establishes diagnosis.

Management of DPH

- Immediate disconnection of patient from ventilator (may require up to several seconds depending upon the volume of trapped gases and the extent of E'PEEP).
- Haemodynamic recovery usually occurs during expiration.
- May require vasoactive medication to support circulation during this recovery period.

Cardiac manipulation

- This is not uncommon during thoracic surgery resulting in brief hemodynamic instability.
- Compression and irritation of the myocardium results in brief and self-limiting hypotension.
- Atrial fibrillation can occur intra-operatively and may require DC cardioversion.
- Myocardial ischemia due to cardiac manipulation is rare and is usually due to underlying ischemic heart disease.

Management of cardiovascular disturbance during manipulation

- Good communication between surgeon and anaesthetist will avoid needless intervention.
- Ask the surgeon to stop what they are doing momentarily if the manipulation is leading to prolonged arrhythmia.
  - If there are repeated recurrences, the surgeon may have to find another approach involving less cardiac manipulation.
- Maintenance of normal electrolyte, acid-base balance and intravascular volume will reduce risk of arrhythmias.
- Consider early per-operative DC cardio-version.

Air embolism

- Suspect where the patient is head up/procedures involve close proximity to large veins.

Management

- Treatment involves 100% O_2.
- Left lateral decubitus (Durant maneuver) and Trendelenburg position.
  - Prevents air traversing into the right side leading to right ventricular outflow obstruction.
- If CPR is required, place the patient in a supine and head-down position.
  - CPR may break up the bubbles into smaller ones which will create less of a haemodynamic insult.
- Fluid resuscitation (to increase intravascular volume, increase venous pressure and venous return).
  - Colloid resuscitation is preferred over crystalloid as the former. may increase any pre-existing cerebral oedema.
- Aspirate the CVP line until air is seen (doesn't always work).
- Vasopressor support.
  - The evidence favours ephedrine boluses.

Spurious hypotension

- Innominate artery (first branch of the aortic arch, supplies blood to the right arm and the head and neck) compression can occur during thorocoscopic procedures, reducing arterial blood flow in the right arm.
- BP monitoring in the right arm may result in false hypotension leading to unnecessary intervention.
- BP monitoring in the left arm and palpation of carotid arteries should be considered.

Further reading

Myles PS, Ryder IG, Weeks AM, et al. Diagnosis and management of dynamic hyperinflation during lung transplantation. *Journal of Cardiothoracic and Vascular Anaesthesia* 11:100, 1997.

Analgesia failure

- Successful thoracic surgical outcome can depend upon good quality post-operative pain relief.
- The thoracic surgical population are rarely straight forward, often with multiple co-morbidities.
- Failed analgesia can lead to:
  - Increased pulmonary complications.
  - Need for mechanical ventilation.
  - Excessive sympatho-adrenal stress responses.
  - Increased mortality.

The gold standard

- A regional block is recommended for all open thoracotomies.
- Thoracic epidural analgesia (TEA) is considered the gold standard for thoracotomy and remains the gold standard for open oesophageal surgery.
- There is however increasing evidence that continuous paravertebral infusions provide equivalent reductions in post-operative complications.
- Occasionally, on awakening, patients are still in significant pain.
- The key is to recognize this, intervene and re-assess the patient once the intervention has been made.
- Patients should not be discharged from recovery until the anesthetist is satisfied that the patient is comfortable.
- The pain team should be made aware of any difficult situations earlier, rather than later.
- Alternative analgesic techniques are discussed below, none without potential drawbacks.

Familiarity of technique is likely to be as important as the technique itself.

Difficult situations

- Running remifentanil infusions intra-operatively mask pain very effectively!
  - One should attempt to make a judgement on the efficacy of the definitive analgesic technique (i.e. TEA, paravertebral infusion) early on during the case so that the patient does not awaken in agony at the end.
  - It is prudent to optimize the analgesia BEFORE you wake the patient up.
  - Giving large top-ups/boluses of analgesics in an awake patient who is writhing around in pain immediately after thoracic surgery is associated with more complications.

- Beware of the patient with multiple co-morbidities.
  - Patients with severe COPD may not tolerate any degree of opiate narcosis; it may be particularly important to optimize pain relief in this patient sub-group using alternative analgesics.
  - Extreme pain and its associated sympathetic response may be enough to trigger peri-operative myocardial ischaemia and/or infarction in patients with coronary heart disease.

Analgesia options
Thoracic epidural analgesia
(See 📖 Thoracic epidurals p. 686).
- Excellent analgesia is achievable in the majority of cases with minimal procedure-related morbidity.
- Infusions may consist of local anaesthetic alone or more commonly a low-dose mixture of opioid and local anaesthetic.
- The effects upon regional blood flow are still unknown, particularly when vasopressors are required to offset hypotension.
- However the use of TEA has been shown to reduce anastamotic leak after oesophagectomy, implying adequate or even enhanced splanchnic flow.

Problems
- Hypotension
  - Particularly intraoperative.
- Motor block
  - Less common with more dilute mixtures.
- Total spinal injection.
- Dural puncture (1–2%).
- Epidural haematoma.
- Infection.
- Pruritis.
  - May be helped by ondansetron/naloxone.
- Urinary retention.
  - Catheterize intra-operatively.
- Failure.
  - Fall-out, misplacement, catheter migration.

Trouble shooting
There are many reasons for poorly performing epidurals; some possible solutions are listed below. The continuous presence of suitably trained personnel until the onset of effective analgesia is recommended.
- No detectable block and pain despite 'adequate' top-up dose:
  - Re-site epidural.
  - If too difficult, consider paravertebral and or opioid PCA.

- Breakthrough shoulder-tip pain. Various approaches to this:
  - Paracetamol 1 g IV.
  - NSAID—paracoxib 40 mg IV or diclofenac 75 mg IM (provided no contra-indications).
  - Direct intra-operative phrenic nerve block or indirect post-operative phrenic nerve block.
  - An interscalaene brachial plexus block—low volume LA used (10 ml 0.5% bupivacaine). Shown to be more effective than NSAID IV. Not without complications (phrenic nerve blockade, complications of block insertion, LA toxicity etc.). Also… may delay discharge from recovery.
- Patchy block:
  - Try high volume, low concentration top-up (i.e. 15–20 ml 0.1% bupivacaine).
- Unilateral block (this is rare):
  - Pull catheter back 2–3 cm and top-up in usual manner.
- Block rapidly recedes after repeated top-ups:
  - Exclude intravascular migration by careful aspiration for blood.
  - Injection of adrenaline (15–20 µg) may result in tachycardia; however, if in pain already, this may not be a sensitive test.
  - Consider changing infusion to higher strength (or higher volume) if available.
- Persistent pain despite epidural re-site:
  - Consider one-off dose epidural opioid (i.e. 2.5 mg diamorphine) or alternative additive (see below) and addition of PCA. (Either abandon epidural or substitute for opioid-free mixture).

Epidural additives

- Many drugs have been given via the neuraxial route and often with reasonably good effects. However, by increasing the complexity of any infusion or through repeated external boluses, drug errors (with potentially catastrophic results) intuitively increase.
- Side effects of such drugs must also be taken into consideration, particularly if more troublesome than the pain itself.
- Agents that have been shown to have analgesic effects include:
  - Clonidine—side effects: sedation, hypotension & bradycardia.
  - Ketamine—side effects: nausea, sedation, psycho-mimetic disturbances.
  - Epinephrine—reduces plasma opioid and LA levels: decreases re-distribution of LA via vasoconstriction and also has spinal cord $\alpha2$ agonist effect → analgesia.

Alternative techniques to consider in event of TEA failure

Paravertebral analgesia

(See 📖 Thoracic paravertebral block p. 692).

- Paravertebral administration of local anaesthetic agents (PVA) represents an alternative to TEA with some studies quoting similar efficacies.

- The unilateral nature of the block avoids side effects from bilateral sympathetic block and the anatomy of this area facilitates low concentration LA infusions (although the block can spread to both sides).
- PVA may either be by single shot injections performed by the anaesthetist before induction; or by infusion via a dedicated catheter that may be inserted intraoperatively by the surgeon.
- The former only has 6–8 hours effect; this is an issue with extensive surgery or for intercostal drain-related pain.
- There are no opioid receptors in the paravertebral space, thus, PCA opioids should be co-administered if an infusion is to be used postoperatively.
- Failure rate of PVA may be higher than with TEA (6–10%)—multifactorial:
  - Inexperienced user.
  - Less well defined end point in achieving access to the space.
  - Inability to use opiates in the infusion.
  - Less well defined changes in haemodynamics with onset of analgesia.

Intercostal nerve blocks
(See ☐ Intercostal nerve block, p. 700).
- The intercostal nerves may be blocked with local anaesthetic however, as for single shot paravertebral injections, their effects are short-lived and repeated blocks are recommended.
- Beware LA toxicity.
- Surgical cryotherapy can improve pain post-operatively but results in an increased incidence of chronic post-thoracotomy pain and can not be recommended.

Intrapleural analgesia
(See ☐ Intra-pleural analgesia, p. 696).
- The placement of an interpleural catheter is used in some thoracic centres.
- After open thoracic procedures in adults intrapleural analgesia is not effective and should not be used.

Oral analgesia
- In keeping with the WHO acute pain ladder, all patients should receive regular paracetamol.
- NSAIDs can be very effective adjuncts to regional techniques however their use must be carefully considered in the elderly or patients with pre-existing renal impairment; relative fluid restriction may contribute to any post-operative renal dysfunction.
- Nefopam may offer additional analgesia however safety data in thoracic patients is currently lacking.
- Newer opiate receptor agonist drugs such as OxyContin® and Oxynorm® are also available and should be considered as part of local protocol in conjunction with discussion and advice of the pain team.

Chronic pain
- Significant acute pain may lead to an increased incidence of chronic pain, which occurs in around 50% of patients and can be extremely debilitating.
- Preemptive analgesia using TEA (with a variety of additives) or PVA have not conclusively been shown to reduce the incidence of chronic pain.
- The use of pre-operative neuromodulatory agents such as gabapentin may show promise for the future.

Further reading

Block BM, Liu SS, Rowlingson AJ et al. Efficacy of postoperative epidural analgesia: a meta-analysis. *Journal of the American Medical Association* 2003; 290:2455–63.

De Cosmo G, Aceto P, Gualtieri E, Congedo E. *Analgesia in thoracic surgery: review. Minerva Anestesiologica* 2008 [Epub—ahead of print: http://www.ncbi.nlm.nih.gov/pubmed/18953284. Accessed 25.11.08.

Joshi GP, Bonnet F, Shah R et al. A systematic review of randomized trials evaluating regional techniques for post-thoracotomy analgesia. *Anaesthsia and Analgesia* 2008; 107(3):1026–40.

Critical care and the post-operative thoracic patient

Immediate post-operative care

- Critical care of the high risk patient should start in the operating theatre.
  - Anaesthetic and surgical care should complement standard ICU, including low tidal volume ventilation, appropriate antibiotics, transfusion triggers and tight glycaemic control.
- Close liaison with the critical care team is required to ensure seamless transition into post-operative care.
- A detailed handover is required including pre-morbid state, pre-operative investigations, anaesthetic technique, intra-op events and details of the surgical procedure.
- Main aims of ITU:
  - Optimize balance between oxygen delivery & consumption.
  - Extubation with chest physiotherapy.
  - Optimize fluid, vasopressor & inotrope therapy.
  - Optimize analgesia.
  - Optimize glycaemic control.
  - Optimize temperature control.

> ⚑ Post-operative complications and death are commonplace in the high risk thoracic surgical patient. A high degree of suspicion is required to optimize patient outcomes by prompt diagnosis and aggressive treatment of post-operative complications in this patient group.
>
> ❶ Any suspicion of sepsis should prompt immediate triggering of the surviving sepsis guidelines.

Handover on ITU

History

- What procedure has the patient undergone?

The anaesthetic

- Pre-operative status?
  - Pre-operative tests results.
  - Other co-morbidities and their impact.
  - Drugs & allergies.
  - Indication of predicted outcome (morbidity/mortality).
- Intra-operative behavior?
  - Airway issues.
  - Respiratory issues, e.g. prolonged desaturation on one lung or difficulty with ventilation.

- Haemodynamics.
- Vasopressors or inotropes.
- Analgesia; any problems with epidural?
- Fluids?
  - Volume & type of IV fluid given.
  - Blood products given.
  - Total blood loss.
  - Urine output throughout procedure
- Intubated or extubated?
- If the patient remains intubated and ventilated reasons as to why?
- Ease of intubation should the patient require re-intubation.

The surgery
- Complex or straightforward.
- Length of procedure.
- Do they need a return visit to theatre for any reason.
- Pathology (benign/malignant/metastases).
- Palliative or probable curative surgery.
- Does the surgical site preclude any ICU procedures.
  - Transoesophageal doppler probes MUST NOT be placed into the oesophagus of an oesophagectomy patient as it will disrupt the anastamosis.
  - Remaining lung volume and ventilation strategies.
  - Tracheal surgery and airway issues.
  - Fistulae (tracheo-oesophageal fistulas and chest drain issues).

Assessment & immediate management
- Trauma patients who have come to critical care require a complete primary survey and secondary survey.

Airway
- Intubated:
  - Reason the patient has been brought to you still intubated
  - Tube size and length.
  - Awake fibreoptic intubation? Pending airway difficulties predicted?
  - ETT position on chest X-ray (should be 1–2cm above the carina provided patient has not had complex tracheal surgery).
  - Cuff pressure.
  - Are you aiming to extubate imminently/next day or will they be intubated long-term? This has implications on the sedation you choose.
- Extubated:
  - Are there any extubation or airway concerns such as retained secretions, vocal cord injury, or airway oedema?

Breathing
- ❶ Thorough clinical examination of chest must be performed
- Record:
  - SpO_2
  - Respiratory rate if extubated.
  - Ventilator parameters if intubated.

- ABGs on immediate return. What are the normal values for that patient?
- Use lung-protective ventilator settings.
- Chest drains:
  - Location
  - Patency.
  - Volume of loss through drain.
  - Bubbling/swinging.
- Surgical site and its implications in further care?
- Raise head of bed 30–45°.
- Initiate chest physiotherapy as soon as possible
- Prescribe nebulizers.
- Devise a weaning protocol if extubation appropriate.
- Consider bronchoscopy if appropriate.

Circulation
- ❶ Thorough examination of the cardiovascular system must be performed.
- Record:
  - HR.
  - BP.
  - CVP.
  - Capillary refill time.
- Record baseline ECG if there are concerns.
- Any requirement for assessment of cardiac output or myocardial function?
- Vasopressors/inotropes:
  - Did the patient return with a norepinephrine/epinephrine infusion?
  - Is it optimized?
  - Is it still required?
- Signs of sepsis?
  - Blood and sputum cultures
  - Antibiotics needed?
  - Further transfusion?
  - Microbiology advice sooner rather than later.
- ❶ Involve surgeons early if there is continued drain losses/tense abdomen/increasing vasopressor/inotrope requirement despite maximization of other parameters.

Drugs
- Sedation
  - Is it required?
  - Dual or single (propofol or midazolam/propofol ± opiate or midazolam ± opiate).
  - Remifantanil → is a viable option for ITU sedation and affords good control—watch for rebound pain on the cessation of infusion!

- Analgesia
  - Epidural/paravertebral; effective?
  - Do you need to re-site/top-up the epidural?
  - PCA needed?
  - Continuous opiate infusion in a patient who remains sedated and ventilated?
- Existent pre-operative medication?
  - Continue or stop certain medications.
- Anti-coagulation for thrombo-embolism prophylaxis
  - Observe guidelines regarding regional anaesthesia and thromboprophylaxis.
- Antibiotics.

Electrolytes and environment

- Glucose
  - Good blood sugar control decreases morbidity and mortality.
  - Aim for BM 8–10 mmol/L—as per NICE-SUGAR guidelines (Sliding scales are modified according to clinician preference).
  - The exact level to achieve still remains controversial, with tighter control increasing the risk of hypoglycaemic episodes. There is now emerging evidence that extremely tight control may be harmful, therefore stick within a sensible range rather than a very narrow one.
  - Feeding regime; continuous vs feed breaks.
- Electrolytes
  - Na^+/K^+/Urea/Creatinine and Mg^{2+}
  - Consider whether IV fluids need to be altered/supplemented.
  - Consider need for rapid electrolyte replacement, e.g. K^+/Mg^{2+}
- LFTs-albumin level particularly important marker of chronic mulnutrition state; particularly in oesophagectomy patients.
- Temperature control (>36˚C; use forced air warmers, fluid warmers).
- Ensure pressure areas and eyes are protected.

Fluid status

- Record and monitor input and output closely
- Many thoracic patients require minimal fluid replacement, as they are often prone to acute lung injury (lobectomy/pneumonectomy/oesoophagectomy).
  - Speak with the surgeon regarding their ideal post-op fluid replacement regime.
- Record urine output.
- Appropriate fluid balance?
- Need for CVVH?
  - Positive/even/negative balance?

Gastrointestinal

- Consider early enteral feeding.
- NG feeding.
  - If NGT becomes dislodged in an oesophagectomy patient, seek surgical advice.
  - ⚠ Do not re-site yourself.

- Anti-emetics?
- Prescribe stress ulcer prophylaxis.
- TPN?
- Record patient weight.

Haematology

- Hb/Hct/Plt/WCC
  - Aim for HCT >30%.
  - Transfusion triggers are controversial (clinician discretion).
  - TRICC trial states a trigger of Hb ≤ 7 g/dl in a previously fit patient; may need to be higher in patients with cardio-respiratory co-morbidity.
- Clotting.
  - Correct coagulopathy.
  - Ensure XM blood available if bleeding.
  - ?other blood components needed.
  - Seek haematology advice early.

Imaging and infection

- CXR.
  - ETT position.
  - Pathology; pneumothorax, haemothorax, pulmonary oedema or atelectasis.
  - CVP line position-ideally tip should be level with the carina.
  - NGT position.
  - Chest drain position.
  - Do they need a repeat CXR?
- Indications for further imaging
  - CT/MRI to assess pathology/collections or blood loss.
  - C-spine imaging if neck remains un-cleared and the patient is still intubated (trauma).
  - Ultrasound to facilitate drainage of collections or to assess intra-thoracic pathology.
- Microbiology
  - Culture results (sputum/urine/swab/blood).
  - Are the correct antibiotics prescribed according to positive results?
  - Stop un-necessary antibiotics.
  - Always involve microbiology early.

Relatives and communication

- Communicate findings/management plan clearly with nurse looking after the patient and the nurse in charge.
- Review surgical operative note and discuss events and current treatment with relatives.

- Discuss patient with multi-disciplinary team. Involve surgeons/ physicians/microbiologists/radiologists/physiotherapists/dietitians etc.
- If there are DNR orders on a patient, ensure daily review of the order takes place and communication of reasoning is clear.

Further reading

Beed M, Sherman R, Majahan R. (2007). *Emergencies in Critical Care*. Oxford University Press.
Brooks A, Girling K, Riley B, *et al. Critical Care for Post Graduate Trainees*. Hodder Arnold 2005.
Bersten A, Soni N, Oh T. *Oh's intensive care manual*. 6th ed. Butterworth-Heinmann. 2008.

Pain management

(See 📖 Management of intra-operative problems, p. 543) regarding analgesia failure).

Pathophysiology of pain after thoracic surgery

- Painful stimuli from the chest wall and pleura are transmitted via the intercostal nerves and from the mediastinum via the phrenic nerve.
- Furthermore, both the vagus and sympathetic nerves may play a limited role in transmitting pain from the thorax.
- Intercostal nerves can be damaged during (prolonged) rib retraction, rib fracture and by position of rib sutures when closing the incision.
- Chest drains and residual pleural blood cause further irritation, inflammation and pain.
- Post-operatively, the movement of respiration aggravates the wound and may lead to diaphragmatic splinting and atelectasis.
- The phrenic nerve is not usually blocked by thoracic epidural blockade
  - Thus, shoulder tip pain is common in patients where epidural analgesia is used in isolation.

Factors affecting pain after thoracic surgery

Surgical technique

- Video-assisted thoracoscopic surgery (VATS) through smaller incisions can reduce post-operative pain, unless large instruments are used through multiple intercostal spaces.
- Sternotomy incisions fixed with steel wires are usually well tolerated
- Classic postero-lateral thoracotomy provides good access, but requires division of many chest wall muscles.
  - This is often considered one of the most painful of all surgical incisions.
  - Muscle-sparing incisions have been described, but these suffer a reduced field of view.

Patient factors

- Patients already receiving chronic opioid therapy develop tolerance making post-operative analgesia more difficult.
- Young age is a predictor of post-operative pain.
- The elderly are more sensitive to systemic opioids.
- Psychological factors such as anxiety and nihilism can accentuate the perception of pain. Good pre-operative communication can mitigate the effect of these influences.

Acute pain management

- Specific drugs are discussed in more depth (See 📖 Immediate post-operative care, p. 570).
- Thoracic epidural infusion is considered the gold standard analgesic technique for thoracotomy, and is discussed along with other regional analgesic techniques. (See 📖 Thoracic Epidurals, p. 690).

Systemic opioids
- For an open thoracotomy, opioids are more effective in combination with other analgesic techniques, particularly regional anaesthesia.
- A balance must be struck between pain relief and side-effects, i.e. respiratory depression in patients with limited respiratory reserve.
  - Currently this is best achieved using patient-controlled analgesia (PCA).

NSAIDs
- Effective adjuncts but present several well known risks.
- Elderly patients with pre-existing renal impairment and peri-operative hypovolaemia are particularly susceptible to renal failure.
- The NSAID inhibition of inflammation may be counter-productive in procedures such as pleurodesis.
- Specific inhibitors of the COX-2 isoenzyme have not found widespread use due to concerns of increased severe myocardial ischaemic events.

Paracetamol
- Probably the safest non-opioid and has been shown to be morphine sparing after major surgery.
- The intravenous prodrug Proparacetamol is increasingly being used.

Gabapentin
- May be useful for providing pre-emptive analgesia, limiting chronic post-operative pain or in patients with opioid tolerance.

Chronic post-thoracotomy pain
- One study quotes an incidence of chronic post-thoracotomy pain after surgery as:
  - Up to 80% at 3 months.
  - Up to 75% at 6 months.
  - Up to 61% 1 year.
  - Up to 36% at 4–5 years.
  - Up to 21% at 6–7 years.
- The incidence of severe pain can be as high as 3–5%.
- Certain factors may preclude chronic pain development:
  - Age.
  - Gender.
  - Analgesia regime; high consumption of analgesics during the first post-operative week is associated with a higher risk of chronic post-thoracotomy pain.
  - Incision type.
- Little is known about the factors responsible for the transition of acute to chronic pain.
- There is conflicting evidence supporting the use of pre-emptive, multi-modal analgesia in prevention of chronic post-thoracotomy pain.

- A relationship between the severity of acute post-operative pain and the development of chronic post-thoracotomy pain has been suggested. Therefore, effective analgesia in the early post-operative period following thoracotomy may reduce the incidence of chronic pain.
- Chronic post-thoracotomy pain interferes with the patient's normal daily life in more than half of patients.
- Anaesthetists and surgeons should be aware of this fact and should look for effective means of preventing and treating this distressing side effect.
- Initiation of thoracic epidural analgesia prior to incision or the use of a muscle-sparing incision does not significantly impact pain or physical activity according to some studies.

Further reading

Cook TM, Counsell D, Wildsmith JA. Major complications of central neuraxial block: report on the Third National Audit Project of the Royal College of Anaesthetists. *British Journal of Anaesthesia* 2009; 102: 179–90.

Davies RG, Myles PS, Graham JM. A comparison of the analgesic efficacy and side-effects of paravertebral vs epidural blockade for thoracotomy–a systematic review and meta-analysis of randomized trials. *British Journal of Anaesthesia* 2006; 96: 418–26.

Delirium

Disorders of consciousness are common amongst ICU patients and range from mild confusion to overt psychotic phenomena.

- Delirium is an acute disturbance of consciousness with loss of cognition, perception and the ability to focus attention, which in itself can contribute towards confusion. It is a purely clinical diagnosis requiring:
  - Impairment of consciousness and attention—withdrawal, inability to converse (easily mistaken for depression).
  - Global disturbance of cognition.
  - Psychomotor disturbance—agitation and combativeness.
  - Disturbance of sleep-wake cycle.
  - Emotional disturbances.
- Occurs in around 10–20% of hospitalized adults.
- Incidence rises with age and pre-existing dementia.
- Up to 80% of patients in ICU have delirium at some stage during their stay and this appears to be an independent predictor of hospital stay, long-term cognitive dysfunction and mortality.
- 4 diagnostic categories:
  - Delirium due to a medical condition.
  - Substance-induced delirium due to intoxication or withdrawal.
  - Delirium due to multiple aetiologies.
  - Delirium not otherwise specified.

There are well-established scoring systems that aim to identify delirium early. However, delirium may be a marker of an unidentified aetiological factor implicated in the increased morbidity and mortality observed.

Aetiology

Delirium involves the prefrontal, parietal, and fusiform (especially right) cortices. The final common neurological pathway may involve:

- Excessive stress response, mediated by the hypothalamopituitary-adrenal axis.
- Imbalance of neurotransmitters: reduced acetylcholine, increased dopamine.
- Immunological factors such as cytokines (increased TNF-alpha, reduced IGF-1, somatostatin).

Metabolic/toxic encephalopathy

- Accounts for the vast majority of cases of delirium in the ICU.
- Usually a mild and fluctuating alteration of consciousness with symmetrical motor abnormalities, involuntary movements and normal pupillary responses.
- Sedative agents used in ICU have clearly been shown to be independent risk factors for the development of delirium (See Table 11.1 for other causes of metabolic encephalopathy).

Table 11.1 Causes of metabolic encephalopathy

System failure:	Drug withdrawal:
Respiratory, i.e. hypoxia ± hypercarbia	Alcohol
Renal	Benzodiazepine
Hepatic	Opioid
Electrolyte imbalance	Hypo/hyperglycaemia
(especially ↑/↓ Na$^+$, ↑Ca^{2+})	Surgery
Sepsis	Toxins, e.g. alcohol
Hyperthermia	Pancreatitis

Septic encephalopathy

- May be diagnosed in the presence of altered mental state, with the exclusion of any other risk factors for delirium (infection in particular).
- The precise mechanism for cerebral dysfunction remains unclear but is thought to involve problems with cerebral microcirculation, generation of inflammatory cytokines, alterations in blood-brain barrier permeability, and abnormal neurotransmitter function.
- Acute neuronal degeneration may also play a role.

ICU encephalopathy

- A distinct syndrome of behavioral disturbance observed in patients several days after admission to ICU.
- Presents as delirium and is thought to occur as a result of sleep deprivation, altered sleep-wake cycles and a noisy environment.
- It is a diagnosis of exclusion and other causes must be actively sought in the first instance.

Differential diagnosis

- Dementia.
- Aphasia (especially Wernicke's aphasia).
- Schizophrenia.
- Depression/mania.
- Attention deficit disorder.

Investigations

Bloods
- FBC, ESR, CRP, Film.
- U&E, glucose, LFTs, thyroid function.
- Ca^{2+}, Mg^{2+}, PO_4^{3-}
- ABG's; ± toxicology.

Septic screen
- x3 sets blood cultures.
- Urinalysis.
- Sputum culture.
- CSF.
  - Cell count, glucose, protein, gram stain; +/– Ziehl-Neelsen stain, culture, oligoclonal bands.

Radiology
- CXR, CT Brain.

Other
- Neurophysiology.
- EEG.
  - Degree of slowing correlates with clinical state.

Management and prevention
A number of strategies have been employed to minimize the risk of delirium outside the ICU and all are unit, patient and staff dependant.

Identify aetiology
- Detailed history and examination are necessary with clinical findings correlated to results of investigation.
- Enquire about alcohol + recreational drug use.
- Check drug chart for possible pharmaceutical causes.

Institute preventatve measures
- Removal of the source while preventing any further harm to the patient and staff.
- Sedation 'holidays'.
- Continuous patient re-orientation.
- Stimulating cognitive activities during daylight hours.
- Early mobilization.
- Use of eye glasses and hearing aids where appropriate.
- Subdued lighting and reduced noise levels at night.
- Nocturnal melatonin therapy.
- Prophylactic anti-psychotic medication.
- Nurse in well lit, quiet and calm environment.

Drug therapy
- No antipsychotic agent has been subject to rigorous randomized controlled trials in ICU delirium. The list below represents a non-exhaustive list of agents that may be used when delirium becomes problematic or poses a threat to safety.

- ❶ All antipsychotics may cause hypotension, extrapyramidal side effects, akathisia, neuroleptic malignant syndrome and prolonged QT interval, which may cause torsades de pointes and VT in susceptible individuals.
- ❶ Antipsychotic agents may have serious drug interactions that should not be overlooked.
- ❶ Beware prescribing agents which you are not familiar with.

Antipsychotics

Haloperidol

- 2.5–5mg PO/IM slow IV QDS (reduce in elderly).
  - Tried and tested agent, probably best first line.
  - May require up to 20 mg acutely.
  - Has a relatively high incidence of extrapyramidal effects.

Chlorpromazine

- 25–50 mg PO QDS
  - Causes marked sedation.
  - Cardiovascular side effects common with parenteral administration.

Trifluoperazine

- 1–6 mg PO daily in divided doses.
  - Extrapyramidal side effects common above 6 mg daily.
  - Can cause pancytopaenia.

Olanzapine

- 10 mg (range 5–20 mg) PO OD.
  - Mild antimuscarinic effects.
  - Metabolism reduced in females, elderly and non-smokers.

Quetiapine

- 25 mg PO BD on day 1, increasing by 50 mg OD to maximum 750 mg/day.
  - Can be useful for negative symptoms, rarely causes neutropaenia.

Further reading

Bersten AD, Soni N, Oh TE. *Oh's Intensive Care Manual*, 5th ed. Edinburgh: Butterworth Heinemann, 2003.

Pun BT, Ely EW. The importance of diagnosing and managing ICU delirium. *Chest* 2007; 132(2): 624–36.

Ely EW, Shintani A, Truman B, et al. Delirium as a predictor of mortality in mechanically ventilated patients in the intensive care unit. *Journal Of the American Medical Association* 2004; 291(14): 1753–62.

Nutrition

A neglected aspect of the overall management of patients is nutrition, but half of all surgical patients suffer protein energy malnutrition. Sepsis, injury and starvation are the main contributors to postoperative morbidity and mortality. Over the past 30 to 40 years advances in enteral feeding techniques, venous access and enteral and parenteral nutritional formulations have made the provision of nutritional support possible for most critically ill patients. There are many specialized formulations available. Nutritional therapy, although considered essential, is limited by evidence base (case reports, meta-analyses and lack of robust study methodology).

Nutritional requirements

It is difficult to isolate the independent contribution of nutritional status on outcome. The average 70 kg man requires about 2000 kcal/day. During starvation the body uses glycogen stores and then muscle protein, to provide this requirement. In illness or after surgery, burns or trauma, the following sequence occurs:
- Energy requirements are increased up to 30%, primarily by altered levels of catecholamines and cortisol.
- An apparent resistance to insulin increases blood glucose levels.
- Fluid balance becomes difficult to assess due to vomiting, diarrhoea, stoma losses, drain losses and third space losses.

Nutritional assessment

Body weight >10% ideal body weight—currently best measure
- Assessment of BMI is essential:

> Body mass index = Weight (kg)/Height (m)^2

The following can be used to assess dietary status:
- Clinical history (e.g. anoerexia, nausea, vomiting, diarrhoea, previous surgery, weight loss).
- Dietary history (types and amounts of food taken, dysphagia).
- Physical examination (weight, body mass index (BMI), general appearance, cachexia).

The following tests are used to gauge the severity of protein energy malnutrition and the subsequent response to nutritional treatments:
- Anthropometric (limited value on ICU)
  - Skin fold thickness/skeletal muscle mass.
- Biochemical
  - Albumin, transferrin retinol binding protein and pre-albumin. (Plasma albumin concentrations are usually not affected by nutritional intake and will not increase in metabolically stressed patients until the cause of the stress is removed. In chronic nutritional depletion, plasma albumin levels may even increase due to a combination of dehydration, decreased protein degradation and movement of extra-vascular albumin into the intra-vascular compartment.

- Muscle function tests; pre-operatively have been shown to predict postoperative complications. Requires an alert/awake patient and is complicated by metabolic derangements such as hypercapnoea, hypoxia, hypophosphataemia and the effect of various medications.
  - Hand grip dynamometry.
  - Respiratory muscle strength (maximal voluntary ventilation, maximal airway pressures and vital capacity).
- Immunological (lymphocyte count, cellular imunity or delayed cutaneous hypersensitivity).
- Impedance and conductance.

Nutritional replacement therapy

- To ensure that the body is well placed to fight infection and undergo subsequent necessary healing processes by:
  - Conserving body protein
  - Maintenance of normoglycaemia.

Step 1—estimate total fluid requirements

- 30–40 ml/kg/24h or 1 ml water/calorie for an adult (supplemented should fluid losses be excessive).

Step 2—estimate total calorie requirement.

- 25 kilocalories/kg/day is the estimate most often used.

Harris-Benedict equation

- Used to calculate resting energy expenditure (REE)
  - Women: REE = 655 + (9.6 × weight in kg) + (1.7 × height in cm)—(4.7 × age in years).
  - Men: REE = 66 + (13.7 × weight in kg) + (5.0 × height in cm)—(6.8 × age in years).
  - Calorie requirements/day = 1.25 × REE (for each 1°C above 37 add 10% extra allowance.

Step 3—assimilate nutrient requirements

- Calories can be given in three forms:

Carbohydrate:

- 30 to 70% of the total calories, usually given as glucose but fructose and sorbitol are used in some countries. Insulin may be required to maintain blood glucose concentration within normal limits, especially since insulin resistance is often seen as part of the response to stress.

Fat:
- 20 to 50% of the total calories can be given as fat. Critically ill patients often utilize fat better than carbohydrate as an energy source. Omega-6-polyunsaturated fatty acid (PUFA) triglycerides should be provided to prevent essential fatty acid deficiency—at least 7% of total calories.

Protein:
- 15 to 20% of the total calories per day can be administered as protein or amino acids depending on route of administration.

Trace elements electrolytes and vitamins:
- 1 mmol/kg of both sodium and potassium needed (altered when to account for excessive losses).
- Magnesium, iron, copper, zinc and selenium are also necessary, but in trace amounts.
- Phosphate replacement is vital as it is pivotal to most metabolic processes resulting in the formation of ATP. Hypophosphataemia is associated with failure to wean secondary to muscle weakness.
- Fat soluble vitamins (A, carotene) and water-soluble vitamins (B, C, D, E) are required but in extremely small amounts.

Step 4—choose route.

Step 5—evaluate effects of regime and maintain it at steady state according to the patient needs.

Enteral feeding
- Mixture of fat, carbohydrate, protein, water, electrolytes, minerals and fibre.
- Feeds have about 1–1.5 kcal/ml.
- Energy is delivered as fat and carbohydrate.
- Start rate normally around 30 ml/hr (varies between institutions), increasing to achieve the caloric requirement.
- Preferred route; abundant evidence to support early institution after major surgery.
  - Preserves the gastrointestinal barrier function that can prevent or decrease translocation of bacteria across the bowel wall which may decrease nosocomial infections.
  - However, it may increase the risk of ventilator associated pneumonia via increases in gastric pH encouraging gastric colonization.
  - The gastric tube (oral/nasal) may compromise lower oesophageal sphincter function so may add to aspiration risk.
  - Requires adequate gastric motility and minimal gastric residual volume.
  - If feeding needs to be stopped periodically to allow gastric emptying, then the calorie target will not be met.

Routes
- *Nasogastric feeding (NG)* is the most commonly used route, but relies on adequate gastric emptying.
- *Nasojejunal feeding (NJ)* avoids the pylorus and is used in patients with gastric stasis.
- *Percutaneous endoscopic gastroenterostomy tube (PEG) or jejunal feeding tube:*
  - An endoscope is passed into the oesophagus, then stomach. A tube is then guided into the stomach or jejunum percutaneously. This technique is applicable to patients who do not tolerate NG tubes and serves as a longer term solution.

Factors that reduce the feasibility of enteral feeding
- Impaired swallowing:
  - Sedation, tracheostomy, oesophageal disease, surgery, cerebrovascular accident, other neurology.
- Reduced gastric emptying:
  - Pain, anxiety, opioids, post-op ileus.
- Protection of surgical site:
  - Suture lines around anastamosis.
- Paralytic ileus
- Abdominal distension (which may be sufficient to result in compromised respiratory function).

Parenteral feeding (TPN)
- Ideally TPN should be administered via a tunnelled subclavian vein central line.
- TPN can be delivered into peripheral veins via very fine-bore catheters.
- Lines used for TPN should be inserted under full aseptic technique and TPN should be delivered through a dedicated part on the line.
- Interruptions and reconnections should be kept to a minimum and again carried out under aseptic conditions.
- TPN solutions should contain a balanced mix of:
  - Protein—(a balanced solution of essential (40%) and non-essential (60%) amino acids).
  - Carbohydrate—glucose (4 kcal/g) is used as the main source of carbohydrate.
  - Lipid—lipid emulsions are used because to supply a large amount of energy in a small volume (9 kcal/g).
  - Water, vitamins, electrolytes and minerals.
- Evidence shows that TPN does not influence the overall mortality rate of surgical or critically ill patients. It may reduce the morbidity, especially in malnourished patients.
- Monitoring of TPN:
  - Regular BM.
  - FBC.
  - U+E's.
  - LFT's.
  - Calcium/phosphate, plasma lipids, trace elements.
  - Signs of line sepsis.

- New research in immunotherapy suggests that the addition of glutamine, arginine and the omega-3 fatty acids, may enhance the immune response during critical illness.
- Blood sugar should be controlled during feeding and evidence suggests aiming for a plasma level <10 mmol/L.
- The most common reasons for parenteral feeding are:
  - Post surgery—if bowel function is likely to be disturbed or if attempts to use the enteral route have failed.
  - Short-bowel syndrome.
  - Gastrointestinal fistulae.
  - Prolonged paralytic ileus.
  - Inflammatory bowel disease.
  - Preoperatively—can be considered for malnourished patients.

Specific situations where nutritional requirements are altered

Sepsis

- Catabolic state—total calorie requirements are increased and rapid net protein breakdown occurs.
- Up to 10–20% increase in calorific requirement.
- Higher nitrogen intakes may be required.
- Micronutrient and electrolyte requirement are also altered— electrolyte concentrations should be monitored frequently.
- Due to the anti-insulin effect of sepsis upon the endocrine system, hyperglycaemia is more common. Higher insulin infusion rates will follow.
- Hypertriglyceridaemia with lipaemic serum may occur and fat intake may need to be decreased.

Liver failure

- Associated liver failure may mean marked pre-existing electrolyte abnormalities. Fluid volume may need to be restricted significantly in order to minimize ascites formation.
- It is common to see hypomagnesaemia and hypokalaemia.
- Severe hyponatraemia, despite high total body sodium concentrations may be observed.
- Rapid correction of plasma sodium concentration should be avoided since total body sodium is often abnormally high and central pontine myelinolysis may result.
- Encephalopathy often results due to accumulation of ammonia secondary to defective urea cycling.
- Administration of certain amino acids may worsen this situation, therefore nitrogen sources with increased branched chain amino acids and reduced aromatic sulphur containing amino acids should be considered.

Respiratory failure

- Respiratory quotient—the ratio of carbon dioxide production to oxygen consumption RQ—and this is normally between 0.85 and 0.90.
  - Metabolism of fat is associated with an RQ of 0.7.
  - Carbohydrate metabolism gives an RQ of 1.0.
- Those with respiratory failure accumulate CO_2, therefore a more lipid based feed regimen will be associated with a lower RQ secondary to lower resultant CO_2 production.
- One should aim for a minimal calorie intake.
- Administration of higher protein feeds is associated with an increase in oxygen consumption, however this is of little practical importance since small increases in inspired oxygen tension overcomes the problem.
- It is unproven as to whether provision of branched chain amino acids (leucine, isoleucine and valine) improves overall outcome amongst the ICU and HDU population.
- The respiratory centre may be stimulated aiding muscle regeneration, which may quicken weaning from artificial ventilation.

Renal failure

- Basically, care is needed not to fluid overload.
- Care is also required, particularly with potassium, magnesium and phosphate administration.
- Low volume/low sodium feeds are available for enteral nutrition in patients with renal compromise.
- Nitrogen intake may also need to be reduced to between 0.5 and 0.8g N_2/kg/day in patients with chronic renal failure.
- A patient who has recently been dialysed, may have lost amino acids, therefore it may be necessary to increase provision.
- Fluids used in peritoneal dialysis usually contain glucose providing a 'hidden' source of calorie intake in such patients.

Immunonutrition

- Arginine is an amino acid which has been given post-operatively in doses of up to 30 g/24hr to adult patients but the benefit remains unclear.
- It is required for a variety of metabolic functions:
  - Urea synthesis.
  - Lymphocyte proliferation and wound healing.
  - Stimulates the release of hormones including insulin, prolactin and growth hormone.
  - Nitric oxide production.
- These effects may be beneficial in the gastrointestinal tract.
- Glutamine (administered as Omega-3 polyunsaturated fatty acids (O3PFA's) has also been used as a nutritional supplement.
- Serious illness may lead to increased requirement.

- It is essential for:
  - Formation of the antioxidant compound glutathione.
  - Use as a substrate for metabolism by leucocytes and enterocytes.
- Augmentation of lymphocyte and macrophage function.
- O_3PFA's are currently being evaluated as both immune modulators and antiinflammatory agents and doses of up to 5 g/24h have been used in critically ill patients with sepsis.
- Studies report trends towards lower multi-organ failure rates, fewer infection-related complications, reduced requirements for mechanical ventilation, and possible decreased length of ICU stay.
- There was however an increased risk of death although this did not reach statistical significance.

▶▶ Nutrition pitfalls and tips

- Be vigilant for signs and symptoms of malnutrition.
- Be pro-active in instituting a feeding regime.
- Agents which promote gastric and intestinal motility such as metoclopramide and erythromycin should be considered:
  - Erythromycin increases motilin, a substance which enhances contractile activity of the gastric antrum and duodenum.
  - Metoclopramide is a selective dopamine-2-receptor antagonist which increases peristaltic contractility of the oesophagus, gastric antrum and jejunum.
  - Neither erythromycin nor metoclopramide have effects that may affect healing in the large bowel.
- Some studies suggest that early post-operative feeding is safe and effective, with reduced hospital stays.
- The absence of bowel sounds or passage of flatus do not preclude enteral feeding, especially when this is instituted distal to the pylorus.
- Diarrhoea during artificial feeding, although usually with a high osmotic load to the colon, may be associated with *Clostridium difficile enterocolitis*.
- Patients on long-term nutritional supplementation should have U&E's checked regularly.
- Feed breaks have been shown to increase morbidity and mortality from all causes through unstable blood sugar readings in the critically ill patient. Continuous feeding minimizes these swings.
- The use of propofol sedation may lead to excessive lipid intake. Therefore, lipid content of feed should be calculated to account for this.
- Higher fibre containing feeds may increase the rate of anastamotic healing.

Further reading

Appelboam, Sair. Nutrition in the critically ill patient. *Anaesthesia and intensive care medicine* 2006; 7(4): 121–3.

Bersten A, Soni N, Oh T. *Oh's intensive care manual*. 6th ed. Butterworth-Heinemann (UK). Chapter 87.

Airways and extubation

- Much of the emphasis during training in anaesthesia is focussed upon tracheal intubation.
  - Complications arising from tracheal extubation are three times more common.
- Double lumen tubes (DLT) are less well tolerated by the awakening patient as they are bulkier, stiffer and more difficult to remove than a single lumen tube (SLT).
  - These features, together with the effects of surgery and the patient's pre-existing pulmonary function make tracheal extubation a potentially challenging intervention.

▶ Immediate extubation in the operating theatre should be the goal. Preparation for extubation is summarized below.

Preparation for extubation (DLT)

- Optimize:
  - Analgesia.
  - Thermodynamics.
  - Haemodynamics—normal as possible without excessive pharmacological support.
- Clear secretions and airway.
  - Endotracheal/bronchial lumens—use fresh suction catheter for each pass down the tube.
  - Upper airway—using Yankeur sucker.
- Reverse any residual neuromuscular blockade.
- Increase FiO_2
  - Avoid prolonged periods of 100% O_2; except in cases of difficult airway, as it will worsen atelectasis and potentially ↑ physiological shunt.
- Deflate endobronchial cuff.
- Sit patient up 45° (if no associated trauma prevents) to ↓ atelectasis and improve respiratory mechanics.
- Consider extubation when the patient has an adequate tidal volume, respiratory rate and respiratory pattern.
- ▶ Consider the patient's gas exchange in the context of their pre-operative state. Hypercapnia and hypoxaemia are not absolute contraindications to extubation.

Awake vs. deep extubation

Answer the fundamental questions below to assist in the decision making:
- Was the patient easy to mask ventilate?
- Was the patient difficult to intubate?
- Is the patient starved (emergencies)/does the patient have gastro-oesophageal reflux?

- ▶ If there has been any difficulty with the management of the airway, or there is a risk of airway soiling, then an awake extubation may be advisable.
- ❶ The uncomplicated pre-operative airway may change during the course of surgery-manipulation may lead to oedema.
  - Thus, the post-extubation airway may be more difficult to manage
  - Ensure there is a leak around the deflated tracheal cuff prior to extubation.

DLT extubation of the difficult airway

- Airway exchange catheter (AEC):
  - Consider applying local anaesthetic to the trachea via the tracheal lumen of the DLT.
  - Pass the AEC down the tracheal lumen of the DLT.
  - Remove the DLT and leave the AEC in-situ until the patient is awake.
  - The patient can be oxygenated via the AEC using a Rapi-fit connector (15 mm).
  - The AEC acts as a bougie (under direct laryngoscopy) if emergency re-intubation is required.
- The DLT may be withdrawn so that the endobronchial tip lies within the trachea.
- Remove the DLT when the patient is awake.

Immediate vs. delayed extubation

Immediate extubation

- Avoidance of invasive ventilation post-operatively in thoracic surgical patients mitigates against the following complications:
  - Nosocomial chest infection.
  - Disuse atrophy of respiratory muscles.
  - Bronchial stump disruption.
  - Persistent air leak.

> 📖 In a case-series of patients requiring right postero-lateral thoracotomy as part of a 2-stage oesophagectomy the following was demonstrated:
> - Factors associated with the need for re-ventilation were:
>   - Prolonged duration of OLV (median 167 minutes vs. 130 minutes [not re-ventilated]; p <0.005).
>   - ↓FEV₁/FVC (63% vs. 73% [not re-ventilated]; p <0.05).
>   - Cigarette smoking, COPD, and neo-adjuvant therapy; p >0.05.
> - Authors concluded that immediate extubation was both feasible and associated with low morbidity and mortality.

- Immediate extubation is both feasible and safe in patients undergoing single lung transplant (re-intubation rate = 24 %) and lung volume reduction surgery.
- ▶ Consider non-invasive ventilation following immediate extubation.

Delayed extubation
- When a patient is ventilated post-operatively, the DLT should usually be exchanged for a SLT.
- In cases of known or suspected difficult airway, this can be facilitated by an AEC (see above).

Difficult extubation
Typically, difficulty in removing an endotracheal tube can be attributed to the following:
- Failure to deflate endotracheal/bronchial cuffs.
- Large cuff catching on the vocal cords:
  - After cuff deflation it acts as a sleeve thus increasing the external diameter of the deflated cuff.
  - ETT too large in first place.
  - Rarely due to a laryngeal abnormality, e.g. sub-glottic stenosis following previous tracheostomy.
- Adhesion of the tracheal tube to the tracheal wall due to a lack of lubricant.
- Rarely, difficult extubation may be caused by surgical fixation of the endobronchial tube.

Strategies to overcome difficult extubation as described above include:
- Ensure all cuffs completely deflated.
- Re-insertion of the tube.
- Rotation of the tube.
- Consider re-inflation of cuff(s) to smooth out any folds that may be catching on the glottis.

- Attempt extubation under direct laryngoscopy.
- Failure to extubate following these interventions should prompt fibreoptic examination of the tube and bronchus.

⚠ Avoid excessive traction on the tube in cases of difficult extubation, as the tube may be sutured to an intra-thoracic structure. In this circumstance, surgical removal of the tube may be required.

Airway morbidity
Aspiration of gastric contents
(See 📖 Pulmonary aspiration in thoracic patients, p. 646).

Upper airway obstruction
- In addition to laryngospasm, other causes of UAO pertinent to thoracic anaesthesia include:
  - Vocal cord injury.
  - Vocal cord dysfunction.
  - Vocal cord paralysis.
  - Laryngeal oedema.

(See later in chapter)

Tracheomalacia
- Chronic extrinsic compression of the trachea can cause erosion of the tracheal rings and subsequent tracheal collapse.
- The patient typically presents with inspiratory stridor, exacerbated by increases in air flow, e.g. coughing during extubation.
- In suspected cases, extubation under deep anaesthesia may be advisable so as to avoid coughing.
  - CPAP can be used to stent the trachea following extubation.
- The patient may need to be re-intubated urgently if the airway cannot be maintained by CPAP.
  - It is important to remember that success is dependent on the tube stenting the narrowed part of the trachea.

Tracheal/bronchial injury
Associated with DLT:
- Up to 0.2% cases.
- Risk factors include using an inappropriately large DLT, and nitrous oxide related cuff distension.
- Tracheo-bronchial rupture typically occurs at the junction of the posterior membranous and lateral cartilaginous walls of the airway.
- Not necessarily associated with difficult intubation.
- Avoid over-inflation of the endobronchial cuff, use the lowest volume of air required to seal the airway.
- Avoid movement of the DLT with an inflated bronchial cuff.
  - Consider deflating the bronchial cuff prior to positioning the patient.
- Cases noted intra-operatively warrant consideration of surgical correction.
- Fibreoptic surveillance and antibiotic cover may be more appropriate for cases discovered post-operatively where there is a small defect.

Lower airway obstruction
- This is usually due to retained secretions and clotted blood
  - Typical clinical signs include wheeze, coarse crepitations and/or reduced/absent breath sounds due to atelectasis.

❶ The operative lung should be suctioned prior to re-inflation so as to avoid blowing debris into the distal narrower airways.

Bronchial stump dehiscence
- This may occur after lung resection and is associated with the formation of a broncho-pleural fistula (BPF). It may occur in the immediate post-operative course (1–7 days) or later. Risk factors include:
  - Main stem or intermedius bronchial stump.
  - Pre-operative chemotherapy or radiotherapy.
  - Previous ipsilateral thoracotomy.
- In the immediate post-operative phase bronchial stump dehiscence presents as:
  - A sudden and large air leak from an intercostal drain.
  - Reduced tidal volume if ventilated.
  - Haemoptysis.
- It is typically the result of inadequate initial closure.
- The diagnosis is confirmed by CXR and/or bronchoscopy.
- Treatment of bronchial stump dehiscence in the immediate post-operative phase warrants surgical correction.

Anastamotic complications
- These occur in up to 20% of patients who have lung transplant
  - Broadly speaking, the anastomosis may become necrotic or blocked.
  - Treatment options include endoscopic stenting, ablation and open repair.

The thoracic patient requiring postoperative ventilation

Ultimately, the decision to leave a patient intubated for a spell of post-operative ventilation is down to the Anaesthetist. There are various factors which may negate immediate post-op extubation (non-exhaustive list):

- Already intubated ICU/trauma/unwell patient.
- Elderly/frail patient.
- Polytrauma patient with other ongoing issues.
- Demonstrable poor ABG profile despite adjudged adequate intra-operative ventilation:
  - Acidaemia.
  - High lactate.
- Hypothermia.
- Failure to spontaneously breathe on emergence, having been reversed adequately
- Poor haemodynamic profile intraoperatively requiring ongoing vasopressor/inotropic support
  - Sepsis.
  - Major blood loss or situation requiring ongoing transfusion which has lead to adverse ABG/haemodynamic profile.
  - Cardiac event intraop/severe arrhythmias.
- Development and or signs of ALI intraoperatively/high risk of development postoperatively.
- Surgical requirement.

Further reading

Chandrashekar MV, Irving M, Wayman J, et al. Immediate extubation and epidural analgesia allow safe management in a high-dependency unit after two-stage oesophagectomy. Results of eight years of experience in a specialised upper gastrointestinal unit in a district general hospital. *British Journal of Anaesthesia* 2003; 90:474–9.

Hartley M, Vaughan R. Problems associated with tracheal extubation. *British Journal of Anaesthesia* 1993; 71:561–8.

Karmarkar S, Varshney S. Tracheal extubation. Continuing education in anaesthesia, *critical care and pain* 2008; 8:214–20.

Airways obstruction

Airways obstruction may occur following thoracic surgery due to:
- Laryngeal or tracheal oedema.
- Vocal cord injury or dysfunction 2° recurrent laryngeal nerve injury.
- Blood, gastric contents or pooling of retained secretions within the small airways.

The net result is atelectasis, increased work of breathing, pneumonia and hypoxaemia secondary to VQ mismatch. This can cause failure to wean from and/or prolongation of artificial ventilation, increased hospital stay and, at worst, death.

Retained secretions
- Natural airway secretions protect the airway epithelium from infection and mechanical damage by trapping foreign particles, including infectious material, and they also act as a transport medium to clear the respiratory system of these threats.
- Mucociliary escalator disruption by the ETT and reduced cough effort, caused by pain and immobility, both serve to reduce the usual clearance of respiratory secretions.
  - Fluid restriction ± drying of the airways compound the problem by making the retained secretions more viscous and thus more difficult to clear.
- Ultimately, these viscous, retained secretions cause atelectasis, and ETT narrowing or complete blockage.

Prevention & management of retained secretions

Early mobilization
- Common sense approach to aid active deep breathing and cough thus preventing or minimising atelectasis.
- Requires optimum analgesia and available physiotherapy.
- No direct evidence of improved outcome but increased time out of bed is associated with a shorter hospital stay.

Humidification of inspired oxygen
- Mucociliary function is inhibited by dry gases and secretions become tenacious and difficult to expectorate.
- HME devices are a minimum requirement during artificial ventilation.
- HME performance varies with ambient conditions such as temperature, fluid status of patient and minute volume.
  - The device may become blocked with secretions and requires regular changing.
- For prolonged ventilation HME devices alone are insufficient and active humidification is required from the outset.
  - They increase the dead space and resistance of the circuit and so increase the work of spontaneously breathing patients.

- Hot water bath humidifiers are most commonly in use and can achieve humidity levels equal to the normal upper trachea
- Complications include condensation within the circuit causing blockage, overheating and infection.

Airway suctioning

- Required in artificially ventilated patients to maintain patency of the airways.
- Catheters are commonly 48–56 cm long allowing the catheter tip to access the mainstem bronchi.
- The tip is usually blunt with side holes to reduce the risk of mucosal damage. Usually transparent to allow inspection of secretions.
- Closed circuit suction catheters are now the norm because:
  - They avoid the need for disconnection of the patient from the ventilator allowing for maintenance of PEEP.
  - They reduce exposure of the nursing staff to infectious droplets
  - They are cheaper as the suction catheter is reused. This is possibly associated with reduced ventilator acquired pneumonia.
  - Secretion clearance is no different to open suction techniques.
  - Ventilator malfunction, episodes of haemodynamic compromise and hypoxia may also be reduced.
- ❶ Only minimally invasive/shallow suctioning should be used where there is an anastomosis or suture line close to the carina:
  - Suctioning only reaches the end of the ETT, thus only clears secretions in the tube.
  - Limited evidence suggests that it is associated with fewer haemodynamic/gas exchange adverse effects, with no change in duration of ventilation.
- Saline is often instilled:
  - Thins down secretions.
  - Causes coughing which aids natural secretion removal, but can be violent resulting in bronchospasm.
  - There is little evidence to support its routine use. It may increase the risk of infection by transporting bacteria from the ETT to the small airways.
- Suctioning should be performed when clinically indicated rather than as a routine.
- Physical examination and a characteristic saw tooth pattern seen on expiratory flow graphics suggest the need to suction.

Mucolytics

- Inhaled acetylcysteine:
  - Reduces mucus viscosity by splitting disulfide bonds linking mucoproteins together.
- Recombinant human DNA-ase:
  - Breaks down DNA strands within mucus causing thinning. This is expensive!

Ventilation techniques/physiotherapy

- Manual hyperinflation commonly involves the use of a self-inflating bag, but can be performed using some ventilators.
  - A large tidal breath is delivered over a prolonged inspiratory time and held momentarily.
  - Rapid release then results in higher peak expiratory flow → enhanced secretion removal (similar to a prolonged natural cough).
  - Caution in patients following lung resection as this maneouvre can result in trauma, staple line disruption and adverse haemodynamic effects secondary to excessive airway pressures.
- Physiotherapy techniques:
  - Hand percussive therapy.
  - Postural drainage—may increase gastro-oesophageal reflux potential.
  - Evidence for these techniques is limited in mechanically ventilated patients and pain may limit effectiveness.

Bronchoscopy

- Ultimately, this may be required in refractory cases where simple measures have failed.

Innovative techniques

- Kinetic beds are also promoted to reduce atelectasis and VAP but have limited evidence for secretion management.
- Specialized ETTs are produced by some manufacturers with in-built supraglottic suction channels:
  - Allows continuous aspiration of secretions from above the cuff or intermittent suctioning timed with expiration below the cuff.
  - The manufacturers claim these tubes reduce the incidence of VAP and remain patent and clean. They are not in common usage currently.
- High frequency chest wall oscillation vests:
  - Being marketed for use in critical care for post-operative thoracic patients, including those receiving mechanical ventilation.
  - The manufacturer claims that secretions are mobilized more effectively, thus reducing ICU stay and morbidity, with good patient tolerance for short intermittent treatment periods.
  - They are currently not in common usage in this patient subgroup and evidence is currently limited.

Vocal cord injury

- Temporary sore throat and hoarseness are seen in up to 65% of patients undergoing intubation for general anaesthetic.
  - Most resolve spontaneously and are of little significance.
- Vocal cord injury may be direct, or dysfunction may occur following neurological damage.
  - Significant injury such as arytenoid dislocation or vocal cord paralysis requires early identification to avoid complications.

Vocal cord redness/haematoma
- Reported bronchoscopic finding in up to 44% cases following DLT intubation.
- Risk increases with difficulty of intubation/extubation, ↑ size of ETT, ↑ duration of intubation, and presence of gastro-oesophageal reflux.
- Achieving OLV using a bronchial blocker rather than a DLT reduces the risk.
- Granulation tissue may develop on the vocal cords even after short term intubation.

Management of hoarseness

- Reassurance and supportive measures are usually all that is necessary.
- Patients with persistent hoarseness 48 hours post-operatively should be reviewed by an ENT surgeon to exclude vocal cord injury.

Vocal cord dysfunction/paralysis
- Vocal cord paralysis may be unilateral, causing hoarseness, or bilateral potentially causing airway obstruction dependent upon degree of damage.
- The patient may present with post-extubation stridor, or may exhibit a poor cough and weak voice.
  - These patients are at risk of aspiration.
- Most commonly caused by direct pressure of an ETT cuff poorly positioned in the larynx, which causes a temporary neuropraxia affecting the external or recurrent laryngeal nerves
  - However, incidences as high as 3% have been reported for permanent voice change in patients undergoing surgery in sites other than the head and neck.
- Patients undergoing aortic surgery and left lung resection are at a greater risk of damage to the left recurrent laryngeal nerve due to its anatomical pathway.
- Vocal cord dysfunction is associated with increased morbidity, i.e. pneumonia, arrhythmias, re-intubation and a longer hospital stay.

Prevention & management of vocal cord dysfunction

Preventative measures
- Avoid cuff over-inflation.
- Monitor cuff pressure during long cases, particularly if N_2O is used.
- Ensuring the cuff is below the cords. Confirm cuff/tube position with fibrescope when using DLT.
- Take particular care where there has been neck extension for surgical positioning as this can cause ETT migration.

Management
- Severe vocal cord dysfunction may require re-intubation and early tracheostomy to allow ENT evaluation and treatment.

Arytenoid dislocation
- A rare complication of direct laryngoscopy and intubation; reported incidence of approximately 0.02%.
- Case reports exist related to uneventful SLT, DLT and LMA insertion.
- Difficult intubation and use of the McCoy laryngoscope, a lighted stylet and DLT are risk factors.
- Associated with laryngomalacia, renal insufficiency, acromegaly and chronic glucocorticoid intake.
- Symptoms include hoarseness, sore throat, dysphagia and stridor.
- Most commonly diagnosed using fibreoptic laryngoscopy but CT may be helpful.
  - Early diagnosis and treatment improves recovery. Operation within 10 weeks of injury is associated with a better chance of return of normal phonation.

Management of arytenoid dislocation
- Surgical closed reduction.
- Symptoms may resolve spontaneously with conservative techniques such as voice training.

Laryngeal oedema
- Incidence following extubation ranges from 2.3% to 22% in those intubated for prolonged periods (>36hours).
- Risk factors include:
  - Female sex.
  - C1 esterase inhibitor deficient patients.
  - Large ratio of ETT size to laryngeal size.
  - High cuff pressures.
  - Traumatic intubation.
  - History of self-extubation and re-intubation/bucking on the tube.
  - Higher severity of illness.
  - Head and neck trauma.

- High ETT cuff pressures limit mucosal perfusion causing swelling and ulceration. This can be significant in hypotensive patients and lead to chronic stenosis.
- In addition, manipulation of the ETT or repositioning of the neck will irritate mucosa and may prevent adequate venous drainage.
- Over aggressive fluid administration should be avoided.
- Stridor usually presents within 30 minutes of extubation, but has been reported to start as late as 6 hours post-extubation.

Management of laryngeal oedema

- Some authors suggest performing a leak test around a deflated cuff prior to extubation.
  - A small or absent leak is said to be predictive of post-extubation oedema; however this is not universally accepted.
- Surgical cricoid splitting has been reported necessary to allow extubation of a DLT following a 5 hour operation.
- Stridor should initially be treated with nebulized epinephrine 3–5 ml of 1:1000.
- Head-up positioning and humidified oxygen.
- In severe respiratory distress re-intubation is required with a smaller ETT.
  - Re-intubation is associated with increased morbidity and the risk of complete airway obstruction if intubation fails.
- The use of prophylactic steroids prior to extubation remains controversial.
  - However, steroids can be considered in those patients at particular risk of oedema and where the benefits of steroids outweigh the risks.

Further reading

Hagberg C, Rainer G, Krier C. Complications of managing the airway. Best Practice and Research. *Clinical Anaesthesiology*. 2005; 19(4): 661–59.

Knoll H, Ziegler S, Schreiber J, *et al*. Airway injuries after One Lung Ventilation: A comparison between double lumen tube and endobronchial blocker: A randomized, prospective, controlled trial. *Anaesthesiology* 2006; 105: 471–7.

Mechanical ventilation in the post-operative thoracic patient

Introduction

- Delayed post-operative extubation may increase peri-operative morbidity, lengthen the post-operative recovery period, increases the cost of care post-operatively and delay early ambulation and rehabilitation.
- Early extubation, particularly after lung resection, reduces the risk of post-operative air leak and reduces pressure placed on lung tissue sutures.

Drawbacks

- Post-operative mechanical ventilation following major thoracic surgery is essential in certain patients; however, its benefit in the failing lung can be readily outweighed by the associated increased morbidity and mortality.
- Non-physiological positive pressure ventilation in the post-operative lung may lead to barotrauma, volutrauma, and increased release of inflammatory mediators.
- Intra-operative one-lung ventilation can injure the dependent lung via hyperperfusion and hyperinflation.
  - This can result in direct physical damage to the alveoli via stress forces, and pro-inflammatory mediator release resulting in an inflammatory diffuse alveolar damage.
- The operated lung is also exposed to direct surgical manipulation resulting in the release of pro-inflammatory cytokines, which in turn may lead to ALI or ARDS.

⚠ These circumstances may lead to the development of ALI/ARDS (2.45% of all lung resections, and 7.9% of pnuemonectomies), which in turn will require prolonged post-operative mechanical ventilation.

⚠ This is associated with a mortality rate of 40%.

Predictors of post-operative ventilation

- Identification of factors that predict prolonged post-operative ventilation allows for appropriate resource management peri-operatively.
- This may reduce the length of time of post-operative ventilatory support.
- Pre-operative and intra-operative factors that predict prolonged post-operative ventilation are:
  - Low pre-operative FEV_1.
  - Higher pre-operative serum creatinine.
  - Intra-operative RBC transfusion.
  - Presence of a thoracic epidural.
  - Volume of lung resected.
  - Co-morbidities.

Protective ventilation strategies

The ARDS Network has shown that the following criteria reduce mortality in patients with ARDS, and a benefit in the post lung resection patient can be inferred.
- Limit tidal volumes to reduce volutrauma.
  - 6 ml/kg.
- Limit airway plateau pressures to reduce barotraumas.
  - <30 cmH_2O.
- Use of PEEP to aid recruitment and oxygenation, and minimize damaging shear forces of small airways opening and closing.
- Tolerate a "relative hypoxia" by using the lowest feasible FiO_2 to achieve target.
  - SpO_2 >90%.
  - FiO_2 <0.6.
- Allow "permissive hypercapnoea", tolerating elevated $PaCO_2$ in presence of reduced tidal volumes.

Impaired ventilation

Physiology

- Ventilation describes how gases move to and from the alveoli.
- Post-operatively, ventilation is typically impaired for a variety of reasons. In broad terms these include:
  - Upper & lower airway obstruction.
  - Mechanical impairment, e.g. thoracotomy pain, pneumothorax, haemothorax, obesity, supine position, diaphragmatic palsy secondary to phrenic nerve palsy.
  - Impaired respiratory drive, e.g. narcosis s opioid.
- Characteristic lung volume/capacity abnormalities include:
  - ↓VC.
  - ↓V_T.
  - ↓FEV_1.
  - ↓FRC.
- Hypoventilation produces a mismatch between pulmonary ventilation and pulmonary perfusion. Thus, the V/Q ratio falls and pulmonary shunt fraction increases → worsening hypoxaemia and hypercapnia.

Presentation

Spontaneously breathing patient

- Dyspnoea; diaphoresis; tachypnoea; agitation; inability to talk normally; sitting upright; subjective exhaustion.

Mechanically ventilated patient

- High or low ventilator pressure alarms; low or high tidal volumes.
- Lack of chest movement.

Associated features

Other features may be present and may aid diagnosis:

- Cyanosis; hypoxaemia; hypercapnia; tachycardia, hypertension or hypotension.
- Pleuritic chest pain; haemoptysis.
- Mediastinal shift; altered percussion note; wheeze; bronchial breathing; reduced air entry; raised JVP/CVP.
- Evidence of sepsis.
- Intercostal chest drainage, e.g. blood, pus, continuous bubbling
- Respiratory/cardiac arrest.

Immediate management

- 100% O_2, ABC, call for help.
- Ensure airway is patent; check patency and position of ETT if intubated. Intubate/replace airway if necessary.
- If patient is spontaneously breathing:
  - Consider bag mask ventilation → non-invasive CPAP/NIV → Intubation + mechanical ventilation.
- If patient already mechanically ventilated:
  - Ensure ventilation possible → check equipment working and connected → switch to bag and mask ventilation if in doubt.
- Ensure intercostal drains are swinging.
- Fluid resuscitate as indicated.
- Establish and treat specific cause.

Investigations

In most cases history and examination will elucidate the cause. Investigations which may aid in assessing severity or determining a diagnosis include:

Bloods

- **ABG.**
  - Essential.
  - Type I/II respiratory failure?
  - Acidosis/high lactate.
- **FBC, U&Es, LFTs, clotting studies, CRP.**
- **Cultures.**
  - Blood and sputum if sepsis is suspected.

Radiology

- **CXR.**
  - Chest drain position/pneumothorax/ haemothorax/ effusions/ pulmonary oedema.
- **Chest ultrasound.**
  - Can aid drainage of acute/large effusion.
- **CT chest.**
- **CT pulmonary angiogram.**
  - Suspected PE.

Other

- **ECG.**
  - Exclude arrhythmias/post operative myocardial events.
  - Especially relevant if pre-morbid cardiac history ort post pneumonectomy.
- **Bronchoscopy ± BAL.**
- **Echocardiogram.**

Specific causes
Treatment will depend on the underlying cause.

Upper airway obstruction
- Thoracic procedures regularly require rigid bronchoscopy and other forms of upper airway instrumentation.
- It is therefore no surprise that upper airway obstruction is commonplace.

Lower airway obstruction
- Atelectasis ± pneumonia.
  - Very common after one lung ventilation
  - Secondary to retention of secretions, splinting, poor lung re-expansion, poor cough.
  - May develop into lobar collapse.
  - ↑ inflation pressures.
- Chronic obstructive pulmonary disease
  - Common in thoracic patients.
  - Already limited respiratory reserve.
- Bronchospasm.
- Foreign body.

Mechanical impairment
- Pain/pneumothorax/haemothorax/pleural effusion/empyema.
- Skeletal deformities.
- Diaphragmatic splinting 2° ↑ intra-abdominal pressure /obesity.

Impaired gas exchange
- ARDS/ALI.
- Cardiogenic pulmonary oedema.
- Pulmonary fibrosis.
- Pulmonary contusion

Problems relating to surgery
- Post-operative air leak.
- Bronchopleural fistula, tracheoesophageal fistula.
- Chylothorax.
- Neuromuscular damage.
- Anastamotic leak after oesophageal resection, pneumonectomy, tracheal resection.

Further management
This should be aimed at the underlying cause:
- Guide oxygen therapy and respiratory support with serial ABG analysis and aim to achieve $PaO_2 > 8$ kPa and $PaCO_2 < 7$ kPa where possible.
  - However, any goal must be set within the context of the patient's pre-operative state.
  - You may need to consider permissive hypercapnia.

- Use lung protective ventilation strategies.
  - Avoid high pressure ventilation following resection surgery.
- Drainage of pneumothorax/haemothorax.
- Regular chest physiotherapy.
- Mini-tracheostomy by skilled operator. This will provide direct route for bronchial suction.
- Consider invasive monitoring of CVP + IABP.
- Antimicrobials.
- Bronchodilators.
- Nutritional support.
- Speak to surgeons early as surgical re-exploration may be necessary.

Pitfalls

- Exclude equipment fault.
- Ensure respiratory depression is not a consequence of inadequate reversal of anaesthetic/neuromuscular blockade or excess opioid.
- Metabolic acidosis may cause dyspnoea and should be corrected with appropriate resuscitation.

Measures to reduce pulmonary complications after thoracic surgery

- Good analgesia.
- Erect body position to ↑ FRC.
- Humidified oxygen.
- Regular chest physiotherapy.
- Incentive spirometry.
- Avoid fluid overload (+ve balance should not exceed 20ml/kg in 1st 24 hours post-operatively).
- Avoid hyperinflation peri-operatively, i.e. VT<10ml/kg during OLV.
- Avoid ↑ RV pressure in presence of RV dysfunction, i.e. avoid hypoxia/hypercapnia.
- Supportive measures include adequate hydration and nutrition.

Further reading

Cardiovascular and Thoracic Anaesthesia. J. Gothard, A. Kelleher, E. Haxby. Butterworth-Heinemann: London, UK.

J. Deslauriers, R. Mehran, editors. *Handbook of Perioperative Care in General Thoracic Surgery.* Philadelphia, Pa: Elsevier Mosby; 2005.

Lung isolation and independent lung ventilation

Lung isolation (LI) and independent lung ventilation (ILV) are fundamental components of thoracic anaesthesia; the technical methods employed to achieve this are discussed elsewhere (See 📖 Techniques for lung isolation, p. 716).

This section discusses the use of LI and ILV within the critical care setting.

- LI is used as a temporary measure until surgical or radiological management are commenced.
- ILV can be useful in the management of unilateral lung disease or injury when conventional modes of ventilation have failed.
- ILV has been used sporadically as a rescue strategy since 1976 and its current use is based on Level 3 recommendations.

Lung isolation (physiological separation)

- Each lung is ventilated as an independent unit after isolating one side from the other.
- The clinician can then chose the appropriate mode of ventilation/strategy tailored to the pathology of the side involved, as each has differing airway resistance and compliance.

Table 11.2 Indications for differential lung ventilation

Strategy	Indication
Lung Isolation (Anatomical separation)	Massive haemoptysis
	Massive air leak (BPF)
	Whole lung lavage
	Lung abscess
	Copious secretions
Independent Lung Ventilation (Physiological separation)	Unilateral parenchymal injury:
	Aspiration pneumonitis
	Pulmonary contusion
	Pneumonia
	Massive unilateral PE
	Post op. complications after single lung transplant
	Bronchopleural fistula
	Unilateral bronchospasm
	Severe bilateral lung disease failed by conventional ventilation

Lung isolation (anatomical separation)

- Temporary isolation of one lung or segments from blood and contaminants from the diseased/affected lung until surgery or embolization can be performed.
- Indications for LI (See Table 11.2).
- LI is usually achieved with the use of a DLT. EBB, spigots and valves can also be used. (See Table 11.3) for the merits of the different LI techniques.

Table 11.3 Methods of lung isolation

	DLT	EBB/Spigot	Valves
Insertion	Can be positioned blindly	Needs a bronchoscope	Needs a bronchoscope
Age & size	Only in adults	Very small adults and children	N/A
Isolation	Lung isolation	Lung, lobe or segment	Lobe or segment
BPF +/– empyema	Up to 10 days, ILV possible	EBB—emergent use in massive air leak	Removable valves
Massive haemoptysis	Best choice	Bronchoscopic positioning difficult	N/A
Whole lung lavage	Only choice	N/A	N/A
ILV	Only choice	Selective ventilation only	Selective ventilation
LVR	Used during surgery	Used during surgery	Non-surgical management
Gas exchange	Potential for optimization	Hypoxia from shunt	Improve V/Q mismatch

Achieving anatomical separation of the lungs

Assessment

- Bronchoscopy is used to assess correct positioning of DLT, EBB etc.
- Auscultatory checks are unreliable, (pathological lungs do not produce 'textbook' signs!)
- Water bubble technique:
  - Tracheal port is placed under water with 40 cmH$_2$O plateau pressure on the bronchial port.
  - Bubbles at the tracheal port denote an air leak around the bronchial cuff.

- Balloon inflation technique:
  - Balloon replaces the underwater seal.
  - Inflation of the balloon at the tracheal port during positive pressure ventilation through the bronchial port denotes an air leak.

Maintenance of isolation
- Precise monitoring of the position of the tube is mandatory and this should be checked fibreoscopically at regular intervals, particularly if any of the monitoring parameters change drastically (changes in PAW, compliance etc).
- 32% will become misplaced during routine care, particularly when turning the patient or changing their position.
- Adequate sedation/paralysis are required in order to prevent or minimize movement of the tube resulting from movement or coughing.

Complications
- Bronchial cuffs generate high pressures (50 mmHg with an inflation of just 2 ml of air.
- Complications commonly result from this:
  - Bronchial ischaemia.
  - Bronchial stenosis.
  - Pneumothorax.
  - Pneumomediastinum.
  - Subcutaneous emphysema
- Deflating the cuff prior to moving the patient can help minimize these.
- Bronchial rupture (0.05 to 0.2%).
- Equipment related risk factors increasing the likelihood of bronchial rupture:
  - Traumatic intubation.
  - Cuff over-inflation.
  - Over-sized double-lumen tubes.
  - Prolonged intubation.
- Patient-related risk factors increasing the likelihood of bronchial trauma:
  - Underlying malignancy.
  - Infection.
  - Chronic steroid use.
  - Prior tracheobronchial surgery.

Ventilation strategies
Synchronous independent lung ventilation
- Can be performed with two-ventilators or a single ventilator
  - Certain ventilators can be connected via an external cable—this creates a master and a slave ventilator.
  - One contains a Y-piece and separate PEEP valves.
  - Each lung and its individual static/dynamic compliances and resistances will determine the flow and tidal volume delivered.

- Respiratory rate of both lungs is kept identical.
- The respiratory cycle can either be in phase or 180 degrees out of phase.
- Selective PEEP can also be added to either lung.
- The clinician chooses the appropriate tidal volumes and inspiratory flow rates.

Asynchronous independent lung ventilation

- Offers greater flexibility.
- Less complicated than synchronized ventilation.
- Evidence shows no disadvantage compared to synchronized ILV.
- Variations of asynchronous ventilation include:
  - Bilateral continuous mandatory ventilation.
  - Continuous mandatory ventilation and synchronized intermittent mandatory ventilation.
  - Continuous mandatory ventilation and high frequency jet ventilation.
  - Continuous mandatory ventilation and continuous positive airway pressure.

Specific strategies for certain conditions

Anatomical separation

Massive haemoptysis

- ILV may be life saving until definitive surgery or embolization is available.
- Once the bleed is isolated, conventional pressure/volume target ventilation should be employed whilst definitive therapy is sought expeditiously!
- DLT's are used in preference to blockers:
  - Offer the added advantage of permitting bronchial toilet.
  - Bronchoscopic therapy is possible.
- ❶ Intubation may be technically difficult in profuse hemoptysis.
- Bronchial blockers and SLT's:
  - Easier to intubate with single-lumen endotracheal tubes, then deploy an endobronchial blocker.
- ❶ Final placement using a bronchoscope will be very challenging and potentially dangerous with copious amounts of blood!
- ❶ After deployment it is impossible to monitor continued bleeding distal to the blocker.

Whole lung lavage

- Sequential lung lavage is the recognized treatment of pulmonary alveolar proteinosis. (See 📖 Broncho-alveloar lavage, p. 288).

Physiological separation

Asymmetric parenchymal lung disease.

- Examples are pulmonary contusion and aspiration.
- The more compliant, disease free lung will receive most of the ventilation via the pathway of least resistance resulting in:
  - Over distension and barotrauma.
  - Diversion of perfusion towards the abnormal side resulting in a large shunt.

- PEEP applied via conventional ventilatory strategy may be inadequate in recruiting diseased alveoli, and may be excessive on the normal side contributing to hyperinflation.
- Initial volumes of 4 to 5 ml/kg per lung can be used and this can then be adjusted according to target plateau pressures.
- Selective PEEP can now be applied to improve recruitment in the diseased lung without overinflating the normal lung; adjusted to gas exchange parameters or mean airway pressures.
- When tidal volumes between the lungs differ by <100 ml and compliance differs by <20%, ILV can eventually be discontinued safely.

Single lung transplant
- ILV may prevent the need for re-transplantation, and can be useful in the management of:
  - Pulmonary graft dysfunction.
  - Acute rejection.
  - Surgical pulmonary contusion.
  - Acute respiratory distress syndrome.
- Management of single lung transplant patients can be similar to management of unilateral parenchymal lung disease, (the transplanted lung has different compliance to the native lung).
- Compliance in the new lung depends upon:
  - The surgical insults to it.
  - The underlying pulmonary pathology (higher in emphysema; lower in fibrotic lung disease).
- ILV with selective PEEP to the transplanted lung will protect the native lung from hyperinflation.
- Risk factors that may predict need for ILV post-single lung transplant for COPD include:
  - Severity of underlying airway obstruction.
  - Peri-operative injury to the donor lung.
  - Size of donor lung.

Bronchopleural fistula
- The management of this condition is further discussed (See 📖 Post-operative air leak, p. 632).
- The mainstay of therapy consists of intercostal drainage with an adequate suction device to prevent tension pneumothorax development.
- Subsequently, positive pressure ventilation and negative pressure from the chest tube suction can delay healing of the fistula site.
- Decreasing air leak from the fistula, and maintaining adequate oxygenation produce conflicts.
- Therefore, ILV is a therapeutic alternative:
  - The patient is intubated with a DLT.
  - The fistula side is ventilated with the lowest possible tidal volume, respiratory rate, PEEP and inspiratory time to minimize air leak.
- An alternative is to use high frequency jet ventilation on the fistula side with conventional ventilation on the normal side.

Unilateral airway obstruction
- The affected side is ventilated with a low respiratory rate, low tidal volume and prolonged expiratory time to prevent the accumulation of intrinsic PEEP.
- The unaffected side is supported with conventional ventilator settings.

Acute bilateral lung disease
- A controversial indication for the use of ILV with little outcome data available at the time of writing.
- Has been reported to be successful in the treatment of ARDS.
- ILV can be combined with placement of the patient in the lateral decubitus position and application of selective PEEP to the dependent side.
- Preferential PEEP should recruit alveoli in the better-perfused dependent side while diverting perfusion to the better-ventilated non-dependent side.

- Any decision to institute ILV must account for the expertize required in double-lumen tube/endobronchial blocker insertion, skilled and intensive nursing, specialized monitoring and ready availability of fibreoptic bronchoscopy
- ILV is technical; potential complications must be carefully weighed against any perceived benefits before proceeding with ILV.

Further reading

Tuxen, D. Independent lung ventilation. In: Tobin MJ., editor. *Principles and Practice of Mechanical Ventilation*. McGraw-Hill; 1994. pp. 571–88.

Brodsky, JB; Mihm, FG. Spit-lung ventilation. In: Hall JB, Schmidt GA, Wood LDH., editor. *Principles of Critical Care*. McGraw-Hill; 1992. pp. 160–4.

Acute lung injury and ARDS (ALI/ARDS)

Introduction
- Acute Respiratory Distress Syndrome (ARDS) continues to be a significant and challenging problem in modern practice of Intensive Care.
- It may affect as many as 10% of intensive care patients and carries a significant mortality, however survivors tend to have few longer term problems.
- In the critically ill patient it is characterized by:
  - Poor oxygenation.
  - X-ray changes.
  - Altered lung compliance.
- It tends to occur in a spectrum of clinical severity, with milder forms termed acute lung injury (ALI), progressing through to the more severe Acute Respiratory distress Syndrome (ARDS).

Definition
(American—European Consensus Conference on ARDS criteria):
- Acute onset of:
  - Bilateral infiltrates on CXR (patchy, diffuse, or homogeneous)
  - Presence of one or more precipitants of ARDS.
  - $PaO_2/FiO_2 \leq 27$ (corrected for altitude).
  - No clinical evidence of left atrial hypertension.

Clinical presentation
- Diagnosis is confirmed clinically and radiologically, firstly by the exclusion of cardiogenic pulmonary oedema, and secondly by meeting agreed criteria (See Table 11.4).
- The conditions manifest as acute hypoxia and a widening alveolar-arterial gradient refractory to supplemental oxygen.
- As alveolar dead space increases hypercapnia begins to develop
- Radiological features of interstitial and alveolar infiltrates lag behind clinical deterioration.
  - It may be difficult to differentiate between ALI, cardiogenic pulmonary oedema, and pneumonia.
  - Indeed the conditions may coexist.
- The multifactorial causation of the condition is reflected in the varied clinical onset and progression.

Table 11.4 ALI vs. ARDS

	Chest x-ray	Oxygenation[1]	PCWP[2]	Onset
ALI	Bilateral Infiltrates	$PaO_2{:}FiO_2$ <40	<18 mmHg	Acute
ARDS	Bilateral Infiltrates	$PaO_2{:}FiO_2$ <27	<18 mmHg	Acute

[1] regardless of PEEP

[2] with a normal LAP

Pathogenesis

- Characterized by diffuse alveolar damage within the affected lungs.
- Alveolar damage results in:
  - Non cardiogenic pulmonary oedema.
  - Surfactant dysfunction.
  - Generation of complex inflammatory exudates.
- This leads to non uniform, heterogeneous lung involvement resulting in impaired gas exchange and oxygenation with marked reduction in lung compliance.
- Neutrophils are thought to play an important role in the pathogenesis of ALI/ARDS, being found in increased concentrations in the epithelial fluid and alveoli of affected patients.
- It is also thought that neutrophil migration into alveoli and subsequent activation triggers an inflammatory response with reactive O_2 species, cytokines and proteases all being released and contributing to ongoing lung damage.
- ALI/ARDS occurs in three phases:
  - Exudative   Day 0–5   Hypoxaemia, CXR Infiltrates, ↓ pulmonary compliance.
  - Proliferative   Day 5 →   ↑ dead space, microvascular. thrombi
  - Fibrotic   Day 14 →   loss of lung architecture, pulmonary fibrosis, ↑ dead space.

Non-surgical precipitants of ALI/ARDS

Divided into pulmonary and extra pulmonary causes.

- Pulmonary:
  - Pneumonia.
  - Aspiration.
  - Lung contusion.

- Fat embolus.
- Near drowning.
- Inhalational injury.
- Reperfusion injury.
- Extra pulmonary:
  - Sepsis.
  - Trauma.
  - Massive transfusion.
  - Pancreatitis.
  - Post cardiopulmonary bypass.

Management

- Aimed at providing oxygenation and limiting any ventilator associated trauma that may worsen existing lung injury.
- There should be exemplary ITU Care:
  - Head up tilt.
  - Gastric protection.
  - Thromboprophylaxis.
  - Glycaemic control.
  - Nutrition.
  - Scrupulous asepsis.
- Treatment should also be directed at the underlying cause, and any complications of ITU management, particularly sepsis, should be aggressively treated.

Ventilation recommendations

- Published by the ARDS network group based on their findings from a multicentre trial in 2000.
- These criteria demonstrated a reduction in mortality in patients with ARDS, and included:

Tidal volume
- Limitation to 4–6 ml/kg to reduce volutrauma.

Plateau airway pressure
- Limitation to <30 cmH$_2$0 to reduce barotrauma.

Respiratory rate
- Respiratory rate should be set initially to cover baseline minute volume < 35 bpm initially.

PEEP
- To aid recruitment and oxygenation.
- To minimize damaging shear forces of small airways opening and closing.

Parameters to aim for
- Tolerance of "relative hypoxia".
  - SpO_2 >88–95%.
  - PaO_2 7–11 kPa.
- Use of lowest feasible FiO_2.
  - FiO_2 <0.6.
- "Permissive hypercapnoea".
  - Tolerating elevated $PaCO_2$ (>8hPd if possible) in presence of reduced tidal volumes.
- pH.
  - 7.3–7.45.
  - Increase RR in attempt to reduce $PaCO_2$ (still aiming to keep RR <35bpm).
  - If not achievable, one can re-increase Vt in 1 ml/kg increments (still aiming to keep plateau airway pressure <35 cmH₂O).

Further treatment options

- In patients with ARDS whose gas exchange is poor despite adherence to the above guidelines, consideration may be given to the following techniques:

Prone ventilation
- Patient is turned from supine into the prone position.
- Improves oxygenation in up to 70% of patients with ARDS via recruitment of dorsal areas of lung and improvement of V/Q matching.
- Care needs to be taken with pressure areas, and adequate sedation ± muscle relaxation as required.
- Patients are usually placed supine again after periods of 12–18 hours.

Corticosteroids
- The role of corticosteroids in management of ARDS remains controversial.
- May reduce the fibrosis and length of recovery period, but timing of dosing and length of treatment is unclear.
- Beneficial effects may be counteracted by problems such as superadded infection, hyperglycaemia and administration of TPN.

Nitric Oxide
(See 🕮 Nitric oxide, p. 72).
- Previously used in severe ARDS to improve pulmonary blood flow through pulmonary arterial vasodilatation in ventilated areas of lung only, hence oxygenation via improved V/Q matching.
- Difficulties with administration (inhaled) and no proven benefits have led to reductions in its use.

Prostacyclin

(See 📖 Nitric oxide, p. 72).
- Improves pulmonary blood flow through pulmonary vasodilatation and leads to improved V/Q matching.
- May be used in patients unresponsive to prone ventilation and is normally nebulized according to unit protocols.

ECMO

(See 📖 Extra Corporeal Life Support, p. 524).

Prognosis and outcomes

- The overall risk of mortality from ARDS is thought to be 40–60%, with the majority of patients dying of sepsis and/or multiple organ failure.
- In survivors, lung function usually returns to normal within 6 to 12 months, although a small minority of patients may be left with residual restrictive lung disease.

Further reading

ARDS Network group. Ventilation with lower tidal volumes as compared with traditional tidal volumes for acute lung injury and the acute respiratory distress syndrome. *New England Journal of Medicine*. 2000; 342:1301–8.

Bernard GR, Artigas A, Brigham KL, *et al*. Report of the American—European Consensus Conference on ARDS: definitions, mechanisms, relevant outcomes and clinical trial coordination. *Intensive Care Medicine*. 1994; 20:225–32.

Post-pneumonectomy pulmonary oedema (PPO) and OLV

This is the combination of pulmonary oedema and refractory hypoxaemia occurring after lung resection (including pneumonectomy, lobectomy and bilobectomy, but not wedge resection.), with no identifiable cause.

Incidence

- Clinically and histologically this condition is identical to ALI/ADRS. The overall incidence of PPO is between 1–7%, occurring more commonly post lobectomy than pneumonectomy.

Mortality

- Mortality from pneumonectomy ↑ from 10% to >30% if PPPO ensues.
- It is seen in 3% of pneumonectomies and can occur in more limited pulmonary resections.

Pathophysiology

- The pathogenesis of PPO is thought to be multifactorial.
- Remember the surgical stress response will itself lead to fluid retention by the action of aldosterone → ↑ Na^+/H_2O retention.
- OLV has been implicated:

The dependent lung

- Is at risk of hyperoxia, volutrauma and barotrauma during OLV; all of which have been implicated in the development of post-operative ARDS.
- In addition, this lung is hyperperfused as it is now receiving the majority of the cardiac output.
  - This may induce shear stresses within the pulmonary vascular endothelium, increasing hydrostatic pressures and increasing the likelihood of pulmonary oedema formation.

The non-dependent lung

- At risk of ischaemia during the intra-operative period.
- The ischaemic period results in direct tissue damage, leading to systemic release of reactive oxygen species during re-oxygenation.
- The ischaemic insult to alveoli during OLV is of particular importance
  - Bronchial blood vessels do not contribute to alveolar blood supply with the alveoli relying solely upon the alveolar oxygen tensions and mixed venous oxygen levels.
- By providing oxygen (insufflated via a CPAP circuit), to the non-dependent lung and ensuring maintenance of a good cardiac output, the thoracic anaesthetist can help minimize these insults.

Prevention

- A restrictive fluid strategy will help protect against but does not eliminate PPPO.
- An intra-op fluid load of >2 l, and a net positive fluid balance of >20 ml/kg/day in the first 48 hour period are independent risk factors for PPPO.
- Management is based on the empirical approach to any ALI/ARDS (See 📖 Acute lung injury and ARDS (ALI/ARDS), p. 616).
- Early recognition and aggressive treatment are key to improving survival.
- (See Table 11.5) for factors predisposing to PPPO.

Table 11.5 Factors associated with PPPO

Operative phase	Predisposition to PPPO
Pre-op	M > F
	Pre op chemotherapy/radiotherapy
	Age >60
	Residual lung perfusion <55%
	↓ serum elastase
Intra-op	Right pneumonectomy
	Return thoracotomy
	Use of blood products
	↑ duration of surgery
	>2L fluid
	PIP >40 cm H_2O
Post-op	Net 24 hr balance >2L
	Non balanced chest drainage system

Mediastinal shift & atelectasis

Introduction
- Mediastinal shift commonly occurs towards the operative side, especially after lobar or pulmonary resection.
- Mediastinal shift is part of a compensatory mechanism for volume loss and is augmented by elevation of the hemi-diaphragm.
- Excessive shift is most commonly due to atelectasis.
- Atelectasis is a reduced volume (collapse) of all or part of the lung.

Pathophysiology
- The triad of general anaesthesia, one lung ventilation and surgical manipulation result in diaphragmatic dysfunction and ↓ surfactant activity → alveolar instability and non-obstructive atelectasis.
- Absorption atelectasis, where gas is absorbed from non-ventilated alveoli, also occurs.
- The lung is re-expanded before thoracotomy closure, despite this, mucus plugging or secretions may cause obstructive atelectasis.
- Atelectasis causes retraction of the lung; the heart and mediastinum shift toward the atelectatic area, the diaphragm is elevated, and the chest wall flattens.
- Perfusion of atelectatic pulmonary segments lowers the V/Q ratio, increases pulmonary shunt and results in progressive hypoxaemia and hypercapnia.
- This may be offset initially by recruitment of contralateral alveolar units caused by the mediastinal shift.

Aetiology of post-operative atelectasis
- Pain
  - Causes chest splinting, inadequate cough and hypoventilation.
  - Results in failure to re-expand collapsed alveolar units.
- Opioids.
  - Cause hypoventilation and impair coughing.
- Haemorrhage into the airways.
- Bronchospasm.
- Pleural effusion.
- Pneumothorax.
- Inadvertent endobronchial intubation.

Symptoms & signs

- Slowly developing atelectasis is usually asymptomatic or causes only minor symptoms.

Rapid onset atelectasis

- Pain on the affected side.
- Sudden onset dyspnoea.
- Cyanosis.
- RS.
  - Dull percussion note over the involved area.
  - Diminished or absent breath sounds.
  - Reduced or absent chest movements.
  - Trachea and apex beat are deviated towards the affected side.
- CVS
  - Hypotension.
  - Tachycardia.

CXR findings

- Displacement of fissures.
- Opacification of the collapsed lobe.
- Hilar displacement.
- Mediastinal shift toward the side of collapse.
- Loss of volume on ipsilateral hemithorax.
- Elevation of ipsilateral diaphragm.
- Crowding of the ribs.
- Compensatory hyper-lucency of the remaining lobes.
- Silhouetting of the diaphragm or the heart border.

Prevention

- Humidified oxygen.
- Careful systemic hydration.
- Bronchodilators.
- Chest physiotherapy.
- Incentive spirometry should be taught and used pre- and post-operatively.
- Early ambulation.
- Analgesia:
  - Adequate peri-operative analgesia is very important as this permits patients to breathe deeply, cough forcefully, and participate in chest physiotherapy exercises.
  - Use of epidural analgesia is a very effective pain control measure.
  - Sparing use of narcotics to avoid suppression of cough reflex and hypoventilation.
- Suctioning.

Management
- The goal of therapy is to ensure adequate oxygenation and ventilation while the collapsed areas of lung are re-expanded.
- In addition to the above preventative measures, the following should be undertaken:
  - Increase the inspired oxygen concentration to achieve an arterial oxygen saturation of greater than 90%.
  - Patients in severe respiratory distress may require intubation and mechanical ventilation.
  - CPAP/NIV may augment oxygenation and re-expand affected lung.
  - Treat any underlying pneumonia with a broad-spectrum antibiotic.
  - Consider fibreoptic bronchoscopy where atelectasis fails to respond to simple measures and/or the patient is intubated.

Further reading
Magnusson L, Spahn D. New concepts of atelectasis during general anaesthesia. *British Journal of Anaesthesia* 2003; 91: 61–72.

Pneumomediastinum & subcutaneous emphysema

Pneumomediastinum (PM) and subcutaneous emphysema (SE) are usually regarded as relatively benign and self-limiting conditions. However, both can be fatal as a result of airway obstruction, respiratory failure or cardiovascular failure.

Definition

- Pneumomediastinum is the presence of air surrounding the mediastinal structures. Also known as mediastinal emphysema.
- Subcutaneous emphysema relates to the presence of gas in the subcutaneous layer of the skin; note, this may not necessarily be air, e.g. gas gangrene.

Pathophysiology

- PM/SE usually occur as a result of an acute rise in intra-alveolar pressure causing extravasation of air into the perivascular interstitial tissues.
- Dissection of tissue planes enable the air to track back towards the hilum of the lungs, into the mediastinum and into the soft tissue of the face, arms, thorax, abdomen and even the lower limbs.
- In the rare situation where the air is under pressure, and causing physiological compromise, some have used the terms "tension pneumomediastinum" and "tension subcutaneous emphysema".

Risk factors

- A recent review of SE after pulmonary resection found that 6.3% of patients had clinically apparent SE.
- A third of these patients had persistent SE despite ICD suction.
- Risk factors for SE were:
  - Pre-operative FEV_1 < 50%.
  - Persistent air leak.
  - Previous thoracotomy.
- SE that persists despite increasing chest tube suction is more likely in patients who have had a lobectomy.

Aetiology

Pulmonary air leak

- Barotrauma to the lungs secondary to positive pressure ventilation (For a more detailed explanation see 📖 Barotrauma, p. 548).
- Post-operative bronchopleural fistula.
- Ruptured suture/staple lines.
- Spontaneous rupture of bulla—may be associated with sudden exertion, coughing, vomiting.

Air leak from other sites
- Perforation of the trachea, bronchus or oesophagus following intubation/surgery/stabbing/gunshot.

Clinical presentation

Pneumomediastinum
- Central/retrosternal chest pain.
- Dyspnoea.
- Crepitus in the suprasternal notch and cervical region.
- Hoarseness.
- Evidence of associated pneumothorax.
- If under pressure, "tension pneumomediastinum" may present with a similar picture to cardiac tamponade due to restricted venous return to the heart. (See 🕮 Traumatic cardiac tamponade, p. 470).
- Mediastinitis and associated sepsis if pneumomediastinum associated with contamination by oropharyngeal or orogastric contents.

Subcutaneous Emphysema
- Generalized swelling, usually with crepitus:
  - Can extend to the face, thorax, abdomen and the extremities.
  - Even when self-limiting, the cosmetic deformity can be distressing.
- Neck swelling can cause sore throat, dysphagia, dysphonia, stridor and dyspnoea
- Neck swelling sufficient to cause airway obstruction is rare; more common after traumatic neck injuries or tracheobronchial surgery
- Chest wall SE can restrict ventilation.

Management
Identify the site of the air leak and appropriately treat it, to alleviate the emphysema and prevent its progression.

Investigations

Radiology
- **CXR**
  - May demonstrate pneumothorax.
  - Pneumomediastinum is associated with a distinct black line running parallel to the heart border, more easily seen on the left, caused by separation of the parietal pleura from the heart border.
  - A lateral CXR may show air beneath the sternum and surrounding the anterior border of the heart.
- **CT thorax**.
  - Will establish the extent of pneumomediastinum and may help identify the location of the air leak.
- **Contrast studies of the oesophagus**

Other
- **Oesophagoscopy** and **bronchoscopy may** establish the site of an air leak.

Treatment options

- High flow oxygen speeds resolution of emphysema by facilitating resorption of nitrogen from the tissues and pneumomediastinum.
- A patent, functioning ICD in the pleural space will usually drain any pneumothorax/persistent air leak.
- If ventilated, weaning of peak airway pressures and alteration of I:E ratios may help prevent extension of SE.
- Surgical exploration may be required:
  - A VATS procedure and pneumolysis can be effective in SE for post-operative patients where the air leak is directed into the tissues, and not into the pleural space.
  - By directing the leak into the pleural rather than subcutaneous space, it can be effectively drained with intercostal drainage.

---

❶❶ *Airway obstruction from severe neck swelling*

- Requires immediate intervention:
  - Expect a narrowed and oedematous larynx on laryogoscopy
  - Use a smaller than normal ETT, and plan for difficult/failed intubation
  - If time permits fibreoptic nasal endoscopy may aid assessment of the airway, and can be used to perform awake fibreoptic intubation
  - The technique of induction will depend on the clinical situation and judgement of the anaesthetist
  - Undertake in theatre with senior anaesthetic and surgical assistance—a potentially difficult emergency tracheostomy may be needed.

- Decompress "tension pneumomediastinum" by needle or anterior cervical mediastinotomy.
  - Tracheostomy incision has been reported to be effective in decompression of the mediastinum and soft tissues of the neck.
- Restricted ventilation due to chest wall emphysema can be relieved by incision, or subcutaneous drains connected to suction.
  - Some advocate small incisions through the skin down to the pectoralis fascia in the infraclavicular region to decompress the subcutaneous tissues in an emergency—referred to as "blow-holes".

Prognosis

- Aetiology dependent.
- If spontaneous/associated with pneumothorax, prognosis is good and emphysema is usually self-limiting.
- If associated with mediastinitis, airway, respiratory or cardiac compromise can be rapidly fatal if not treated urgently.

Summary

- Pneumomediastinum and subcutaneous emphysema are usually self-limiting, but morbidity/mortality from pressure effects is possible.
- Identify and treat the cause early to reduce morbidity or mortality.
- Tension pneumomediastinum, though rare, is life-threatening and should be decompressed by emergency cervical mediastinotomy.
- Massive subcutaneous emphysema can lead to airway or respiratory compromise, requiring emergency intubation/tracheostomy and release of pressure with tissue incisions.

Further reading

Williams DJ, Jaggar SI, Morgan CJ. Upper airway obstruction as a result of massive subcutaneous emphysema following accidental removal of an intercostal drain. *British Journal of Anaesthesia* 2005; 94(3):390–2.

Cerfolio RJ, Bryant AS, Maniscalco LM. Management of Subcutaneous Emphysema After Pulmonary Resection. *Annals of Thoracic Surgery* 2008; 85:1759–65.

Herlan DB, Landreneau RJ, Ferson PF. Massive spontaneous subcutaneous emphysema. Acute management with infraclavicular "blow holes". *Chest* 1992; 102:503–5.

Post-operative air leak

- Post-operative air leak is common, with an approximate incidence of 15% after pulmonary resection.
- The usual cause of an air leak is an alveolar-pleural fistula occurring between a small bronchiole or alveolar unit and the pleural cavity.
- Post-operative bronchopleural fistulae are less common (5%) but have an associated higher mortality and are more difficult to treat.
- Post-operative air leak may necessitate prolonged chest drain insertion and hospital stay and may increase the risk of pulmonary infection.
- The risk of an air leak can be minimized by using stapling devices, tissue sealants and techniques such as pleural tenting at the time of resection.
- Air leaks should be checked for at the end of surgery by inflating the lung under water and looking for air bubbles.

Alveolar-pleural fistulae

- Chest drains inserted at the end of surgery drain air from these small air leaks and encourage full lung expansion.
- As the lung expands adhesions form between the resection margin and the pleura, thus sealing the fistula.
- The majority seal with complete expansion of the lung over 3–5 days.

Risk factors

- Non-anatomical resection.
- Emphysematous lung resection.
- Poor nutritional status.
- Previous radiotherapy.
- Infection.
- Trauma.

Clinical presentation

- Recognized by incomplete lung expansion on CXR and ongoing air loss from chest drains.
- Digital pleural drainage systems can quantify the size of the air leak.

Management

- Reposition the chest drain and/or insert further drains; application of adequate low pressure suction (-10 to -20 cm H_2O) via the chest drain promotes lung expansion.
- If the lung remains inflated upon discontinuation of suction, the drain can be safely removed.
- If the air leak persists in the absence of a pneumothorax, the drain can be connected to a flutter bag and the patient managed in the outpatient setting. Most leaks resolve in 1–3 weeks.
- If the lung collapses then pleurodesis may be required.
  - Tetracycline or talc is injected through the chest drain.
  - Drain is clamped and the patient nursed in different positions.
- Surgery is rarely indicated for persistent leak.

Anaesthesia

- Normally straightforward as the leak is small and significant infection unlikely.
- A double lumen tube is usually required to permit one lung ventilation.
- Suitable analgesia including a thoracic epidural may be needed depending on the surgery undertaken.
- An Asherman chest seal may be useful in cases where the chest drain has fallen out and further chest drain insertion is considered high risk.

Bronchopleural fistulae (BPF)

- These arise from a larger bronchus and are managed according to the timing of presentation.
- Mortality and morbidity can be high (20%).
- Usually present 7–15 days post-operatively.
- Can present several months after primary surgery associated with recurrence or infection.

Risk factors

- Increased age.
- Poor wound healing.
- Poor nutritional status.
- Previous chemotherapy or radiotherapy.
- Pneumonectomy.
- Excessively long bronchial stump.

Clinical Presentation

- Cough ± haemoptysis (this may be confused with pulmonary oedema).
- Sepsis 2° pneumonia/empyema.
- Respiratory distress proportional to the size of fistula.
- Persistent large air leak or a sudden increase in size of air leak.
- Tension pneumothorax.
- Falling air-fluid level in a hemithorax following pneumonectomy.
- Subcutaneous emphysema.

Management

- Intercostal chest drains required in all cases; suction may be required but excessive suction may cause loss of tidal volume if air leak very large.
- Bronchoscopy often needed to confirm diagnosis.
- Nurse operative side down to avoid contamination of unaffected lung.
- Early presentation (within 7 days post operatively) associated with technical difficulty at the time of lung resection; leak is often large and urgent surgical management usually required
  - The stump may need to be re-sutured or clos.ed with an intercostal muscle flap.
- Late presentation is usually associated with empyema and abscess formation.
  - This requires drainage and treatment with intravenous antibiotics prior to any definitive surgery.
  - May also be associated with recurrent tumour.
- Fistulae after lobectomy are very rare; usually associated with bi-lobectomy
  - Conservative management usually recommended.
- 20–30% of small bronchopleural fistulae close with chest drainage alone.
- Patients may be septic and extremely unwell.

Anaesthesia

- (See 📖 Anaesthesia for lung transplantation, p. 364).
- Anaesthesia for BPF is high risk and should be undertaken by experts
- Principles of anaesthesia for BPF:
  - Prevent spillage of empyema into the normal bronchus and contamination of the unaffected lung.
  - Control distribution of ventilation.
  - An increase in the air leak from a non-isolated fistula reduces alveolar ventilation, increases pulmonary shunt, and could cause a tension pneumothorax, e.g. during IPPV.
- Protect the good lung can be achieved by:
  - Appropriate patient position, i.e. semi-sitting ± lateral tilt (affected side lowermost).
  - Endobronchial intubation of the main bronchus contra-lateral to the BPF using DLT/SLT, or by placement of a bronchial blocker in the main bronchus of the affected side.
- The size of the air leak is dependent on a pressure gradient between the mean airway pressure at the site of the fistula and interpleural space. Spontaneous ventilation or high frequency jet ventilation (HFJV) can be used to minimize the pressure differential.
- A functioning chest drain with under water seal (no suction) is required in all cases.

- Suitable anaesthetic techniques include:
  - Rapid intravenous induction with muscle paralysis and fibreoptic placement of double lumen tube (DLT). Manual ventilation with small tidal volumes will be required until lung isolation achieved.
  - Deep inhalational anaesthesia and maintenance of spontaneous ventilation until lung isolation achieved.
  - Awake intubation with single lumen tube and subsequent bronchial blocker placement.

Chylothorax

Definition

The uncommon, but potentially fatal presence of chyle within the thorax.

Physiology

- Chyle is produced at up to 4 l/24h and contains a combination of gut-derived and lymphatic constituents including lymphocytes, immunoglobulins, enzymes and digestive products.
- Usually discovered after it manifests itself as a pleural effusion.

Causes

(See Table 11.6)

Table 11.6 Causes of chylothorax

Mechanism	Pathology
Obstruction	INTRINSIC:
	Neoplasm
	Developmental abnormality
	Filariasis
	EXTRINSIC:
	Neoplasm (70% lymphoma)
	Infection (TB)
	Subclavian vein occlusion
	Aortic aneurysm
Trauma (20%)	Blunt trauma
	Penetrating wounds
	Surgical procedures
	Coughing
	Hyperextension of spine
	Weight lifting
Iatrogenic (80%)	Post oesophagectomy
	Post lung resection
	Post mediastinal surgery
	Aortography
	Left heart catheterization
	Idiopathic
Inflammatory	Sarcoidosis
	Amyloidosis
	Cirrhosis

Presentation and assessment

Symptoms
- Dyspnoea/tachypnoea.
- Low grade pyrexia.
- Cardiovascular collapse.

Signs
- Dullness to percussion.
- Tracheal shift.
- Tension chylothorax (rare).
  - Similar in presentation to tension pneumothorax.
- High output from chest drains, especially after introduction of enteral feed.
  - In any post-thoracic surgical patient, especially after introduction of enteral feed, should be highly suggestive of a chylous leak.
- Visibly milky chest drain loss.

Investigations

Bloods:
- **FBC**
  - Immunosuppression?
- **U&E, LFT**
  - Hypocalcaemia.
  - Hypoproteinaemia—low serum albumin.
  - Hyponatraemia.
- **ABG**
  - Acidosis.
  - Hypoxia denotes large chylothorax.

Radiology:
- **CXR**.
  - Mediastinal shift.
  - Pleural effusion.
- **CT chest /abdomen**.
  - If malignant aetiology suspected.

Other:
- **Lymphangiography**.
  - If anatomical origin is not obvious.
- **Drain fluid triglyceride level**.
  - >110 mg/dL reflects a 99% chance that the fluid is chyle
  - <50 mg/dL reflects only a 5% chance that the fluid is chyle
  - 50–110 mg/dL, use lipoprotein analysis to inspect the pleural fluid for chylomicrons or cholesterol crystals
  - A ratio of pleural fluid cholesterol to triglyceride of <1 is also diagnostic.
- **Drain fluid lymphocyte count**
  - Higher than plasma.

❶ Enteral placement of "cream" or methylene blue is not advocated.

Differential diagnosis
- AIDS related complex.
- Congestive heart failure.
- Exudative pleural effusion.
- Malignant pleural effusion.
- Pseudochylothorax.

Management

Conservative
- Minimize straining and position patient slightly head-up.
- Insert intercostal chest drain connected to underwater seal
- Thoracocentesis/drain fluid analysis.
- Consider parenteral feeding.
- Enteral feed may offer protection against bacterial translocation but consists of medium chain triglycerides. This can lead to essential fatty acid deficiency.
- Somatostatin analogues may have some effect in reducing the flow of chyle.
  - The proposed mechanism being either reduction in gastric secretions and hence chylous volume, or reduction in lymphatic losses by increasing tone in lymphatic vessels.
- Chemoradiation may promote resolution of chylothorax and should be used in patients with malignant chylothorax who are not surgical candidates.
- 50% resolve with conservative management alone. Reported mortality stands at between 10 and 50%.

Surgical
- Chyle leak greater than 1 L/24h for 5 days, or a persistent leak for more than 2 weeks despite conservative management.
- Nutritional or metabolic complications, including electrolyte depletion and immunosuppression.
- Loculated chylothorax, fibrin clots, or trapped lung.
- Post-oesophagectomy chylothorax
  - Patients with this carry a high mortality rate if treated conservatively.
- Thoracic duct ligation is the criterion standard.
  - The duct is usually ligated between the eighth and twelfth thoracic vertebrae, just above the aortic hiatus.
  - The approach is usually through the right chest, either by an open right thoracotomy or through a thoracoscope.

- A pleuro-peritoneal shunt can be successful for refractory chylothorax but can be complicated by infection and obstruction.
- Pleurodesis is often used for malignant chylothorax, but it will not work in a case of loculated chylothorax or a trapped lung.
- Surgical pleurectomy is a treatment option.

▶▶ Traumatic cases do better if left to conservative management. This is usually due to the fact that there is an identifiable single lesion; Vs. potential multiple/unidentifiable lesions in other cases.

Further reading

Merrigan BA, Winter DC, O'Sullivan GC, et al. British Journal Of Surgery 1997; 84(1): 15–20.

Wemyss-Holden SA, Launois B, Maddern GJ. Management of thoracic duct injuries after oesophagectomy. British Journal Of Surgery 2001; 88(11): 1442–8.

Dugue L, Sauvanet A, Farges O, et al. Output of chyle as an indicator of treatment for chylothorax complicating oesophagectomy. British Journal Of Surgery 1998; 85(8): 1147–9.

Post-operative pneumonia

Respiratory complications account for almost half of all post-operative morbidity in thoracic surgical patients. Thoracic surgery is second only to open abdominal aortic surgery with respect to the risk of developing pneumonia post-operatively.

Introduction

- Patients scheduled for thoracic surgery may be at risk of developing post-operative pneumonia (POP) for various reasons:
  - Malnourished.
  - Pre-existing impaired pulmonary function.
  - They may have undergone radiotherapy or are immunocompromised as a result of peri-operative chemotherapy.
- The pathophysiological effects of a thoracotomy further increase the risk of developing post-operative POP.

> ### POP definition & diagnosis
>
> Post-operatively, the patient should satisfy one of the following two criteria:
>
> ***Crepitation or dullness to percussion on chest examination plus any of the following***
> - New onset of purulent sputum or change in character of sputum.
> - Isolation of organism from blood culture.
> - Isolation of pathogen from specimen obtained by trans-tracheal aspirate, bronchial brushing, or biopsy.
>
> Or...
>
> ***CXR demonstrating new or progressive infiltrate, consolidation, cavitation, or pleural effusion plus any of the following***
> - The above 3 factors.
> - Isolation of virus or detection of viral antigen in respiratory secretions.
> - Diagnostic single antibody titer (IgM) or fourfold increase in paired serum samples (IgG) for pathogen.
> - Histopathological evidence of pneumonia.

❶ There are several definitions of post-operative pneumonia.

Severity indicators

- 'CURB-65'.
  - **C**onfusion.
  - **U**rea >7 mmol/l.
  - **R**espiratory rate >30 bpm.
  - **B**lood pressure systolic <60 mmHg.
  - Age >**65**.
  - Hypoxaemia PaO_2 <8 kPa.

POP key points

- Incidence of POP in thoracic surgery is procedure dependent:
  - 54% of bronchoplasties
  - 42% of bi-lobectomies
  - 30% of extended resections
  - 29% of lobectomies
  - 20% of pneumonectomies.
- ☠ Associated overall mortality 10—30%.
- For comparison:
  - 1.5% incidence post major non-cardiac surgery.
  - 21% associated 30-day mortality in this setting.

Patient related risk factors

- >70 years old.
- Weight loss >10% in preceding 6 months.
- Moderate to severe COPD.
- BUN level <2.86 mmol/l.
- Cigarette smoking.
- Chronic steroid use.
- Pre-operative chemotherapy.

Typical causative organisms

- *Haemophilus.*
- *Streptococcus sp.*
- *Pseudomonas.*
- *Serratia.*
- *Candida albicans.*
- Enteric organisms.
- Multiple organisms in a third of cases.

Prophylaxis & prevention of POP

Antibiotics

(See Table 11.7) for suggested regimes and ALWAYS consult microbiology for advice).

- Approximately 23% of patients have microbial colonization of the bronchial tree pre-operatively.
  - *Haemophilus* and *Streptococcus* colonies most frequent; *Pseudomonas* and enteric gram negative colonization of bronchial tree is less common.
  - Approximately half of patients colonized pre-operatively develop POP despite antibiotic prophylaxis.
  - There does not appear to be a relationship between the degree of colonization and the likelihood of POP.
- It is believed that the majority of POP is due to micro-organisms found in the patient's oral cavity, pharynx and hypopharynx post-operatively.
- There is some evidence to support the use of amoxicillin-clavulanic acid (Augmentin) prophylaxis over 2nd generation cephalosporins.
  - In a non-randomized controlled trial, augmentin reduced the overall incidence of POP by 45% in patients who had pneumonectomy/lobectomy for a non-infectious indication.
  - This reflected a decrease in infection due to *Haemophilus*, *Streptococcus*, and other B-lactamase producing micro-organisms.

❶ The ideal antibiotic prophylaxis against POP in thoracic surgery patients remains to be found.

Table 11.7 Suggested anti-microbial regimes for pneumonia (may vary according to institution)

	Condition	Likely organisms	Antibiotic suggestion
(a)	Acute exacerbation of COPD	Viruses	1st—amoxicillin 500mg PO TDS
		Strep. pneumoniae	2nd—erythromycin 500mg PO QDS
		H. influenzae	3rd—doxycycline 200mg PO stat then 100mg OD
		Moraxella catarrhalis	
(b)	Post influenzal pneumonia	*Staph. aureus*	Flucloxacillin 1g PO/IV QDS ± in addition to the above
(c)	Aspiration pneumonia		Antibiotic not needed unless symptomatic with new CXR changes
			Augmentin 1.2g IV TDS

(Contd.)

Table 11.7 (Contd.)

Condition	Likely organisms	Antibiotic suggestion
(d) Community acquired pneumonia	H. influenzae S. pneumoniae S. aureus	Mild—amoxicillin 500mg-1g PO TDS (penicillin allergic: doxycycline 200mg PO OD or erythromycin 500mg PO QDS
		Moderate—Mild + erythromycin 500mg PO QDS (clarithromycin 500mg IV BD if PO not possible)
		Severe—Augmentin 1.2g TDS IV + erythromycin 500mg PO QDS (clarithromycin 500mg IV BD if PO not possible)
(e) Hospital acquired	H. influenzae S. pneumoniae S. aureus	Mild—same as (a). Moderate—augmentin 1.2g IV TDS Severe—piperacillin/tazocin 4.5g IV TDS
(f) Ventilator acquired pneumonia	Enterobacteriae Acinetobacter Candida MRSA Pseudomonas	An aminoglycoside such as gentamicin 5–7 mg/kg IV OD *plus, either* … An anti-pseudomonal penicillin such as piperacillin/Tazocin 4.5g IV TDS or … An anti-pseudomonal cephalosporin such as ceftazidime 1g IV BD or … A monobactam such as aztreonam 2g IV TDS or … Certain quinolones such as ciprofloxacin 500mg IV BD
TB		Seek micro. advice (See 📖 Antibiotics, p. 130).

If known MRSA colonization; add in teicoplanin 200–400mg IV OD.

Non-invasive pressure support ventilation (NIPSV)
- Pre-operative NIPSV improved respiratory spirometry and gas exchange in patients scheduled for elective lobectomy compared to controls.
  - IPAP 10–14 cmH$_2$O.
  - EPAP 2–4 cmH$_2$O.
- Elective NIPSV post-operatively maintained this advantage.
- Lobar collapse in the NIPSV group was 14.2% compared to 38.9% in the control group.

- The study was underpowered to pass comment on the benefit of NIPSV on POP.
  - However, it did demonstrate a significant trend in the reduction of post-operative atelectasis.

Analgesia & chest physiotherapy

- The inability to cough, deep breathe and expectorate thick respiratory secretions places the post-operative thoracic patient at a huge risk of developing POP.
- Strategies to mitigate this risk include:

Analgesic strategies (see 📖 Analgesics, p. 118).
- Thoracic epidural (local anaesthetic ±opioid).
- Paravertebral block.
- Intercostal blocks.
- Parenteral patient controlled analgesia (opioid).

Physiotherapy
- Deep breathing techniques.
- Manual techniques (dependent on adequate analgesia):
  - Chest wall compression.
  - Chest clapping/percussion.
- Positioning to achieve drainage of secretions.
- Nasopharyngeal suctioning.

Surgical approach
Video-assisted thoracoscopic surgery (VATS)
- Major thoracic surgery may be achieved by a thoracoscopic. approach which utilizes a small "utility" thoracotomy without spreading the ribs.
- Approximately 10% converted to open thoracotomy.
- Incidence of POP after thoracoscopic wedge resection reported as 2.8 %.

Treatment
Antibiotics
- Ensure that samples are taken for microbiological examination and culture, e.g. sputum, trans-tracheal aspirate, blood (See Table 11.7).
- Initial broad spectrum cover; refer to your institution's microbiological guideline for the treatment of hospital acquired pneumonia.
- Subsequent antibiotic therapy may be tailored according to patient response and antibiotic sensitivities.

Respiratory failure
- Humidified oxygen via face mask.
- Regular chest physiotherapy.
- Adequate and appropriate analgesia.

NIPSV
- ↓ requirement for sedation.
- ↓ intubation rate in post-thoracotomy patients with acute respiratory failure from 50% to 20.8%.
- ↓ mortality in these patients from 37.5% to 12.5%.

Invasive ventilation
- Associated with significant morbidity:
  - Respiratory muscle atrophy.
  - Exacerbation of POP.
  - Bronchial stump disruption.
  - Bronchopleural fistula.
  - Persistent air leak.

Further reading

Arozullah AM, Khuri SF, Henderson WG, et al. Development and validation of a multifactorial risk index for predicting postoperative pneumonia after major noncardiac surgery. *Annals of Internal Medicine.* 2001; 135:847–57.

Schussler O, Dermine H, Alifano M, et al. Should we change antibiotic prophylaxis for lung surgery? Postoperative pneumonia is the critical issue. *Annals of Thoracic Surgery.* 2008; 86:1727–33.

Perrin C, Jullien V, Venissac N, et al. Prophylactic use of non-invasive ventilation in patients undergoing lung resectional surgery. *Respiratory Medicine.* 2007; 101:1572–8.

Pulmonary aspiration in thoracic patients

- Aspiration refers to the entry of foreign material into the lungs. Post-aspiration morbidity relates to:
  - The amount and nature of the aspirated material.
  - The pre-morbid status of the patient.
  - The ability of the patient to mount a defensive response.
- It is a serious complication of anaesthesia
- Incidence of 1:1,100 to 1:14,000 amongst patients undergoing any form of anaesthesia.
- Thoracic surgical patients are at a higher risk, especially those having oesophageal surgery.
- Certain thoracic surgical conditions predispose to aspiration of infected material.
- General risk factors for aspiration are shown (See Table 11.8). * Those of particular importance among thoracic patients.

Table 11.8 Risk factors for aspiration of gastric contents

Risk Factor	Example
Increased volume of material with regirgitant potential	Non-fasted patient.
	Impaired gastric emptying:
	• *Trauma*
	• *Opioid usage*
	• *Autonomic neuropathy e.g. Parkinson's disease*
	• *Physical obstruction e.g. gastric tumour*
Surgical conditions providing reservoir for fluids	*Oesophageal:
	• *Web/pouch*
	• *Stricture/tumour*
	• *Achalasia*
	*Pharyngeal pouch
	*Tracheo-oesophageal fistula
	*Pus from:
	• *Bronchiectasis*
	• *Lung abscess*
	• *Broncho-pleural fistula*
	• *Empyema*
Increased intra-gastric pressure	*Tense surgical pneumoperitoneum
	Obesity

(Contd.)

Table 11.8 (*Contd.*)

Risk Factor	Example
Lowered oesophageal sphincter tone	Pregnancy
	*Surgical conditions:
	• *Post oesophagectomy*
	• *Tumours involving GOJ*
	• *Hiatus hernia*
Loss of upper airway reflexes	Lowered conscious level
	*Surgical conditions predisposing:
	• *Topical anaesthesia of airway*
	• *Dysphagia*
	• *Neurological disease; thymic surgery and myasthenia*
	• *Laryngeal nerve palsy 2° Pancoast tumour*

Pathophysiology (pneumonitis vs. pneumonia)

- Half of the adult population aspirate during sleep—normally completely cleared by natural defense mechanisms including ciliary action and phagocytosis by alveolar macrophages.
- Chemical pneumonitis (CP).
  - If the pH of aspirate is <2.5 and the volume >0.3 ml/kg, then sterile pneumonitis (ALI) will ensue irrespective of other factors
  - Antibiotics are therefore not indicated.
  - CP may progress to ARDS or bacterial pneumonia (BP).
  - If signs of infection develop after 48 hours treat with broad spectrum antibiotics.
- BP can result acutely from gastric aspiration when there is:
  - Small bowel obstruction.
  - PPI, antacid treatment.
  - Enteral feeding.
- This will require antibiotics from the outset.
- Thoracic patients prone to chronic aspiration (CAP) tend to have *Strep. pneumoniae, Staph. aureus, H. influenza, enterobacteria* induced pneumonia.
- Barium is inert and does not produce ALI; but large amounts may mechanically interfere with gas exchange → hypoxia.
- Massive haemoptysis (See 📖 Massive pulmonary haemorrhage, p. 484).

Prevention of aspiration in thoracic anaesthesia

- Aspiration is a two stage process:
  - Accumulation of gastric contents or infected material in the pharynx or the large airways.
  - Failure of airway isolation.
- Where possible the amount of infected material should be reduced (e.g. draining empyema with a chest drain before DLT intubation for BPF).
- Position the patient appropriately to reduce the risk of aspiration from lung abscess etc. before intubation.
- Meticulous care in positioning the endobronchial tube, particularly on final positioning of the patient prior to knife-to-skin.
- Make sure the endobronchial and tracheal balloons are fully inflated.
- Tumours blocking airways lead to infection and accumulation of infected secretions distally. Surgical manipulation will squeeze the secretions into the proximal bronchus and risk aspiration into the dependent lung, therefore:
  - Suction secretions from the ipsilateral bronchus frequently.
  - The endo-bronchial tube placed into the contra-lateral bronchus should minimize risk of aspiration into this side.
- Aspiration rates are similar in nasogastric and gastrostomy fed patients.
- Aspiration following oesophagectomy (lack of gastro-oesophageal sphincter) can be minimized by nursing patients at 45°.

Presentation & assessment

- Desaturation that remains un-resolved after a dislodged tube is re-positioned is highly indicative of aspiration.
- A definitive diagnosis of pulmonary aspiration, when not witnessed, can only be made by the finding of gastric contents within the tracheobronchial tree, either on direct observation by fibreoptic bronchoscopy or upon suctioning.
- Many cases of aspiration pre and post-operatively will be silent.

Clinical signs

- Tachypnoea.
- Pyrexia.
- Hypoxaemia.
- Coarse lung crepitations.
- Wheeze.
- Signs of severe sepsis and shock within hours of aspiration of infected material.

Investigations

Radiology
- **CXR**.
  - Pulmonary infiltrates may take hours to become visible.
  - May progress to consolidation of the affected lobe.
- **Pulmonary scintigraphy and ventilation-perfusion imaging**.

Immediate management

Once recognized, the priorities are oxygenation of the patient and prevention of further contamination of the airway.

During barium study
- Intubation and ventilation if severe hypoxia
- Bronchoscopy to extract as much barium as possible
- ▶ Do not lavage; barium will spread further.

During OLV
- Suck out secretions from both bronchi and pharynx before re-positioning DLT.
- If large aspiration → hypoxia; replace DLT with ETT and use a bronchoscope to suck out secretions.

Empyema and lung abscess
- Bronchoscopy and suck out infected material.
- Severe ALI and pneumonia may ensue.
- Critical care management and surviving sepsis protocol.

Aspiration at or before induction of anaesthesia
- Administer 100% oxygen.
- If the patient's upper airway reflexes are present:
  - Turn to the left lateral position.
  - Place head down and suction the oropharynx.
  - If tracheal suction is required, intubate the trachea. If possible tracheal suction should be performed prior to the commencement of mechanical ventilation.
- If the patient has depressed or absent airway reflexes:
  - Position as above and intubate the trachea.
  - Cricoid pressure should be used unless the patient is actively vomiting (due to the risk of oesophageal rupture).
  - Once the airway is secured, tracheal suction should be performed; using either a catheter or through a bronchoscope.
- Particulate aspiration may require bronchoscopy and lavage to remove obstructing particles.
- There is no evidence to show that the use of antacids, H_2 receptor blockers, proton pump inhibitors or prokinetics decrease the incidence or alter the outcome of pulmonary aspiration.
- Antibiotic therapy should be considered in those patients who fail to improve within 48 hours and is definitely indicated in those patients who subsequently develop pneumonia.
- Corticosteroids are of no proven benefit.

Further management

- Close observation of the patient is necessary to detect the development of hypoxaemia and secondary pulmonary infection. If the patient is asymptomatic after 2 hours, then respiratory problems are unlikely.
- Chest physiotherapy may be of benefit.
- CPAP (or the addition of PEEP in the mechanically ventilated patient) may improve oxygenation.

Further reading

Marik PE. Aspiration pneumonitis and aspiration pneumonia. *New England Journal of Medicine.* 2001; 344:665–71.

Engelhardt T, Webster NR. Pulmonary aspiration of gastric contents in anaesthesia. *British Journal of Anaesthesia.* 1999; 83:453–60.

The role of bronchoscopy on the ITU

Bronchoscopy and bronchoscopic anatomy are discussed elsewhere in this book (See 📖 Bronchoscopy, p. 282.).

Flexible fibre-optic bronchoscopy has therapeutic and diagnostic indications. Bronchoscopy requires an experienced operator and trained assistance. As patients are often intubated (tracheostomy or COETT), the assistant should support the tube to reduce trauma to the trachea and scope.

Indications

Diagnostic

- Collection of microbiological ± cytological specimens by broncho—alveolar lavage, brush specimens or biopsy.
- The presence of lesions of unknown etiology on the chest radiograph film or the need to evaluate recurrent pneumonia, persistent atelectasis or pulmonary infiltrates.
- To assess patency or position of endotracheal tube/tracheostomy tube.
- The need to assess patency or mechanical properties of the upper airway.
- The need to investigate haemoptysis.
- Identify the location and extent of injury from inhalation or aspiration
- Diagnose ruptured trachea/bronchus, tracheo-oesophageal fistula, broncho-pleural fistula.

Therapeutic

- Clearance of secretions, mucus plugs, vomitus, clots or foreign bodies to allow lung re-expansion.
- To aid placement of tracheostomy tube or double lumen tube.
- The need for aid in performing difficult intubations or percutaneous tracheostomies.
- To localize and control haemoptysis by directed placement of balloon catheter.
- Cleansing; removing soot and other toxins.
- Therapeutic management of endobronchial toilet in ventilator associated pneumonia.

Absolute contraindications

- Absence of consent from the patient or his/her representative unless a medical emergency exists and patient is not competent to give permission (consent ♂ must be filled out).
- Absence of an experienced bronchoscopist to perform or closely and directly supervise the procedure.
- Lack of adequate facilities and personnel to care for such emergencies as cardiopulmonary arrest, pneumothorax, or bleeding.
- Inability to adequately oxygenate the patient during the procedure.
- Patients with certain conditions that would usually be considered to be absolute contraindications unless the risk-benefit assessment warrants the procedure:
  - Coagulopathy or bleeding diathesis that cannot be corrected.
  - Severe refractory hypoxemia.
  - Unstable hemodynamic status including dysrhythmias.

Pre-use checks

- Check scope has been leak tested and disinfected.
- Check the control lever and tip move in harmony.
- Ensure a patent suction port and adequate suction is available.
- Ensure image is adequate, focused and white balanced if required.
- Ensure microbiological sample trap, sterile gloves, syringes and flushes are available.
- Obtain adequate trained assistance.
- Ensure emergency drugs and intubation equipment are readily available.

Procedure

- Pre-oxygenate with 100% O2 for 10 mins and fully monitor throughout.
- IV sedation may already be in place as the patient is most likely already sedated to allow mechanical ventilation. Consider analgesia ± paralysis and increasing the basal sedation rate.
- If un-intubated, apply local anaesthetic to nose and pharynx.
- Lubricate scope with gel/saline.
- Insert scope through the endotracheal/tracheostomy port and direct scope to examine individual bronchi/bronchopulmonary segments.
- Perform a broncho-alveolar lavage by instillation of 20 ml sterile saline and aspirate contents with suction in to a microbiological trap.
- Irrigate lungs with sterile saline till clean to remove carbonaceous debris in cases of inhalational injury.
- If SpO_2 <90% or cardiovascular instability occurs, remove scope and re-oxygenate patient before considering continuing.
- After procedure, reset ventilator as appropriate.
- Perform CXR afterwards in all cases.

Pitfalls and tips

- ↑ tip angulation will increase difficulty in advancing towards image.
- Keep scope straight for easy rotation.
- Keep view of where you want to go in the centre of the image.
- If you loose the image, withdraw scope till you recognize the anatomy.
- Ensure that the small arrow indent on the camera/scope viewfinder sits at the 12o'clock position to allow for optimal orientation.
- Consider the use of glycopyrolate/atropine to dry secretions (care in patients with cardiovascular instability).

Cleaning and sterilization

- Manual cleaning includes washing outer surface with soapy water.
- Use a brush to clean the working channels.
- Flush the working channels and suction with sterile water.
- Scope should be leak tested before sterilization with 2% glutaraldehyde or 10% ethylene oxide.

Further reading

Singer M, Webb AR (2004). *Oxford Handbook of Critical Care.* p. 38.

Jolliet PH, Chevrolet JC. Bronchoscopy in the intensive care unit. *Intensive Care Medicine* 1992: 18;160–9.

Leibler JM. Fibre-optic Bronchoscopy for diagnosis and treatment. *Critical Care Clinics,* 2000: 16(1);83–100.

Low cardiac output state

Definition

- Occurs when the cardiac output is unable to match the metabolic demands of the patient.
- It is important to recognize and treat low cardiac output to prevent further deterioration in the patient's condition.

> Cardiac output (l/min) = Heart rate (bpm) X Stroke volume (ml)

- Cardiac Index (CI) can be calculated by dividing CO by the body surface area of the patient in m^2.
- Determinants of stroke volume are: preload, afterload, myocardial contractility.

Aetiology

- There are many causes, which vary due to the clinical situation and often co-exist:

Heart rate

- Bradyarrhythmias.
- Heart block.
- Tachyarrhythmias.

Preload

- Hypovolaemia.
- Haemorrhage.
- Pulmonary hypertension.
- Right ventricular failure.
- Pericardial constriction/tamponade.

Afterload

- Overt vasoconstriction.
- Profound vasodilatation.

Myocardial contractility

- Ischaemia or infarction.
- Myocardial stunning.
- Electrolyte abnormalities (K^+, Ca^{2+}).
- Metabolic disturbance ($\downarrow$ pH).
- Negatively inotropic drugs.

Recognition of low cardiac output

- History and clinical examination are important.
- Additional information from laboratory investigations and haemodynamic monitoring may also be useful in diagnosing the presence of a low cardiac output state.

Clinical features
- Falling BP on trending.
- Decreased urine output (<1 ml/kg/hr).
- Altered cerebration or reduced conscious level.
- Cool peripheries/increased toe to core temperature difference.
- Symptoms and signs of cardiac failure (e.g. breathlessness, crackles on auscultation).

Metabolic features
- Raised serum lactate (4 mmol/L).
- Mixed venous saturation <65%.
- Metabolic acidosis.

Haemodynamic parameters
- Cardiac Index <2.4 L/min.
- Reduction in MAP >25% below baseline.

Immediate management

- 100% O_2/ABC approach.
- Ensure patent airway and adequate respiration.
- Increase FiO_2 to 1.0.
- Treatment should then be directed to the underlying cause(s).

Optimize heart rate
- Treat bradyarrhythmias with anticholinergics:
  - Atropine 300–600 mcg increments/IV.
  - Glycopyrrolate 200–600 mcg increments/IV.
- ❶ If resistant may require external pacing or temporary pacing wire.
- Treat tachyarrhythmias with an appropriate agent:
  - Digoxin, beta blockers, amiodarone, adenosine.
- ❶ Beware polypharmacy and drug interactions.
- ❶ If drug unresponsive tachyarrhythmias or patient unstable, consider synchronized DC cardioversion.

Enhance preload
- Increasing venous return to the heart will increase preload.
- Lay patient flat and raise legs to increase venous return; give rapid fluid boluses of 125–250 ml.
- Avoidance of caval compression in supine patient.

Afterload manipulation
- Cautious use of vasodilators in patients with high SVR.
- Cautious use of vasopressors in patients with low SVR to increase. SVR and also improve myocardial perfusion and oxygen supply.

Myocardial contractility
- Correct electrolyte abnormalities.
- Treat ischaemia and enhance myocardial oxygen supply.
- Consider use of positive inotropic agents in conjunction with cardiac output monitoring.
- Cessation of any negatively inotropic agents.

Intra aortic balloon pump
- Balloon placed into thoracic aorta via femoral artery.
- Cyclical inflation (during diastole) and deflation (during systole) to increase coronary perfusion and improve afterload.
- Thus increases myocardial O_2 supply and reduces myocardial work and O_2 demand.
  - ❶ Only indicated if potentially reversible LV impairment is causing low cardiac output.

Cardiac output monitoring
- A number of different systems are available for monitoring the patient with a low cardiac output state.
- Clinical parameters can be used to assess cardiac output and monitoring via a central venous catheter and arterial line will provide information on HR, MAP and CVP (a surrogate for RAP).
- However information on variables such as LAP and PAP (or surrogates of these) requires further cardiac output monitoring, which may be helpful to guide therapy in the patient whose condition is not improving despite treatment.

Available methods include
Pulmonary Artery Flotation Catheter
- Seen as "gold standard" for measurement of CO.
- Utilizes thermodilution technique.
- Requires skill for insertion, use and interpretation.
- Invasive with significant morbidity.

Lithium Indicator Dilution Cardiac Output Monitor (LiDCO)
- Less accurate than PAFC.
- Requires peripheral arterial catheter.
- Frequent recalibration of equipment required.
- Quaternary ammonia ion in some muscle relaxants (mainly atracurium) can artificially increase the sensor sensitivity.

Transoesophageal doppler
- Easy insertion, however very movement sensitive.
- Inaccurate measurements; uses surrogate measures of cardiac output.

Transthoracic echocardiography
- Non invasive.
- Does not accurately measure determinants of cardiac output; gives overall picture of cardiac function.
- Poor views in ventilated patients.

Impedence cardiography
- Largely experimental; not widely used in current practice.

Further reading

Bersten A, Soni N, Oh T (2003). *Oh's Intensive Care Manual*, 5th Edition, Butterworth Heinemann.

Jhanji S, Dawson J, Pearse RM. Cardiac output monitoring: basic science and clinical application. *Anaesthesia* 2008 Feb; 63(2): 172–81.

Post-operative fluid management

- Peri-operative fluid management of the thoracic patient provides both a quantitative and qualitative challenge.
- The thoracic cavity has no third space favouring a restrictive fluid strategy.
- The ideal strategy maintains intravascular volume for an adequate cardiac output, without accumulation of excessive lung water to the detriment of gas exchange.
- Peri-operative fluid delivery needs to be tailored to both surgical and patient factors, taking into consideration deficit, anticipated loss, and maintenance requirements.

Pathophysiology

- The principle aim of peri-operative fluid management is to maintain vital organ perfusion.
- 60% of total body weight is water—2/3 intracellular and 1/3 extracellular (plasma and interstitial).
- Hydrostatic and oncotic forces govern the dynamic Starling equilibrium between these compartments.
- The physiological response to thoracic surgery has both endocrine and inflammatory effects in this equilibrium. The net effect:
  - ↑ capillary permeability.
  - ↑ aldosterone, ↑ ADH, ↑ ANP.
  - Conservation of Na^+ & water → ↑ in capillary hydrostatic pressure.
  - ↑ excretion of K^+.
  - ↓ serum oncotic pressure.
  - ↓ functional ECV.

Consequences of over hydration

- Rightward shift of the Starling myocardial performance curve → ↑ cardiac work and may potentiate post-op cardiac morbidity.
- RV strain due to ↑ pulmonary vascular resistance will be accentuated by any ↑ in venous return (a major issue with post R pneumonectomy patients—they are prone to RV infarction).
- Fluid accumulated in the lungs predisposes to pneumonia and compromises the blood alveolar interface (↓ diffusion capacity)
- FRC and FVC are also compromised.
- ↑ in capillary hydrostatic pressure favours extravasation of fluid, predisposing to tissue oedema with adverse consequences on gastric motility, tissue oxygenation and wound healing.

Consequences of under hydration

- Beyond compensatory mechanisms, cardiac output will fall compromising microcirculatory flow and tissue oxygen delivery.
  - A 10% reduction in intravascular volume will ↓ CO by 20%.
  - A 20% reduction in intravascular volume will ↓ CO by 40%.

- Reduction in tissue oxygen availability is the final common pathway leading to shock, with accumulation of products of cellular metabolism and ↓ cellular ATP.
- The susceptibility of different tissues to hypoxia and ischaemia will determine the extent of end organ damage.
  - Splanchnic and renal tubular circulations are particularly vulnerable
  - Immune function is impaired and the systemic inflammatory response to thoracic surgery is increased.

Table 11.9 Quantitative considerations in delivery of peri-operative IV fluid

Category	Factor	Result
Pre-op deficit	Fasting/anorexia	Intravascular volume depletion
Co-morbidity	CVS function	Needs cardiac replacement
	Renal function	
Anaesthetic technique	Central neuraxial blockade	Vasodilated vasculature → excessive fluid administration
	Pharmacology	
Patient positioning	Lateral decubitus vs. supine?	Venous pooling?
Thermoregulation	Increased or decreased temperature	Contracted vs. dilated circulation
Duration of surgery	Short vs. long procedures?	Increased losses
Surgical technique	Size of surgical plane	Evaporative losses
	Haemostasis	
	Open or VATS	
Capillary integrity	Endotoxaemia/sepsis	Vasodilated hyperdynamic, leaky circulation
	Pro-inflammatory cytokines	

- The quantity of fluid administration is of primary importance, but the choice of fluid will also govern the physiological response.
- Intravenous fluids are categorized by their ability to traverse cellular boundaries between body fluid compartments.
- Qualitative considerations influencing choice of peri-operative fluid administration:
  - Oxygen carrying capacity.
  - CVS/Renal function—dependent oedema.
  - Plasma oncotic pressure.
  - Coagulopathy.

- Electrolyte balance.
- Nutrition.
- Acid-Base status.

Fluid management for specific thoracic procedures

Lobectomy

- Limited pulmonary resections have no third space losses and therefore require restoration and maintenance of blood volume only.
  - 1.5 ml/kg/hr crystalloid intra-operatively with rapid restoration of normal diet will negate the need for meticulous fluid management.

Pneumonectomy

- These patients have a specific susceptibility to the complications of fluid overload.
- ↑ in capillary hydrostatic pressure, as the whole cardiac output passes through the remaining lung, favours ↑ alveolar lung water and predisposes to pulmonary oedema.
- There is a clear association between excess peri-operative fluid and PPPO but the aetiology of this ALI is multi-factorial.

Oesophagectomy

- Peritoneal and intestinal third space losses ↑ peri-operative fluid requirement.
- Once any ileus resolves (usually day 3–5) these interstitial losses will shift back into the IV space with a resultant diuretic phase.
- Quantifying this third space loss is difficult, making any peri-operative fluid strategy challenging.
- Achieving an adequate urine output (0.5 ml/kg/hr) must be balanced against an escalating +ve fluid balance that risks anastomotic oedema and breakdown.
- Half the daily fluid requirements can be given via a jejenostomy entereal feeding tube and half IV as balanced salt solution.
- The jejenostomy feed is then increased to achieve the patient's caloric requirements (1 cal/kg/hr). The IV component is proportionally tailed off, particularly once the diuretic phase of gut recovery ensues.
- Oral intake can commence by day 5–7.

Further reading

Slinger PD. Perioperative fluid management for thoracic surgery: The puzzle of post pneumonectomy pulmonary oedema. *Journal of Cardiothoracic and Vascular Anaesthesia* 1995; 9(4):442–51.

Powell-Tuck J, Gosling P, Lobo DN, *et al*. British consensus guidelines on intravenous fluid therapy for adult surgical patients (GIFTASUP).

Pulmonary embolism

- Obstruction to circulation in the pulmonary arterial bed by a foreign substance.
  - Leads to a failure of the blood supply to lung tissue, creation of shunt and eventual infarction.
  - May be small and therefore asymptomatic and undetected or may be massive (causing obstruction to greater than 50% of pulmonary circulation) and fatal.
- Associated with a high mortality rate, despite advances in medical management.
- Management requires a multi-disciplinary approach spanning radiology, medical and surgical specialties.
- Early diagnosis is the key to minimising mortality.
- Anticoagulation and thrombolytic therapy has lowered mortality from haemodynamically stable PE.

This topic discusses the presentation, tests and surgical management, but does not discuss medical management.

Pathophysiology in thoracic surgery

- Virchow's triad describes 3 main factors contributing to thrombus formation:
  - Haemodynamic changes (stasis, turbulence).
  - Hypercoagulability.
  - Vessel wall inflammation.
- The thoracic surgical population is an at risk group.
- Many have underlying co-morbidities predisposing to venous thromboembolism (malignancy, coagulopathy, and poor mobility pre-op/post-op).
- Thrombosis nearly always starts in the calf veins, which are involved in virtually all cases of symptomatic spontaneous lower extremity DVT.

Symptoms

- Fever.
- Chest pain, haemoptysis, shortness of breath (classic triad but only occurs in <20%).
- Chest wall tenderness.
- Back pain/shoulder pain/upper abdominal pain.
- Pleuritic or respirophasic chest pain (often considered pathognomonic—21% presenting with this symptom alone will have PE).
- Syncope.
- Pleuritic chest pain (worse on inspiration).
- New onset wheeze.
- Productive cough.
- New cardiac arrhythmia.
- Of patients who go on to die from massive PE.
  - 60% had dyspnoea.
  - 17% had chest pain.
  - 3% had haemoptysis.
- Patients may be completely asymptomatic.

Signs

General

- Fever
- Diaphoresis
- Lower limb oedema and thrombophlebitis.

CVS

- Right heart strain (↑JVP, ↑CVP, pulmonary regurgitation, loud P2, RV heave, murmur)
- Hypotension in acute massive PE
  - Results from acute cor pulmonale.

RS

- Atelectasis and alveolar infiltration
  - 24–72 hours later.
- New wheezing
- Pleural rub
- Tachypnoea
- Rales on auscultation
- Cyanosis.

Hypoxia in PE

- Results from an increase in alveolar dead space, right-to-left shunting, ventilation/perfusion mismatch and low mixed venous O_2.
- Hypocarbia results from hyperventilation in an attempt to compensate for increased dead space and hypoxia.
- Blood flow is diverted away from the embolized area, overperfusion of the un-embolized area results.
- Atelectasis develops distal to the embolus, further worsening V/Q mismatch.
  - Loss of surfactant and alveolar haemorrhage also contribute to the atelectasis.
- Platelet laden emboli release humoral mediators, further propagating thrombosis.

Massive PE

- The definition comprises the size of the clot and the effect upon the patient's cardiovascular system.
- Frequently presents with profound hypotension (systolic BP <90mmHg).
- Mortality 30%–60% depending on the study cited.
- Majority of deaths occur in the first 2 hours of care.

Non-massive PE

- Systolic arterial pressure greater than or equal to 90 mmHg (95% of patients).

Investigations

Bloods

- **FBC**.
  - WBC may be normal or elevated. Counts as high as 20 are not uncommon in patients with PE.
- **U+E, Glucose**.
- **Clotting**.
  - Normal in most patients.
  - ↑PT/↑APTT/↑clotting time have no prognostic value. PE can still occur in fully anti-coagulated patients.
- **D-dimer.**
  - Unique degradation product produced by plasmin-mediated proteolysis of cross-linked fibrin.
  - Considered positive if the level is greater than 500 ng/ml.
  - D–dimer may be raised in sepsis, malignancy and the post-operative patient so is non-specific.
- **ABG**.
  - PaO_2 has a zero or even negative predictive value in a typical population of patients in whom PE is suspected clinically.
  - Other diseases that manifest themselves in a similar manner to PE will also lower PaO_2.
  - May see hypoxaemia, hypocapnia or hypercapnoea, metabolic acidosis.

Radiology

- **CXR**.
  - Virtually always normal initially.
  - May show the Westermark sign (dilatation of the pulmonary vessels proximal to an embolism along with collapse of distal vessels, sometimes with a sharp cutoff).
  - Over time, atelectasis, which may progress to cause a small pleural effusion and an elevated hemidiaphragm.
  - After 24–72 hours, one third of patients with proven PE develop focal infiltrates that are indistinguishable from an infectious pneumonia.
  - The Hampton hump may be observed (classic textbook description); a triangular or rounded pleural-based infiltrate with the apex pointed toward the hilum, frequently located adjacent to the diaphragm.
- **Contrast-enhanced spiral CT chest**—in the stable patient!
  - Can immediately confirm the presence of a proximal PE.
  - Excludes an aortic dissection—inadvertent administration of thrombolytics or anticoagulants in this case could have lethal consequences.

- More sensitive than TOE because it can reliably assess distal branches of the pulmonary artery down to the level of segmental vessels.
- In suspected massive PE, spiral CT is reported to have 100% sensitivity and specificity.
- However, patients with intermediate-probability V/Q scan, this falls to 63% sensitivity and 89% specificity.
- **CT pulmonary angiography (CTPA).**
  - More invasive and harder to perform than spiral CT.
  - A positive pulmonary angiogram is foolproof there is an obstructtion to PA blood flow.
  - A negative pulmonary angiogram provides greater than 90% certainty in the exclusion of PE.
  - Emboli in vessels smaller than third order or lobular arteries are not seen however.
  - Tiny emboli in these vessels can still be seen at PM, even when angio was negative.
- **V/Q scan.**
  - Remains an important part of the evaluation when multidetector CT angiography is not available or not appropriate for the patient.
  - Most institutions will always report V/Q scans as abnormal, no matter what the actual pattern of perfusion.
  - A normal perfusion scan is the pattern with the highest predictive value.
  - You may see, 'indeterminate, intermediate, or low probability' which is not of much use.
  - (See Table 11.10 for V/Q results).

Other
- **ECG.**
  - $S_1Q_3T_3$ pattern (pathognomonic but rare).
  - Non-specific ST changes and sinus tachycardia (commonest).
  - Classic right heart strain and acute cor pulmonale—tall, peaked P waves in lead II (P pulmonale), right axis deviation, right bundle-branch block, an $S_1Q_3T_3$ pattern, or atrial fibrillation.
- **TOE.**
  - Inexpensive and rapidly performed at the bedside.
  - Heavily user-dependent and not readily available.
  - Can detect emboli in the main pulmonary arteries in approximately 70% of patients with haemodynamically significant PE.
  - Ineffective in detecting emboli within peripheral vessels.
  - Unlike CT, may provide additional information regarding homogeneity and mobility of emboli, their relation to the vascular lumen in cross-sectional planes and resultant flow disturbances.
  - This information may be useful to evaluate the age of the embolus and its susceptibility to thrombolysis.
- **Duplex ultrasound scan.**
  - Worth ruling out DVT if lower limb is phlebitis and history points to it.

Table 11.10 V/Q results, actual proven PE existence and next step management

V/Q result	Existence of PE	Plan
Normal	4%	Do nothing
Non-diagnostic (Low probability)	14%	Consider pulmonary angiography/HRCT
Non-diagnostic (Intermediate probability)	40%	Needs pulmonary angiography/HRCT
High	87%	Diagnosis—treat

Research
- Research has correlated a link between elevated brain-type natriuretic peptides (BNP) and right ventricular function in patients with PE, leading to an increased risk for complicated in-hospital course and 30-day mortality.
- A potential alternative to D-dimer is ischemia-modified albumin (IMA) level, which data suggest, is 93% sensitive and 75% specific for PE. IMA in combination with other probability scores appears to positively impact overall sensitivity and negative predictive value. The positive predictive value of IMA, in particular, is better than D-dimer. However, it should not be used alone and, apparently, is still unable to confirm a PE diagnosis with further investigation.

Treatment
The aim of treatment for PE is to relieve symptoms, to prevent recurrence and death and to reduce the risk of developing chronic pulmonary hypertension.

General management

- ABC assessment (suspect massive PE if severe haemodynamic compromise).
- 100% O_2.
- Obtain IV access and start fluid resuscitation (judicious as RV is already overloaded).
- Analgesia as necessary.

Management of massive PE

- Depending on the stability of the patient consider:
  - Anticoagulation (heparin or LMWH) if no contra-indications exist
  - Thrombolysis (e.g. Alteplase). Contra-indications should be sought
  - Surgical embolectomy depending on hospital protocol and availability. For details on the anaesthetic considerations for pulmonary embolectomy. (See 📖 Pulmonary embolectomy, p. 370).
- Institute invasive monitoring (arterial and CVP).
- Patient will require fluid resuscitation and in case of refractory hypotension-consider inotropic or vasopressor support.
- Patients may require ventilatory support.
- Treatment may need to be commenced on clinical grounds alone if cardiac arrest is imminent.
- Most deaths secondary to massive PE occur within 1 hour.

Management of non-massive PE

- In cases of high probability of PE start anticoagulation and then seek confirmation of the diagnosis.
- In cases of intermediate to low probability of PE perform D-dimer. If positive, start anticoagulation and proceed with confirmatory investigations (V/Q scan or CTPA). If D-dimer negative look for alternative diagnosis.

Pharmacological therapy

Un-fractionated heparin

- IV un-fractionated heparin is the initial anticoagulation of choice in PE.
- The advantage of heparin is that it has a short half life (useful if patient is likely to have to undergo surgery) and is easily reversible with protamine.

LMWH

- This group of anticoagulants have many advantages over un-fractionated heparin.
- They require no blood level monitoring, have a greater bioavailability, a longer half life and a more predictable dose response.

Warfarin

- Oral anticoagulation should only be started in confirmed cases of PE.
- It should be overlapped with un-fractionated heparin or LMWH for five days to prevent the early pro-coagulant effect of un-opposed warfarin.

Post-operative arrhythmias

Arrhythmias in critical Illness

- Unsurprisingly the combination of severe illness, metabolic stress and acutely deranged physiology is a potent stimulus for arrhythmias.
- These are most commonly supraventricular (SVT) and frequently require treatment.
- AF occurs in up to 25% of patients after thoracic surgery.
- Ventricular arrhythmias occur in up to 15% of patients and appear to be associated with AF.
- They are associated with increased morbidity, hospital stay and mortality.
- Through reductions in cardiac output and oxygen delivery, they have a variety of detrimental effects on organ function.

More benign rhythms have already been discussed (See 📖 Low cardiac output state, p. 656). This section aims to tackle the more life-threatening post-operative arrhythmias.

General prevention

- Maintain normal cellular homeostasis and correct physiological disturbances pre-emptively.
- Avoidance of cellular hypoxia and consequent ion channel dysfunction is of paramount importance.
- Pharmacological prophylaxis has been studied, predominantly in cardiac surgery; agents with class II (β-adrenergic antagonist) action (including amiodarone) appear the most useful.
- Other agents that may reduce peri-operative arrhythmias include diltiazem, verapamil and magnesium.

Adverse signs

- Any of the following accompanying the arrhythmia warrants intervention:
  - Hypotension.
  - Chest pain.
  - Signs of heart failure.
  - Reduced level of consciousness.

Treatment

- It is essential to establish:
  - The effect of the rhythm on the patient.
  - The diagnosis (in broad terms).
  - Any identifiable precipitant.
- A thorough history and examination is mandatory.
- Treatment algorhythms such as those utilized in ALS can help guide emergency treatment (beyond the scope of this text).

- In general, tachyarrhythmias causing adverse signs should be electrically cardioverted and pharmacological treatment of severe bradyarrhythmias serves to buy time before definitive electrical pacing.

Immediate treatment of any severe arrhythmia

- High flow 100% O_2, ABC approach.
- Ensure adequate breathing/ventilation.
- Intubate as necessary.
- Establish continuous monitoring (ECG, SpO_2, NIBP).
- IV access.

Investigations

Bloods
- **FBC, U+Es, Cardiac Enzymes, TFTs, Mg^{++}, Ca^{++}.**
- **ABGs.**

Radiology
- **CXR.**

Other
- **12-lead ECG +/– rhythm strip.**
- **Echocardiogram.**
  - TOE if anaesthetized and skilled operator.

Specific life-threatening arrhythmias

Ventricular tachycardia (VT)

- Monomorphic (most common), or polymorphic (associated with prolonged QT syndrome).
- If lasts >30s, classified as sustained.
- Often symptomatic and can degenerate into VF.
- Broad complex tachycardia should be considered VT until proven otherwise; inappropriate treatment for SVT can be fatal.
- The most common mechanism is via micro re-entry through ischaemic/scarred myocardium.
- AV dissociation is diagnostic, but difficult to visualize with fast rates.
- Capture and fusion beats confirm AV dissociation.
- If a typical bundle branch pattern is seen in the chest leads and there is no AV dissociation, then the rhythm is supraventricular with bundle branch block.

Treatment

Monomorphic VT

- If adverse signs → DCCV.
- If haemodynamically stable → amiodarone 300 mg initial dose, followed by 900 mg over the proceeding 24 h.

Polymorphic VT

- A variant that causes QRS complexes to vary both in axis and amplitude, giving rise to the name Torsades de Pointes.
- It may occur secondary to prolonged QT syndrome or myocardial ischaemia.
- If adverse signs → DCCV.
- If haemodynamically stable → magnesium.

Ventricular Fibrillation (VF)

- This rhythm is not compatible with a cardiac output and so rapid loss of consciousness ensues.
- It is often fatal but has the best outcome of all cardiac arrest rhythms if witnessed and treated rapidly with pre-cordial thump DCCV.
- The ECG shows disorganized and chaotic electrical activity of varying amplitude.
- In general, the greater the amplitude the better the prognosis.

Treatment

- Immediate DCCV.
- If sustained/shock resistant → amiodarone (as above).

SVT

- Rate control of SVT is rarely accomplished with digoxin alone and β-blockade is often inappropriate.
- Electrical cardioversion may be warranted but arrhythmias commonly recur.
- Amiodarone has proven a valuable agent in this setting due to its predictability and relatively good short-term side-effect profile.
- Magnesium is probably underused as a rate-controlling agent.
- Risks of systemic anticoagulation often outweigh any perceived benefits in these patients.

AV nodal re-entry tachycardias (AVNRT)

- The re-entry circuit is confined to the AV node itself.
- Patients often present with palpitations.
- They are not often associated with structural heart disease.

Treatment

- If adverse signs (rare) and no adenosine → DCCV.
- If haemodynamically stable → vagal maneuvers, adenosine (can use flecainide, sotalol or verapamil).
- Long-term → radiofrequency ablation ± surgery.

AV re-entry tachycardias

- An accessory pathway exists (most commonly the Bundle of Kent), bypassing the AV node.
- Patients with WPW can develop AVRT or AF, which itself can deteriorate into VF if untreated.
- In this variant of AF, rapid and (variably) wide QRS complexes are seen, commonly causing haemodynamic compromise.

Treatment

- If adverse signs (rare) and no adenosine → DCCV.
- If haemodynamically stable → vagal maneuvers, adenosine (can use flecainide or sotalol).
- Long-term → radiofrequency ablation ± surgery.
- ! Digoxin and verapamil are absolutely contraindicated in suspected WPW with tachycardia, as these drugs may precipitate fatal VF.

Atrial fibrillation (AF)

- The most common arrhythmia in the post operative thoracic patient.
- Associated with increased risk of stroke, other arrhythmias and prolonged hospital stay.
- It may be asymptomatic or present with palpitations, heart failure or embolic phenomena.
- It may be chronic or paroxysmal.
- The risk of intra-atrial thrombus increases with time and thus it is important to establish the duration of AF.

Fast AF treatment

- If adverse signs → synchronized DCCV ± amiodarone.
- If stable + >48 hrs → control rate (β-blocker, magnesium, digoxin).
- If stable + <48 hrs consider amiodarone.

Atrial flutter

Anticoagulation in AF

- Risks must be balanced against those of bleeding, particularly in the perioperative setting.
- Age and other medical co-morbidities are other important considerations.
- Incidence of stroke in AF is between 5–8% per year.
- Systemic anticoagulation reduces this by about 50%.
- TOE may assist clinical decisions to attempt cardioversion, whether electrical or chemical (exclusion of intra-cardiac thrombi).

Cardioversion in AF

- Many anti-arrhythmic drugs are associated with significant side effects, particularly with long-term or in the presence of structural heart disease.
- Advice from cardiology can be extremely helpful.
- Sustained cardioversion is likely to be unsuccessful if LA diameter >45 mm or in the context of ongoing critical illness.

- Due to retention of atrial contractility, it causes haemodynamic compromise less commonly.
- It may deteriorate into AF.
- Drugs prolonging AV node conduction will slow ventricular rate but rarely revert to sinus rhythm.

Treatment

- If adverse signs → synchronized DCCV.
- If haemodynamically stable → control rate (β-blockers, digoxin, amiodarone, verapamil).
- AVOID class I drugs (can cause 1:1 conduction).

Atrial Flutter (AFl)

- Due to retention of atrial contractility, causes haemodynamic compromise less commonly.
- It may deteriorate into AF.
- Drugs prolonging AV node conduction will slow ventricular rate but rarely revert to sinus rhythm.

Treatment

- Cardiac pacing is necessary in symptomatic patients and anti-arrhythmics for patients with brady-tachy syndrome.

Sick sinus syndrome

- May be associated with congenital and ischaemic cardiac disease.
- A variety of arrhythmias occur including sinus bradycardia, SA arrest and bradycardia-tachycardia syndrome.
- AF and or AFl may also occur, typically episodically.
- It may present as syncope, near-syncope or cardiac arrest.

Further reading

Amar D, Zhang H, Roistacher N. The incidence and outcome of ventricular arrhythmias after non-cardiac thoracic surgery. *Anaesthesia and Analgesia* 2002; 95(3):537–43.

Sedrakyan A, Treasure T, Browne J, Krumholz H, Sharpin C, van der Meulin. Pharmacologic prophylaxis for postoperative atrial tachyarrhythmias in general thoracic surgery: evidence from randomized clinical trials. *Journal of Thoracic and Cardiovascular Surgery* 2005; 129(5):997–1005.

Bersten AD, Soni N, Oh TE. (2003) *Oh's Intensive Care Manual*, 5th ed. Edinburgh: Butterworth Heinemann.

Cardiac herniation

- A rare but potentially fatal complication of intrapericardial pneumonectomy.
  - Case reports after lobectomy and after closure of the pericardial defect.
  - Cardiac herniation can also occur following traumatic rupture of the pericardium, particularly after blunt chest trauma.
  - Can occur secondary to congenital pericardial defects.
- Herniation occurs through the pericardial defect created during surgery. It is more likely if the defect is large and has been left open.
- There is an increasing incidence as a result of more radical procedures being performed for the treatment of lung cancer.
- A high index of suspicion is required to successfully diagnose this complication.
- Emergency re-operation offers the only chance re-survival. Overall mortality is between 30–64%.
- Cardiac herniation can be effectively prevented by patching the pericardial defect with tissue such as fascia lata or an artificial Teflon patch at the time of primary surgery.

Signs and symptoms

- Signs and symptoms of cardiac herniation are related to the location of the pericardial defect.
- A right sided herniation causes kinking or torsion of the SVC and IVC resulting in a dramatic fall in cardiac filling with subsequent hypotension, tachycardia and raised CVP.
  - Right sided herniations are more common than left.
- A left sided herniation causes compression or strangulation of the ventricular wall resulting in sudden hypotension, dysrrhythmias including VF, and myocardial infarction.
- ❶ There should be a high index of suspicion of cardiac herniation after pneumonectomy in any patient with sudden onset of a low cardiac output state in the absence of haemorrhage or cardiac failure.
- 75% of cases present before completion of surgery usually during repositioning or extubation of the patient.
- Cardiac herniation is very rare >24 hr post operatively due to the formation of adhesions between the heart and pericardium.
- There is a single case report of cardiac herniation occurring six months after a right intrapericardial pneumonectomy.

Risk factors

- Repositioning onto the operated side.
- Coughing.
  - This causes a large increase in thoracic pressure directly affecting the exposed pericardium after pneumonectomy.
- Positive pressure ventilation
  - During re-operation efforts should be made to minimize peak airway pressures.
- Applying excessive suction to chest drains.

Investigations

No single imaging modality is diagnostic of cardiac herniation.

Radiology
- **CXR.**
  - May show a distorted cardiac shadow characterized by a snow cone appearance, particularly in right sided herniation.
  - A left sided herniation may only be visible on a lateral film.
- **CT imaging.**
  - May be helpful but is rarely practical in the emergency situation.

Other
- **TTE/TOE.**
  - May show obstructed pulmonary arterial flow and impaired filling.
  - It may be helpful in excluding other causes of sudden post-operative shock.
- **ECG.**
  - May show ST-T wave abnormalities or abnormal rotation of the axis.

Treatment
- Re-operation and return of the heart to its normal position is the only treatment available.
- Patch closure of the pericardial defect is then required.
- While waiting for re-operation, simple steps can be taken to limit the cardiovascular sequelae of the herniation.
  - The patient should be turned onto the non operative side.
  - Suction of the chest drains should be discontinued.
  - The patient should be allowed to continue spontaneous ventilation for as long as possible in order to reduce intrathoracic pressure.
  - If the patient if ventilated, peak pressures should be reduced to the minimum possible and the ventilatory rate increased to compensate.
  - Efforts should be made to reduce any coughing e.g. if the patient is intubated, sedation should be increased or muscle paralysis used.

Techniques in thoracic anaesthesia

Total intravenous anaesthesia (TIVA)

TIVA involves the use of a combination of intravenous drugs (anaesthetic agent and analgesic agent), in the absence of all inhalational anaesthetic agents including nitrous oxide, to provide general anaesthesia

The pharmacodynamic and pharmacokinetic properties of newer intravenous anaesthetic agents like propofol, and short-acting opioids such as remifentanil, render them inherently suitable for administration via continuous infusion.

Sophisticated computer models, and subsequently software incorporating these into infusion devices, have been developed relatively recently. Consequently, the delivery of intravenous anaesthesia has become more practical, user friendly and readily applicable to thoracic anaesthesia.

Basic concepts involved in TIVA

Target controlled infusion (TCI)

- Allows delivery of a pre-determined blood concentration of a particular drug, based on a patient's sex, age and weight, by automatically adjusting the rate of infusion of the drug, until the anaesthetist enters a different "target" concentration.

Pharmacokinetics

- A three compartment is used.
  - Central compartment—into which the initial bolus of drug is injected.
  - Second compartment—receives drug from the central compartment first, consisting of well-perfused tissues with a high rate of drug uptake.
  - Third compartment—final compartment; has a much slower rate of uptake, representing the poorly-perfused tissues in the body.
- Once the target value, is set an initial bolus is calculated and delivered according to estimation of the volume of the central compartment
- The device then modifies the infusion rate to maintain the target value, allowing for the redistribution and elimination of the drug
  - If the anaesthetist increases the target value, the device delivers a rapid infusion to reach the new target concentration.
  - If a lower target concentration is required, the system pauses, allowing the effect site concentration to fall, and then restarts at a lower infusion rate.

Context sensitive half time

- This concept refers to the fact that a relationship exists between a drug's rate of elimination from the body and its duration of infusion.

- It is defined as the time plasma concentration takes to fall to 50% of the value after discontinuing an infusion.
- Following a prolonged infusion there will be more drug to redistribute from the peripheral compartments back into the central compartment, which will tend to maintain the plasma concentration and duration of action.

Practical issues

- Secure intravenous access is required that can be readily visualized by the anaesthetist.
- The EC50 (effective concentration required to prevent 50% of patients moving in response to a painful stimulus) has been measured as 6–7 µg/ml with an oxygen: air mix and 4–5 µg/ml with 67% nitrous oxide in ASA I and II patients.
- There are large variations between individual patients pharmacokinetic and pharmacodynamic characteristics. The administration of other drugs such as opiates and benzodiazepines will reduce propofol requirements.
- The target concentration will therefore be determined according to the patient's response and the clinical situation.

Dosing schedule

- Induction with propofol.
  - 4–8 µg/ml is usually selected (although concurrent administration of other drugs may modify this).
- Maintenance
  - 3–6 µg/ml is adequate under most circumstances. In the elderly or high-risk patient a lower initial target should be set, and increased incrementally until the desired effect is achieved.
- Sedation
  - 0.5–2.5µg/ml are usually required.

For concurrent remifentanil dosing schedule (See 📖 Analgesics, p. 118).

Advantages in thoracic anaesthesia

- Beneficial in circumstances where accurate delivery of inhalational agents may be difficult e.g. laryngoscopy, bronchoscopy.
- Propofol does not attenuate the hypoxic pulmonary vasoconstriction response, in contrast to inhalational agents, and therefore there is a potential benefit of using the technique in thoracic surgery, in patients undergoing one lung ventilation.
- Avoids unwanted side effects of volatile agents and nitrous oxide.
- Safe in malignant hyperpyrexia susceptible patients.
- Use of remifentanil via TCI allows for ease of analgesia control (particularly for acutely painful/stimulating situations).

Disadvantages

- Cost.
- Perceived increased risk of awareness; there is an inherent feedback mechanism during delivery of inhalational anaesthesia to a spontaneously breathing patient to regulate the depth of anaesthesia.
  - If the spontaneously breathing patient is in too light a plane of anaesthesia, their minute volume will increase and consequently so will the delivery of anaesthetic agent.
  - Conversely, a patient's minute volume will tend to fall as they enter a deeper plane of anaesthesia, therefore reducing drug delivery.
  - This offers a degree of protection against the possibility of awareness.
  - Cardiovascular, renal or hepatic impairment may affect pharmakokinetics.
- If remifentanil is turned off too early, the patient will awaken in pain unless other longer acting forms of analgesia are in place.

Patient positioning

General protective measures

Principles are the same as for any other kind of surgery:

- Do not to over extend joints (usually not >90 degrees).
- Pad areas in direct contact with metal or hard surfaces.
- Keep eyes closed and/or pad appropriately.
- Minimize objects/cables touching the patient.
  - Protect all pressure areas as procedures can be lengthy.

The lateral decubitus position (see Fig. 12.1)

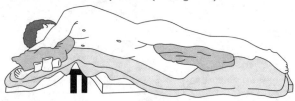

Fig. 12.1 The left lateral decubitus position.

Terminology

- When positioned in the left lateral (decubitus) position the patient lies on his left side to provide access for a right sided procedure (thoracotomy).
- The uppermost side is referred to as the non-dependent side.
- The lowermost side is referred to as the dependent side.

The position

- Arms are placed above the axilla in order to facilitate surgical access.
- ⚠ Brachial plexus traction—take extra care to prevent weight bearing on the arm or axilla.
- Ensure most of the weight of the body is borne by the chest, supported by a vacuum splint or pads.
- ⚠ Dependent arm compression—particularly in the deltoid region.
- Move arm from under the chest into a flexed position underneath the non-dependent arm support.
- ⚠ Dependent iliac crest is also vulnerable on the dependent side
- It is advisable to pad the area.

Physiological changes

- Moving to the lateral position alters the ventilation perfusion relationships. (See 📖 One lung ventilation and the lateral decubitus position, see p. 14).
- Lower lung receives increased perfusion and decreased ventilation due to gravity.

- Upper lung receives reduced perfusion and increased ventilation.
- ⚠ Ventilation perfusion mismatch can occur. Positioning of the patient should take account of the need for the dependent lung to expand. If pads or bolsters are placed directly under the chest rather than below the axilla or the hip then the mechanics of ventilation will be further impaired.

The 'Table Break" position

- Opens the thoracic cavity more easily for the surgeon.
- Can cause compression of the great vessels in the chest/abdomen leading to reduced venous return and arterial outflow obstruction, both of which can cause hypotension.

Special points

- Cardiorespiratory compromise is common during patient positioning.
- Monitoring must be rapidly re-established after transfer.
- If cardiorespiratory compromise occurs, the table break should be removed first, then if necessary, the patient placed in supine position.
- Double lumen tubes WILL move! Remember to check that position is optimal using a fibreoscope. Particularly if right sided DLT.
- Check all monitoring and lines are secure, accessible and untangled and position of patient is optimal with stable vital signs.

Further reading

Cucchiara R, Faust J, Patient Positioning In *Anaesthesia* 5th ed. Miller D. Oxford: Churchill Livingstone; 2004.

Servant C, Purkiss S. *Positioning Patients for Surgery*. Greenwich Medical Media; 2002.

Anderton JM, Keen RI, Neave R. *Positioning the Surgical Patient*. Butterworths; 1988.

Thoracic epidurals

It is well known that post-operative pulmonary complications often have a greater impact upon mortality and morbidity in the thoracic surgical population. Thoracic epidural anaesthesia (TEA) is considered to be the gold standard.

Aims

- Pain free coughing and deep breathing.
- Bilateral sensory block of surgical site/s.
- Selective thoracic sympathectomy.
- Minimal motor involvement.

Indications

- Analgesia following thoracic or upper gastrointestinal surgery.
- Analgesia following thoracic trauma (flail chest, rib fractures).

Contraindications

Absolute
- Patient refusal.
- Uncorrected coagulopathy (INR>1.5, platelets <50).
- Therapeutic anticoagulation.
- Local skin infection.
- Raised ICP.
- Uncorrected hypovolaemia.

Relative (risk v_s benefit)
- Neurological disorders.
- Fixed cardiac output state.
- Abnormal spinal anatomy.
- If platelets <80, consider further investigation and risk:benefit consideration.
- Antiplatelet medication (clopidogrel in particular).
- Prophylactic anticoagulation; requires careful planning to ensure epidural performed during a safe time period.

Benefits of epidural analgesia

- Strong cough and deep breathing:
  - ↓ post-operative pulmonary complications.
- Early, un-impaired mobilization:
  - ↓ thromboembolism risk.
- Selective sympathetic blockade:
  - ↓ post-operative ischaemic events in at risk groups.
  - Coronary sympathetic input → lower maximal heart rate, coronary vasodilation and improved myocardial oxygen delivery.
  - ↓ post-operative stress response (↓ circulating catecholamines).

- Gastro-intestinal:
  - Minimization of post-operative ileus.
  - Protein sparing.

Thoracic spine anatomy

- 12 vertebrae.
- The thoracic spine is kyphotic.
- Spinous processes steeply aligned in the high/mid thoracic region, and less so in the lower thoracic spine.
- Borders:
  - Antero-lateral: Pedicles and anterior neural arch.
  - Postero-lateral: Laminae and ligamentum flavum.
- Thoracic nerve roots are half the diameter of lumbar roots, and thus are preferentially blocked.
- Preganglionic sympathetic fibres exit via T1-L2 roots.

Technique

- Loss of resistance to air or saline is used. Saline is associated with a reduced dural puncture rate.
- It is arguable that ALL epidurals should be performed in the awake patient as:
  - Shooting pain/paraesthesia may denote wrong placement.
  - One can assess sensory block before GA.
- The approximate bony level can be identified from surface anatomical landmarks:
  - The spine of the scapula lies at T3.
  - Inferior angle scapula lies at T7.
  - Tuffier's line is at the level of the anterior, superior iliac crests (about L3/4).

Approach

Midline

- Straightforward in lower thoracic spine. Steep angulation of the spinous processes in the mid and upper thoracic spine requires a variable degree of cephalad angulation of the needle.

Paramedian

- Often preferred because of the steep oblique angle of the thoracic spinous processes.
- For a paramedian approach, the Tuohy needle is inserted 1–2 cm lateral to the spinous process of the more cephalad vertebra.
- The needle is advanced perpendicular to the skin until the lamina or pedicle is encountered, and then redirected 30° cephalad and 15° medially.
- The needle is then "walked off" the lamina, at which point the needle should be approaching the ligamentum flavum.
- The needle is then advanced using a loss of resistance technique. Note that the thoracic ligaments are less dense and a false loss of resistance is not uncommon.

- Approximately 4–5 cm of catheter may be left in the epidural space. Too short and it may fall out. Too long and the tip may lie in an inappropriate position.

Insertion site

- More cranial spread of LA occurs after low/mid thoracic epidurals, than higher ones.
- Therefore, mid/low epidurals should be sited at a bony level that corresponds roughly to the midpoint of the surgical incision; higher epidurals should be sited more cranially to the incision to provide optimal wound coverage.

Suggested regime

- Local protocols vary; an example is described below:
  - 3 ml 0.25% L-bupivacaine test dose; presence of a subarachnoid catheter should become clear at this point.
  - Fentanyl 50–100 mcg bolus.
  - Further 2–5 ml increments of 0.25% L-bupivacaine intra-operatively to establish block.
  - Commence infusion of 0.1% L-bupivacaine + 2 mcg/ml fentanyl or 0.1 mg/ml diamorphine; infuse at 0–10 ml/hr.
- In the elderly it may be necessary to reduce the loading dose by up to 40%.

Benefits of epidural LA + opioid mix over LA or opioid alone

- Best analgesia during mobilization.
- Less hypotension.
- Minimal duration of ileus.
- Increased time to first analgesic rescue.

Side effects

Technical

- Failure to site epidural.
- Problems with block achieved (inadvertently high, inadequate height, unilateral, or patchy).
- Dural puncture headache (dural puncture rate is 0.4%; lower rate of headache with higher thoracic epidurals).

Drug related
- Hypotension, (may present with dizziness, nausea and vomiting).
- Local anaesthetic toxicity.
- Total spinal.
- Itching, nausea, respiratory depression (opioid related).
- Urinary retention.
- Bradycardia (high thoracic block).
- Reduced respiratory function (opiate related).
- ❶ Rare, but can cause potentially catastrophic neurological impairment
  - Epidural haematoma.
  - Epidural abscess.
  - Spinal cord injury.
  - Anterior spinal artery syndrome.

Evidence

- Isolated, self limiting nerve lesions have been reported in about 1:200 patients following thoracic epidural insertion.
- The 3rd National Audit Project (NAP 3).
  - 1:24,000–1:54,000 (0.002%) patients suffered permanent neurological injury.
  - 1:50,000–1:140,000 (0.0007%) resulted in death or paraplegia.
- Few randomized controlled studies exist directly comparing epidural to PVB. The data available does suggest that paravertebral blockade provides comparable analgesia with a better side-effect profile.
- In spite of this, studies have not been able to consistently demonstrate a mortality benefit.
- For this reason the risk to benefit ratio of insertion should be carefully evaluated and discussed with the patient. Many anaesthetists obtain specific consent prior to inserting an epidural.
- Failure fall-out rates vary widely and are dependent on the institute, but are probably around 15%.

Guidelines for patients receiving anticoagulation

- Due to the relative infrequency of complications, guidance regarding anti-coagulation and thromboprophylaxis is based largely on consensus, and local practice, rather than data from trials.
- ❶ All patients receiving epidural analgesia should be closely monitored for signs of neurological deficit suggestive of vertebral canal haematoma or abscess. This includes:
  - Back pain, sensory changes and in particular, loss of motor function.
  - Conventional regimes with dilute local anaesthetic for should not precipitate motor block.

Anti-coagulation
Warfarin

- Before thoracic epidural analgesia warfarin should be discontinued for at least 4–5 days. The INR should be within normal limits prior to placement. Warfarin therapy should not be re-instituted until after removal of the epidural catheter and the INR should be <1.5 prior to catheter removal.

Anti-platelet agents

- There is considerable variability in patient responses to antiplatelet agents. Thrombocytopenia is a relative contraindication dependent on the circumstances. There may yet be a role for testing of platelet function prior to neuraxial block.
- NSAIDs (including aspirin).
  - In isolation do not appear to increase the risk of vertebral canal haematoma in patients undergoing neuraxial blockade.
- Thienopyrdine derivatives including Clopidogrel and ticlopidine.
  - Potent antiplatelet agents causing irreversible inhibition of ADP.
  - Clopidogrel should be discontinued at least 7 days and ticlodipine at least 10–14 days prior to neuraxial blockade.

Anti-platelet agents and coronary stents

- After insertion, patients with bare metal stents require aspirin and clopidogrel for at least 4 weeks. Patients with drug eluting stents require aspirin and clopidogrel for at least 12 months.
- ❶ Stopping one or more anti-platelet agents may make epidural analgesia safer, but significantly increase the risk of peri-operative stent thrombosis.

Thromboprophylaxis

- Options include multiple daily dosing of subcutaneous unfractionated heparin, or once-daily low-molecular weight heparins (LMWH).
- Local guidelines vary but in general an epidural should not be sited or removed within 4 hours of s/c heparin, 3 hours after IV heparin and 12 hours of LMWH adminstration.

Pitfalls

- Lumbar epidural is unsuitable for thoracic/upper abdominal surgery:
  - Poor analgesia due to inadequate sensory block height associated with a dense motor block which restricts mobilization.
  - Resultant hypotension and pain can lead to tachycardia and coronary vasoconstriction (sympathetic outflow to coronary circulation is not blocked), potentially causing myocardial ischaemia.
- However, complete cardiac sympathetic block does not always occur with high thoracic epidurals.
- Unilateral block may result from poor technique, inadequate LA volume, or passage of the catheter through an intervertebral foramen.
- Hypotension:
  - Epidural infusion + GA may result in profound hypotension.
  - Exclude surgical bleeding as the cause of intra-operative hypotension BEFORE attributing it to epidural infusion.
- Trained staff must manage epidurals peri-operatively to ensure maximum benefit.
- Securing methods are NOT uniform amongst clinicians:
  - Using sutures/tunneling may be associated with a higher rate of local infection.
  - UK fall-out rates vary enormously.
  - Histoacryl® skin adhesive has been used to secure the catheter to the patient's back. Benefits are a reduced fall-out rate, antimicrobial action and speed of use.

Further reading

McLeod G and Cumming C. Thoracic epidural anaesthesia and analgesia. Continuing Education in Anaesthesia, *Critical Care and Pain* 2004; 4:16–19.

Cook TM, Counsell D, Wildsmith JA. Major complications of central neuraxial blocks: report on the 3rd National Audit of The Royal College of Anaesthetists. *British Journal of Anaesthesia* 2009; 102:179–190.

Wilkinson J, Chikhani M. The use of Histoacryl® skin adhesive to secure thoracic epidural catheters: a volunteer study. *Regional Anesthesia and Pain Medicine.* 32(5):148.

Thoracic paravertebral block

- Paravertebral block is the introduction of local anaesthetic into the space lying just lateral to the vertebra.
- Local anaesthetic penetrates the spinal nerves as they emerge from the intervertebral foramina.
- Provides potent unilateral analgesia and sympathetic blockade over several dermatomes adjacent to the level of injection.
- It may be administered via single or multiple shot injections, or via a continuous infusion catheter. Injections can also be made bilaterally.

Indications

Postoperative analgesia
- Thoracic surgery.
- Upper abdominal surgery.
- Breast surgery.

Surgical anaesthesia
- Breast surgery.
- Chest wound exploration.

Trauma
- Fractured ribs.

Contraindications
- Patient refusal.
- Infection at insertion site.
- Emphysema.
- Tumour in the paravertebral space.
- Anticoagulation/coagulopathy relative contraindication.

Advantages
- Less hypotension compared to epidural.
- Comparable postoperative analgesia to epidural when given by continuous infusion.
- Provides superior analgesia to intrathecal, intercostal, extrapleural blocks and standard intravenous analgesia.
- Possibly less risk in anticoagulated patients than epidural insertion.

Technique

Landmark
- Patient positioned lateral or sitting.
- Strict aseptic technique.

- Palpate spinous process corresponding to desired level of incision; usually spinous process of T5 or T6.
- Mark needle insertion point 3 cm lateral to the cephalad edge of the spinous process.
- Raise a weal of lidocaine at insertion point, and then advance a 16–18G Tuohy needle perpendicular to the skin in all planes until the transverse process is contacted at ~3cm depth.
- Withdraw the needle slightly and re-angle cephalad. "Walk" off the bone in a cephalad direction and advance up to 1 cm further.
- Some practitioners recommend a loss of resistance technique (air/ saline). Loss of resistance is felt as the needle passes through the superior costo-transverse ligament.
  - This endpoint is not as distinct as that found with epidural insertion.
  - Some authors suggest the needle should simply be stopped 1 cm deep to the transverse process.
- Aspirate prior to injection to check for air/blood/CSF and slowly inject local anaesthetic in 5 ml aliquots with repeated aspiration.
- A catheter may be inserted via the Tuohy needle, or intra-operatively under direct vision by the surgeon.

Local anaesthetic dose

- Single shot technique:
  - 15–20 ml 0.25%-0.5% bupivacaine (± epinephrine 1:200,000); can spread up to 3–5 dermatomes .
- Infusion.
  - Single shot injection followed by catheter infusion of 0.25% bupivacaine at 0.1 ml/kg/hour.
- Multiple single shot technique:
  - 5ml 0.5% bupivacaine with epinephrine (2.5 µg/ml) at each level required can provide analgesia for an average of 22 hours.

Ultrasound-guided

Distance to space guidance

- Ultrasound is now being used to measure depth to transverse process prior to insertion of the needle with the landmark technique.
- Though the technique of needle insertion remains the same, the information about depth to paravertebral space is thought to reduce inadvertent overshoot.
- The long axis of the ultrasound probe is placed in line with the spinal column, 3 cm lateral to the spinous processes. Parietal pleura and transverse processes are identified as hyperechoic structures and the distance from the skin measured.
- Thus, the operator knows how far to advance the needle before expecting contact with the transverse process.

Continuous in plane technique
- "In plane" techniques have been described which aim to enhance safety by continuous visualization of the needle tip until the paravertebral space is reached:
  - Place the ultrasound probe on the back of the patient with the long axis lying on the horizontal plane, and the medial edge of the probe on the spinous process at the desired level.
  - Move the probe slightly cephalad to visualize the transverse process and the paravertebral space beneath it.
  - Advance the needle in a lateral to medial direction within the ultrasound beam until the costo-transverse ligament is passed.
- ⚠ While visualization of the needle theoretically reduces the risk of pleural damage, it is self-evident that the needle tip will still pass close to the same structures as with any paravertebral block and the same degree of caution should be used.

Complications
- Pneumothorax.
  - Avoid lateral angulation of the needle.
  - Transverse process must be contacted prior to advancement into the paravertebral space. If it is not contacted the needle may be between transverse processes and further advancement may overshoot and puncture the pleura.
- Inadvertent epidural/subarachnoid injection—avoid medial angulation of the needle.
- Inadvertent intravascular injection of local anaesthetic.
- Nerve injury.
- Spinal cord damage.
- Local anaesthetic toxicity.
- Haematoma.
- Infection.

Further reading

Karmakar M. Thoracic paravertebral block. *Anesthesiology* 2001; 95(3):771–80.

Joshi G, Bonnet F, Shah R, *et al.* A systematic review of randomized trials evaluating regional techniques for post-thoracotomy analgesia. *Anesthesia and Analgesia* 2008; 107(3):1026–40.

Pusch F, Wildling E, Klimscha W, *et al.* Sonographic measurement of needle insertion depth in paravertebral blocks in women. *British Journal of Anaesthesia* 2000; 85(6):841–3.

Intra-pleural analgesia

Intra-pleural block requires injection of local anaesthetic into the space between the parietal and visceral pleura, to produce ipsilateral somatic blockade of multiple thoracic dermatomes. The terms "intra-pleural" and "inter-pleural" are used interchangeably.

▶ The efficacy of intra-pleural block following thoracotomy is inconsistent.

Indications

- To provide unilateral analgesia following thoracic surgery, breast surgery and upper abdominal surgery.
- To provide analgesia for non-surgical pain e.g. chronic pain syndromes, herpes zoster and pancreatitis.

Contraindications

Absolute
- Patient refusal.
- Allergy to local anaesthetic agent.
- Localized infection at insertion site.

Relative
- Emphysema.
- Bullous lung disease.
- Recent pulmonary infection or empyema.
- Pleural adhesions or pleurodesis.
- Haemothorax.
- Coagulopathy.
- Contralateral phrenic nerve paralysis.

Anatomy

- The intercostal space has 3 muscle layers:
  - External intercostal muscle.
  - Internal intercostal muscle which becomes fibrous posteriorly at the angle of rib to form the posterior intercostal membrane.
  - Innermost intercostals muscle (intercostalis intimus).
- Intercostalis intimus is incomplete and freely allows fluid to pass into the sub-pleural space. Thus, intra-pleural analgesia can be achieved by 2 routes:
  - Placing LA either between the visceral and parietal layers of pleura.
  - Placing LA deep to the internal intercostal muscle but superficial to parietal pleura.
- In either case, LA will diffuse around adjacent intercostal nerves.
- LA tends to accumulate in the paravertebral space and block the sympathetic chain.

Technique

(See Fig. 12.2)

- Position the patient as for epidural catheter insertion.
- The insertion point lies anywhere between a point 8 cm lateral to the spine (T_4 to T_8), and the mid-axillary line.
- A continuous pressure, loss-of-resistance technique using saline, as opposed to air, is advocated to reduce the risk of pneumothorax.
- The patient's breath is held at end-inspiration if spontaneously breathing or end-expiration if ventilated with positive pressure. This ensures maintenance of maximal negative pressure during needle insertion.
- A Tuohy needle is "walked off" the superior border of the rib. A "pop" may be felt as the needle pierces the posterior intercostal membrane. A loss of resistance indicates the pleural space.
- An epidural catheter is commonly inserted by 5–6 cm, but single-shot injections can be used.
- Alternatively a catheter can be placed under direct vision by the surgeon during the procedure.

Doses and infusions

- One shot injection:
  - 5–30 ml bupivacaine 0.5% ±1:200,000 epinephrine.
- Continuous infusion:
  - 0.1–0.5 ml/kg/hr bupivacaine 0.5%.

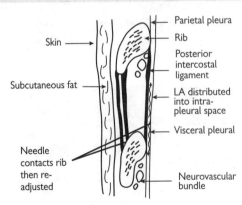

Fig. 12.2 Approach for intra-pleural analgesia.

Practical issues

- The number of nerves affected depends upon:
  - Level of the catheter.
  - Volume and concentration of drug used.
  - Effects of gravity.
- Following thoracotomy, most patients will have a chest drain inserted. LA injected into the intra-pleural space WILL drain from the chest via the ICD and thus reduce any benefit.
- The presence of blood in the thoracic cavity may also reduce the effect.

Complications

- Pneumothorax.
- Systemic local anaesthetic toxicity.
- Phrenic nerve paralysis.
- Recurrent laryngeal nerve paralysis.
- Horner's syndrome.
- Haemorrhage.
- Ipsilateral Bronchospasm.
- Intra-bronchial injection.
- Pleural effusion.
- Bronchopleural fistula.
- Infection.

Further reading

Kambam JR, Hammon J, Parris WC, et al. Intrapleural analgesia for post-thoracotomy pain and blood levels of bupivacaine following intrapleural injection. *Canadian Journal of Anesthesia* 1989; 36:106–9.

Murphy DF. Interpleural analgesia. *British Journal of Anaesthesia* 1993; 71:426–34.

Intercostal nerve block

Indications

- Post-operative analgesia for thoracic/upper abdominal surgery.
- Fractured ribs.
- Placement of intercostal chest drains.
- ▶▶ Intercostal nerve block is inadequate for intra-operative analgesia.

Contra-indications

Absolute

- Patient refusal.
- Sensitivity or allergy to local anaesthetic.
- Infection at the injection site.

Relative

- Emphysema or bullous lung disease.
- Contralateral pneumothorax.
- Ipsilateral empyema.
- Coagulopathy.

Anatomy

Intercostal nerves

- Emerge from the ventral rami of T1 to T11.
- Run in the intercostal groove along the inferior border of the rib, lying between the internal and innermost intercostal muscles.
  - Within the intercostal groove the intercostal vein/artery/nerve lie superior-inferior. **V.A.N** mnemonic.
- At the mid-axillary line each nerve gives off:
  - Lateral cutaneous branch, which further divides into anterior and posterior branches supplying the muscles and skin of the posterolateral thorax and abdomen.
  - Anterior cutaneous branch continues to supply the muscles and skin of the anterior thorax and abdomen.
- The 3rd to 6th intercostal nerves supply the muscles and skin of the thorax.
- The 7th to 11th intercostal nerves pass under the costal margin and supply the muscles and skin of the abdomen.

Technique

- Informed consent.
- Standard monitoring; resuscitation equipment should be available.
- I.V. access.
- The blocks can be placed with the patient either sitting, prone or lateral—whichever gives best access to the area to be covered.

Landmark
- Palpate the angle of the rib ~7–10 cm from the midline, immediately adjacent to the erector spinae muscles.
- A block anterior to the mid-axillary line reduces the likelihood of blocking the lateral cutaneous branch.

Needle technique (see Fig. 12.3)
- Aseptic technique.
- Hold the rib between two fingers of the non-needling hand.
- Insert a 20–24G short-bevelled needle through the skin with approximately 20 degrees cephalad angulation, to contact the lower border of the rib.
- Walk the needle off the lower border of the rib and advance until a loss of resistance is felt; usually 3–5mm deep.
- Aspirate gently and inject 5 ml of local anaesthetic e.g. 0.5% Levobupivacaine.
- Catheter insertion is possible using a 16–18. Gauge Tuohy needle with the above technique.

▶▶ Blockade 2 levels above and below the dermatomal level of surgical incision is required.

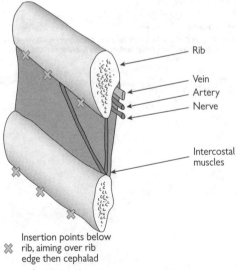

Rib

Vein

Artery

Nerve

Intercostal muscles

✖ Insertion points below rib, aiming over rib edge then cephalad

Fig. 12.3 Needle points for intercostal block.

Complications

- Systemic local anaesthetic toxicity.
- Intravascular injection.
- Pneumothorax.
- Solid/hollow abdominal organ injury.
- Haemorrhage (including haemothorax).
- Spinal anaesthesia; dural cuff extends up to 8 cm lateral from midline.
- Infection.

Practical points

- Cross innervation from adjacent spinal nerves means multiple level injections are often required for complete analgesia.
- Systemic absorption of local anaesthetic from the intercostal space is the highest in the body. It is extremely important to calculate a safe dose of local anaesthetic.
- Consider epidural/paravertebral blockade if multiple level bilateral blocks are required.
- Intercostal nerve block above T7 can be difficult due to the position of the scapulae; consider epidural block.
- Supplemental analgesia is often still necessary.

Further reading

Joshi GP, Bonnet F, Shah R, et al. A Systematic Review of Controlled Trials Evaluating Regional Techniques for Post-thoracotomy Analgesia. *Anaesthesia and Analgesia* 2008; 107:1026–40.

Patient controlled analgesia (PCA)

Concept

The patient titrates their analgesia to a value above the minimum effective analgesic concentration, but below the minimum toxic concentration. The overall result should be a near optimal state of analgesia that can be maintained with minimum sedation and side effects.

Note that post-thoracotomy, patients require dynamic analgesia i.e. analgesia that permits coughing, deep breathing and movement, in order to minimize respiratory complications.

PCA for post-operative pain

- Epidural.
- Intravenous.
- Intranasal.
- Transdermal.

Analgesic efficacy

- Epidural administration of local anaesthetic ± opioid provides the best analgesia:
    - Continuous epidural infusion (CEI) is superior to patient controlled epidural analgesia (PCEA).
    - CEI causes more nausea, vomiting and motor block that PCEA.
- Intranasal diamorphine/fentanyl and inontophoretic transdermal fentanyl provide equally effective analgesia as IV opioid PCA.

Practicalities

- Avoid PCA if:
    - Patient confused/impaired cognition.
    - Physically incapable of pressing handset.
- Pre-operative and post-operative patient education to allay fears of overdose and addiction.
- Follow hospital prescription guidelines, standardized observation and side effect protocols.
- Consider consulting the acute pain team for further advice in cases of:
    - Chronic Renal Impairment (consider Fentanyl/Oxycodone).
    - Morbid Obesity.
    - Obstructive Sleep Apnoea (OSA).
- Titrate analgesia to achieve patient comfort prior to starting PCA.
- Prescribe NSAIDs and paracetamol if no contra-indications.
- Prescribe oxygen, anti-emetics and rescue naloxone.

Administration

Epidural

> **Regime**
>
> - 0.125% L-Bupivacaine + 4 mcg/ml fentanyl.
> - 3–5 ml bolus.
> - 10–15 min lockout.
> - No background infusion.
> - If a background infusion is used, the bolus dose may be decreased ± lockout increased.

Intravenous

- Used where epidural analgesia is contra-indicated/refused/difficult to insert or not required.
- Commonly used in combination with paravertebral and intercostal nerve blocks.
- ❶ Systemic opioid side effects may limit dosage, leaving the patient with suboptimal dynamic pain relief → pulmonary complications in thoracotomy patients.

> **Regimes**
>
> - No evidence that one opioid is superior.
> - PCA boluses should aim to provide the minimum dose required to produce analgesic effect:
>   - Morphine: 1–2 mg.
>   - Fentanyl: 10–20 mcg.
>   - Pethidine: 10 mg.
>   - Diamorphine: 0.5 mg.
>   - Tramadol: 10 mg.
>   - Oxycodone: 1 mg.
> - Lockout time.
>   - 5–8 mins.
> - Background infusion:
>   - Little evidence improves analgesia.
>   - May increase risk of respiratory depression.
>   - Useful in opioid tolerant patients; start with same dose as bolus in mg/hr.
>
> ❶ Patient response may vary dramatically with different opioids.
>
> ❶ Potential risks/complexity of multiple opioid regimes.

Intranasal
- Uses high concentration/low volume lipid soluble opioid, e.g. fentanyl or diamorphine.
- Rapid absorption with no hepatic first pass effect.

Regimes

- Intranasal PCA fentanyl 25 mcg every 5 min PRN.
- Intranasal PCA pethidine 27 mg every 5 min PRN.
- Intranasal PCA diamorphine 0.5 mg every 5 min PRN; equally as effective as IV PCA for post-operative pain.

Transdermal
- Fentanyl HCl ionotophoretic transdermal patches use an imperceptible electrical field to deliver a controlled dose of drug.
- This system overcomes problems of potential needle stick injuries, infections, pump errors and failures whilst enabling patient mobility.

Regime

- 40 mcg fentanyl.
- 10 mins lockout.
- Patient can initiate 6 doses/hr per 24 hours.

❶ Opioid induced respiratory depression

- IV opioid PCA risk: 0.1–0.8%.
- Increases to 1.1–3.9% if background infusion used.
- Risk Factors:
  - Background Infusion.
  - Bolus doses >1 mg.
  - Elderly patients.
  - Respiratory disease/OSA.
  - Concomitant sedatives.
  - Operator error.
  - Equipment error.
- Rescue Naloxone 400 mcg IV bolus repeated to effect. Patient may require continuous infusion due to short half-life of naloxone.

Further reading

Macintrye PE, Ready LB. *Acute pain management: a practical guide*, 2 edn. London: WB Saunders; 2001.

Dale O, Hjortkjaer R, Kharasch ED. Nasal administration of opioids for pain management in adults. *Acta Anaesthesiologica Scandinavia* 2002; 46:759–70.

Power I. Fentanyl HCl iontophoretic transdermal system: clinical application of iontophoretic technology in the management of acute postoperative pain. *British Journal of Anaesthesia* 2007; 98:4–11.

Management of the shared airway

- Many thoracic surgical procedures require the anaesthetist and surgeon to share the patient's airway.
- Bronchoscopic examination in the anaesthetic room before proceeding to surgery is a common example.
- Patients who require airway surgery present a unique problem as to how to secure and share the airway safely, while providing adequate surgical access.
- No one anaesthetic technique exists to cover the wide range of "shared airway cases" in thoracic surgery.

Principles for successful management

Communication

- Paramount to successful and safe team working.
- Establish with the team exactly what each person is going to do, what equipment and access is required, and what is going to happen in case of difficulty with the airway.

Pre-operative assessment

- Patients who require shared airway management to facilitate airway surgery typically have intrinsic or extrinsic airway pathology.
- A major focus of the anaesthetic assessment is on the location and extent of any airway lesion and how this affects the patient.
  - This information allows planning for airway management and tracheal intubation. (See 📖 Tracheal resection and reconstruction, p. 322).

Induction

- ▶▶Avoid airway irritation and coughing. This may worsen an already critically narrowed airway.
- IV induction and rapid paralysis is often the technique of choice as local anaesthetic techniques and gas induction increase the likelihood of airway obstruction in patients with airway pathology requiring surgery.
- Sometimes the balance of risks favours a spontaneously breathing technique.
- ❶ In patients with severe respiratory distress who are unable to lie supine, the use of neuromuscular blocking agents may eliminate the only muscular tone which is keeping the airway patent.
  - However, the application of IPPV and PEEP may stent the airway open and actually improve tidal volume.
- (See Table 12.1) for a summary of the anaesthetic considerations for rigid and flexible bronchoscopy.

Airway management & tracheal intubation

- Some patients may obstruct their airway when supine. Allow these patients to optimize their own position themselves prior to induction of anaesthesia.

- Partial tracheal obstruction and collapse following induction of anaesthesia may render bag-mask ventilation and tracheal intubation very difficult or impossible.
  - A rigid bronchoscope and an able operator must be present during induction of anaesthesia.
- SVC obstruction may make airway management more challenging.
- If there is suspicion/CT evidence of a lesion occluding the airway, care should be taken to limit gas trapping distal to the obstructing lesion by limiting inspiratory pressures and allowing time for expiration.
- Depending on the procedure, access to the airway may not always be possible.
- Good communication and team working are paramount to allow access and observation of the patient at appropriate times.

Table 12.1 Anaesthetic considerations for bronchoscopy

Rigid bronchoscopy	Flexible bronchoscopy
Intense surgical stimulus	Less stimulating
Requires NMB	Spontaneous breathing or with NMB
IV maintenance	Volatile anaesthesia possible
No control of inspired oxygen	

Specific hazards
Airway obstruction
- Beware obstruction of endotracheal tubes and catheters by surgical equipment, surgical manipulation, debris, secretions and blood.

Bleeding and soiling
- Airway tumours bleed easily
  - It is the surgeon's responsibility to ensure the patient's airway is clear of debris and blood after rigid bronchoscopy. Maintaining a high index of suspicion will prevent disaster.

Extubation/recovery
- Complete central airway obstruction may occur intra-operatively or in the early post-operative period as a result of retained sputum and/or blood clots.
- Worsening hypoxia and hypercarbia can progress to cardiovascular collapse without prompt treatment.
- Re-intubation with the rigid bronchoscope and suctioning is required and hence the surgeon and rigid bronchoscope should remain with the patient until satisfactory spontaneous respiration is well established/

Key points

- Clear communication and team work is paramount.
- Understand the surgeon's aims and the planned surgical procedure.
- Maintain a patent airway to ensure oxygenation and ventilation.
- Maintain anaesthesia with volatile or intravenous agents.
- Provide a clear surgical view and unhindered access.
- Protect the airway from soiling, e.g. blood.
- A rigid bronchoscope and surgeon should always be immediately available in case of catastrophic intrinsic/extrinsic airway obstruction.

The fibreoptic bronchoscope and the difficult airway

Introduction

Fibreoptic bronchoscopes (FOB) have been used to facilitate thoracic anaesthetic practice since the early 1980s. Currently FOBs are widely used and have several uses during thoracic anaesthesia.

Uses of the flexible bronchoscope

- To confirm position of DLT.
  - Accepted as gold standard.
  - Almost mandatory in Western practice.
  - 30% of DLT's will be misplaced without direct visualization.
- To guide endobronchial intubation with:
  - DLT.
  - SLT + Bronchial blocker.
  - Univent SLT (incorporates bronchial blocker).
- Difficult direct laryngoscopy.
- Pulmonary toilet.

Preparation

Equipment

- Sterilized, leak-tested, and lubricated (water soluble) intubating bronchoscope with an OD <4 mm.
  - FOBs with OD >4mm likely to stick in the narrow lumens of a DLT.
- ❶ When working with DLT's below 37 french, FOBs are particularly prone to sticking.
- Working light source.
- Camera and video stack (useful for learning).
- ± difficult airway trolley if appropriate.

Routine

- Wipe tip of intubating bronchoscope with alcohol wipe to clear any residue from sterilization process.
- Confirm movement of bronchoscope tip.
- Confirm patency of the working channel e.g. inject some sterile saline down it.
- Focus bronchoscope.
- Ensure camera is white-balanced.
- De-fog bronchoscope tip with commercial solution. Alternatively, wipe the tip of the bronchoscope on the patient's tongue.

- Ensure the triangular indentation on your circular field of view is placed at 12 O'clock position. This is done by rotating the camera head clockwise or anticlockwise.

Practical use

The insertion and positioning of DLTs and BBs are discussed in later sections of this chapter. The use of FOBs in critical care is discussed (See 📖 Pulmonary aspiration in thoracic patients, p. 646).

Difficult laryngoscopy

- An in-depth discussion of difficult airway management and local anaesthesia for awake fibreoptic intubation is without the scope of this chapter.
- Patients with anticipated or unexpected difficult laryngoscopy pose an especially difficult problem in thoracic anaesthesia as DLTs tend to be more difficult to insert and position even in patients where direct laryngoscopy is easy.
- Fibreoptic techniques to achieve endobronchial intubation and lung separation in a patient with a difficult airway predominantly focus on the exchange of a SLT with a DLT.

▶ The use of a SLT + BB or a Univent tube may be preferable to a DLT in patients with a difficult airway, especially when it is expected or likely that a period of post-operative intubation is required, i.e. it removes the need for exchange of DLT with SLT at the end of the procedure.

Awake oral fibreoptic intubation—options

- SLT inserted in awake patient, then anaesthetized
  - SLT exchange with DLT over AEC
- Univent ETT inserted awake and endobronchial blocker advanced when anaesthetized
- SLT + BB
  - If not able to pass DLT or if limited mouth opening
- Awake tracheal DLT intubation is possible, but requires excellent local anaesthesia ± sedation. Advancement of the endobronchial lumen is achieved after induction of anaesthesia.

Asleep oral fibreoptic intubation

- SLT + AEC → DLT in anaesthetized patient.

GA

- LMA + fibreoptically placed AIC → SLT.
  - SLT exchange with DLT over AEC.

Tips & trouble-shooting

Fibreoptic intubation

- Unable to visualize glottis:
  - Ask patient to take deep breath.
  - Protrude tongue/anterior tongue traction.
  - Jaw thrust.
  - Change patient position e.g. supine to sitting.
  - External laryngeal manipulation (uncomfortable in awake patient).
  - Trans-illuminate the larynx using the tip of the fibrescope. If the light is not visible or dull, it is likely that you are in the oesophagus; withdraw the fibrescope until you recognize structures.
- Unable to pass SLT/DLT past glottis:
  - Typically caused by hang-up of ETT on posterior elements of glottis or tip of ETT abutting vocal cords.
  - Aim to pass fibrescope through the anterior half of the glottis.
  - Ensure bevel of ETT faces posteriorly before it is railroaded.
  - Try to keep fibrescope tip in midline.
  - Ask the awake patient to take a deep inspiration while the ETT is advanced i.e. vocal cords abduct.
  - Withdraw ETT slightly and twist through 90° anti-clockwise; advance and re-attempt passage through the glottis.
  - ⚠ Do not twist the ETT against the vocal cords as this can result in injury.
  - Other maneuvers include neck flexion/extension, application/ removal of cricoid pressure.
- Fibrescope sticking within ETT:
  - Ensure adequate lubrication.
  - You may have to use a fibrescope with a smaller OD.

AIC/AEC assisted intubation

- Ensure fibrescope and external surface of catheter are adequately lubricated to prevent sticking.
- Oxygenation and ventilation may be achieved with both devices in the trachea by using the appropriate "Rapi-fit" 15 mm luer lock adapters which can be connected to a standard breathing circuit or jet ventilator respectively.
- AIC can be used with ETT ID ≥7 mm.
- AEC can be used with ETT ID as narrow as 4 mm (dependent on catheter chosen). Ensure the use of soft tipped AEC eg Cooks soft-tipped extra-firm exchange catheter.

❶ At 56cm in length, the AIC is too short to reliably facilitate SLT exchange with a DLT. Adult AEC vary in length between 70–100 cm dependent on manufacturer.

Further reading

Patane PS, Sell BA, Mahla ME. Awake fibreoptic endobronchial intubation. *Journal of Cardiothoracic Anesthesia* 1990; 4:229–31.

Arndt GA, Buchika S, Kranner PW, *et al*. Wire-guided endobronchial blockade in a patient with limited mouth opening. *Canadian Journal of Anaesthesia* 1999; 46:87–9.

Techniques for lung isolation

The most common technique for lung isolation is the use of a double lumen tube (DLT). Bronchial blockers (BB) are however increasingly used. Lung isolation enables one lung ventilation (OLV) to be performed.

Indications

- Can be considered absolute and relative.
- Protection from contamination and severe asymmetrical lung disease are absolute.
- Lung isolation for surgical access is considered relative.

Absolute
Protection from contamination

- Abscess.
- Haemorrhage.
- Bronchopulmonary lavage.
- Bronchiectasis.

Unilateral or asymmetrical lung disease

- Bronchopleural fistula.
- Bronchial disruption.
- Bullous lung disease.
- Trauma.

Relative
Surgical access.

- Thoracoscopy.
- Lobectomy.
- Pneumonectomy.
- Thoracic aortic aneurysm.
- Lung transplantation.
- Cardiac surgery.
- Oesophageal surgery.
- Spinal surgery.

Double lumen tubes

- PVC disposable (Mallinckrodt type), based on the original Robertshaw design.
- Latex based red rubber type (Robertshaw).
- Mallinckrodt types—largest 41F gauge to smallest 26F gauge (FG; external circumference in millimeters).
- Left and right-sided types.

- DLTs have a tracheal and bronchial lumen; the bronchial limb has a distal bronchial cuff, whilst the tracheal cuff is above the tracheal opening.
- Right sided bronchial tubes have a lateral slot to enable ventilation of the right upper lobe. Malpositioning may result in occlusion the RUMB with resulting morbidity.

Advantages
- Permit selective ventilation of either lung without requiring tube reposition.
- Permit suction of either lung.
- Allow application of positive end expiratory pressure (PEEP) to ventilated lung.
- Allow application of continuous positive airway pressure (CPAP) or insufflations of oxygen to non-ventilated lung.

Left DLT
- Can be used for most situations.
- Left sided tubes offer greater margin of safety compared to right sided tubes, as less precise positioning required.

Right DLT
- Required when there is distortion, rupture or tumour of the LMB, preferred/required for surgery involving the LMB.
- A school of thought is that R tubes should be used for ALL left thoracotomies, to provide additional protection to the R lung.

Disadvantages
- Difficult to use in patients who are difficult to intubate.
- Difficult/impossible to place if lower airway narrowing distortion.
- Cannot be used in small children.
- Relatively contraindicated in the critically ill, as insertion takes longer.
- May require tube change after operation if post-operative ventilation required.

Complications
- Malposition.
- Trauma and bronchial rupture.

Size and depth selection
- Average man 39/41F.
- Average woman 37/39F.
  - Size reflects the patient's height better than other parameters.
- Can use tracheal width at inter-clavicular line on CXR as a guide—e.g.
  - >18mm use 41F.
  - >16mm use 39F.

- • >15mm use 37F.
- • >14mm use 35F.
- Select the largest size that will comfortably fit through the glottis
- Average depth placement for a 170 cm tall person = 29 cm
  - For every 10 cm increase in height advance tube 1cm
  - For every 10 cm decrease in height withdraw 1cm.

Tubes are usually placed blindly and then position confirmed with fibreoptic bronchoscopy (FOB).

Double lumen tube (DLT)

Insertion

- Check cuffs and connections.
- Once a view of the cords is obtained, orientate the tube so that the tip concavity faces upwards.
- Pass the tube through the vocal cords:
  - Remove the stylet then advance and rotate 90°, left for a left sided right for a right sided.
  - Advance until tube meets gentle resistance (typically at 29 cm for 170 cm tall patient).
- Confirm ability to selectively ventilate the appropriate lung clinically.
- Use a FOB to adjust position tube appropriately.

Clinical checking of DLT position

- Clinical checking is a skill all thoracic anesthetists should be happy with:

Ventilate through both lumens and auscultate

- Inflate the tracheal cuff until no leak can be heard at the mouth.
- Chest wall should rise equally on both sides with bilateral breath sounds.
- ❶ If unilateral ventilation observed, it is likely that both lumens are lying in a mainstem bronchus.
  - Deflate cuffs.
  - Pull back tube 1–2 cm and re-assess.

Ventilate via the bronchial lumen and auscultate

- Clamp off the tracheal portion of the Cobb's connector.
- Open the lumen cap so it is open to the atmosphere.
- Now, gas leaking around the bronchial cuff can be heard at the open tracheal connection as it passes up the tracheal lumen.
  - Inflate the cuff GENTLY (about 2 ml) until the leak stops.
- Breath sounds should be heard and the chest should only rise on the side intubated with the bronchial portion of the tube.
- ❶ If bilateral breath sounds are heard and bilateral lung inflation is seen, the tube has not been advanced far enough.
- ❶ If the lower lobe appears to inflate > upper lobe, the tube may have been advanced too far.
- ❶ L tube—if R lung isolates, tube is in R main bronchus.
- ❶ R tube—if L lung isolates, tube is in L main bronchus.

Always verify tube placement with fibreoptic bronchoscopy!

- (See 📖 The fibreoptic bronchoscope and the difficult airway, p. 712.).
- ❶ Be aware; clinical checking alone →
  - Incorrect positioning 38%.
  - Wrong main stem intubated 20.8%.
  - Double-lumen tube above the carina 38.7%.
  - Therefore, fibreoptic checking should be mandatory.

Tips

- DLT's are more bulky then endotracheal tubes, use a generous amount of lubricant to help insertion.
- The tracheal cuff lies near the teeth during intubation be careful of damaging it.
- It is often beneficial to increase the anterior bend on the DLT tip, with the stylet still in situ. This aids passage through the cords.
- Maintaining laryngoscopy during rotation on DLT enables free 90 degree turn and reduces possibility of twisting, kinking, or the endobronchial lumen finishing against bronchial wall.
- If there is significant resistance whilst attempting to pass the tube through the cords; do not use further force! Use the next size tube down.
- As the stylet is removed from the DLT- keep a tight hold of the tube as the whole tube can become dislodged easily.
- Tubes with a carinal hook can cause a significant amount of trauma to the airway if placed without due care.
- It is often helpful to rotate the head AWAY from the side to be intubated, as the tube is turned and advanced toward the appropriate main bronchus.

Fibreoscopic insertion techniques

- (See 📖 Bronchoscopic anatomy, p. 40).
- Correct visualization requires passing the FOB down both lumens.
- Via the tracheal lumen:
    - The carina should be clearly visible.
    - Withdraw the tube if tracheal lumen is too close to the carina.
    - Insert the tube further if bronchial cuff herniating.
- Via the bronchial lumen:
    - Check bronchial tip clear of secondary carina.

Right sided tube

- The lateral slot should be aligned with the opening of the RUL.
- When visualized through the tracheal lumen, the proximal edge of the right sided bronchial cuff should usually be at or just below the carina.

Railroading

- Alternatively, one can place the fibreoscope through the bronchial lumen just after the tube is placed below the vocal cords.
- The scope can then be maneuvered down the side to be intubated.
- Once this is achieved, the DLT can be advanced over the scope, thus railroading the tube into the correct side under direct vision.

- ❶ Fibreoscopic checking of tube position **must be performed**, both after initial placement and after moving the patient, or at any time if there is doubt about the tube.
- Movement of the patient results in the need to adjust the position of double-lumen tube position up to 83% of cases.
- Distal displacement is more common than proximal displacement.
- Movements of 16 to 19 mm of a left double-lumen tube and 8 mm of a right double-lumen tube can compromise functional lung separation.

For management of misplacement of DLT (See 📖 Techniques for lung isolation, p. 716).

Monitoring

- Bronchoscopy is essential to exclude double-lumen tube displacement and to re-position it if necessary.
- Pulse oximetry, end-tidal capnography, peak and plateau pressures, as well as continuous spirometry can be used for non-invasive monitoring, but cannot replace readily available bronchoscopy.

Bronchial blockers

Discussed in more depth (See 📖 Use of a bronchial blocker, p. 722).

Fogarty occlusion catheter

- Balloon size range from 0.5 to 3 ml of air.
- Fine plastic catheter with wire stylet with inflatable balloon at end.
- Passed down or outside standard tube and moved into position by shaping wire in tip. Guided with fibreoptic visualization.

Advantages

- Can be used in critically ill.
- Can be passed nasally.
- Come in small sizes so can be used in small children.

Disadvantages

- No hollow lumen.
- Lung deflates slowly by absorption atelectasis.
- No oxygen insufflations.
- No CPAP.
- No suction.
- Can migrate easily.

Conventional endotracheal tube

- Used in dire emergency such as massive pulmonary haemorrhage.
- Normal uncut tube placed blind beyond the carina.
- Usually goes down right main bronchus.
- Turn head to right to encourage passage down left main bronchus.

Further reading

Campos JH. Current techniques for perioperative lung isolation in adults. *Anesthesiology* 2002; 97:1295–301.

Eastwood J, Mahajan R. One-lung anaesthesia. *British Journal of Anaesthesia*. CEPD Reviews 2002; 2:83–7.

Gothard J, Porter H. Controversies in thoracic anaesthesia. In: Ghosh L, Latimer RD, editor. *Thoracic Anaesthesia: principles and practice*. Oxford: Butterworth-Heinemann; 1999.

Use of a bronchial blocker

What is a bronchial blocker?

A fine catheter that will pass through the lumen of an ETT, with a balloon (the blocker) attached just proximal to the distal end. When inflated in a main bronchial lumen, the chosen lung is thus isolated from ventilation which continues to the contra lateral lung via the ETT. The bronchial blocker may be a built in component of an adapted ETT or used via a multiport adapter with a standard ETT. Techniques have been described for passing a BB outside the lumen of the ETT rather than through it.

Advantages of using a bronchial blocker

- A more simple approach in the difficult Airway.
- Can be passed nasally (except Univent®).
- Ventilation may continue during placement.
- Appropriate sizing usually not an issue.
- Lobar isolation and selective ventilation possible.
- Avoidance of ETT changes (good for use in ICU patient already intubated).
- Reduced incidence of laryngeal trauma (smaller tube).
- Reduced incidence of sore throat compared to DLT.
- Possibly improved recognition of tracheobronchial anatomy (better visualization).
- Can be used in children.

Disadvantages/risks of using a bronchial blocker

- Increased time to position compared with DLT.
- FOB essential for positioning.
- Unable to bronchoscope isolated lung.
- More likely to dislodge and need repositioning during surgery.
- If dislodges into trachea, inflated cuff may prevent ventilation to either lung and result in hypoxia.
- Right bronchial anatomy can make right sided placement difficult.
- Inferior suction to isolated lung.
- Increased time required to collapse isolated lung.
- To encourage lung collapse, suction is often applied, if this is excessive, lung injury may ensue.
- High pressure low volume balloon design require care to prevent potential over-inflation and bronchial injury/rupture.
- More difficult or less effective when applying CPAP to the isolated lung.
- Requires repositioning if collapse of the other lung is required.
- Contamination of non operative lung more likely.
- Case reports of blocker shearing on removal through a side port, or being included in staple lines during sleeve resection.
- Currently BB's are 2–3 times more expensive than DLT's.

When to use a bronchial blocker

Although a BB can be used for most indications for OLV, there are situations when a BB may be the preferred option.
- The difficult airway.
  - Restricted mouth opening, protruding teeth, Mallampati grade 3 or 4 and limited neck extension may make the passage of a DLT difficult.
  - When awake fibreoptic intubation indicated.
  - C spine immobilization in the trauma setting.
  - Following radical neck surgery, anatomy may be altered and passage of a DLT may be impossible or cause damage.
- When Nasal Intubation is required/necessary.
- To avoid a tube change.
  - Those who arrive already intubated eg trauma setting.
  - When post-op ventilation planned, particularly if surgery involving the neck raises concern of airway swelling and a potentially difficult tube change.
- When the bronchial anatomy is altered.
  - Following lung resection, residual lung expands and fills the space created. This may alter the angle between the trachea and main bronchus thus making placement of DLT difficult. A CXR pre-op may indicate a possible problem.
  - In the presence of tracheal stenosis.
- Patients unable to tolerate OLV
  - Selective lobar blockade had been described in patients with severe respiratory compromise. The entire operative lung is not collapsed and non operative lobes participate in gas exchange.
- In children/very small adults, when DLT's are not available/too large.
- Use of the BB in low risk elective situations to become familiar with the equipment and technique.

When not to use a bronchial blocker

- When protecting the healthy dependant lung from pus, blood or fluid is vital.
  - The BB has greater potential for movement with resultant loss of adequate seal.
  - Preventing infected secretions contaminating the dependent lung when the BB in the operated lung is deflated is also difficult.
- During therapeutic bronchopulmonary lavage (not possible with BB).
- When rapid lung collapse required (less good for VATS procedures).
- For right sided procedures (placement of BB in RMB more difficult).
- Discussion should occur with the surgeon. Some surgeons may have particular preferences with regard to certain procedures. This is of importance during pneumonectomy/sleeve resection where surgery is occurring close to chosen airway device.
- When one is unfamiliar with the equipment or technique. The DLT still remains the most common first choice. There is a learning curve associated with the use of a BB. If the clinical situation dictates the use of a BB and one is unfamiliar, experienced help should be summoned.

Types of bronchial blocker

- Three types of independent BB are currently available.
  (See Table 12.2).

Table 12.2 Types of bronchial blocker

	Arndt	**Cohen**	**Fuji**
Size	5F, 7F, 9F	9F	9F
Balloon Shape	Spherical or Elliptical	Spherical	Spherical
Guidance Mechanism	Nylon wire loop that is coupled with the FOB	Wheel device to deflect the tip	None, pre-shaped tip
Smallest recommended ETT for coaxial use	5F (4.5 ETT), 7F (7.0 ETT), 9F (8.0 ETT)	9 F (8.0 ETT)	9F (8.0 ETT)
Centre channel	1.4mm internal diameter	1.4 mm internal diameter	2.0mm internal diameter

Generic insertion technique

- Correct technique requires visual demonstration and then time and opportunity to practice in controlled circumstances.
- Manufacturer's websites often provide useful teaching aids and videos for the equipment they produce and should be referenced when learning.
- Successful placement of a BB will be optimized by thorough pre-op assessment of the upper airway, the lower airways as visualized on the CXR, and good knowledge of tracheobronchial anatomy as visualized using the FOB.
- Ensure equipment sizes are compatible before commencing.
- Test the balloon still works after the BB has been inserted through the adapter port.
- When positioned, inflate the blocker balloon under direct vision whilst using a method of ensuring the least volume is used to achieve a seal.
  - Attaching the suction port of the BB to a capnograph and inflating slowly until the CO_2 trace plateaus is a suggested method.
  - Using the FOB confirm correct balloon positioning with no herniation.
  - Record depth of BB insertion and volume used to inflate the balloon.
  - Deflate balloon before positioning patient.
  - Repeat procedure when OLV is required.
- During lung collapse, ensure BB suction lumen port is open. The central wire, if present, needs to be removed.
- When removing the blocker, remove with the whole adapter to avoid shearing of blocker balloon leaving debris in the airway.

Type specific techniques

Arndt bronchial blocker

- Use the multiport adapter provided by the manufacturer.
- Make sure the blocker cuff is fully deflated and lubricated before passing through the adapter.
- Lubricate the FOB adequately.
- Pass the blocker and FOB through their respective adapter ports and advance the blocker so that the loop may be visualized.
- Advance the FOB into and through the loop so that the FOB is coupled with the blocker.
- The guide loop should be adjusted appropriately. If to loose BB may enter the contralateral main bronchus and jam. Too tight and advancement along the FOB is difficult/impossible.
  - NB. The last 3 steps may be carried out in isolation with the assembled adapter placed into the breathing circuit.
- Advance the FOB into the bronchus of lung to be blocked.
- Keeping the FOB stable advance the BB till the loop is seen to be free of the end of the FOB.
- Retract the FOB keeping the blocker tip in view.
- The tip of the blocker may need further advancement or retraction to achieve correct position in the desired bronchus.
- Tighten the connecter to fix the BB relative to the multiport adaptor
- Once the balloon is positioned, the guide wire can be removed from the lumen of the blocker, however it cannot then be replaced.

Cohen bronchial blocker

- This BB uses the same adapter port as the Arndt BB.
- Place the BB through the adapter first before the FOB.
- Advance the tip beyond the tip of the ETT, followed by the FOB to facilitate easy passage of both.
- Deflection of the tip is in one direction only, by counterclockwise rotation of the wheel at the proximal end.
- Right sided insertion is generally easier as the BB tends to naturally select the right main bronchus.
- To block the left main bronchus, the blocker should be inserted with the wheel facing to the left.
- The distal end of the blocker has a black arrow on it indicating the direction of deflection. Again for left bronchus intubation, this should be facing the left.
- If difficulty is encountered in guiding the tip into a bronchus, an external plastic sleeve or gripper at the proximal end provides a means of manipulating by transmitting torque along the blocker.

Fuji (uniblocker)/univent tube

- This is a single lumen ETT that has a BB as a built in component, using a dedicated channel; separate to the main lumen of the ETT.
- Available in sizes 3.5–9.0 mm (ID), for ages 6 to adult
  - Relatively larger than corresponding standard ETT's to accommodate the blocker channel.

- • This must be taken into account when choosing the size, particularly in those with a difficult airway.
- No guidance system so placement relies upon rotation of the angled tip as it is advanced under direct vision.
- The shaft is re-enforced with a metallic mesh which affords the transmission of torque along the blocker to the tip.
- The tip of the blocker is placed in the desired bronchial lumen and the cuff inflated.
- A quick release component of the multiport adapter allows removal of the blocker without disconnecting the whole adapter from the ETT once the blocker cuff is deflated. The ETT may then be used for post op ventilation.

Further reading

Campos JH. 'Which device should be considered best for lung isolation: Double lumen endotracheal tube versus bronchial blockers?' *Current Opinion in Anaesthesiology* February 2007; 20:27–31.

Cohen E. 'Pro: The new bronchial blockers are preferable to double lumen tubes for lung isolation' *Journal of Cardiovascular and vascular Anaesthesia* December 2008; 22(6):920–4.

Slinger P 'Con: The new bronchial blockers are not preferable to double lumen tubes for lung isolation' *Journal of Cardiothoracic and Vascular Anaesthesia*. December 2008; 22(6): 925–9.

Jet ventilation

Introduction

Provides a means of gas insufflation at high velocity, directly into the patient's airway. Exhalation is completely passive relying upon an airway which is completely open to the atmosphere, with no obstruction to expiratory flow.

Its provision does not require an ET tube; thus allowing unhindered examination of the airway, operative procedures to the airway and the ability to use lasers without the risk of igniting flammable tubing are possible.

Jet ventilation has been shown to reduce ventilator induce lung injury by as much as 20%.

Physiology of gas flow

- HFJV utilizes tidal volumes that may be smaller than combined anatomical and equipment dead space.
- During normal laminar flow (small airways) airflow is most rapid in the centre of the airway and slower at the periphery.
  - HFJV exaggerates this pattern, such that gas moves very rapidly down the centre and gas at the periphery is drawn out of the lung.
- This exaggerated flow causes further gas mixing due to the creation of a relative concentration gradient between gas molecules.
- Regional differences in compliance and resistance amongst different lung units are also exaggerated resulting in gas flow between alveoli.
  - This increases deadspace and CO_2 rebreathing occurs.
- This effect is exaggerated by high-frequency breaths and facilitated by the higher mean airway pressures seen in HFJV, leading to extensive pendelluft with recirculation of gas between different regions.
- Smaller gas volumes effectively reach more respiratory units than similar volumes generated during conventional ventilation.
- Simple molecular diffusion and cardiogenic mixing also contribute. The latter is due to the tiny oscillations/agitations that occur where the heart is in close proximity to the lung (this can often be seen on a capnograph trace during apnoea).

Modes of access

- The connection between the ventilator and the patient's airway can be established via:
  - Translaryngeal-infraglottic access.
  - Transtracheal-infraglottic access.
  - Supraglottic access.

Low-frequency jet ventilation (e.g. the anaesthetic room Sander's injector)

Gas exchange

- Physics.
  - Ventilation is achieved by means of convective ventilation or bulk flow (i.e. the mass flow of gases into and out of the lung) in a manner similar to spontaneous respiration.
- Parameters.
  - The alveolar ventilation (V_A) generated is calculated by the formula: $V_A = f \times (V_T - V_D)$ where V_T and V_D are tidal volume and dead space, respectively; f is the ventilatory rate.
  - Tidal volume is the sum of the injected and entrained volumes.
- A jet frequency of 8–10/min allows adequate time for exhalation by passive recoil of the lung and chest wall and prevents trapping of air and build up of increased pressure in small airways.

O_2 supply

- Direct from the high-pressure wall-piped oxygen at 4 bar.
- When used during surgical procedures, the effective FiO_2 in the trachea is 0.8–0.9 because of dilution by entrainment of ambient air.

Uses

- Short investigative procedures.
  - Laryngoscopy.
  - Bronchoscopy.
  - Important role in the management of a difficult airway or the 'can't intubate, can't ventilate' scenario via a cricothyroidotomy cannula.

High frequency jet ventilation

General

- Involves the use of very high respiratory rates (>60 breaths per minute) with very small tidal volumes, usually below anatomical dead space.
- Minimizes the degree of bronchial and mediastinal excursion compared with conventional ventilation.
- The fine jet catheter can be passed through the surgical field, bridging the defect or pathology and manipulated by the surgeon during the operation.
- Airway resection and end-to-end anastamosis can be accomplished around the fine catheter.

High Frequency Oscillatory Ventilation (HFOV)

Gas exchange

- High respiratory rates up to 15 Hz (900 breaths per minute).
- Pressure oscillates around a constant distending pressure (equivalent to the PEEP).
- Gas is pushed into the lung during inspiration, and then pulled out during expiration.

- Generates very low tidal volumes; generally less than the dead space of the lung.
- Tidal volume is dependent on:
  - Endotracheal tube size.
  - Power.
  - Frequency.

Uses

- Often used in patients who have hypoxia refractory to normal mechanical ventilation:
  - Severe ARDS (the OSCAR trial-High Frequency Oscillation in ARDS is being concluded; results should be available soon).
  - ALI.
  - Other oxygenation.
  - Neonates.

High Frequency Flow Interruption (HFFI)

- High Frequency Flow Interruption is similar to HFJV but the gas control mechanism is different.
- A rotating bar or ball with a small opening is placed in the path of a high pressure gas and as the bar or ball rotates, the opening lines-up with the gas flow and a small, brief pulse of gas is allowed to enter the airway.
- Frequencies for HFFI are typically limited to a maximum of about 15 Hz.

High Frequency Positive Pressure Ventilation (HFPPV)

- High Frequency Positive Pressure Ventilation is utilized by using a conventional ventilator at the upper frequency range of the device (90–100 breaths per minute).
- A conventional breath is used and tidal volumes are usually higher than (HFOV, HFJV and HFFI).
- HFPPV is rarely used now.

Common set parameters

Tidal volume

- A function of driving pressure, cannula resistance, inspiratory time, entrainment volume, and the impedance of the respiratory system.
- Increasing driving pressure leads to increased V_T and airway pressure and a resultant reduction of $ETCO_2$.
- However, large increases in driving pressure (DP) may lead to CO_2 retention if the set frequency is too high to allow time for adequate expiration in the shortened respiratory cycle (stacking).

Pressure

- HFJV is a form of time-cycled, pressure-limited ventilation.
- If ventilator parameters are held constant, a decrease in chest wall or lung compliance will result in a reduction in minute ventilation.
- The driving pressure is most influential for CO_2 elimination.
- Modern jet ventilators are equipped with a second airway measurement line, which monitors the airway pressure continuously and independently of the jet insufflation line.

- **❶** HFJV causes rapid buildup of pressure if there is inadequate egress of air during expiration.
  - A ventilator high-pressure alarm and an automatic shut down facility is a necessity for safe utilization of this ventilation modality.

Intrinsic PEEP
- An important component of HFJV; it is inversely related to expiratory time and so increases with the frequency.

Oxygenation
- Can be improved by increasing driving power, FiO_2 or inspiratory time, but CO_2 retention may occur if the latter is set too high to allow adequate expiration.

Indications
Elective
- Management of the anticipated difficult airway using pre-emptive placement of a trans-tracheal jet cannula, direct laryngoscopy, and vocal cord surgery.
- Airway and thoracic surgery (e.g. major conducting airway surgery such as carinal resections, resection of tracheal stenosis, and tracheal reconstruction).
- During one-lung ventilation, HFJV applied to the non-dependent lung during surgery, can help in carbon dioxide elimination and improve oxygenation, reducing the ventilatory stress on the dependent lung
- Management of broncho-pleural fistula and tracheo-bronchial tree disruption, HFJV results in a smaller gas leak through pathological low-resistance pathways.

Emergency
- LFJV via a trans-tracheal cannula as an interim life saving measure in the 'can't intubate, can't ventilate' scenario (with an assured gas egress pathway).

Intensive care
- The physiology of HFJV makes it ideal for patients with acute lung injury or ARDS.
- The current lung protective strategies employed using conventional ventilation include; PEEP at a level above the lower inflection point to maintain recruitment of alveoli and low tidal volumes to reduce peak airway pressures.
- High-frequency ventilation uses very small tidal volumes allowing the use of higher end-expiratory lung volumes to achieve greater levels of lung recruitment, while avoiding injury from excessive end-inspiratory lung volumes.
- The high respiratory rates allow preservation of near normal $PaCO_2$.
- These are good reasons to employ HFV in ARDS, but advantages over conventional ventilation have not been validated by clinical trials (OSCAR trial results pending).

Complications

- Barotrauma.
- Inadequate gas exchange (hypoxaemia, hypercapnia) in patients with severe lung pathology.
- Pneumothorax.
- Pneumomediastinum.
- Pneumopericardium.
- Subcutaneous emphysema.
- Gastric distension and rupture.
- Dysrhythmias.
- Necrotising tracheo bronchitis and enterocholitis especially in neonates.

Techniques for improving hypoxia

Physiological causes of hypoxia during one lung ventilation

- Hypoxaemia is a complication that affects 9% to 27% of patients undergoing one lung ventilation (OLV) and is influenced by several factors.
- Most thoracic procedures will involve selective ventilation of the dependent lung with the patient in the lateral decubitus position.
- Approximately 20–25% of the cardiac output will continue to pass through the non-dependent lung this increased shunt may result in a reduced PaO_2.
- Hypoxia is more common when the right lung is collapsed.
- It usually occurs after a few minutes as the oxygen in the non-ventilated lung is absorbed.
- It is common to see the oxygen saturation dip, but then rise again a few minutes later as the non-ventilated (non-dependent) lung collapses more completely and blood flow through it decreases.
- For a detailed description of the physiological changes that occur during (OLV). (See 📖 One lung ventilation and the lateral decubitus position, p. 14).

Causes of desaturation

Changes in lung function and impaired oxygen delivery

- Ventilatory issues.
  - Oxygenation and shunt.
  - Lobar or segmental bronchial obstruction by secetions of the dependent lung.
  - Re-absorption of residual oxygen from non dependent lung leading to increased shunt.
- Cardiac Output.
  - Position, vasodilatory effect of GA and use of epidurals.
  - Impaired hypoxic pulmonary vasoconstriction (high MAC of volatile agents).
- Oxygen transport.
  - Low haemoglobin.
- Oxygen delivery.
  - Inadequate FiO_2.

The placement of double-lumen tubes

- Misplacement of double lumen tubes and displacement during surgery.
- Minor changes of tube position cause more episodes of hypoxaemia than the other physiological factors put together!
- Always maintain a high index of suspicion!

Physiological changes during OLV

(See 📖 One lung ventilation and the lateral decubitus position, p. 14.)

- During OLV, when ventilation is interrupted, the blood flow to the non-dependent lung takes no part in gas exchange = Shunt → hypoxia.
- The shunt is minimized by:
  - Gravity favoring flow to the dependent lung.
  - Surgical compression and lung retraction squeezing shunted blood out of the non-ventilating lung.
  - Surgical ligation of non-dependent blood vessels (especially if a pneumonectomy is being performed).
- Once hypoxic pulmonary vasoconstriction commences blood flow to the non-dependent lung decreases from around 50% to around 30% and may reduce shunt from ~50% to 30%.
- However, the dependent lung loses volume due to compression and hypoxic vasoconstriction, which may divert some blood back to the non-dependent lung.
- Secretions may pool in the dependent lung causing impaired ventilation.

Techniques for improving hypoxia during one lung ventilation

General

- Don't forget to look for and treat the usual causes of hypoxia from disconnection to tension pneomothorax.
- Increase FiO_2 to 1.0.
- Confirm/correct the position of the DLT using a fibreoptic bronchoscope.
- Regular suctioning of dependent (and non-dependent) lung.
- Ensure adequate cardiac output.

Non-operated (dependent) lung

- Ensure adequate ventilation.
- Recommended tidal volumes are 6–8 ml/kg.
- Apply PEEP
  - PEEP can increase FRC:VQ ratio and improve lung compliance.
  - ❶ High levels of PEEP can have deleterious effects on PaO_2 due to the diversion of blood flow through the non-dependent lung
  - ❶ Emphysematous patients often exhibit auto-PEEP. This results in a 'stacking' phenomenon resulting in excessive PEEP compromising cardiac output.

Operated (non-dependent) lung

- Apply 2–10 cmH_2O CPAP with FiO_2 1.0 to the non-dependent lung.
- Intermittent re-inflation of non-dependent lung or return to bilateral lung ventilation.
  - Following discussion with surgeon consider intermittent inflation of the non-dependent lung (it is important to have optimal operating conditions with a deflated, immobile lung). However, this should not be achieved to the detriment of adequate oxygenation of the patient!

- • A single inflation will temporarily oxygenete shunted blood. The lung will eventually re-collapse due to absorption atelectasis and therefore must be re-expanded approximately every 5 min.
- • Occlusion of pulmonary artery by surgeon.
  - • If all other attempts to improve oxygenation fail, it may be appropriate as a last resort to partially or completely reduce blood flow to the non-dependent lung by occlusion of the pulmonary artery (clamping, ligation or with pulmonary artery catheter).

Other measures
- • Pharmacological manipulation of pulmonary vascular resistance to improve blood flow to dependent lung (iNO/aerosolized PGI$_2$).
- • Reduce blood flow to non-dependent lung (IV almitrine).
  - • iNO alone to the dependent lung has little supportive evidence … however, in combination with a potent vasoconstrictor targeted to the non-dependent lung, there is evidence for benefit.
- • Ventilatory measures (e.g. HFJV).

Further reading

Ferreira HC, Zin WA, Rocco PRM, et al. Physiopathology and clinical management of one lung ventilation. *Journal of Brasilian Pneumology* 2004; 30:566–73.

Benumof, Jonathan L. MD One-Lung Ventilation and Hypoxic Pulmonary Vasoconstriction: Implications for Anesthetic Management. *Anesthesia and Analgesia* 1985; 64:821–33.

Silva-Costa-Gomes T, Gallart L, Vallès J, et al. Low vs high dose almitrine combined with nitric oxide to prevent hypoxia during open chest one-lung ventilation. *British Journal of Anaesthesia* 2005; 95:410–16.

Central venous catheters

Introduction

Central venous access with monitoring of central venous pressure (CVP) is highly desirable for pneumonectomies, oesophagectomies and resections of large tumours.

> * ❶ CVP reflects the net effect of venous capacitance, vascular tone, blood volume, and right ventricular function; consequently, it is only a rough guide to fluid management.
> * Shifts in fluid volumes during thoracic procedures are usually small, and values recorded may be difficult to interpret due to the physiological effects of the lateral decubitus position and lung collapse.

As well as their use intraoperatively, they are particularly useful for postoperative fluid management; particularly following pneumonectomy/oesophagectomy where it is essential to avoid fluid overload.

Indications

* Monitoring and guidance.
  * Fluid balance/estimation of circulating volume/monitoring acute circulatory failure (especially where vasopressor, inotropic support are being used).
* Drug administration
  * Long term antibiotics/chemotherapy/irritant drugs (many vasopressors, inotropes).
* Devices
  * Placement of trans venous pacing wires/pulmonary artery flotation catheters.
* Dialysis
  * Post operative haemodialysis/haemofiltration.
* Laboratory tests
  * Particularly, mixed venous oxygen saturation levels.
* Replacement
  * Fluids, TPN.
* Access
  * Situations where poor venous access exists.

Contraindications

* Severe coagulopathy.
* Thrombocytopenia.
* Local skin sepsis.
* Distortion of landmarks.

Insertion

- Potential sites for insertion.
  - Internal jugular vein.
  - Subclavian vein.
  - Femoral vein.
  - Peripherally inserted central catheter (PICC) lines.
- Most common site for placement peri-operatively is the internal jugular vein on the ipsilateral side to the surgical procedure
  - The subclavian approach carries a higher associated morbidity relating to insertion, but may pose less of a catheter related infection risk.
- NICE (National Institute for Clinical Excellence) guidelines from 2005 state 2-D imaging ultrasound guidance should be considered in most clinical situations where central venous catheter insertion is necessary (See below).
- Following the placement of monitoring and establishing full asepsis the 'central' vein is visualized with ultrasound and the needle placed within the vein. The procedure then follows a standard catheter over a guide wire (Seldinger technique).

X–ray confirmation of position

- For the placement of central lines in the chest, the tip of the central line should be at or above the level of the carina on the post-operative check x-ray.
  - This coincides with the correct position above the tricuspid valve within the SVC.
- ❶ Be aware that catheters within the carotid artery may give the above X ray appearance and be considered fit for usage
  - However, this could result in catastrophic consequences secondary to intra-arterial drug/TPN placement.

IF IN DOUBT

- Connect to a transducer and ensure the trace is not arterial
- Perform a blood gas analysis
  - If PaO_2 reading is >10k Pa/saturation is >75% it is likely to be arterial!.

Summary of nice guidelines (NICE 2005)

- 2-D imaging ultrasound guidance should be the preferred method when inserting of central venous catheter into the internal jugular vein in adults and children in 'elective situations'. ('Elective situation' means that the operation, or other treatment, has been planned—that is, it is not an emergency).
- 2-D imaging ultrasound guidance should be considered in most clinical situations where CVC insertion is necessary, whether the situation is elective or an emergency.
- Everyone who uses 2-D imaging ultrasound guidance to insert central venous catheters should have appropriate training to ensure they are competent to use the technique.
- Audio-guided Doppler ultrasound guidance is not recommended for use when inserting central venous catheters.

Complications

- Pneumothorax or haemothorax (for central lines inserted in IJV and subclavian veins).
- Infection.
- Air embolus.
- Arrhythmias (if line or wire comes into contact with endocardium/ valves).
- Haematoma.
- Vascular (venous or arterial) damage.
- Malposition of the catheter.
- Indwelling catheter related sepsis.
- Catheter embolism.
- Thrombosis.
- Cardiac tamponade.

Further reading

National Institute for Health and Clinical Excellence (September 2002).Technology appraisal: the clinical effectiveness and cost effectiveness of ultrasonic locating devices for the placement of central venous lines.

Arterial catheters

Arterial catheters are required for the majority of thoracic procedures.

Indications

- Pre-operative assessment indicates a significant lack of cardiac and/or respiratory reserve.
- Procedures associated with significant haemodynamic variability:
  - Pneumonectomy.
  - Bronchial carcinoid resection.
  - Oesophagectomy.
- NIBP measurement is difficult:
  - Obese patients.
  - Patient position.
- To facilitate cardiac output monitoring:
  - LiDCO®.
  - PiCCO.
- Frequent venous/arterial blood sampling.
- Patients receiving vasopressor/inotropic support.

Contraindications

- Local infection.
- Coagulopathy is a relative contraindication.

Insertion

Site

- Most commonly the radial artery:
  - Predictive value of Allen's test to assess contra-lateral ulnar artery blood flow to the hand is not proven.
- Also brachial, ulnar, dorsalis pedis, posterior tibial, axillary and femoral arteries may be cannulated.
- ⚠ Consider insertion site with regard to accessibility during surgery.

Technique

- An in-depth description of arterial cannulation is outside the scope of the handbook.
- Troubleshooting tips are summarized below.

Complications

- Embolism, e.g. air, thrombus.
- Infection:
  - Incidence similar to central venous catheter related infections.
  - Risk increases with time in-situ.
  - More common in femoral site and when sutures are used to secure in place.

- Inadvertent bleeding:
  - Ensure all connections are secure and taps turned off.
- Inadvertent intra-arterial drug administration:
  - Can cause distal ischaemia and tissue injury, e.g. thiopentone.
  - Consult vascular surgeon.
- Distal ischaemia 2° arterial thrombosis:
  - 0.09% (radial)—0.2% (axillary/femoral).
  - Risk increases with multiple insertion attempts, in-situ >3 days, use of non-teflon coated catheters, and low cardiac output states.
  - Consult vascular surgeon; management options include intra-arterial vasodilator therapy with heparinization or surgical thrombectomy.
- Aneurysm and pseudoaneurysm formation.

Troubleshooting

Difficult insertion

- Repeated attempts at the same site may cause vasospasm and further difficulty in cannulation.
- Use ultrasound to visualize artery and guide needle insertion.
- When using a simple cannula, attach a 2 ml syringe, plunger removed, into the cannula hub. This provides a reservoir that will slowly fill when the needle enters the artery.
- If the wire will not thread into the artery, gently rotate the needle 180° and flatten out the needle; re-attempt having performed these steps.
- Try a different artery.

Inaccuracy

- Damped trace:
  - Under-reads systolic, over-reads diastolic, MAP unchanged
  - Obstruction in tubing between arterial line and transducer, e.g. air bubbles, blood clot, kink in connecting tubing.
  - Tubing too long or too elastic/compliant.
- Resonance or under damped:
  - Over-reads systolic, under-reads diastolic, MAP unchanged.
  - Stiff, non-compliant tubing or diaphragm.
- Transducer not zeroed or not placed at level of heart.
- Distal limb catheters (foot) produce higher peak systolic pressures than more central catheters (femoral/radial).

Further reading

OHB Emergencies in Anaesthesia: *Intra-arterial Injection* p. 344–5.

Craft T.M., Nolan J.P., Parr M.J.A. *Arterial cannulation* in Key Topics in Critical Care. 2nd ed. Iowa: Taylor and Francis Group; 2004. p.35–6.

Insertion of intercostal drains

Indications

- Drainage:
  - Persistent/recurrent pneumothorax after simple aspiration.
  - Simple pneumothorax in a positive pressure ventilated patient.
  - Malignant pleural effusion, pus (empyema), blood (haemothorax) or lymph (chylothorax).

- ❶ Simple pneumothorax without drainage may evolve into a tension pneumothorax (especially when the patient is mechanically ventilated

---

- Thoracotomy:
  - Placed under direct vision during surgery.
  - Often two drains placed for lung resection.
  - Apical tube drains air and basal tube drains fluid.
  - Alternatively anterior and posterior drains are placed towards the lung apex, and side holes provide basal drainage.
- Patient with multiple rib fractures:
  - These patients are at risk of developing pneumothorax.
  - Prior to inter-hospital transfer, especially by air.
  - If they are to receive positive pressure ventilation.

▶▶ Tension pneumothorax is a clinical diagnosis. Needle thoracocentesis should be performed before ICD insertion.

▶▶ Delay in decompression of tension pneumothorax can be fatal

Contraindications

Absolute

- Lung adherent to chest wall.

Relative

- Unclear clinical/radiological picture.
  - Seek radiological opinion if differential diagnosis is unclear between bullous disease and pneumothorax, or between collapse and pleural effusion.
- Coagulopathy.
  - Correct prior to insertion if the situation permits
- Drainage of post-pneumonectomy space.
  - Consult thoracic surgeon.
  - Suction is not applied as this may cause mediastinal shift and obstruct venous return.

Insertion

Equipment
- Local anaesthetic ± sedation.
- Scalpel and blunt dissection forceps.
- Sterile drapes, syringes and needles, silk suture, swabs, dressing.
- Drainage:
  - Closed, low resistance and uni-directional.
  - Usually consists of connecting tubing and closed underwater seal bottle.
  - ⚠ Water will be drawn into the pleural cavity if the underwater seal is raised above the level of the chest.
  - One-way flutter valve may also be used if clinically appropriate.

Drain size
Broadly speaking, the BTS recommends narrow bore drains as they are more comfortable.
- Acute haemothorax.
  - Wide bore (28–30 F) drains recommended; this allows for more accurate assessment of further blood loss and mitigates risk of clot obstructing drainage.
- Pneumothorax.
  - Debate continues about the optimum sized catheter for drainage of pneumothorax.
  - Up to 87 % pneumothoraces can be drained by 9 F drains.
  - Air leak may exceed the capacity of smaller catheters.
- Effusion/empyema.
  - Narrow bore (8–14 F) drains recommended.
  - Smaller incisions reduce leakage of blood/fluid from insertion site.
  - Wide bore catheter may be required for thick malignant or infected fluid to reduce the risk of blockage.

Site
- Traditionally placed in the mid-axillary line, 5th intercostal space.
- The BTS recommends insertion in the "safe triangle".
  - Posterior border = latissimus dorsi.
  - Anterior border = pectoralis major.
  - Inferior border = line above the horizontal level of the nipple.
  - Apex below the axilla.
- Occasionally a drain is inserted in the mid-clavicular line, 2nd intercostal space to treat apical pneumothoraces.
- Insertion site may have to correspond to position/level of collection/ locule; ultrasound guidance useful in this context.
- Site immediately above the rib to avoid damage to the neurovascular bundle which lies immediately beneath the inferior border of the rib.

Technique
- Confirm side/site of tube placement (CXR ± US).
- Secure IV access.

- Position patient supine or sat up with arm abducted over head.
- Full asepsis.
- Infiltrate LA down through skin and muscle to rib periosteum; consider supplemental sedation/analgesia.
- Aspiration of pleural air/fluid should be possible during LA infiltration
  - ⚠ Further imaging should be sought if air/fluid cannot be aspirated at this stage. Do not proceed further.

Open insertion (16–24 F; >24 F drains)
- Make incision (slightly larger than tube diameter or operator's finger, whichever is the largest) parallel and superior to rib.
- Insert wound closure suture and then dissect bluntly down to pleural space. A purse string suture is not recommended for wound closure as it causes an unsightly, painful scar.
- Insert finger into pleural cavity and sweep finger around to ensure viscera are not adherent.
- Guide chest drain into pleural cavity using your finger or forceps mounted onto the drain. Direct apically for air and basally for fluid if possible. Ensure all drainage holes are well inside the pleural cavity.
- Connect to underwater seal or flutter valve and clinically confirm position by fogging of drain, drainage of fluid, bubbling of underwater seal, respiratory swing, or fluttering of the valve.
- Secure in place with a skin suture tied around the tube.

Seldinger insertion (8–14 F; 16–24 F drains)
- Insertion under direct vision using ultrasound is recommended.
- Fixation as above.
  - ▶ Never use substantial force.
  - ▶ Never use a trochar.

Ultrasound
- Useful to localize empyema, effusions and diaphragm, and to define loculations or pleural thickening.
- Real time scanning can help to ensure accurate placement especially if initial blind aspiration fails.

CXR following ICD insertion to assess drain position, complications, and success/failure of procedure.

Clamping drains
- ❶ Never clamp a bubbling chest drain—risk of tension pneumothorax.
- Clamping a drain for pneumothorax should only be done in consultation with a thoracic surgeon/respiratory physician, and should be unclamped if there is any clinical deterioration.

- Drains for large pleural effusions may be clamped under supervision to control drainage rate, and therefore to reduce the risk of re-expansion pulmonary oedema.

Removal
- Lung re-expanded or pleural cavity drainage complete, no air leak.
- Remove during expiration or a Valsalva manoeuvre—this maintains a positive intrapleural pressure to prevent the influx of air. Have an assistant available to close the skin with the previously inserted suture.
- Repeat CXR only necessary if changing clinical signs or ABG indicate.

Troubleshooting

Lung not expanding/inadequate drainage
- Reassess tube position—?respiratory swing,CXR.
- Loculated effusion—consider US guidance.
- Consider high volume, low pressure suction (10–20 cmH$_2$O).
- Increase tidal volume or PEEP if ventilated.
- Consult thoracic surgeon.

Persistent air leak
- Reassess tube position—may have migrated out of chest cavity.
- Minimize airway pressures and PEEP. Wean to spontaneous breathing modes if possible.
- Accept relative hypercapnoea.
- In trauma consider bronchoscopy to exclude airway rupture.
- Consult thoracic surgeon.

Complications
- Painful insertion; use sedation and LA unless contraindicated.
- Lung trauma causing persistent air leak.
- Subcutaneous emphysema secondary to air leak around drain at skin insertion.
- Intra-abdominal organ laceration.
- Neurovascular bundle trauma.
- Vagal stimulation.
- Malposition, kinking, disconnection.
- Pulmonary oedema 2° rapid lung re-expansion.
- Infection; antibiotic prophylaxis recommended in trauma patients requiring chest drain insertion (incidence 7 2.4%).

Further reading

Laws D, Neville E, Duffy J. On behalf of the British Thoracic Society Pleural Disease Group, a subgroup of the British Thoracic Society Standards of Care Committee: British Thoracic Society guidelines for the insertion of a chest drain. *Thorax* 2003; 58(II):53–9.

Craft TM, Nolan JR, Parr MJA. *Chest tube thoracostomy in Key Topics in Critical Care.* 2nd ed. Taylor and Francis Group 2004. pp. 111–13.

Index

CW00745698

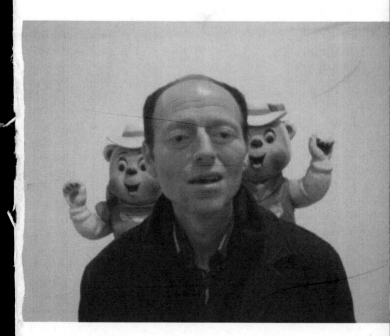

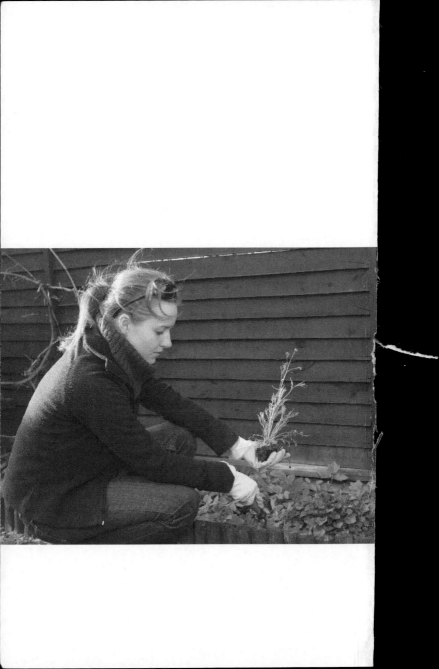

Baruch Solomon

Earn a Living as a Self Employed Gardener

How to Tell the Difference between Weeds and Flowers

Published by Lulu Publishers

www.lulu.com

Copyright © Baruch Solomon 2010

The right of Baruch Solomon to be identified as the author of this work has been asserted.

ISBN

978-1-4457-2168-2

Printed and Bound by Lulu Publishers

www.lulu.com

CONTENTS

Page

CHAPTER 1 - INTRODUCTION

Why Become a Gardener?

Well for starters, it has all the advantages of being your own boss
with few of the risks. You work the hours you like, where you
like and for whom you like. If you're having trouble paying the
bills, you can always work a bit extra and if you want to disappear
for a couple of days you won't need a sick note from your doctor.

Forget about having to suck up to the boss or fit in with a
corporate ideology. All kinds of people become gardeners, and
you can adapt the job to fit around your personality. Nobody
minds if their gardener is a bit eccentric. You can be male, female
or transgender. You can look and act like a Greenpeace
campaigner, white van man or someone who does interior design.
You can be silent and phlegmatic or the touchy feely type who
goes into ecstasies over clematis. You can be a bit simple or have
a PhD in rocket science. If someone asks you about greenfly, you
can dispense advice in a West Country accent while leaning on
your spade or do a Google search on your BlackBerry. Whatever
the image you wish to project, your customers will love you for it,
and it will give them something to talk about at dinner parties.

The job is seasonal, but for eight or nine months of the year you'll
have no trouble finding all the work you want. Very little happens
between Christmas and March however. You may find a few jobs
if you put enough effort into advertising, but is it really worth the
time and expense? It's probably a better idea to save a bit of
money during the summer months. Then you can use the time to

catch up on daytime TV, write your novel or get yourself a sun tan in Tenerife.

Your starting costs are minimal. A medium sized rucksack with a few tools shouldn't set you back more than a hundred pounds. Best add another hundred or so for advertising. As for overheads, mine consist of little more than replacing lost tools, bus fares and the odd bacon sandwich between jobs.

You don't have to deal with endless paperwork, difficult employers, office backstabbing or having your talents unappreciated. If someone gives you a hard time, you can walk away. If a customer sacks you, there are plenty more fish in the sea. Generally speaking, you can act according to your commonsense rather than the suffocating requirements of health and safety and political correctness. If a ladder seems dodgy, don't go up it. If an attractive customer kicks you in the shins, it means you're staring at her boobs. Strange to say it, some customers will actually thank you for using your own judgment and initiative.

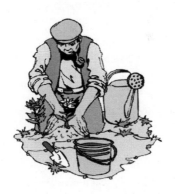

But most of all, what's special about gardening is that you can live in a city and still go to work in the great outdoors, in the wind and the sun; feeling and smelling and working with plants and soil and leaves. Even now, I still get a brilliant feeling starting work on sunny mornings and a sense of contentment and satisfaction walking home in the twilight at the end of a long day.

But is Gardening for You?

Gardening isn't for everybody though, at least not as a job. If you're terrified of creepy crawlies or freak out when you see a bit of dog poo on the lawn, then expect a few unpleasant surprises. You'll also find it tough if you're not used to being physically active. Gardening is manual work. Its one thing to stroll up and down the lawn with a Flymo for ten minutes before collapsing on a recliner with an iced drink and a Sunday paper. If you garden for a living however, you'll need to keep going for eight hours or more, with maybe a lunch break and the odd cup of tea which you sip as you're working. Not all gardening is heavy work but some is, and you do get your hands dirty. Then there's the weather to contend with. Nobody expects you to work through a downpour but you can't pack up and go home at the first sign of drizzle either. Sometimes it's miserable and damp and clammy; other days, the weather can't make up its mind. If you are working in winter, you've the cold to worry about as well, which isn't as bad as you'd think, since you warm up surprisingly quickly when you're physically active.

Gardening is a lonely job. Some of your customers will like a natter, especially the older ones; but you'll need to get used to being on your own most of the time. You can work with a friend of course, but it'll have to be the kind of friend you can handle being alone with for long periods. If you thrive on office gossip or the camaraderie of the workplace, then self-employment may not be for you. If you still want a job in gardening, then you might want to consider working at a park, garden centre or city farm.

As a gardener, you'll never be out of a job, but you don't get looked after. You won't get sick pay or fringe benefits, and you have to save for the winter. If it rains, you won't get paid. If you go on holiday, you don't just have to budget for the holiday but for the fact that you're not getting a wage while you're away.

And it's not as if you'll make a fortune either, unless you reach the stage where you can employ other gardeners to do the work. However many people want to employ you, you can only charge so much an hour and you can only work so many hours a day.

What this Book Will Tell You

There are plenty of things that this book won't tell you. It won't tell you how to win a marrow competition, grow the best dahlias in the county or have your garden listed in the celebrated Yellow Book. You'll learn some basic things about plants, weeds, soils, seasons and so on, but if it's specialised or detailed information you're after, then there are plenty of excellent books already written that cater for all levels of expertise.

This book isn't about getting a job as a gardener either. You can do that of course. You can get a job cutting grass on council estates or dispensing advice in garden centres. You can work for a professional landscaper or travel the world acquiring strange and wonderful species for the Eden Project. Depending on what you go for, you'll need anything from a failed GCSE in metalwork to a Royal Horticultural Society qualification to a PhD on the implications of global warming for Venus fly traps in Laos. If any of the above sound like your cup of tea, then good luck to you, but you're on your own, since the only reason I came into gardening in the first place is that I'm completely unemployable.

You won't learn anything in this book about garden makeovers like they do on the telly. Everyone seems to want to be a designer or landscape gardener these days and a few people actually try to make their dreams a reality. There is money to be made, but it's a very risky and competitive business, and the market isn't that large. Unless people are well to do, they either do their own landscaping or leave their garden as it is. Even those people who can afford to pay a professional aren't likely to do so again for several years; probably when they move house again. Keeping gardens tidy and well maintained, on the other hand, requires regular work. Many people don't want to be bothered with it and are happy to pay you to do it for them.

What this book will do, more or less, is to equip you with the knowledge, confidence and know how you will need in order to find regular self-employment and not make too much of a pillock of yourself while you're doing it. You'll learn how to advertise and get customers. You'll learn which tools you need to buy for yourself, which ones you can borrow and which ones to avoid using at all costs. You'll learn how to charge in such a way that both you and the customer feel you've got a fair deal. You'll learn basic gardening tasks, etiquette and that most important secret of all; how to tell weeds from flowers!

I have included some basic gardening knowledge. I have tried, however, to reduce this to a few simple rules. I will be introducing you to some of the most common weeds and plants, but all you really need to know about them to start with is what they look like. In order to keep the price of the book down, I haven't included any colour illustrations. When I get to the sections on plant species however, I will be direct you to some excellent web resources that can be used in conjunction with this book to help you recognise them.

I don't pretend you won't encounter problems. You'll have days when there's mess all around you and you're convinced the owner will come out and sack you on the spot. (That's only happened to me twice!) You'll leave weeds and pull out flowers. You'll step back to admire your handiwork and find you've squashed a begonia. You'll knock over the odd terracotta pot or pretentious artefact that passes for modern sculpture. But don't forget that when I started I was a bigger clot than you'll ever be, and I never had a book like this to help me.

CHAPTER TWO - GETTING STARTED

This book is about two things. It's about becoming a gardener and it's about starting a business. To be a gardener, you need to use tools. To start a business, you need to think about how you are going to get customers.

If you've ever seen Gardener's World, you may think that you have to know all about delphiniums, black spot and why home grown artichokes taste better than the ones you buy in Sainsbury. If you've never been self-employed before, you may have the idea that to start a business you need a white van and your own shop or office.

What you will learn to do in this book is far simpler and much more manageable. It's also a bit less glamorous than going on Dragons Den though it can, in its way, be every bit as rewarding. You've probably worked out by now that you don't need business premises. Gardens aren't portable and you can't take them down the high street to have the grass cut. You may be forgiven for thinking that you need a van, or at least a hatchback, but this is definitely not the case. I've never even passed my driving test, and being a gardener hasn't made me want to. Most of your customers will have their own lawnmowers and large tools. I travel between jobs by bus, carrying everything I need in a medium sized rucksack.

Landscaping is a little different, but I've known at least two landscape gardeners without cars who operate by having everything delivered to the place they're working at. In these days of concern about the environment, not driving can only boost your green credentials.

Equipment Worth Investing in

In theory, you could become a self-employed gardener without any financial input at all. You could rely entirely on the customers' tools and drum up trade by knocking on peoples' doors. Realistically though, you'd want to spend around a hundred pounds on tools and about the same again on advertising.

I recommend the following equipment and tools.

A Mobile Phone

No doubt you have one of these already, unless you're over eighty five. If you're not always able to answer it, make sure the voicemail is working and that you've recorded a polite, personalised greeting. If someone is phoning for the first time, they want to be reassured that they've called the right number.

A Medium Sized Rucksack for Your Tools

It doesn't need to be large enough to travel the world during your gap year but it should be both bigger and stronger than a knapsack and cost between £20 and £30. When I buy a new rucksack, I bring my shears and loppers with me to check whether I can fit them inside before I buy it.

A Pair of Garden Shears/Hedge Clippers

These are used for a variety of jobs and are one of your most important pieces of equipment. They need to be reasonably sharp, which is one reason not to rely on borrowing them from your customer. I have to confess I've never had any success at sharpening shears myself, although people tell me you can do wonderful things with sandpaper. I tend to replace mine every couple of months; usually I lose them before they have a chance to get blunt. A cheap pair will normally cost between five and ten pounds.

Secateurs

These are the small things you use to prune roses, but like shears, they have a multiplicity of uses. I have to replace mine about once a week. It's not a good idea to spend more than a fiver on them therefore, unless you're confident you're not going to lose them.

Loppers

These have blades like secateurs but long handles like shears. They can normally cut branches more than an inch thick and make a lot of jobs, especially, bagging up waste, a lot quicker than they would otherwise be. You can get a cheap pair for between five and ten pounds. Make sure the handles aren't too long to get into your rucksack.

A Small Fork

This is essential for weeding, especially when you have to go carefully around areas where there are delicate plants. Be prepared to pay between five and ten pounds and don't be tempted to buy a cheaper, plastic fork or one with flimsy blades. They may be alright for containers with fluffy compost in them but when you try and dig dandelions out of heavy, dry, clayey soil, they will bend back and become useless. If the blades don't look like they can take a bit of punishment, they probably can't.

A Clearaway Sheet

This normally costs about £9 and is excellent for chucking garden waste on to. It's often as good as a wheelbarrow for carting stuff around the garden and together with loppers, makes bagging up waste a lot easier. They're not always on sale in DIY places. If they aren't, they'll almost certainly sell the sheets you put into the back of estate cars to protect the floor from spillages and messy children. These work just as well.

Gloves

A pair of basic gardening gloves costs about two to five pounds. They're good for handling prickly stuff like brambles, roses, stinging nettles and pyracantha, but they have two defects. They get wet in the rain and they make it difficult to move your fingers around freely. If you simply want to keep your hands clean and handle yucky stuff, you'll be much better off with washing up gloves, or the disposable latex gloves you can buy in the chemist.

Something Waterproof

A light mac will do, and it doesn't have to be made out of anything expensive like Gor-Tex. It's for drizzly days or days when the weather can't make up its mind whether to rain or not, and you have to contend with the odd light shower, or days when you're in the middle of something and it's more trouble to pack up than to carry on working in the rain. If it's really chucking it down you won't do yourself or your customers any good by trying to play the hero. It's almost impossible to work efficiently when you're soaked to the skin and you'll get mud everywhere. Some kindly females may go "oh you poor wet gardener!" and want to mother you, but it's far more likely they'll think you're a complete pillock.

A Roll of Bin Bags

Some councils supply free bags or bins for garden waste. Others make you buy garden waste bags from the library for a pound each, and then when they're full you have to phone the relevant department to arrange for them to be picked up. If I were uncharitable, I would say that some local authorities want to claim they have a recycling scheme while ensuring that as few people as possible put them to the inconvenience of operating it.

So where does that leave you? In the interests of the environment, you should be extolling the benefits of compost

Some Garden Tools You May Want to Carry With You (Not to Scale)

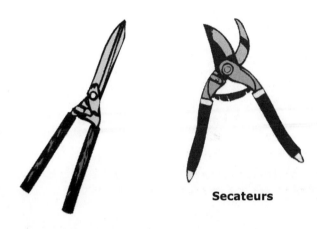

Secateurs

Shears/Hedge Clippers

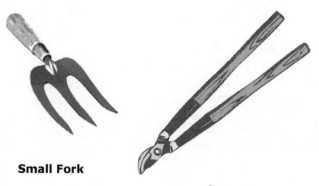

Small Fork

Loppers

heaps to your customers, but most still opt for stuffing their waste into black bin bags. Hopefully they will be taken to the recycling centre rather than smuggled past the bin men.

A Plastic Lunch Box

I ought to invest in one myself; then I wouldn't waste money on bacon sandwiches.

String or Twine

It's useful to carry some of this with you as you never know when you'll need to tie branches back to a trellis or a plant to a stake.

A Radio

If you feel you need one, I suggest getting something bulky and cheap that you can hear up to ten feet away. Forget I-pods or personal stereos. If it involves headphones or sticking anything in your ears, then you can guarantee that the reception will go wrong the moment you make a sudden movement. You'll spend more time fiddling around with it than you will do working.

A Power/Circuit Breaker

A power breaker is a safety device you can use with a lawnmower, hedge trimmer or other electrical tool. As the name suggests, it cuts the power off when you do something stupid like accidentally chopping through the wires.

You have to be reasonably daft to go over the flex with the lawnmower; even I've only done it once. The electric shock wasn't a pleasant experience, any more than explaining it all to the nice old lady whose mower it was, but I did live to tell the tale. Keeping the flex out of the way of a hedge trimmer blade can be a real headache; just one reason to choose ordinary hedge clippers.

Let's have a look at the bill we've run up so far. The following is based on what I normally expect to pay. Depending where you shop, you may pay a little less or more for these items.

Rucksack	25.00
Loppers	7.50
Shears	7.50
Secateurs	4.00
Small fork	5.00
Gardening gloves	3.00
Kitchen/Latex gloves	2.00
20 Bin bags	1.50
String/twine	2.00
Plastic lunch box	2.00
Portable radio	10.00
Power breaker	8.00
Total	**£77.50**

This budget includes several non-essentials, and unless you're really on your uppers, constitutes a pretty minimal outlay. What's more, nearly all the above items are obtainable from DIY superstores, your local hardware retailer, or the place on the high street that sells stuff that's fallen off a lorry for 99p. For rucksacks, if you can't find what you want on a market stall, then Argos is quite a good bet.

That takes care of the tools of your trade, but what about being a businessperson?

Getting Business/Advertising

If you are going to earn a living as a gardener, you will need to attract customers. This shouldn't be a problem unless you live in a steel or mining town where everyone's unemployed or a remote village where outsiders aren't welcome and Ebenezer Longways has kept everyone's garden immaculate since 1927. Generally speaking, there are plenty of people who will happily pay for a cheap, cheerful, flexible person like you. All you have to be able to do is to let your potential customers know that you exist, and that you can be trusted not to make a pig's breakfast of their herbaceous border. You need in other words, to advertise.

It's surprising how many people are apparently oblivious to this basic fact about setting up any business. How many people do you know with plans to offer aromatherapy sessions, open art galleries or sell homemade pottery on the internet? I bet they haven't thought out a coherent marketing strategy. Advertise your gardening business properly and you'll be up and running while they're still whingeing over croissants and cappuccinos that the world doesn't appreciate their potential.

So what's your first step? One obvious place to start is to tell all your friends and relatives that you're becoming a gardener, and hope that they'll all tell their friends and relatives. No doubt you'll land yourself a couple of jobs here and there and when people see how brilliant you are, they'll recommend you to more people. It'll work probably, provided you don't mind waiting a few years to develop a clientele.

If on the other hand, you plan on having a full time job this summer, you're going to have to speed things up a little. In my experience, the most effective method by far is door to door leafleting. A simple, cheap, friendly looking leaflet offering to tidy peoples' gardens will definitely generate a response. If you put these out during the gardening season, you can expect a phone call for every 50-100 leaflets, and about two thirds of the people who call you will actually use you. Say you decide to get your business going over a two or three months, try ordering five thousand leaflets and start putting out around five hundred of them each week (about 3 hours work). You may well find, as I did, that you soon have as much business as you can cope with and still have leaflets to spare.

Designing the Leaflet

You don't need a professional designer to produce an acceptable leaflet. If you know the rudiments of desktop publishing or even word processing you can probably do it yourself on your home computer. And it definitely doesn't need to be in colour. A black and white leaflet on A5 paper is fine, and very cheap to produce. What you put on it, however, and how you express yourself, is crucial. You need to show your customers that you're a nice reliable person who's not afraid of hard work and who, while perhaps not an expert is intelligent enough to be left on their own. It should also include at least one image to do with gardening on it which, if nothing else, will relieve the monotony of print. The illustration on the next page provides an example of such a leaflet.

Once you've designed the leaflet, the next stage is to send it to a professional printer who does leaflets. You can shop around on the internet and printers often advertise in publications like Loot. Some companies are more reliable than others so it's important that you have a look at their web site and talk to them on the phone to see whether they sound like they know what they're doing before you part with your cash. Hopefully, you'll be able to email your leaflet to the printer, although you may prefer to send it in the post with a cheque. You should also be able to have the leaflets delivered to you, especially since your printer may be in a different town. Before sending anything to your printer, make sure you're both agreed on full costs, including delivery charges; as well as on when you can expect your leaflets to arrive.

Printing costs vary enormously according to the type of leaflet being printed and the sort of printing the company specialises in. As already noted, the leaflet doesn't have to be superior quality or professionally designed. All you need is a simple black and white leaflet on A5 paper, and some printers will happily turn out 5,000 of these for less than £50.

An Example of a Leaflet Advertising Gardening Services

Need Help With Your Garden?

I offer a reasonably priced, friendly gardening service in your area.

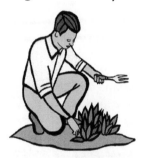

I may not be up to Royal Horticultural Society standards but I've a good deal of commonsense and I'm happy to do all those jobs like digging, weeding, mowing lawns, clipping hedges and bushes etc that you may not have the time for.

If you want to know more about the service I offer, then give me a call on;

12345 678910

I look forward to hearing from you.

Once your leaflets have arrived, you can start putting them out without any more ado. I wouldn't deliver them all at once however, as you may get more calls than you can handle, and you want to take some time building up your business so that you can gain some skills and experience without feeling under too much pressure. As for where to deliver them, semi-detached leafy suburbs are best, but any area where houses have gardens will do.

There are certain basic manners when it comes to leafleting. Don't put more than one leaflet through a letterbox however many doorbells there are, and make sure you put the leaflet all the way through the box so that it lands on the mat. When doing so however, it's a good idea not to stick your fingers all the way through as it's not unknown to get quite badly bitten by an angry dog. You'll see a lot of notices saying "no leaflets" or "no circulars" while you're out doing your deliveries. Respect them but don't take the criticism personally. In many areas people are inundated by leaflets advertising pizzas and takeaways; some companies leaflet the same areas every couple of weeks. You're advertising something different, which many people actually want. I've never had any complaints when delivering gardening leaflets.

In fact, leafleting can be quite a pleasant activity, especially on a sunny day. While you're out and about have a look at people's front gardens. Can you name any of the plants or shrubs growing there? Can you tell the weeds from the flowers? Invent your own names for things that you see. The more excruciating they are the more likely it is that you'll remember them next time you see them.

So there you are on the first warm sunny day in spring, your bundle of leaflets in your hand. You've been shopping for your equipment and now it's all carefully packed into your brand new rucksack. All that remains is to find some customers. As you stride confidently up and down people's front drives, pausing occasionally to admire the daffodils and crocuses, you can't help feeling that it's good to be alive. You start humming a tune; something you haven't done in years. You feel a vibration in your pocket. It's your phone ringing. Then, just as you're about to take a call from your very first customer, it suddenly hits you. *Wait a minute; I don't know a ruddy thing about gardening!*

CHAPTER THREE – BASIC GARDENING SKILLS
TOOLS AND THEIR USES

So you've got your tools. You've advertised and somebody has phoned up wanting you to come and do a job. You turn up on a bright April morning with a pale blue sky and a watery sun that feels pleasantly warm on your back. The customer shows you her garden. She apologises profusely for not having kept it in immaculate condition and worries about saying the wrong thing because she thinks you know more than she does. "My Brian always leaves the edges," she'll sigh, before asking you how often you think she should cut the grass. "And is it too late to prune the roses? And should I cut my Forsythia back? Oh, and could you dig over the vegetable patch but mind my seedlings. I don't know where all these weeds come from, and this sticky stuff gets everywhere! Do you know what it's called? And careful of the clematis next to the fence. Oh yes, the hedge needs doing as well. Don't worry; I've got an electric trimmer. And what about getting rid of the waste; do you take it away with you?"

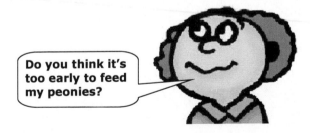

Do you think it's too early to feed my peonies?

Believe it or not, I'm only exaggerating slightly. A seasoned indecisive garden enthusiast can keep going in this vein for several minutes with very little encouragement. I find it quite endearing, a bit like the nervous contestants you see on "Who Wants to be a Millionaire". It can be a bit daunting for the beginner though. You haven't a clue how to mow a lawn, never mind use a hedge trimmer. The only thing you know about forsythia is the bloke on the telly who goes "nice to see you" and "points make prizes". No doubt you've sailed breezily through your entire life without a moment's thought for how people get rid of weeds, clippings, grass cuttings and the like if they aren't allowed to put them in the dustbin.

Suddenly it occurs to you that you have bitten off more than you can chew. You used to help Daddy mow the lawn when you were a child but how exactly did Daddy get it going? When and how do you cut bushes or prune roses? Most worrying of all, *how do you tell the difference between weeds and flowers?*

What you Will Learn in Chapters Three and Four

In this chapter I will introduce you to the garden tools and items of machinery you'll most commonly come into contact with. Then in Chapter Four, I will take you through some garden jobs you'll frequently be asked to do. I'll be working on the assumption that you don't have a van in which to cart around heavy, petrol driven machinery, and that you rely on the customer for anything you can't get into your backpack.

Reading a book about how to do something is no substitute for experience however, and if you haven't done any gardening at all, then it's probably best to find an environment where you can practice the tasks you read about without doing any damage. You may have a garden where you live. If not, you've probably got friends and family who'll be grateful to have you practise on theirs. You can contact your local voluntary service and say you're wiling do a bit of gardening for senior citizens. This can be a particularly good way to start. Not only will you be doing a kindly act but many elderly people will have been enthusiastic gardeners in their time and only too glad to pass on their knowledge.

Garden Tools and What They're For

Everybody has their own preferences tools wise. I like to keep things simple, largely because I'm limited by what the customer has and what I can carry on my back.

The following tools are ones that I use on a frequent basis.

Shears/clippers	Small fork	Lawn rake
Secateurs	Large fork	Broom
Loppers	Hoe	Dustpan & brush
Handsaw	Lawn mower	

I use the following tools only occasionally; sometimes as a substitute for something on the first list.

Trowel	Spade	Shovel
Soil rake	Edging shears	Strimmer
Hedge trimmer	Garden vacuum	

You'll see all sorts of gadgets and gizmos in garden centres that are supposed to make life easier. Long metal tubes attached to gas canisters for scorching weeds on the patio. Shredders for getting rid of garden waste that need to be unblocked every few seconds. Scissors straight out of a conceptual art exhibition intended for edging the lawn extremely slowly and painfully. Zimmer frame like contraptions to take the pain out of digging that get stuck fast in anything that isn't already light and crumbly. Presumably, most people who buy these contraptions only get to use them a couple of times a year and so never get round to asking for their money back.

I'm not saying that there aren't any new inventions that work, but until you're ready to make your own judgements, there's a lot to be said for simple, honest tools that have stood the test of time.

Shears/Hedge clippers

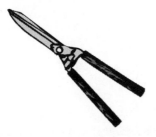

I mention these first because even if you buy nothing else, it is absolutely essential that you have your own pair. Your customers may or may not own shears, but if they do they will almost certainly be blunt. The main tasks they are good for are trimming bushes and hedges and cutting grass that the mower can't get to, such as the edges of the lawn. Many people nowadays prefer to use electric strimmers and hedge trimmers for these jobs, but hand shears are far more versatile, and in your average sized garden, a lot less hassle. You don't have to waste time plugging them in or worry about chopping through the flex, and you can get into all sorts of awkward spaces. It's much easier to shape bushes the way you want them with shears, and best of all, they don't make a horrible, ear splitting noise.

You don't need an expensive pair. You can usually buy something quite adequate from a DIY store for six or seven pounds. Bear in mind that however much you pay for them; if they're being used constantly they'll go blunt in a couple of months and unless you have more success at sharpening them then I have, they'll need to be replaced.

Secateurs

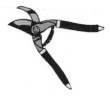

Secateurs are both smaller and sharper than shears. You can make a neater cut with them, but you can only cut one stem at a time, which isn't much use when trimming a hedge. They are used for careful, "close up" cutting, such as in pruning roses and deadheading flowers.

It's best to bring your own, if only because they're very easy to lose. Losing customers' tools is generally a lot more embarrassing than losing your own.

Loppers

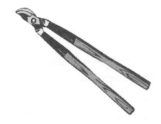

Loppers are like a cross between secateurs and shears. That's to say, they have long handles like shears and blades like those on a pair of secateurs. The result is a tool that can slice easily and neatly through thick branches. Not only does that make them useful for bushes and trees but also for quickly chopping up garden waste. They're an excellent labour saving device but most of your customers won't have them, so it's definitely worthwhile to buy your own. They'll cost approximately the same as a pair of shears.

Hand Saw

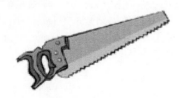

If you have a pair of loppers you won't need one very often, but they do come in useful occasionally. The saw should have long teeth and be small, so that you can get into awkward spaces. DIY stores sell folding saws that look like large penknives for around £10. These are ideal.

Small Fork and Trowel

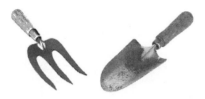

These are used for digging and weeding when you're working in small spaces or where you need to be close up in order to avoid doing any damage. I generally find small forks more useful than trowels. They're less likely to do damage to things that you can't see underground, such as bulbs. They're also better at getting weeds out, because you've more chance of getting the whole root instead of merely slicing through it. Trowels are good for digging holes for planting though, as well as for scraping lawnmowers clean and digging around roots.

As with secateurs, it's best to buy your own, because they're easy to lose. You need to make sure that they are made of metal and strong, otherwise they will bend back as soon as you apply a bit of pressure, rendering them almost useless. Generally speaking, be prepared to pay at least a fiver.

Large Fork and Hoe

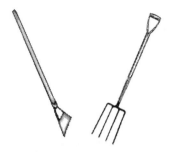

These are for digging, weeding or breaking up the ground in larger spaces. With a fork, you can dig out deep rooted weeds and turn the soil over. You're thus more likely to use it on beds that have been neglected for some time. If a border is in reasonably good nick, then it's often quicker and easier just to break the soil up with the hoe and in the process slice the heads off any annual weeds that are popping their heads above the soil.

The hoe in the above illustration is a Dutch hoe. The other kind of hoe is called a draw hoe, which is indispensable to many millions of small farmers in Africa and other parts of the Global South, but which you don't get to use a lot in an English domestic garden.

Nearly all your customers will have a large fork and many will have a hoe as well. You don't want to carry these tools with you unless it's absolutely necessary. If you have to take them on the bus, put a carrier bag round the prongs or blade, or the driver might claim that it's an offensive weapon and not let you on.

Spade and Shovel

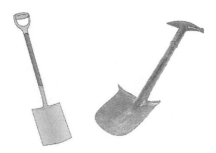

It's surprising how many people can't tell a spade from a shovel. A spade is designed for digging, which is why it has a straight blade that will go easily into the ground. A shovel has curved edges, making it useless for digging, but ideal for moving stuff about, be it earth, manure, coal or snow.

Just as with a small fork and trowel, I use a spade a lot less often than a large fork. If you're using prongs instead of a wide blade, you're less likely to do damage or slice weeds in half when you want to get them up by the roots.

I use a spade chiefly for digging holes or as a substitute for a fork or shovel when the customer doesn't have one available.

Lawn Mowers

You've probably noticed that I'm not too keen on garden machinery. It usually takes time to set up, frequently goes wrong, is useless for getting into nooks and crannies and the noise is not conducive to having beautiful, lofty thoughts. If you disagree, then you might want to consider getting a job drilling holes in the road.

Thankfully, most machinery isn't really necessary in a domestic garden, but you will have to become familiar with lawnmowers. Most people have electric mowers which are much simpler to operate and don't go wrong very often. Petrol mowers are meant for very large gardens but tend to be kept as status symbols by men with postage stamp lawns and even smaller penises.

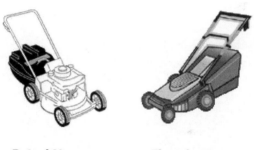

Petrol Mower   **Electric Mower**

If you don't have transport, you'll need to get used to using a variety of mowers. I will be giving more detailed descriptions of mowers in subsequent chapters.

Rakes

There are two basic kinds of rakes; lawn rakes and soil rakes. I use a lawn rake a lot more frequently than I do a soil rake. You can use it for sweeping up grass cuttings if your mower hasn't got a grass box or more frequently, for sweeping debris and rubbish on lawns, soil and gravel paths; anywhere where it does a better job than a broom.

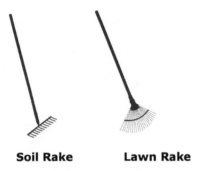

Soil Rake   **Lawn Rake**

In late autumn, you'll spend a lot of time sweeping up leaves and unless you have a good garden vacuum, a lawn rake is indispensable.

A soil rake is more likely to be used for moving or levelling soil, or for tilling the surface e.g. when sowing grass seeds. It's stronger than a lawn rake, but sharper and less pliable, so if you do find yourself using it on a lawn, you need to be careful not to tear the grass up in the process.

Mechanical Hedge Trimmer

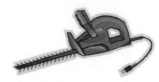

It's difficult to find anything nice to say about hedge trimmers. A lot of customers will offer to let you use theirs, and you should try to save their feelings by letting them down gently. Granted, you'll occasionally find that you can trim a hedge a bit quicker with one than you can with a pair of shears. This in no way alters the fact that they are a pain in every way, and to be avoided if it's at all possible.

They're difficult and dangerous to use at awkward heights and angles and the cheap ones your customers own will generally be unable to cut through anything thicker than a couple of millimetres. They also spread clippings everywhere, which makes sweeping up the mess a much bigger job.

Worst of all they're a death trap. When mowing a lawn, it's relatively easy to avoid going over the flex. When trimming a hedge, the flex has a habit of constantly getting in front of the blade. Accidents with a hedge trimmer are quite common so whatever you do, never use a hedge trimmer without a power breaker.

Strimmer/Grass Cutter

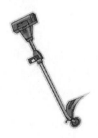

In large areas of grassland, e.g. the grounds of housing estates, you'll see people cutting the grass with petrol strimmers, usually wearing protective glasses and ear muffs. The garden equivalent is usually electric, less powerful and mainly for cutting the edges of lawns or places you can't get to with the lawn mower.

Inside the bottom is a coil of plastic wire. There's a hole through which the end of this protrudes and when the strimmer is used, this bit cuts the grass by revolving at high speed. When the end of the wire gets broken, say by hitting a stone, there is usually a mechanism by which the coil unwinds slightly, feeding more wire through the hole.

They have their uses, but you can't beat a good old fashioned pair of hand shears.

Garden Vacuum

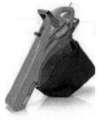

You're only likely to need this in late autumn, when there is a serious amount of leaves to pick up. Again, if your customer has one, it will probably be electric. You can put it on blow and suck – as the actress said to the bishop - and each is extremely powerful. The bottom bit, which sometimes looks like a pelican's pouch, is detachable and you take it off in order to throw the rubbish away. Some vacuums shred the leaves, so that they take up a lot less space than when you simply rake them up.

That covers the garden tools you need to know about. In the next chapter, we will look at how to use them to do some of the more common garden tasks.

CHAPTER FOUR – BASIC GARDENING SKILLS
COMMON GARDEN TASKS

Things you'll be Asked to Do

Below are the most common tasks you'll be required to do in a garden.

Mowing and edging lawns

Trimming, chopping, pruning and deadheading

Clearing overgrown areas

Digging/turning soil over

Planting and sowing seeds

Sweeping up leaves and other debris

Tying plants to walls, fences or stakes

Clearing up the mess

Last but not least, you'll be expected to do weeding, weeding and more weeding. This is dealt with in a separate chapter.

Mowing and Edging Lawns

Some of your customers will want you to cut the grass. Others, who spent their formative years in households where mowing the lawn was a "Daddy job"; consider it their bounden duty to drag their men folk away from the footie on a Saturday afternoon to do it. Either way you can expect to have to trim the edges. There's about as much chance of "Daddy" trimming the edges as there is of his leaving the toilet seat down.

Hand mowers almost invariably give the least hassle, provided the grass isn't too long. They're safer to use than petrol or electric mowers. They don't pollute the environment, hardly ever go wrong and are generally quicker, at least in a small garden. It's a great shame that hardly anybody uses them any more.

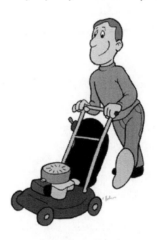

Your customers' mowers will either be electric or petrol driven. They also come in a variety of shapes, sizes and configurations, which it will be up to you to familiarise yourself with. I will be giving a description of some of the more common ones later on in this book, as well as a brief step by step guide on how to use them. This book is not a technical manual however, and the best way to familiarise yourself with different mowers is to get some hands on experience.

Starting the Mower

There are exceptions, but generally speaking, you start an electric mower by holding down the safety button while you press the start lever. You start a petrol mower by holding down the start lever and pulling the ripcord.

The Actual Mowing

There's not really much to say about this. Where there's room, you simply push the mower up and down the lawn, and when you have irregular edges, you'll need to use it like a Hoover or vacuum cleaner in order to get into awkward nooks and crannies.

Some customers like to see a "cricket pitch effect" i.e. alternate sections of light and dark looking grass. This impression is created by the way the sun shines on newly cut grass if it has been cut in regular rows. No doubt people like stripes because they're traditional but to get them, you usually need a petrol mower and the lawn has to be spacious enough for you to be able to walk up and down it in straight lines. Speaking for myself, I prefer a lawn to look like a patch of reasonably short grass than a pair of striped pyjamas.

Sometimes, particularly if the grass is long and/or damp, the blades will get clogged up with grass and you will have to remove this by hand. Make sure you unplug the mower first, just in case it starts accidentally. If it's a petrol mower, then disconnect the spark plug.

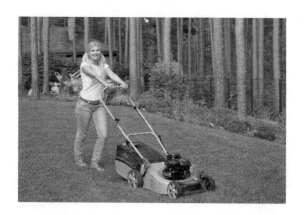

Cleaning a Mower

Some people take great pride in their tools and carefully clean their mower every time they use it. If you're really sad, you can even sign up for courses to learn how to do it properly. I just use a trowel or gloved hand to scrape the blades and the underside. The mowers' innards won't exactly gleam, but let's face it; you're only going to get everything dirty again in a week or two. With petrol mowers, bear in mind that when trying to get to the underside, it's probably not a good idea to turn the machine too far onto its side in case oil or petrol leaks out somewhere.

Safety

There are a few safety issues when using electric or petrol mowers. As I pointed out above, make sure they are switched off before putting your hands near the blades, either to unblock them or clean them afterwards. It's not likely that a mower will switch itself on again, but it has been known, and the consequences of getting your hands caught in the blades don't bear thinking about. With an electric mower disconnect it and with a petrol one, try to pull the spark plug out, though this may not be practicable, since it expands when hot and doesn't come off easily.

The next point, which applies to electric mowers, is to make sure you don't go over the flex. You could do so at some point though, which is why you should carry a power breaker with you so that the electricity cuts off as soon as you're in danger of being electrocuted.

Don't try and mow the lawn in the rain. This applies especially to electric mowers as you can get electrocuted. It's unwise to cut very wet grass anyway, as the mower gets clogged up constantly and the lawn looks as if it's had an extremely bad haircut.

Edging

It's usually difficult to get right to the edge of the lawn with a mower, which is why edging is regarded as a separate task. Depending on how formal the lawn is and the type of customer you're working for, you may simply need to clip the really sticky out bits with your shears or you may need to go round carefully giving the edge a manicure. Either way, your shears are probably the best tool for the job provided you don't mind kneeling down. They're versatile for getting into nooks and crannies, and if the grass cuttings are conspicuous, you're already on your knees so you can pick them up as you go along.

Edging with Strimmers

Your customer may have an electric strimmer or grass cutter, which is often quicker if less accurate than using shears. I briefly described strimmers in the last chapter. When using a strimmer, you need to watch what you're doing and not let the cutting wire get too close to the grass or edge; otherwise, you can create ugly dents or bald patches.

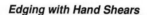

Edging with Hand Shears

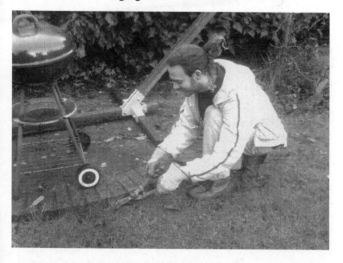

For safety reasons, make sure you don't cut the flex and that you use a power breaker. It's also a good idea not to get the cutting wire too close to your feet, especially if you don't want to slice your toes off.

Edging with Long Angled Shears

Your customer may have special edging shears, which means that you don't need to kneel down to cut the edges. They can do an excellent job given the right conditions, which are;

a. They're not blunt, which they usually are.
b. The edge of the lawn is higher than the ground next to it.

In gardening, you rarely get the right conditions for anything.

Raking the Lawn

Most but not all mowers have a grass box which collects the clippings as you cut the grass. Some mowers however, especially hover mowers, don't. Even where there is a grass box, the mechanism doesn't always work very effectively and a lot of grass ends up on the ground. A few grass clippings on the lawn - say if the grass was already quite short before you cut it - won't do any harm, but if there are enough to be clearly visible, you will need to sweep them up with a lawn rake. If the customer doesn't have one, you can either use a hard broom or a soil rake (very gently).

Trimming, Pruning, Deadheading and Other Forms of Cutting

Many people think pruning is a highly skilled activity and that you're a real gardener if you know how to do it properly. To be fair, you do need to have some idea of what you are doing but generally speaking; you can keep your customers happy and avoid harming plants by the application of a few simple rules.

I'm going to start with pruning roses. These are what most people think of when they think of pruning, and if you understand how and when to prune them you will not only impress your customers but be able to apply the principles to almost anything else you might be called upon to prune.

How to Prune Roses

When to Prune - Roses should be pruned after they have finished flowering and before the new growth starts on which next years flowers will appear. It's also a good idea not to prune them when it's too cold. Usually, the best time is late autumn or early spring.

What and How Much to Prune – Firstly, cut out stems that are dead, damaged or diseased. A stem is usually diseased if it is badly discoloured. You should also cut out old stems so that the plant concentrates its energy on young, healthy ones.

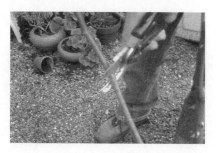

As for cutting back the plant as a whole, it varies with the kind of rose. With climbing roses and miniature roses for example, you don't take off very much at all. With most bush roses however, which are the usual sort you see growing in flower beds, you cut the whole rose back to around a third of it's original height, and then thin out the remaining branches, leaving the youngest, healthiest, strongest looking shoots for next year's flowering.

How to Cut Rose Stems

This point is very important, not just for the health of the plant, but because if you don't do it properly you will have proved to your customer that you don't know a thing about pruning.

Stems must be cut just above a node; that's to say, either to where there is a leaf or branch growing out of it, or where there is a bud on the stem indicating that one is intending to start doing so (see diagram below).

***Nodes on a
Rose Stem***

]

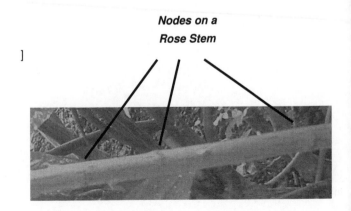

Some General Rules for Pruning

The above guidelines are for pruning roses, but if you understand the principles behind them, you can often make a good guess about pruning other plants.

We learned for instance, that you need to cut a rose stem at a node, or at a point where there is either a bud or new stem growing out of it. The same is true with other plants. With bushy plants of course, this wouldn't be possible as there are so many stems that it would take you all day. But if it's a plant that you would instinctively cut with secateurs or loppers rather than with shears, then you should aim to cut every branch at a node.

We also learned that most roses should be pruned in late autumn or early spring. That's because (a) it's after they've done most of their flowering, (b) the stems on which next year's growth will flower haven't grown yet and (c) the weather isn't at it's coldest. Other plants are pruned at different times of the year. Ceanothus for instance, which flower in May, are best pruned in June. Hydrangeas, which flower through most of the summer, are normally pruned, if they need pruning, in early autumn. Again, the times may differ but the principle that you prune after flowering, before the new growth starts and while it's not too cold still holds.

As regards what plants need pruning and how much to take off, every plant is different. There exist any number of gardening books and internet sites that can give information about pruning individual plant species, but this book isn't about boring you with copious detail. The point about the relatively simple rules and guidelines I'm giving here is that you'll keep your customers happy, won't harm anything and have an easier time of it generally than I did when I started.

As with roses, it is a good idea to cut out dead, damaged or diseased stems from any plant. You have to use your common sense here of course. If all or most of the plant is suffering from disease, then if you cut off all the diseased branches you'll have no plant left.

It goes without saying that you don't want to cut back anything that's in flower or looks as if it's about to flower, though you can sometimes gingerly trim a few corners or sticky out bits to improve the shape. As for how much to cut off, my rule - which you need to apply with a little commonsense - is to cut off no more than you need to make the plant look tidy unless the customer tells you to or you know it won't hurt the plant to do so. You aren't, after all, going to seriously harm a plant by chopping off too little. It's also worth remembering that most customers are more into how their garden looks than the finer technicalities, and this brings me to the subject of trimming with shears.

Trimming Bushes and Hedges

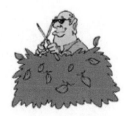

For trimming you will need a pear of shears and a lawn rake or broom to clear up the clippings. You may also need a step ladder.

What's the difference between trimming and pruning? The way I see it, pruning might be best thought of as what you do with secateurs to keep the plant healthy while trimming is what you do with shears to get bushes and hedges into nice shapes. There is quite a bit of overlap between the two activities however. When pruning roses, you also want to get them into a pleasing shape, and when trimming bushes, you need to keep some of the pruning guidelines in mind so as not to harm the plant.

As noted above, one thing that's invaluable when trimming bushes is a sense of aesthetics. What customers generally want, even though they can't always articulate it, is for you to get them into nice round shapes that blend harmoniously with one another. Why do you think Edward Scissorhands was such a popular film? If you have good artistic sense and/or a sense of proportion, this really comes in handy here. It's lovely when someone tells me "you got the garden looking exactly how I envisaged it". Every now and again, you'll need to stand back to see if what you're doing looks right, and you'll have to think "I need a little bit more off this one to match the one at the back" etc. It may take you longer than you thought to achieve the right effect but believe me, it's time well spent. It's the sort of thing that distinguishes you from some of the people who drive around in vans loaded with petrol mowers, strimmers and garden vacuums. They're often efficient, and some of them even charge a reasonable price. They chop everything back and keep the garden under control yet somehow not looking quite right, and your customers know the difference.

Hedge trimming is pretty much the same as bush trimming, except that hedges are usually bigger and take longer than bushes. It's still nearly always the case that they're better done with shears. If, in spite of my invectives and dire warnings, you decide to use your customer's hedge trimmer, then it is imperative that you use a power breaker, and that you are extra careful about not getting the blades near the flex.

Using Step Ladders

This is may be a good place to say something about safety on step ladders. You'll sometimes need to borrow one to get at high bushes or hedges. Some people seem to have a natural sense of balance and feel as comfortable on a wobbly ladder as most of us do on a bicycle. I don't, which is why I follow some simple rules.

If a ladder feels like it's going to give way under you if you go up any further, it probably is. I used to force myself to climb too far up wobbly step ladders because I was afraid people would think I was a wuss if I didn't. After one or two accidents and several near misses, I know differently. For most jobs, you only need to go up a few steps to be high enough to do what you need to do. Obey your nervous system. You'll feel even more of a wuss if you end up paralysed from the neck down.

If you do need to go further up the ladder than feels safe, don't be shy to ask the customer to hold it. Also, always make sure you've got something to grab on to in an emergency, such as the hedge you're cutting.

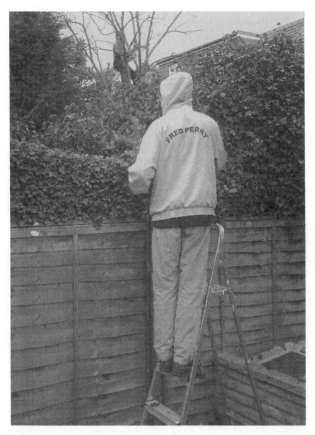

Ignore the tree surgeon in the background; he's showing off.

Make sure your ladder is properly upright. It may feel perfectly safe because all four feet are touching the ground, but it could be leaning at an angle. If you lean in the same direction as the ladder, you'll go flying.

Finally, leave anything more than about eight feet high to a tree surgeon. They can do it a lot more safely, cheaply and quickly than you can and save you a lot of unnecessary stress and irritation.

Using Extension Ladders

These are the sort of ladders that window cleaners and workmen use. They need to be sited safely, i.e. they should be leaning against the wall, tree or whatever at a safe angle, not wobbling at all and not leaning to the right or left. Also, unless someone is holding it, the ladder needs to be the right kind of ladder for the job with appropriate safety attachments. If it isn't, the bottom might slip away, sending you flying. Needless to say, you have a lot further to fall than on a step ladder, and your survival chances will diminish accordingly. I always insist that someone holds an extension ladder when I climb up it, and unless you're au fait with ladders, I strongly recommend that you do the same.

Deadheading

You will need a pair of secateurs. As with pruning, it involves cutting stems at the node. That's where the similarity ends however.

Deadheading, unlike pruning, is done when a plant is in flower. The main reason for it is to stimulate the growth of more flowers. Flowering for plants is a bit like dressing up to go to a party. The pretty colours attract bees who cross pollinate them. This is how plants produce seeds and reproduce. Once a plant has been pollinated, it thinks "great, no need to waste money on party clothes anymore". It may flower less abundantly or stop doing so altogether. The point of deadheading is to fool the plant into thinking "oh dear, something went wrong with my last attempt to attract bees and become pollinated. I'd better have another go". There are many plants, such as roses, dahlias, geraniums, petunias, marigolds and a host of summer flowering annuals; that will keep going all through the summer and most of the autumn provided they are deadheaded regularly.

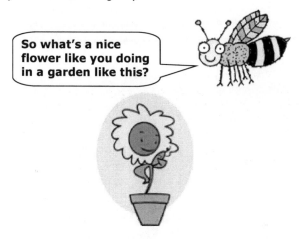

So what's a nice flower like you doing in a garden like this?

To deadhead, cut back the flower head to the nearest node, which as discussed above is the nearest place where you can see that a new stem and thus flower is likely to grow from.

Cutting Away Dead Stuff

As you go through the year, a lot of foliage dies and needs to be cut off or removed. During the middle of summer, especially if it's a dry one, you'll often get the impression that the garden looks tired and withered. At times like these, going carefully round the garden and cutting away all of the brown, dead, withered or twiggy stuff can really freshen up its appearance. Your customer will be impressed with the result and will often wonder how you did it.

It's pretty obvious when something is dead or nearly dead. It snaps or comes away easily in your hand. Sometimes, it means a plant or part of it is unhealthy, aged or dehydrated. Plenty of plants, especially those with bulbs, tubers, corms or rhizomes, die back each year and send up new shoots in the following year. With these, it's better for the plant if you don't cut away decaying stems until they are nearly brown, since the nutrients from them go back into the plant, strengthening it for the following year. You will need to check this with your customer though, since a lot of people are more concerned about short term tidiness than the long term health of a plant.

Chopping Down Overgrown Areas

If you feel your virility has been compromised by not wanting to break your neck on step ladders, then clearing away jungles is your chance to regain your macho credentials. Sometimes you'll get called to a property where the garden hasn't been touched for years. There may be large areas covered in grass, brambles and Japanese knotweed taller than you are. It can look daunting at first sight. That's why the customer is paying you to do it.

For chopping down overgrown areas, you will need the following tools;

A pair of shears

A pair of loppers

A rake or lawn rake

A clearaway sheet

Loads of bin bags (if the customer wants the waste removed).

Sometimes, the customer will want the whole area dug over, with as many of the weeds extracted by the roots as possible. This can range from moderately hard work, if the soil is crumbly and the weeds are the right kind; to virtually impossible if it is almost pure clay and full of thick or intractable roots. I will deal with digging below. A lot of people with seriously neglected gardens however, are more than happy if you simply cut down and dispose off all the stuff above ground level. They aren't particularly interested in using their garden as a rule. They just want to prevent their neighbours from complaining and to be able to see out of the kitchen window.

Chopping down overgrown gardens is hard work, but not nearly as impossible as it looks. Furthermore, if you're fit and your technique is right, it should rarely if ever take you more than a day to get any job done.

My practice is to kneel down on the ground with my shears - or loppers if appropriate - and chop through everything at ground level. Once I've cleared a reasonable area. I rake everything up onto my clearaway sheet. Sometimes the customer will have a heap for garden waste, in which case I just chuck the stuff on it. Otherwise I chop up any brambles; hard branches etc. with my loppers into pieces about a foot long, then roll them up in the clearaway sheet and tip the contents into a garden waste or black bag. If it's a big job, it's easy to fill twenty or thirty bags.

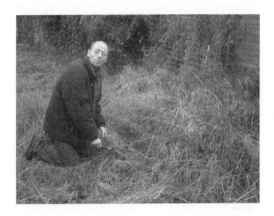

If you feel you'll never finish the job, a trick to encourage yourself is to mentally divide the area to be cleared into individual units of one square metre. Then you can challenge yourself to see how long it takes to clear each one. As a guide, you'll rarely have to clear an area of more than a hundred square metres.

Digging

As far as you're concerned, digging means turning over soil with a large fork, pulling out the weeds in it, or as many of them as you can, and then if necessary, breaking up the soil. It's generally thought to be very hard work and sometimes is, though this largely depends on the soil and what's growing in it.

Reasons for Digging

Unless you're growing vegetables in a serious way, digging isn't actually of that much importance to the health of the soil or the plants growing in it. If an area has been neglected for several years, then it should be turned over, but it's not something you need to do on a regular basis. Some people think that when you put compost or fertiliser onto flower beds, you need to dig it in. This isn't really necessary. Just spread it over the top of the soil and the rain will do the rest.

You need to dig out weeds if you can because that stops them from growing again, but turning over and breaking up the soil has a lot more to do with aesthetics, and with convincing your clients that you've done a thorough job. Despite the impression you may get from garden makeover programmes, most of your customers have quite conventional tastes. They love nothing better than to see their favourite plants standing in a sea of uniform, weed free, freshly dug, crumbly earth. Sometimes, depending on the soil and what's in the way, it is more appropriate to achieve this effect by breaking up the earth with a hoe or small hand fork.

If soil is clayey, it will be more difficult to dig. If the weather is dry it will make the ground very hard. When digging in hard ground, it generally helps to wiggle the fork in a bit with your foot as you push it into the ground. Conversely, if clayey soil is wet, it will stick to everything, slowing you down and making you feel as though you are working in a mud bath; which indeed you are. Clayey soil doesn't break up easily either; and it's much harder to separate the soil from the weeds. Sometimes the only way to do this is by wearing a pair of rubber or latex gloves, kneeling down and going through every bit of the soil by hand or with a small fork as you turn it over. It's a slow, yucky job and if there's a lot to do, you'll need to make this clear to the customer, so that they can decide whether they really want you to do it.

What you absolutely must not do is to take a quick look at an overgrown garden, think "I'll have that done in a jiffy" and quote accordingly. If "having it done" involves digging out all the weeds, you could easily end up taking the best part of a week to do it, and if the customer is paying a fixed price, they might be exacting enough to demand that you go over everything with a toothcomb. My policy is to say "why don't you hire me for a day, and I'll get the garden looking as best as I can in that time". Once they see me roll up my sleeves and get to work, they know I'm not out to double cross them and they're usually delighted with the result.

Planting

Occasionally, you'll get a customer who wants you to take charge of planting. They want you to go down to the garden centre, order everything and then plant it as you think appropriate when it gets delivered. More often than not though, it's a case of them giving you stuff and telling you where to put it. You'll spend a fair amount of time in spring planting out half hardy annuals like marigolds and begonias. In summer, your customers will go down to Devon – all garden enthusiasts seem to spend their summer holidays in Devon - and come back with whatever's the latest fad at the Eden Project. In autumn you will be given tons of bulbs to stick in the ground.

Plants or seeds need to be stuck in soil, either in the ground or in a pot or other container, and to grow they need food, water, sunlight and drainage.

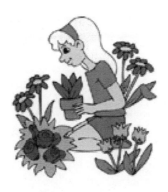

Provided you plant it in the appropriate spot, God will take care of the sunlight. As for water, unless the ground is seriously damp, it's necessary to water anything you plant immediately. Use a watering can, and adjust the amount of water to the size of the plant, the size of the leaves – leafier plants are thirstier - how dry the soil is and the time of year. It's difficult to say how much water you should give each plant but as a general rule, the ground around it should be moist rather than waterlogged. It doesn't matter if you get it slightly wrong. Plants are like children; they're surprisingly tough and they often grow up despite their parents'

mistakes. Two tips though. Don't pour the water out too quickly, and if it's a hot sunny day make sure you don't get water on the leaves. You've probably tried to burn a hole in a piece of paper with a magnifying glass by concentrating the sun's rays on one spot. Well a drop of water on a leaf can have much the same effect.

Food, generally speaking, consists of manure or compost, though some customers will supplement this with fertilisers and/or blood, fish and bone meal. Some plants, such as dahlias or tomatoes, are particularly hungry and require a lot of feeding. Conversely, a number of plants, such as buddleias, lavender and some ornamental grasses; often thrive in poor soils.

If the customer has compost suitable for what you're planting (see below) then use it. If not, then if the soil looks at all fertile go ahead and plant anyway. If it doesn't, offer to nip down the road and buy some. You can get bags of compost from most DIY or hardware stores, and sometimes from pound shops and the like; especially during spring and summer.

Different Kinds of Compost

Compost is basically fertile soil. If it is organic, it will be made up of degraded plant and/or animal waste. If not, it may also contain chemical fertilizers.

If you go to a garden centre, you'll see various kinds of compost on sale; John Innes, mushroom compost etc. Stick to general multipurpose compost for the time being, except with ericaceous or acid loving plants.

I should say a word about soils here. You may have remembered from your science lessons at school that substances can be acid, alkaline or neutral. You may not really know what it means but have a general idea that oranges are a little bit acidic and sulphuric acid is very acidic, which is why it's not a good idea to go around squirting it in peoples' faces.

Just like everything else, soils can also be acid, alkaline or neutral and this is important because different plants have different preferences. If you live in an area where soil is more or less neutral, such as London, or positively alkaline, such the Downs or the Chilterns; then if you want to grow ericaceous or acid loving plants like rhododendrons, camellias, heathers, azaleas and skimmias, you need to make the soil more acidic

One way to do this is to use ericaceous compost. By the same token, ericaceous compost shouldn't be used on the majority of plants that aren't particularly into acidic soil. There's a good chance your customer won't know what kind of compost they have in the shed so you should check what it says on the bag and point it out to them if they have the wrong kind.

Some compost will contain peat, which as well as being good for acid loving plants is used to improve drainage. Peat is extracted from bog lands, mainly in the North and West of the British Isles. Many people have reservations about using it as there is a risk that peat bogs will become endangered. As a result, its use has declined.

How to Plant

If a plant comes from a shop or garden centre, there'll usually be instructions on the seed packet, pot or other container. It's generally a pretty simple business however. If sticking a plant in the ground, you dig a hole that's about one and a half times deeper and wider than the roots of the plant, stick in a bit of soil or compost, stick the plant in, put more compost and soil round the sides until the hole is completely filled up and then pat the soil down. Finally, you water it as described above.

When planting in pots or other containers, it's a similar procedure, except that you don't dig a hole. It's also customary to put gravel, shards from a broken pot or other material at the bottom of the pot to help drainage. There's no reason why you shouldn't use stones for drainage when you stick plants in the ground and some gardeners do, but it's not something to worry about at this stage.

When planting bulbs, you don't really need any water or compost, though it won't hurt. You do have to stick them in the ground at approximately the right depth though. The general rule is that the depth at which the bulb is planted should be two and a half times the height of the bulb. Thus if the bulb is four centimetres tall, it should be planted so that the bottom of the bulb is at a depth of 10cm. If you get it a bit wrong, it's not the end of the world. When I'm gardening, I'm always accidentally digging up bulbs and sticking them back in and I don't take exact measurements every time.

In your early days as a gardener, that's probably all you need to think about. Customers don't normally expect you to be responsible for plant care and when they do they'll usually give you the plant food or weed killer or slug pellets or whatever and tell you what they want done. If you see plants are looking parched, give them a drink of water. If you see some obviously diseased branches on an otherwise healthy plant, cut them off. Other than that, don't worry too much till you're more experienced.

Sweeping and Raking

Sometimes you'll make a mess when gardening. Sometimes there's just a lot of debris lying around. Either way, if you get into the habit of habitually sweeping up on sight without being asked, your customers will appreciate it. From about mid-October till Christmas, the ground will be covered in leaves and raking them up, as well as cutting down dead and wilting stalks, will take precedence over weeding and mowing lawns.

For sweeping and raking you will need;

A lawn rake, especially if you're working on grass.

A broom to sweep up paved areas.

A dustpan and brush

A clearaway sheet

Gloves, for picking leaves from around plants with your hands

A garden vacuum, if the customer has one.

I find raking up leaves a therapeutic but surprisingly time consuming activity, so much as I dislike doing so, there is a case for using garden vacuums when they're available. They work in much the same way as the vacuum cleaner you use inside the house. You can either have it on suck or blow and if you're skilful you can use the blower to get all the leaves in the garden into nice neat little piles and then use the sucker to gobble them up. In my case, I usually just blow the leaves all over the place and make an even bigger mess than I started with.

Happily for me, most customers don't have vacuums and I generally resort to using a lawn rake, broom or my gloved hands. Pretty much everybody has a broom of some kind and most customers have a lawn rake. Just to remind you, a lawn rake is different from a standard or soil rake. The head is shaped like a fan and springier (see illustration in previous chapter), so it doesn't do too much damage to the lawn. You can be a little bit rough with it in the autumn however, as this encourages root growth and some people do it on purpose. The technical term is scarifying.

If I have to tell you how to sweep up, it means your mother didn't bring you up properly. One or two things about leaves though. They continue falling over a period of months. Check with your customers whether they want them swept up on a constant basis or simply one big job in late November/December. If the former, don't be too thorough as new leaves will have started falling even before you've finished sweeping. Also, check whether they want the leaves taken off the flower beds. Most customers do, but they don't actually look bad there and they offer some protection to the soil during the winter, so it's not necessarily a good idea. It can also be a lot of work, since you often have to pick up leaves with your (hopefully gloved) hands to avoid damaging the plants.

Tying Plants to Fences or Stakes

There are two reasons for tying plants. The first is that some plants are climbing plants and you want them to climb in the right direction. The other is that some plants are a bit fragile and need to be tied to stakes to stop them falling over.

There are a number of things that can be used for tying plants. Ordinary string isn't bad, and neither is twine, which has the advantage of being green and thus less noticeable. There is also a stronger metal kind of twine coated in green plastic that needs to be cut with pliers (or loppers at a pinch) or which comes in short pieces. As for which type to use when, as a general rule, use the metal stuff when you're dealing with heavy branches and you don't want the cord to snap, and use stringy stuff when you're dealing with more delicate plants that you don't want the metal wire to cut into.

As regards what to tie it to, if the plant isn't next to a wall and you're not trying to train it up a wall, then you'll usually need to tie it to one or more canes or sticks in the ground. When using a stick, you need to knock it in well, preferably with a hammer and preferably in a place where it's unobtrusive - e.g. behind rather than in front of the plant - and then tie the plant to it. If tying a plant to the fence on the other hand, you may find something on the fence to tie it to, e.g. a nail sticking out or a fence post that you can get the cord round. Failing that, you may need to knock in a few screws or nails yourself. On a wooden fence, make sure you don't split the wood. With a brick or stone wall, you'll need wall plugs/Rawlplugs and an electric drill; more of a DIY sort of job really.

Plants that I find habitually need tying to stakes or fences include wisteria, climbing roses, clematis, passionflowers and peonies.

And Finally – Clearing up the Rubbish

When I started gardening, if the customer didn't have a compost heap to put the rubbish on, I'd end up spending ages stuffing rubbish into bin liners which invariably broke. Since then I have worked out a simple way of bagging up stuff which saves me a lot of time.

Firstly, sweep a pile of debris onto your clearaway sheet. Then get your loppers and chop up any significant branches. Finally, roll the rubbish up in the clearaway sheet, tip the clearaway sheet into the bin bag or garden waste bag and empty the stuff in.

Clearaway Sheet

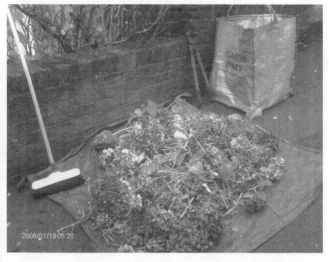

It's a simple technique, but given how much time is spent chopping and bagging, it's one that will save you a surprising amount of time.

That brings us to the end of Chapter Four and covers most of the main tasks you'll be expected to do. Chapters Five and Six will introduce you to the things you see growing in your customers' gardens, be they weeds to get rid of or plants that the customer expects you to protect and nurture, or at the very least to leave alone.

CHAPTER FIVE – WEEDS AND WEEDING

Weeding deserves a chapter to itself. It's something you're going to be spending a lot of time doing, in one form or another. When I started gardening, this was the part that scared me the most.

"I'm not an expert gardener", I'd confess sheepishly over the phone when somebody new rang up "Oh, don't worry," they'd reply cheerfully; "I just wanted you to do the lawn and the hedge and a bit of weeding. I'm sure you know the difference between weeds and flowers."

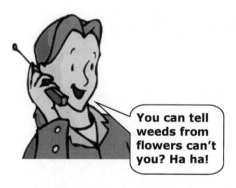

> You can tell weeds from flowers can't you? Ha ha!

The implication of this is that it's something any twit would know. But how exactly do you tell weeds from flowers without knowing the name of every single plant? It's all very well for customers to think it's no big deal. They only have to worry about their own gardens. They know what plants they planted and which ones turned up and started growing in their gardens uninvited. They know what they want to keep and what to throw away. And of course, if they do make a mistake they don't have to answer to anybody for it except themselves.

Don't expect much help from your standard gardening book either. They're designed to tell you how to do your own garden; not other peoples. "Make sure you dig them up by the roots" they advise glibly, assuming your garden is well kept and you can catch dandelions and dock weeds while they're only a few weeks old. As to what is or isn't a weed, most books just fall back on the old cliché that "a weed is a plant in the wrong place". Fine if you want to sound in touch with nature, but try getting away with it when you've pulled up somebody's prize delphiniums.

"If in doubt, ask" is another unhelpful attempt at reassurance; alright if there are one or two things you aren't sure about. But what if nearly everything you see in a customer's garden is a complete mystery to you? Well, perhaps not everything. You may know what brambles and dandelions look like, and I'm sure you've had the odd brush with a stinging nettle. All of these are weeds; so is grass for that matter, if it isn't on your lawn. Then what about buttercups and daisies? And have you ever looked for a four leaved clover? You probably won't have found one but you'll have learned what clover looks like in the process. Maybe you're not as ignorant about weeds as you thought you were.

Some General Guidelines

In this chapter, I'm going to introduce you to a number of common weeds and what they're like, but first of all I'm going to give you some tips on how to expand your knowledge of weeds, as well as what to do if you're not sure whether something is a weed or not.

Learning what weeds you can pull out is like a survival exercise where you're in parachuted into a remote area and have to live on the things you see growing wild, such as roots, berries, nuts, leaves or fungi. How do you learn what's edible and what's poisonous without a degree in botany? Well let's say you find out that one particular leaf or mushroom is safe to eat, then you know that as long as you stick to that, you're fine. Then you spot some brambles with blackberries on them and you think, "Great, I can eat those as well!" Another twenty or thirty lessons like that and you should have little trouble foraging a meal anywhere outside the Sahara Desert.

It's the same with weeds. You don't have to know what everything growing in a garden is to know what is a weed and what is a plant. You just have to learn to identify about twenty or thirty weeds that you can safely pull out. You don't even need to know them by name; just so long as you can recognise them when you see them. You may still come across the odd thing that could be a weed but you're not sure. You can check that with the customer or leave it in to be on the safe side.

So how do you expand your weed repertoire? Later in this chapter, I will be introducing you to a number of the more common weeds you will encounter and their basic characteristics. I will also refer you to some places on the internet where you can see excellent illustrations of any weed you are likely to encounter.

Your first step however, to building up your "rogues gallery" of weeds, is to take a look at what you see growing in peoples' gardens. You don't need to wait until you get a job; an ideal time to start is when you're delivering your advertising leaflets door to door. There will be some things that you just "know" are weeds. In order to memorise them, it's a good idea to make up your own names. The more childish or cringeworthy these are the better. An ex-colleague, who wanted to remember the name of a friend of mine called Pascal, came up to me the following week and asked how "Push Bovine" was. He'd reckoned first of all, that Pascal sounds like "pass cow". He then noted that "bovine" means "cow-like" and decided for no apparent reason that "push" is similar to "pass". I'm no longer on speaking terms with the gentleman concerned but his mnemonic was so excruciating that I've never been able to get it out of my head.

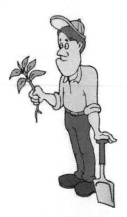

Another thing you can do is to take a look at a few seriously neglected gardens, woodland areas or patches of wasteland. The plants you will see growing there are the things that self seed and grow without any help from a gardener; which after all, is what weeds are. Of course there are some things that self-seed that can look quite nice in a garden, and which your customer may want to keep, such as Ivy or bluebells; but more of that presently.

While you're going through this critical learning phase, there are a couple of strategies to you can employ to minimise the damage you're likely to cause. For instance, if you're not sure whether something growing in a flower bed is a weed or a flower, have a look to see whether it is growing somewhere it wouldn't have been planted; such as on the lawn or through the cracks in the patio. If so, it's more likely to be a weed. It's by no means certain though, since it could have spread from its original location.

It's also worth getting an idea of the customers you're working for. Do they like unusual or wild looking plants? Would they put in a load of seedlings without telling you? Do they automatically bin anything that turns up in their garden uninvited?

Follow the adv ice given above and you'll be surprised how quickly you learn to identify most common garden weeds. Below are some basic guidelines on how to weed, followed by a description of some of the more common weeds you'll encounter.

How to Weed

The only thing your customers know about getting rid of weeds is that you're supposed to pull them up by the roots. Gardening books say the same and it stands to reason. It's very cathartic for one thing. We always like to think we're getting to the "root" of a problem, and if people are paying you good money to get the weeds out, they don't want them back again next week.

As with most of life's problems however, weeding isn't so simple. If you're getting weeds out from between paving stones it isn't possible to dig out roots and if they don't come out by hand, the best you can do is scrape out what you can with a small fork or trowel and spray the area with Pathclear. Some annual weeds don't always need to be got out by the roots. Sometimes it's enough to chop their heads off with a Dutch hoe. Others, such as dandelions, alkanet or potentilla, are virtually impossible to get out entirely if they're been growing for a long time and are well established. Then you have weeds like clover and allium that you can dig out, but which spread so prolifically that the job may take forever. As for ground elder or bindweed, once it's got a toehold, the most you can hope to do is to keep it down.

Even if you do get weeds out by the roots, it doesn't mean they won't come back again. New seeds get carried by the wind and by birds and animals. That's nature; if there is a bare patch of earth it will get colonised.

I'll be looking at how to deal with individual weeds shortly, but there's one general rule that is crucial to keeping in your customers' good books. When weeding any area that hasn't been done for a long time, especially if it's seriously overgrown, always turn over the soil. Two things that never fail to impress customers are sensitively trimmed and shaped bushes (see previous chapter) and newly cleared, freshly turned over earth. As I already mentioned, you don't have to dig too deeply, since this is more about looks than providing a healthy growing environment. A hoe or small fork is often the most appropriate tool. As long as the customer can see generous expanses of crumbly, weed free, fertile looking soil at surface level you can do no wrong.

Bear in mind though, that it can harm plants if you loosen the soil around their roots, so don't dig too close to them. If you want to give the soil immediately around plants the "freshly dug over" look there are two ways to do it. You can use a small hand fork, making sure you don't dig deep enough to affect the roots. If this isn't practicable, you can take some freshly dug soil from elsewhere and sprinkle it around the plants in question.

Finally, a word or two about weed killer. Most of the weed killers you can buy in the shop are not that harmful to the environment or garden, and they don't harm the soil. In fact, if you're not going to go in for composting, I think there's quite a strong moral case for using them. Weeds, when they grow, take up nutrients from the soil. If you let the dead weeds decompose back into the soil, then the nutrients they contain will be returned from whence they came. That seems to make far more sense than having your weeds carted away, then driving to the garden centre in your big thirsty hatchback to pick up organic compost in plastic bags that don't biodegrade.

Whatever your ethical position may be though, the fact is that most weed killers aren't an awful lot of use. They are admittedly, quite effective during spring and early summer when plants are growing most vigorously. The way many weed killers work is that as the plant grows, it drinks the stuff in through its leaves, hopefully poisoning itself. This means that if you chop the weeds down first they won't die, since they won't have any leaves to drink the weed killer with. So you have to leave the weeds as they are while they're going brown and decaying, and this doesn't look very pretty.

Most weed killers furthermore, are not that effective on perennial weeds with well established roots; you may need several applications to kill them. Weed killers containing glyphosate do tend to be more powerful, and while there has been some controversy surrounding them; my own researches have given me little reason to believe that they do serious environmental damage when used domestically.

Pathclear and other weed killers designed for paved or gravelled areas are different, in that they not only kill existing weeds but prevent new ones coming up for – in theory at least – several months. This wouldn't be much use on the soil though, even if it worked; since if you stopped everything growing you'd lose your flowers as well as your weeds.

All this is good news for you. As a gardener, pulling out weeds is your main source of income. Luckily, the demand for your services isn't likely to end anytime soon.

Categories of Weeds

Different weeds need to be dealt with in different ways. We are now going to look at some common classifications and varieties of weeds. In order to keep the price of this book down, I have not included any colour photographs, and therefore cannot provide meaningful illustrations. There are several excellent resources on the internet however, providing graphic illustrations of all the weeds I will mention as well and a good many that I won't. I recommend the following, which can be used in conjunction with the remainder of this chapter. On each of these web sites, it is possible to type in the name of a weed and get one or more illustrations of it. Hopefully all of the URLS will be the same as at the time of writing.

Google Images – *www.google.com*

Down Gardening Services - *www.dgsgardening.btinternet.co.uk*

Bayer Crop Science UK – *www.bayercropscience.co.uk*

Annuals and Perennials

Plants can be divided into annuals, lasting for one year or less, perennials, lasting several years, and the much smaller category of biennials, which die after around two years. You'll hear a lot about annuals and perennials when talking about plants that you want to grow, but here we're concerned with their significance as weeds.

As a general rule, perennials are harder to dig out than annuals but it's important to get all of a root out if you can. I say "if you can"; often this is almost impossible, especially if the weed has been around long enough to develop tenacious roots. It's also important not to put perennial weeds in the compost bin, since if the compost ends up on the soil, even a tiny bit of root is enough to grow a new weed. Bear in mind though, that few of your customers are into real composting. Most will just have a heap of garden waste in a corner and wonder why it doesn't rot down.

Annuals, be they weeds or plants, are so named because they don't live for more than a year. On the one hand, they are generally a lot easier to pull out than perennials because their roots don't go so deep. At the same time, it's less important for you to do so, since they're less likely to grow again if they are cut down to ground level. While they're less tenacious individually however, they often self seed and grow a lot quicker than perennials. Some reproduce up to four times in a season, taking over your garden if they aren't checked. It's usually safe to put annuals on the compost heap if they haven't started flowering yet. If they have, the compost may end up containing seeds, which could end up back in the soil.

It will often be possible to pull out annuals, including the roots, by hand or with a small fork. If there are a lot of them, it may be a better idea to simply spear them with a hoe and then rake, sweep or pick up the severed heads lying on the surface of the soil. All of the following weeds are reasonably easy to pull out or deal with (though with nettles, you need protective gloves).

Willowherb	Wild cranesbill	Nettles
Deadnettle	Groundsel	Shepherd's purse
Daisies	Chickweed	Wild spurge
Geum	Fat hen	Cleavers
Plantain	Hairy bittercress	Thistles

Weeds with Tenacious Tap Roots

A number of perennial weeds, notably dandelions, alkanet, dockweed, comfrey and potentilla; have one main root, often carrot shaped, which is called a tap root and goes down quite deep, in many cases splitting into smaller roots as it nears the bottom. Any gardening book will tell you that you have to get the tap root out, and if the weed is less than a few months old, you can usually do this by digging a bit deeper. In practice, many of the weeds you will be asked to clear have been growing for several years and are much too well established, so you'll just have to get as much of the tap root out as you can. My practice is to try and lever it up with a large fork. If that doesn't work, then I reach down into the newly dug earth as far as I can and pull out anything I can get hold of.

Prolific Perennial Weeds

Generally, perennial weeds don't multiply as quickly as annuals, though some, as we shall see shortly, spread very quickly by developing underground root networks. Three important exceptions to this rule are allium, clover and celandine.

Most things that grow from bulbs are flowers. One important exception however, is allium, or wild onions. They're easy to recognise because on the one hand, they're not really like the spring onions you'd buy in the shop, but on the other hand they do smell like onions. There are also varieties of allium that are cultivated for their flowers but these don't smell like onions, so all in all there isn't much chance of getting it wrong.

The bad news is that they multiply prolifically, have lots of tiny little bulbs and getting them all out can be a very time consuming and almost impossible activity. As with other weeds that are almost impossible to get completely out, make sure you have an understanding with your customer about how much time he or she wants you to spend on them.

Clover is reasonably easy to get out in small quantities. They have interesting roots that are a bit like translucent crystals. Again though, clearing a large patch of them can be a time consuming job. With both allium and clover, if there is a large quantity to get rid of, there may be a case for using weed killer.

Celandine generally isn't worth spending much time over, firstly because it's quite pretty and secondly because it doesn't last very long. It grows in March and early April and has small, violet like leaves and yellow flowers. As soon as it starts to die down and look messy, you can pull out what's on the surface; but it's generally not worth bothering about the roots because they won't be giving you any trouble for the rest of the year.

Brambles

Brambles are big prickly things that you get tangled up in when trying to make your way through thick undergrowth. In mid to late summer, blackberries grow on them which you can stuff your face with while you're working. Be careful not to get them mixed up with raspberries though, which the customer has usually put there on purpose. The best way to tell the difference is that raspberries, while they look similar, aren't prickly. The best way to deal with brambles is simply to hack at them or chop them down with your shears and loppers. When it comes to the roots, you won't be able to dig them all out. Get down as low as you can with your large fork and then use your loppers to cut off anything you can get to.

Hand Weeding

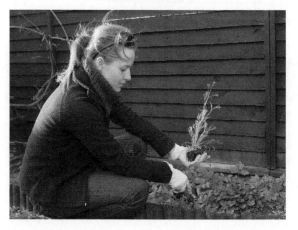

The Worst Offenders

There are four weeds that spread prolifically and are almost impossible to get rid of. These are couch grass, bindweed, Japanese knotweed and ground elder. Unless you manage to get hold of them before they've started spreading, there's little you can do about the roots. I simply get rid of them down to ground level, then if I want to give the soil a dug over look, I pull out the roots I can see, but I don't kid myself that I'm doing anything more than a cosmetic exercise to keep the customer happy.

Japanese knotweed is so pervasive that councils tell you not to put it out with the garden waste. It manifests itself in thick, fast growing stems which can reach waist height in a few weeks and must be chopped to ground level as soon as they appear.

The one you'll hear everyone complain about most though is bindweed. It's a pity, because they have beautiful white flowers and I've seen some creative things done with them, like spreading them over a pink flowering lavatera in July. They do however, grow extremely prolifically and get tangled up with anything in their way. If you don't deal with them quickly, then it can be a job to extricate them from other plants.

Plants that are Sometimes Weeds and Sometimes Flowers

Few customers want to hold on to their dandelions, brambles or bindweed. Fewer still will thank you for pulling out their delphiniums or petunias. There are some plants however, that often self-seed but your customers may like them, and you need to check with them before pulling them out. It's largely a matter of understanding your customer and anticipating his or her wants. You can generally tell very quickly whether you're working for someone who just wants everything looking tidy or someone who's willing to be a bit unconventional in the name of creativity. Here are some of the most common plants that fall into the "sometimes weeds sometimes flowers" category.

Celandine

We discussed this above. They are small, yellow, cottagey flowers
that grow prolifically in early spring. They don't look bad but can
take over your garden. Luckily, they're already withering in April
and are pretty much gone by May.

Forget Me Nots.

These are also of the cottagey variety. They grow in late spring
and while they are prolific, nearly everybody loves them, including
myself. You may be asked to thin them out but rarely to get rid of
them completely.

Corydalis

This has yellow flowers and tends to grow well in cracks, often
next to the side of the house. I find that most customers like it
although it does grow rather prolifically. The roots can also be
damaging to brickwork in the long term. If you do have to pull a
corydalis up, you'll discover that this is because the roots are
surprisingly large and tenacious.

Bluebells

These are bulbs that flower in mid-spring. You can buy them in
shops and most people think of them as flowers. The ones you
see in gardens have usually seeded themselves however, and can

grow very prolifically. Customers will frequently ask you to thin them out.

Ivy

Ivy grows prolifically and attaches itself to things. Customers usually want it, but in moderation. They'll ask you to cut it back and sometimes to peel it off walls and fences. This can leave trails like a snail makes and you should warn your customer of this. Also with fences, you have to be careful not to damage the fence when you peel it off. Sometimes, the ivy is holding up the fence rather than the other way around and you'll have to leave part of it there rather than have the fence come down.

Foxgloves

These are sometimes cultivated but often seed themselves. They are biennials, usually only flowering in the second year of growth and often not surviving beyond that. They look rather like comfrey and alkanet, which your customer will almost certainly want you to treat as weeds, but the edges of the leaves are more serrated. If you're having difficulty telling whether it's a foxglove or not, there's a simple test. Dig it out. If it comes out easily and has little flimsy roots, then it's a foxglove. If it has tenacious, carrot like roots, then it's a weed. Now I think about it, it's a bit like those witch trials they used to have where you'd tie the suspect up and throw her into the village pond. If she floated she was a witch, but if she drowned she was innocent and you were free to try and resuscitate her. Luckily, hastily replanted foxgloves have a better survival record than drowned women. While we're talking about gruesome subjects however, it's worth bearing in mind that foxgloves are deadly poisonous. Even a couple of leaves can be fatal.

Wild Cranesbill/Geraniums

These grow quite prolifically and have little pink dots. They can look very beautiful in the right place and are one of my favourites, but most customers aren't keen on them. They come out easily.

Veronica/Speedwell

These are tall, and spiky with blue to purple flowers. Most customers will like them once they've flowered

Willowherb

These are tall with purple flowers. They're normally classified as weeds and I normally pull them out but sometimes, when they're growing in the right place at the right time, they can look really beautiful. Kenneth Grahame mentions them a fair bit in "The Wind in the Willows".

Feverfew

These are also one of my favourites. They're cottagey plants with daisy-like flowers and you can identify them because they have a distinctive smell; neither especially fragrant nor rank, but once experienced, it's never forgotten.

Michalemas Daisies

These look pretty scraggly until they begin flowering in late summer. They have yellow and purple daisy-like flowers and this will persuade some customers to give them a stay of execution.

That wraps up weeding, weeds and pseudo weeds. I haven't mentioned every weed you'll encounter but we've covered quite a few of the most common ones. If you've taken on board what I have said about them, and gone online to see what they look like, you'll be well on your way to knowing what to pull out and what not to pull out in other peoples' gardens.

CHAPTER SIX - AN INTRODUCTION TO SOME COMMON GARDEN PLANTS.

I'm not going to go into any great detail about plant care or horticulture in this chapter. You'll learn a lot more once you start the job. Those of your customers who know about gardening will be more than happy to share their knowledge with you, and there is a whole industry devoted to producing gardening books that can provide comprehensive information on the subject, adorned with lots of pretty pictures. The purpose of this book however, is to get you started at earning a living tidying peoples' gardens. You don't need to be a plant expert for that. You just need to know enough to distinguish them from weeds and keep them looking tidy without doing any harm. Of course, if you know enough to converse eloquently about flowers for five minutes at a time, your customers will be delighted.

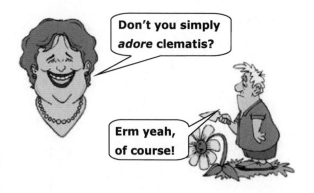

It's worth mentioning a few things though, just so that you have some idea what people are talking about. It's also helpful to be able to identify some of the more common plants you see. As with weeds, I'm not including coloured illustrations in order to keep the price of the book down. I recommend the following web sites however, for use in conjunction with this chapter. On all of these web sites, as with those I recommended for weeds; it is possible to type in the name of a plant and get one or more illustrations of it.

Google Images – *www.google.com*
Shoot – *www.shootgardening.co.uk*
BBC Gardening - *www.bbc.co.uk/gardening/plants/plant_finder/*

I mentioned annuals and perennials when discussing weeds. The distinction is important for plants as well, especially flowers. Annuals are sown each year from seed, or more often in your case, you or the customer buys them in trays from the garden centre during late spring or early summer. Then all you have to do is stick them in a sunny spot in the ground with a bit of water and compost. Many annuals are what are known as half-hardy annuals, which means they aren't really very hardy at all. They are native to a warmer climate than in the UK and will have trouble surviving out of doors before late spring.

Here is a list of some common annuals

Geranium/pelargonium	Wallflower	Petunia
Marigold	Coreopsis	Impatiens
Begonia	Celosia	Verbena

Dianthus/carnations	Cosmos	Lobelia
Nasturtium	Nicotiana	Nigella
Salvia	Sunflower	Phlox
Antirrhinum/snapdragon	Alyssum	Pansy

You can recognise the plants that are most likely to be annuals by the fact that they don't have woody stems or grow from bulbs, tubers or rhizomes. They are particularly colourful, with a high ratio of flower to leaf. Go to any park and you'll see beds full of them. Every few weeks a gang of labourers who know sod all about gardening come along in a lorry, pull them out and stick in a load of new ones.

There's a reason why annuals are so colourful. You'll recall from Chapter Four that plants grow flowers to attract bees that will pollinate them so that they can produce seeds. Annuals have only one year to do this so it's important that they put on a good show. As with other flowers, it's important to deadhead most annuals regularly. That way, there's a good chance they'll carry on being colourful well into autumn.

Apart from foxgloves, which generally self-seed anyway, not many biennials are popular as plants. The reason for this is that in the first year, you don't get any flowers and they die in the third. Two years' growing for one season's flowering doesn't seem a good investment of time and effort in today's busy world.

As we noted in the previous chapter, perennials are plants that last several years; in other words, anything that is not an annual or biennial. But whereas some perennials are woody, taking the form of shrubs and bushes, others such as daffodils or dahlias die back at the end of the season and sprout new growth in the following year. The plants aren't really dead during the winter of course; they're just dormant underground in roots, usually taking the form of bulbs, tubers, corms or rhizomes.

Bulbs, Tubers, Corms and Rhizomes

You probably know what a bulb looks like. They're onion shaped, which isn't a complete coincidence since onions are indeed bulbs. If you can distinguish corms, tubers and rhizomes though, you're cleverer than me. It's probably best think of them all as things that live underground and look like root vegetables, even if they're inedible or poisonous. Every year, new growth in the form of leaves and/or stems will sprout. Later they will flower. After the flowers die, the leaves or stems will start to wither away until all that's left is whatever is underground, ready to send up new shoots next season.

Flowers that grow from bulbs, vegetable like objects or perennial roots play an important role in the garden throughout the growing season. The first to appear in the early spring are often crocuses and snowdrops, shortly to be followed by daffodils and tulips. These give way in mid-spring to bluebells and in late spring to irises. Peonies put on a spectacular display during May. Summer is the season for montbretias, gladioli and day lilies. Dahlias and anemones come out sometime in July and keep going through October, by which time autumn crocuses and nerines will have come and gone.

I've already covered planting bulbs. Rules about depth vary with other perennials but usually, all you need to do is follow the instructions on the packet or plant container. Be careful if anyone asks you to plant or transplant their peonies. If they're not planted at exactly the right depth, they will grow very healthy leaves but won't flower. With dahlias and other half hardy perennials, some people dig up their tubers etc. in late autumn and bring them indoors for the winter. If your customer wants you to do this, he/she will probably be the sort who knows how to give you precise instructions.

Decaying Monbretias in Late Autumn

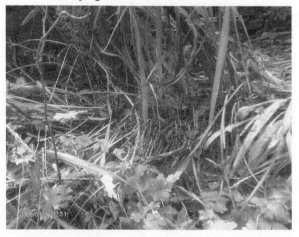

When bulbs *et al* have finished flowering, you should check with the customer when they want the leaves cut back. It's better for the plant to wait until the leaves and stems are almost dead, but some customers will want you to cut them back earlier because the decaying matter can look messy.

Other Common Perennials - Roses

Roses are one of the most common types of garden perennial. It's very easy to recognise them but there are several different types and hundreds of varieties. Most are unlikely to be of interest to you unless you're a retired colonel from Tunbridge Wells who enters them in horticultural shows. As I emphasised in Chapter Three however, you should have a basic grasp of the main categories and some idea of how to prune them and provide basic care. As far as you are concerned, roses fall into five basic types.

Miniature Roses

These are easy to recognise as they are petite. They need regular deadheading, as do most roses but not much pruning..

Tea Roses

These, along with floribundas, are the most common type of roses in domestic gardens. They vary in size, but they don't climb or ramble like climbing and rambling roses. That's to say, they're "rose shaped"; they look like you'd think a rose should look.

Tea roses are distinctive in that they have big single flowers. With regular deadheading they are often still flowering at Christmas.

Dedicated gardeners argue passionately about whether to prune them in late autumn (around November) or early spring (around March).

Floribundas

The difference between tea roses and floribundas is that instead of having single big flowers, floribundas have clusters of little flowers. The times and rules for pruning floribundas are the same as those for tea roses. When deadheading, follow the stem on which the cluster of flowers is growing at least as far as the first node.

Climbing Roses

Unlike the roses we've so far covered, they only usually flower a couple of times in a season. You can prune them back once you've established that they aren't going to flower again. They shouldn't be pruned far back, however. Normally, you'd find a node about a foot from the end of the main branch, and when cutting smaller stems, just go back two or three nodes. Use your commonsense to get it looking reasonably neat. If a branch is very old and/or diseased however, it can be cut out completely.

Rambling Roses

The rules for pruning are different from those for climbing roses. You're supposed to cut the branches that have flowered all the way back to where they begin. However, I've never managed to tell the difference between a climbing and rambling rose and I doubt you will be able to either. What I do know is that you can do a lot less harm pruning a rambling rose like you'd prune a climbing rose than you could the other way round, so it's probably best to treat them all as climbing roses and behave accordingly.

Other Considerations with Roses - Suckers

Often, you'll see straggly rose like stems growing near to or around the sides of roses. These are suckers and you are supposed to cut them off as near as possible to the base. In order to understand what suckers are you need to know something about the roses you buy in garden centres.

Most cultivated varieties of roses are the result of careful breeding over years, decades and centuries. Unfortunately, as with people, the most beautiful are not always the hardiest or the most robust. In order to get a rose that is going to both grow vigorously and look beautiful therefore, the beautiful, cultivated rose is grafted onto the rootstock of a more vigorous but coarser kind of rose. Often however, the rootstock produces its own rose stems and these are the suckers.

If you're not sure whether a stem is a rose or a sucker, there are two ways to tell, though neither is fully reliable. The first is that the stem of a sucker will have seven leaves on the end instead of five. The second is that the leaves on a sucker are less waxy and a lighter green than those on a cultivated rose.

Pests and Diseases

Finally, roses are subject to pests and diseases such as greenfly and black spot. If you have time, cut out diseased stems and leaves (you can tell they're diseased because they're discoloured) but don't go too mad about this as you might end up cutting away most of the plant. Your customer may ask you to spray their roses for them. If they don't have any spray, you can buy stuff from any garden centre or DIY shop. Most customers however, do sod all about pests and diseases and their roses do fine anyway.

Ericaceous Plants

We briefly mentioned these earlier. They include heathers, rhododendrons, azaleas, camelias and skimmias. All you need to know about them is that they need ericaceous compost or plant food on them, and that if a bag of compost says ericaceous you don't put it on anything else.

Ground Cover

If you have expanses of bare earth and want to deter weeds from them or simply make them look more interesting, there are lots of plants that make good ground cover. Examples include;

Bogenias (elephant's ears)	St John's wort	Ivy
Vinka	Campanula	Alyssum

Saxifrage.   Lillies of the valley   Grass

Plants that make good ground cover are likely to grow and spread quickly. They will look reasonably OK but often relatively boring,, since they're intended as background rather than as a centrepiece. For the same reason, they usually require little maintenance and some of them do well in shady conditions. You don't need to know much about ground cover plants at this stage, except that you mustn't pull them out unless they're spreading out of control.

Alpines

Alpines are small plants that look nice in rockeries. Being able to identify alpines is one of the tests of being a real gardener as opposed to someone who calls himself a gardener because he makes a living doing gardens. You've probably realised by now that I belong in the latter category. Alpines tend to be miniature or "petite" plants, so named because you'd expect to see them growing in mountain areas where being small is a protection against strong winds. Many in fact, are smaller versions of things you see in other parts of the garden, such as dianthus, iris, saxifrage, primroses or sedum. You don't need to know too much about them when you're starting out. Stick them in the ground with a bit of compost and water if the customer tells you to. Pull out the weeds around it. Deadhead anything that looks like it needs deadheading and so on.

One thing you should bear in mind with rockeries is that you have to be careful when watering any plants in soil that's sloping, which it usually is in a rockery. The water is apt to run down, taking soil with it. Not only does this make an awful mess, but if the soil isn't put back, this robs the plants you are watering of nutrients. One solution is to create little embankments or mounds of earth in front of the plant you're watering to stop the water flowing downhill.

For the same reason, it's not a good idea to loosen the soil too much when weeding rockeries or sloping beds. The "freshly dug over" look I kept harping on about in previous chapters will result in rapid soil erosion. If you do turn over or loosen the soil, make sure you pat it down again so that it's firm.

Climbing Plants

We've already mentioned climbing roses and Ivy. There are a number of other climbing plants that are common in gardens and although you won't have to worry too much about caring for them, it's useful if you know what they are.

Clematis

If you see a couple of very flimsy looking stems growing up next to a wall, usually during early spring, watch out. It's probably clematis, and as such, needs to be treated with respect. Women go wild about clematis and you accidentally cut them at your peril. Their enthusiasm isn't entirely without justification. They only flower for a couple of weeks but boy, when they do, you'll know what all the fuss is about. You don't have to know too much about them except that you mustn't be fooled into thinking they're nothing important and if you do decide to cut away the dead bits, make sure they really are dead. The best test is whether they snap away in your hand.

Passionflowers

Anyone who has taken the trouble to look at a passionflower will come away with a new appreciation of the expert craftsmanship that nature is capable of. The leaves are nothing to write home about, but the flowers give the impression that they've been hand knitted to an intricate design. When the flowers go they are replaced by big orange fruits like rose hips that are colourful in their own right (though not particularly edible). For such a beautiful plant, they need surprisingly little maintenance, though they do need to be watered in dry weather.

Wisteria

Wisterias have thicker, woodier stems and people often grow them around their front doors. They sport large, purplish lantern like flowers in May and they sometimes flower a second time in July. The foliage grows quickly and needs to be cut back, but it's important not to do so when they're about to flower.

Honeysuckle

Honeysuckle flowers are more charming than exciting. As the name would suggest though, they have a lovely scent.

Jasmine

There are two types; summer jasmine which has white flowers and winter jasmine – a bush rather than a climber - which has yellow flowers. Be very gentle when pruning summer jasmine. It doesn't actually need much pruning but you may need to cut little bits off to give it some shape.

Virginia Creeper

This is a bit like ivy, but is only noticeable later in the year. In the autumn it turns purple and can look really splendid in the right context.

Other Perennials

There are innumerable varieties of these, which is hardly surprising since they include nearly all plants that are not annuals. Some, such as sedum, chrysanthemums and anemones, are made of soft plant matter that dies back in the winter; to be replaced by new shoots in the following season. Others, such as hydrangeas, rhododendrons, hyperciums and fuchsias, to name but a few, are made of more woody material and are best thought of as shrubs or bushes. I'm not going into any detail about their individual care here, since it is beyond the scope of this book. You can look them up on the internet and apply the general rules I've already given you about plant care.

Trees

These are generally not your problem, especially if they're big ones. A customer may want you to prune their apple tree. There are specific techniques which I'm not going to go into here. Suffice it to say that if it's a decent size, then anything involving higher branches is best left to tree surgeons. It will take you ages, give you a crick in the back of the neck and you'll probably fall of your ladder in the process.

My rule for chopping trees or branches down is that if you can catch and hold a branch in one hand, then it's safe to saw it off. Otherwise, don't attempt to cut anything off unless you can be sure that there's nothing it can damage as it falls down; not least yourself.

There is a tool on the market which is like a pair of loppers on a pole with a saw on the other side. This can be useful for getting at very high branches but it does have its drawbacks and isn't suitable if there are a lot of branches to be cut. It's difficult to manoeuvre so you have to try about ten times to cut the branch you want. The other problem is that on most models, it is operated by pulling a sting and the string constantly gets caught on the other branches in the tree.

This is as much as I'm going to say about individual plants in this book. I don't pretend for a moment that this chapter is a comprehensive guide; it isn't intended to be. There is no shortage of beautifully illustrated books and web resources that can provide you with far more

detailed information. All that this chapter is intended to do is to give you a few pointers to set you on your way. If it helps you to identify some of the things you see and not to look completely blank when a customer mentions perennials, tubers or Black Spot, then it has served its purpose.

CHAPTER SEVEN – MOWERS IN A LITTLE MORE DETAIL

A lawn mower is the one piece of mechanical equipment that you will be expected to use on a frequent basis. The main purpose of this chapter is to familiarise you with the more common types of mower, their salient features and how to deal with some potential problems. A few generalisations will be necessary, since with all the basic kinds of mowers, there are different models and makes. Ultimately, the only way you will become conversant with their individual idiosyncrasies is through experience.

Some Considerations Regarding all Electrical Machinery

Since electrical goods normally run off the mains, they have a long flex at the end of them that needs to be plugged into a socket. Many customers have outside plug sockets, normally on the wall of the house or shed, which means that you don't have to go into the house to plug the mower in. Outside plug sockets have a protective cap to keep rain out. To open the socket, it is generally necessary to squeeze the sides or bottom of the cap and lift it up.

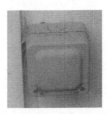

An Outside Plug Socket

Long though the flex on your appliance may be, it may not be long enough to get you all the way down the lawn or to where you need to be in the garden, and you may have to ask the customer for an extension lead. I used to carry one around with me, but it isn't really necessary, since nearly all customers have them.

You will need to carry a power breaker though. This is most important with a hedge trimmer, since the flex is always getting in the way of the blade, making accidentally chopping through it a real likelihood. It's probably least important with garden vacuums, since they don't have blades or cutting mechanisms, though I suppose you could suck the wire up into the machine if you're stupid enough.

Power or circuit breakers can be bought from DIY stores and electrical shops. To use one, plug it into the electricity socket, then plug the mower or hedge trimmer or whatever into the back of the power breaker. Most power breakers have two buttons on the back. One is the "test" button, which you use to make sure the power breaker is working. The other is the "reset" button, which you press before switching on your appliance. Should anything cut the wires or otherwise affect the electricity flow, the power breaker will shut off the supply, preventing short circuits, electric shocks and the like.

It's still a good idea not to let any blade get near the wire, since even if you don't electrocute yourself, you could make a big gash in the flex, creating a future safety hazard. Some people, when they accidentally cut through the flex, tie black insulating tape around it. I don't know whether this is effective protection against electric shocks but it's not a guarantee against short circuits. If you use an appliance that's been patched up in this way, then a power breaker is all the more important.

Most electrical appliances, unless they are very old, will have some form of starter lever and a safety button, which is to prevent you from switching on the appliance by accident. In order to start any appliance, it is necessary to hold the safety button down before pressing the starter lever.

Two final pieces of safety advice are not to use anything electrical in the rain and to always disconnect any appliance before putting your hands near a blade. It is unlikely that a machine will start without being deliberately switched on, but I have known it to happen, and should your hands be in the wrong place at the wrong time, the outcome could be both mangled and bloody.

Safety Button and Starter Lever on an Electric Mower

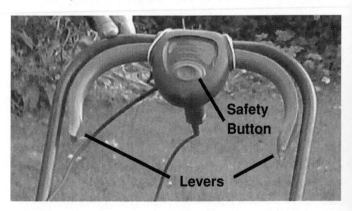

Electric Lawn Mowers

Electric mowers are much easier to use than petrol ones, but
tend to vary widely in their design. In the illustration below, I have
located the main features of electric mowers that you need to
familiarise yourself with.

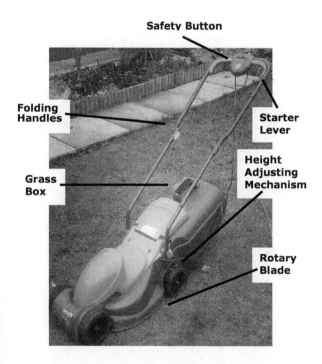

Safety Button

Folding Handles

Starter Lever

Height Adjusting Mechanism

Grass Box

Rotary Blade

Some of the features highlighted in the above illustration are
common to all or nearly all electric mowers. Others are specific to
certain models.

Common Features

Nearly all electric mowers have a safety button and a starter lever. As indicated above, you start the mower by holding down the safety button while you press the starter lever. The other thing they all have in common is that you can fold the handle. This, as you'd expect, is to make it easier to cram it into an often crowded tool shed.

Grass Boxes

Not all electric mowers have a box for collecting grass cuttings. If a mower does have a grass box, it is usually on the back but sometimes in front or on the top. It goes without saying that you need to check if it's full occasionally while you're cutting the grass and empty it when it is.

Generally speaking, if a mower has wheels it will have a grass box, which is likely to be at the back if it's a rotary mower and at the front if it's a cylindrical mower (see below). Hover mowers (see below) will often have no grass box at all. Where they do have one, this will usually be situated on top of the rotary blade, making the mower feel quite heavy to push.

If the mower you are using doesn't have a grass box, or if the grass box doesn't work very well, then you may need to go over the lawn afterwards with a lawn rake to sweep up the worst of the cuttings.

Height Adjusting Mechanisms

Almost all mowers with wheels have height adjusting mechanisms, which are nearly always located around one or more of the wheels. Their purpose is to adjust the cutting height of the mower in accordance with how short you want the grass to be. They vary from model to model and are almost impossible to describe without making what are simple mechanisms and procedures seem convoluted and confusing. Just fiddle around with a few mowers and you'll soon get the hang of it.

If you really get stuck, the chances are that the mower is at the cutting height the customer likes because they probably left it at that height the last time they cut the grass. You can always of course, swallow your pride and ask the customer how the mechanism works.

It's virtually impossible to put a serious height adjusting mechanism on a hover mower. Just assume, for practical purposes, that they don't have them.

*Common Height Adjusting Mechanisms
on Wheels of Mower*

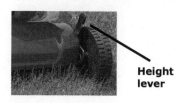

**Height
lever**

Rotary Blades

Both petrol and electric mowers can either have rotary or cylindrical blades. Hover mowers however, will always have rotary blades. Again, any descriptions of the difference will appear convoluted so I have included pictures of rotary and cylindrical blades below.

Generally speaking, mowers with rotary blades are a lot less hassle. Rotary mowers are better at cutting the grass when it has grown too long or when if is a bit damp (it's both dangerous and pointless to cut grass if it's raining or really wet). They are easier to clean and don't get stuck nearly as often as cylindrical mowers. Cylindrical mowers however, have the edge over rotary mowers if you want to cut the grass very short.

Rotary Blade   *Cylindrical Blade*

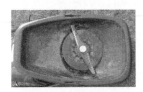   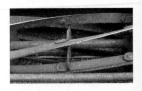

It is worth mentioning here that there are two types of rotary blades. The most common is a single metal blade that screws on and looks like a propeller (see above). Cheaper models however, often have little plastic blades that you fit onto a rotating disk thing inside the mower. Plastic blades constantly fall off the mower and are best thought of as disposable items; I usually get through at least one a session. Your customer should have a supply of spare blades. If not, you can usually buy them at DIY superstores like Homebase or B&Q.

Hover Mowers

You'll probably have worked out by now that whether or not a mower has certain features is largely dependent on whether the mower has wheels or is a hover mower. Hover mowers are very common and always electric. They work on the same principle as a hovercraft. Instead of moving around on wheels, they float on a cushion of air. It can be a pleasant feeling gliding over the lawn with one, but they do have they're defects. As mentioned above, they usually only have one cutting height. They're less likely to have a grass box. They're also not as good as mowers with wheels for going right up to the edge of the lawn.

What to do if Your Electric Mower isn't Working

Electric mowers are generally pretty reliable, but they do have a habit of getting clogged up, especially if the grass is long and damp and/or it isn't depositing cuttings in the grass box properly. Sometimes, you'll have to get down on your hands and knees to pull the grass out of the blade area.

If the grass is seriously long it may be impossible to cut it effectively with a mower, especially a cylindrical one; and you will have to go over it first using a pair of shears or a strimmer, if the customer has one that works properly.

Hover Mower with *Grass Box* on Top

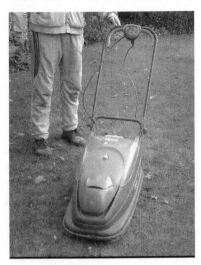

Why Your Electric Mower Doesn't Start

You don't usually encounter problems when starting electric mowers. Should you do so, it may be for one of the following reasons.

* You've used a power breaker but forgotten to press the reset button.

* The plug has loose wiring or needs a new fuse.

* You are using a faulty extension lead. Try plugging the mower lead directly into the mains. If it works, you'll know it's the extension lead that's faulty.

If none of the above work, then there may be a faulty connection or other fault inside the mower. Unless you're good at tinkering with electrical machinery, then leave it alone.

Petrol Mowers

Petrol mowers tend to be more powerful than electric ones and much heavier. They're great fun when they work properly but they can present a few problems to the novice. Many of the features of petrol mowers have their counterpart in motor vehicles. I don't drive, in case you haven't noticed, which is why it feels little short of a miracle to me when I get one going.

With the exception of the choke, all petrol mowers will have all the features in the illustration overleaf. If these are properly understood, this will go a long way to preventing or dealing with the majority of problems encountered when trying to start one.

The Petrol Tank

Petrol mowers, as you'd expect, need to be filled with petrol on a regular basis. They invariably have a petrol tank which, like a petrol tank in a car, has a protective screw cap which must be removed in order to put in the petrol and screwed back on afterwards. A customer who owns a petrol mower will normally have a green plastic petrol can from which to fill it. On top of the petrol can, there should be a funnel which can be detached and screwed on to the nozzle of the can to help you pour petrol into the tank without making a mess.

Petrol Mower

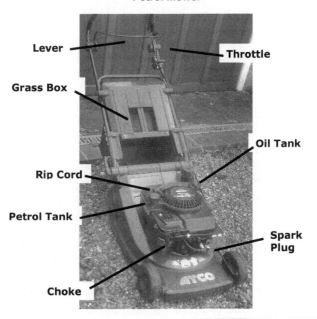

Lever

Throttle

Grass Box

Oil Tank

Rip Cord

Petrol Tank

Spark Plug

Choke

Petrol Canister with Funnel

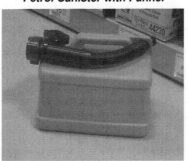

The Oil Tank

Whatever you do, don't get the petrol tank mixed up with the oil tank. I'm not sure exactly what would happen if you poured oil into the petrol tank or petrol into the oil tank but it must be pretty gruesome; noxious gases perhaps, or huge explosions. It should say on the mower which is which, but here are a couple of ways to distinguish the two.

Petrol smells different from oil; more petrolly, if you know what I mean. If you can clearly smell the difference between the two, then you should have no problems telling which is which.

The cap on the oil tank will usually have a dipstick, consisting of a long strip of metal, attached to it. It is important to make sure that the oil tank doesn't contain too much oil or too little. You can tell how much there is by taking out the dipstick and seeing how far up the metal strip the oil has come. If you need to put oil in, the customer should have a bottle of the stuff in the shed.

Choke

Like a car, most but not all petrol mowers have a choke. This is frequently a button, often red, which if you're looking at the mower from the front, is either on the front or the left hand side of the mower. As with a car, you need to use it when the engine is cold. In practice, this means that you should press the button a few times before starting the mower up.

Spark Plug

The spark plug is at the front of the mower and is easy to recognise because it's a rubbery thing on the end of a rubbery wire. It needs to be slotted in to the mower, and while it's difficult to describe, it's pretty obvious where it goes. The mower will not start without the plug being inserted, and it's a good idea to unplug it if you want to put your hands anywhere near the blades.

Choke and Spark Plug on Front of Mower

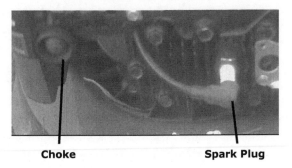

Choke   **Spark Plug**

Rip Cord

You pull the rip cord to start the mower. It normally just takes a few sharp tugs. Before pulling the ripcord however, make sure that it isn't stuck or tangled by holding down the lever (see picture of lever below) and pulling it slowly. If you feel an obstruction, try pulling the cord gently a few times and the problem should usually sort itself out. If not, it may be because you are trying to start the mower on long grass that is getting caught up in the blades. Try moving the mower to a spot where the grass is shorter.

The Rip Cord

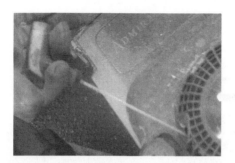

Throttle

The throttle is used to set the mower speed. It looks like a gear lever and you can change the speed by moving the lever. When starting the mower from cold, it should be in start mode.

The Throttle

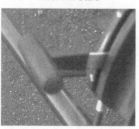

Lever

The lever is normally on the front of the top of the handle and you hold it down while doing the mowing. Sometimes, there will be another lever on the back which, when held down, moves the mower forward so you don't have to push it. On most models, the mower will stop if you let go of the lever.

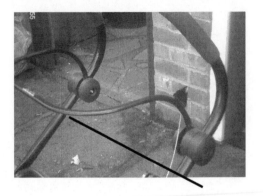

Start Lever

That wraps up the main features of most electric mowers that you are likely to use. Below is a step by step guide to getting a petrol mower going.

How to Start a Petrol Mower

1. Make sure that there is enough petrol in the petrol tank.

2. Make sure that the spark plug is in.

3. Press the choke several times

4. Make sure the throttle is in starting mode.

5. Hold down the lever/s and check that the rip cord is moving freely.

6. Keeping the lever/s down, give the rip cord several sharp tugs.

Hopefully, the engine should start up. If it doesn't, it may be due to one of the following reasons.

a. There is either too much or not enough oil in the oil tank.

b. You haven't inserted the spark plug.

c. You need to press the choke a few more times.

d. The throttle is in the wrong position.

If you've checked all these things and the mower still isn't working, give it a break and go on to something else. Then have another try later. If it still doesn't work, then maybe it's a fault with the mower rather than you.

Cutting the Grass with a Petrol Mower

Once you've got the mower started, cutting the grass is relatively trouble free. People prefer you, where possible, to go up and down the lawn in straight lines to get a "striped effect". You can move the throttle to adjust the engine speed and when you need to switch off the mower, it's usually enough to let go of the lever, though on some models, it's necessary to move the throttle to an "off" position. Once the engine has warmed up, you don't usually need to use the choke to restart it, and you don't normally need to move the throttle back into the start position, though it's useful to have it on a high speed..

Cleaning the mower is pretty much the same as with an electric mower, though you should be careful when turning it on its side that petrol or oil doesn't leak out anywhere. Before putting your hands anywhere near the blades, make sure you pull the spark plug out. That way there's no risk of the mower accidentally restarting.

Finally

I've probably made mowing seem more complicated than it is in this chapter. That's because I've tried to introduce you to a wide variety of mowers. It's best to treat this chapter as reference. If you practice with a friend's mower once or twice, you'll probably know enough to see you through most situations, and if you come across an unfamiliar mower and have to ask the customer for advice, it's not the end of the world.

If you do have problems, they will almost certainly be with petrol mowers. Again, don't be afraid to ask the customer if it refuses to start. If they're unable to get it going, they're hardly likely to blame you for failing to do so.

Chapter Eight – The Gardening Year

Understanding seasons isn't just necessary in order to know what to do when. It is central to understanding what gardening is all about and what makes it so worthwhile.

If you spend most of your life indoors, you may have surprisingly little appreciation of weather. You've probably got an idea of the seasons of the year. You'll be aware that it gets colder in winter and hotter in summer. You'll know that in spring, things start flowering and in autumn, leaves tart falling off the trees. If you're unfortunate enough to suffer from hay fever, you might know there's a lot of pollen around from about May to the end of July. If you're under 30, you'll have had it drummed into you that summers are hotter and winters milder than they used to be, and that by 2020 the UK will either be reduced to semi-desert, under six feet of water or battered by tornadoes at least once a week.

As a gardener you'll be far more conscious of the weather. You'll be checking the weather forecast before going out in the mornings. You'll learn to anticipate a shower, and to decide when it's best to carry on working, shelter in the tool shed or pack up and go home. You'll learn to appreciate that it's OK working on a dull day but nothing bucks you up like a blue sky and a sun with a bit of warmth in it.

You'll also be aware of what's happening to the plants around you. You'll start noticing what flowers and fruits at what time of the year. You'll realise that gardens don't simply look more colourful in summer than in winter, but that the flowers and foliage change from month to month. You'll discover that autumn isn't simply the beginning of the winter, but a panorama of colourful leaves and berries. Even between December and February, when everything looks dead or dormant, there's actually quite a lot going on behind the scenes if you take the trouble to look.

In this chapter, I'm going to try and present what goes on in the garden in a seasonal context, as well as telling you what customers might expect you to do at various times of the year.

Winter

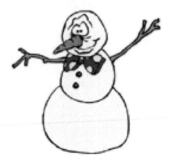

As far as you're concerned as a gardener, it's best to think of the winter as beginning about two weeks before Christmas and carrying on into early March. You aren't going to get a lot of work at this time. If you do, it will mainly be jobs that you or your customers simply haven't got round to. There might be one or two regular customers who like you to keep coming right round the year, but generally speaking, if you want work during the winter; you have to advertise for it, and quite determinedly.

I find that if I put leaflets out in the summer I get roughly one phone call for every fifty. In the winter it's more like one in two hundred and fifty. Not every call ends up in a job either, and most of the work you do get will consist of small, "one off" jobs. If you seriously intend to keep working through the winter therefore, you'll need to be putting out leaflets on a fairly constant basis. Fair enough you say, but for every customer who phones you up, another two or three will hang on to your leaflet and phone you in June when you've already got far more work than you can handle.

You may find it better to adapt your work schedule to the seasons. Be prepared to put in overtime in late spring, early summer and during late August/September, with a view to putting a little money by to tide you over. Then you can use the winter to write your novel, backpack round the world or simply sign on the dole and lie in bed watching the Jeremy Kyle Show.

If you do decide to brave the outdoors, it may not be the most pleasant season for working but neither is it as uncomfortable as you might think. Take a look at people digging up the road or working on building sites. They don't usually look as if they're shivering. It is important to remember that when you're doing manual work, you feel far less cold when you are standing at a bus stop. I normally wear a heavy jacket but on a mild day, I may take it off at some point and work in my shirt sleeves. You may suffer a bit with your hands though, since it's almost impossible to find a pair of gloves that are suitable for gardening, keep your hands warm and allow you to do intricate jobs with your fingers. The worst is if you're doing something like weeding first thing in the morning when your hands are in constant contact with the cold ground.

If the earth is literally frozen, then there's not really much point in going to work. You can't do anything with the soil and it's not too good for the grass to walk on it. During your average British winter though, mud is much more likely to be a problem. The water table is much higher in the winter and so the ground is much wetter. Expect to get covered in the stuff and have a spare pair of shoes and trousers for going home in. This applies especially if you plan on using public transport between three thirty and five in the afternoon. Do you really want hordes of school kids wondering why a filthy, smelly, homeless person is sharing a bus with them?

Surprisingly, there are things that either flower or look beautiful at this time of the year. Cyclamen, primroses and pansies for instance, often flower right through the winter, as do winter flowering vibunums and winter jasmines. This is also the season for pampas grass, which makes a splendid display and dogwoods, whose bare branches come out in beautiful glowing red, yellow and orangey colours.

Look carefully, and you'll notice other plants getting ready for spring. Bulbs are already sending up shoots in December. There are also buds growing on shrubs and trees, such as camelias and magnolias, ready for early spring flowering.

Winter is also a good time for putting in new bushes and shrubs. That's because they're not growing much at this time of the year, so they're not doing too much drinking and eating and don't mind being disturbed so much.

It varies from year to year but usually, sometime in mid-February, the first signs of spring flowering appear. Crocuses are often among the first flowers to come up. Daffodils are also early starters, and in some years have come up as early as January. Kerria comes out in yellow flowers in early February, followed some weeks later by forsythia, both of which flower before they start growing leaves. You might also start to see celandine appear during this period.

Spring

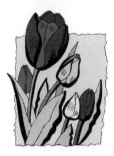

March is when the action starts. They say March comes in with a roar and goes out with a whimper. Most of the time, it feels indistinguishable from winter, but you usually get those first five or six days of bright weather when you can actually feel the warmth of the sun and people say lame things like "oh, spring really is here at last". It may not amount to much, but it's enough to make the garden erupt into a blaze of colour. This is the season for many of your bulbs, such as crocuses, tulips, daffodils, hyacinths and grape hyacinths. Cherry trees erupt into blossom and magnolia trees are covered in striking pinkish white flowers. Just as impressive are camelias, whose buds finally open into large red blossoms. Neglected paths and lawns become covered in celandine, while at eye level, forsythia comes out in dazzling migraine inducing yellow.

It isn't just the flowers either. The weeds and the lawn start growing as well. Your phone will start ringing too, but not as much as it ought to. You'll get a few jobs here and there but things don't really pick up yet. They ought to of course; because the sooner you get a handle on things the easier it is to keep the garden under control, but unfortunately, that isn't how human nature works. Most of your customers will prefer to wait till everything's impossibly overgrown, then try to make you feel guilty because you're booked three weeks solid.

Business really starts to pick up in April. The weather may not seem brilliant to you. Sometimes it will be stereotypical April weather; showers alternating with pale blue skies, so you never know whether or not to get the lawnmower out. Other times it will simply be foul or just plain dull. But it's getting warmer and the grass and weeds are growing in earnest. Leave the lawn for more than a fortnight and the mower may start to struggle. Your phone is ringing constantly. By the end of the month you'll be wondering how to put off your customers rather than trying to attract business. The clocks have changed and it doesn't get dark much before eight. If you're not good at saying "no", you can end up working twelve hour days or seven day weeks. Things will stay that way for the next few months. This is the time of year to cancel all social engagements and pay off your winter overdraft.

Daffodils and tulips are starting to wither and droop, to be replaced by bluebells. Most customers like bluebells but they can be very pervasive, and customers will sometimes ask you to thin them out. Celandine also starts to recede, to be replaced by blue forget me nots and aquilegia. Cherry blossoms will have long disappeared, but apple trees are about to put on an equally magnificent show of their own.

You'll also get stuff to plant out at this time of year, and late April is when you start putting out summer bedding like marigolds, petunias, geraniums and busy lizzies.

When bulbs have finished flowering, it's a good idea to deadhead them. The leaves will start to wither and look straggly, and it will be tempting to cut them off. If your customer is happy, it's best not to do so until they're almost brown. The reason for this is that a lot of nutrients from the leaves go back into the bulb so cutting the leaves off too early weakens next year's flowering ability.

It's also a time of year when you have to be particularly careful when it comes to chopping back stuff and knowing the difference between weeds and plants. When something is flowering or fully grown, it's generally pretty obvious whether you're supposed to pull it out or not, but in spring, lots of things are in their early stages, and if you get a load of seedlings, they're probably from a nearby tree but they could be the annuals that the customer has planted. Sometimes I still have to swallow my pride and ask.

Early Summer

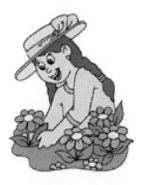

It's barely two months since you were sitting at home waiting for the phone to ring. Now you have to struggle to get a day off or even an early night. It doesn't get properly dark till ten or eleven and believe me, there'll be plenty of work to keep you going till then. You won't be doing yourself or your customers any favours by overworking though. If you come home knackered and doze off in front of the telly, it means you've done an honest day's work. If you still feel physically drained when you leave the house next morning, then you're overdoing it. However busy I am, I try not to do more than two ten hour days in succession and to get a full day off at least once a week. If people whinge that their garden is urgent and please, please can you come this Thursday, you'll just have to be tough. Where were they when you were struggling to pay the rent last January? My customers tend to resort to flattery, which I'm ashamed to say often works.

Exhausting it may be, but it also feels great to be outdoors. You finally get some proper warm weather. The grass is still fresh and green and the garden is full of scents and bees and everything growing at a frantic rate. May highlights include wisteria, with its lantern like purple blooms. They include ceanothus, a hedge like bush that bursts into hundreds of tiny blue flowers. Last but not least, it is the season for of the magnificent, if rather short lived peony. There is also a rather strange kind of weed that grows extremely quickly at this time of the year, covering whole flower beds with ease. It's called a cleaver, is slightly sticky to the touch and is very easy to get rid of. You just grab the stuff in handfuls. It's more or less gone by June anyway, to be replaced by the much more problematic bindweed.

June is the most colourful season of all. It's when all the summer bedding plants come out in earnest, like marigolds, petunias, begonias, penstemon, osteospermum and countless others. It's when clematis is most likely to be flowering, along with shrubs such as hypercium and lavatera, and small, cottagey stuff like campanula, alyssum and lobelias. It's mainly the weeds and the grass that will keep you busy though. They grow at an alarmingly fast rate and all the customers who put off phoning you earlier in the year suddenly find that their gardens have become completely unmanageable. Most of your work therefore, involves weeding, mowing and trimming things back into shape. This is the season for bindweed, which you should deal with as soon as you see it. If you leave it, it will entangle itself with everything else in the garden and be a nightmare to get rid of. Hedges don't need to be done as often as lawns. You need to trim a privet hedge about every four to six weeks during the peak season. When trimming bushes, go easy on anything you aren't sure about. My practice is to cut off no more than I need to in order to get it into a nice shape. Generally speaking, if something is going to flower, then if you cut much off it, you'll prevent it from doing so. If it is flowering, you can see whether or not you're cutting off too many flowers. If it's already flowered, you're probably OK but there are always exceptions.

With experience, you'll get to know what most of the things in the garden are, and how to treat them. In the meantime, check with the customer and failing that, take the precautions suggested above.

Midsummer

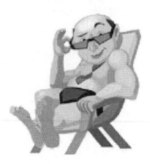

You'll usually have cleared the backlog of work by about the second week of July. This is also the time when your customers start going on holiday. Some of them will want you to come while they're away but others will wait till their garden is overgrown again before they call you. How much things quieten down largely depends on what kind of summer it is. If it's really hot and dry, the lawn and weeds don't grow so much and business can drop quite sharply. You can always put out more leaflets but it may be worth having a few days away yourself. You're probably knackered from the last couple of months and do you really want to work in thirty degrees trying to dig soil that's bone dry? If there's a reasonable amount of rain however, things will carry on growing and you'll probably have a reasonably full schedule.

Whatever the weather, the vegetation is no longer as fresh and green as it was earlier, and a lot of your work will consist of deadheading roses and other flowers, and cutting away dying and withered stalks and leaves. Even if customers don't ask you to do this, they will really appreciate the result.

And you do have to take the sun seriously. I go in for a strong sun cream and a floppy hat which I like to think makes me look loveable. You'll also need to ensure a steady water supply on hot days. Some customers will take great pleasure in constantly plying you with iced drinks, never thinking for a moment that you may want the toilet. Others come out with a thimbleful of orange juice when you're about to collapse from heat exhaustion. I normally keep an empty plastic bottle with me and fill it from the customer's kitchen or the outside tap. I generally find that if I don't drink enough or protect myself from the sun, I end up with a massive headache. I'm told that the cure is to force a couple of pints of water down you. I've tried it with varying results.

Although the most colourful season of the year is over, most bedding plants will continue to flower provided they have plenty of water and are regularly deadheaded. There are some new kids on the block too; dahlias and Japanese anemones for instance, and Miclaelmas daisies. July - August is also the season for blackberries, which make a nice snack while you're trying to get rid of brambles.

Late Summer Early Autumn

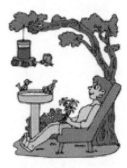

Business perks up again at the end of the summer, especially if it's been a dry one. Once you get a bit of rain everything turns lush green again. Your customers come home from their holidays and from late August you'll find yourself almost as busy as you were in May and June. You'll be finishing work earlier though, as it's getting dark now by eight o clock. Many summer bedding plants are still flowering, as are roses, while others, such as pyracantha, are already sporting red and orange autumn berries. There are some plants that are specific to this time of year, such as golden rod and autumn crocuses. My favourite early autumn plant however, has to be sedum. You hardly notice it in summer, but the heads turn into an absolutely beautiful pink at around this time.

I find September a particularly pleasant month to be working in. It's often almost as colourful as June and the sun feels pleasantly warm without being oppressive. The fact that the warm days are nearly over only gives them a poignancy that makes me appreciate them all the more.

Late Autumn

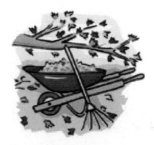

Business declines slowly after the onset of October. At the same time, the number of daylight hours suitable for working in decreases, especially after the clocks change. Your customers start talking about giving the garden a final mow and tidy up. You'll find the ground is a lot damper. The grass, in particular, is never dry, so don't worry if the lawn doesn't come out as nicely as it did in the summer. If your customer wants to get dandelions out of the grass, this is the time to do it, as it won't matter if there are a few temporary holes. Put some compost in the holes and chuck down some new grass seed. If you're seriously into lawn care, this is the time of the year to scarify, aerate and fertilise your lawn. Most of your customers won't know this, and you'll rarely be asked to do it.

There'll be an increasing amount of dead stuff to cut; often, it's rotted enough for you to pull away with your hand. But a surprising number of flowers are still going strong. Dahlias, Michaelmas daisies, roses and lots of summer annuals will make it well into October and even November. Primroses, cyclamen and pansies also do well at this time of the year, but the real beauty of the season comes from autumn berries and the changing colours of the leaves. This is the season for Virginia and Boston creeper, which just look like a boring kind of ivy during the summer, but now come into their own as they turn through graceful shades of pink and purple.

Autumn is the time of year for putting in spring bulbs. They're normally planted in October and November and there's not much to it, except to get them at roughly the right depth. There will be instructions on the packet but a general rule is that the bottom of the bulb should be buried to a depth of two and a half times the height of the bulb. If that sounds like a mouthful, let's say the bulb is two inches high, then dig a hole five inches deep and stick it at the bottom.

Just when you think it's time to pack up for the winter, the leaves start falling in earnest and keep you occupied for a good month or more. Customers you think you've said goodbye to until spring will call you for a final visit, which sometimes turns out to be two or three. With any luck, you'll be working well into December.

After that of course, there won't be much happening for the next two or three months, so put your tools away and start on the Christmas decorations.

CHAPTER NINE – YOUR PERSONAL SURVIVAL

As I indicated in Chapter Two, this book is both about gardening and about running a business. As a gardener you have to know how to get gardens looking aesthetically pleasing and how not to do too much damage. As a business person, you have to know about handling money and dealing with one or two legal formalities. You also need to know about interacting with people. You need to understand what is involved in creating the right impression. You also need to know how to tactfully communicate your own needs and expectations while simultaneously anticipating the customer's. This chapter attempts to address some of the above issues.

Money

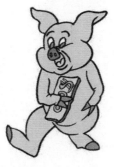

If you expect to be paid for your work, you have to charge your customers money. This brings a whole host of questions. How much should I charge? Do I charge by the hour or give quotes?

When should I expect to be paid? Will it be cash? Do I need to do any paperwork? What if the customer decides not to cough up?

What to Charge

With garden maintenance, it's generally easiest to charge by the hour. As to what the hourly rate should be, there is no simple answer. There are too many variables, such as how skilled you are, your level of physical fitness and the geographical region you live in.

I live in South London where, provided you've got some idea what you're doing and are reasonably fit, you can charge at least ten pounds an hour; possibly more. If you live in Sunderland or Pontypool however, you may have to adjust your prices accordingly. The same goes if you're just starting and you're not yet confident, or if you have a bad back and can't do digging or heavy lifting. As a general rule, if nobody ever complains and lots of people are tipping you, you're probably not charging enough. If more than a small minority express their dissatisfaction however, you're almost certainly overcharging. Few customers like to feel they're being ripped off but most people are willing to pay you fairly for an honest day's work.

Giving Quotes and Estimates

Sometimes, a customer just wants you to give their garden a "once over" and they may ask you to give them a fixed quote for the whole job. This can lead to problems for the novice, since any job invariably takes twice as long as you think it's going to take. Furthermore, if customers know they are only paying a fixed price however long it takes; a minority will exploit the situation by demanding a much more thorough job they'd otherwise expect.

From a customer's point of view however, it's understandable why they may be reluctant to pay you for this sort of job by the hour. If you can't tell them how long the job will take, they can't predict what the bill is going to be.

I have a formula that I have found to work well for both parties in the great majority of situations. I "estimate" that I'll be able to do the bulk of the job in either half a day, a full day or two days, depending on the job. "I should be able to break the back of it" I say; "then we can decide whether you're happy with it as it is or whether you want me to come back to attend to any outstanding details".

What this means is that both you and your customer are on the same side. The customer has peace of mind but won't be too fussy about the details, provided you're using the time as productively as possible. You on the other hand, know you're getting paid properly for your time, so you won't resent doing your best for the customer.

A word about the difference between quotes and estimates; quotes are binding, in that if you give a quote, you have agreed to do a job for a particular price. An estimate, on the other hand, is only an educated guess as to how much the job will cost, and as such can be revised if the job takes longer than expected. Your customers will not always be aware of this distinction, so if you're only giving an estimate and not a quote, you need to spell that out.

Clarity

However you agree to be paid, you do need to make sure that the customer is clear about what he/she will be expected to pay. This is especially important if there are two of you working together. Let's say you charge ten pounds an hour for working on your own, you and your friend will want £10 each. Fair enough, you'd think, since in theory at least, you're getting the job done twice as quickly. Customers don't always see it quite that way however. They often only have a fuzzy idea how long a job takes but they do know what they're shelling out per hour and £20 is a lot of money to them. If you don't explain things at the outset, you could be in for a few unpleasant scenes later.

You and the Law - Benefits

If you want to become a gardener because you are currently not working, you will probably be claiming one or more benefits, be they unemployment, housing, pension, disability, income support or whatever. While you can, as a gardener, ultimately expect to earn full-time wages, it will probably take you a few months to generate a decent clientele. In the meantime, if you are earning money, either as an employee or on a self-employed basis, you are normally obliged to declare your earnings to whatever agency your benefits are coming from.

Many people, of course, don't declare their earnings, and generally speaking, they get away with it since most customers are quite happy to pay in cash. I don't, as a matter of course, condone claiming benefits one is not entitled to, I do feel however, that it is my duty to make you aware of the possible consequences of your decision to declare or not declare your earnings.

If you keep quiet about your activities, there is a small risk of your getting caught, either as a result of an undercover operation or more likely, somebody - usually with a personal grudge against you - reporting you to the relevant authorities. This can lead to prosecution for benefit fraud but in most cases will only result in your benefits being stopped.

Should you decide to declare your earnings, this will usually, depending on the benefit and amount earned, result in the bulk of your earnings being deducted from your benefits; so much for encouraging the long term unemployed to earn an honest bob.

But that's not all. If you're not very careful, you could end up embroiled in a bureaucratic nightmare, involving demands for earnings verification that would overwhelm an accountant and gross financial errors in calculating your new benefit entitlements. A friend of mine, who was both scrupulously honest and frugal in his spending habits, was recently threatened with eviction from his council home after his rent got stopped. So before you open your mouth, be sure what you're letting yourself in for.

Once you're off benefits, you have to consider your legal obligations as a self-employed person. While nobody likes paying

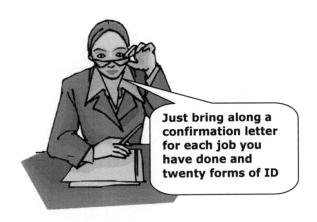

Just bring along a confirmation letter for each job you have done and twenty forms of ID

tax or national insurance, the bureaucracy is a lot easier to cope with. You don't need to be a limited company and you don't even need a business bank account. You simply need to go along to your local tax office, tell them what you're doing and ask to register as a self-employed person. You'll need to make regular but small national insurance contributions, and every year, you will have to fill in a form declaring how much you've earned and how much your expenses were. If you submit it by September, they will work out the tax for you, whereas if you work it out yourself, you don't have to submit it till the following January. It's not a lot of work at all, since you don't need to submit receipts or audited accounts or anything until your annual turnover is quite substantial.

Of course, if you don't declare your earnings to Social Security, and then go and register your business with the Inland Revenue while you're still on benefits, then I regret to say you're a complete and utter idiot and there's noting I can do or say to save you from yourself.

Basic Needs

Gardeners aren't immortal. They need to eat, drink, go to the toilet and protect themselves from the elements. Your customers are only dimly aware of your requirements, though thankfully, most realise that a hot steaming brew every few hours is a British worker's God given right.

Food

If you're working somewhere for half a day or more, some customers will offer to make you a sandwich; a few will even give you a hot lunch. But this is generosity over and above the call of duty, for which you should show gratitude accordingly. More often, it's up to you to make sure you don't go hungry. If like me, you're too lazy to makes sandwiches, you can always nip out for a bacon butty. If you're working somewhere all day, your customer will expect you to take a lunch break, though it would be the height of impertinence to charge for it.

Driink

If you haven't done manual work in seriously hot weather before, you won't know how thirsty you can get; neither will the people you work for. I've had more than one well meaning customer

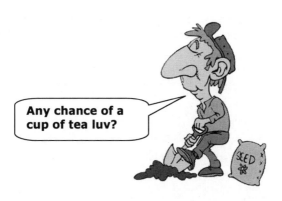

Any chance of a cup of tea luv?

gape at me open mouthed while I down a pint glass of water or orange juice in seconds. If you're seriously thirsty, your work will suffer and even if you think you're OK, you can easily get dehydrated on a hot day and end up with a massive headache.

My normal practice is to keep one or two small plastic soft drinks bottles filled with water in my rucksack. They don't add much weight and it's easy to fill them up again at work. Many houses have an outside tap, which suits me fine, but if you don't want to catch germs and things, it's perfectly reasonable to ask to fill your bottle from the kitchen. Of course, if you're one of those people who only drink bottled water, then you'll have to make your own arrangements.

The Call of Nature

Of course, having enough to drink leads to another slight problem; at some point you will have to use the toilet. If you are bashful about this, then you could be in for some difficult times. Let me state firmly and categorically that it is perfectly acceptable to knock at the door and say to the customer "excuse me, can I use your loo?" No customer is likely to refuse this basic request or think it in any way odd. Many actually go to the toilet themselves.

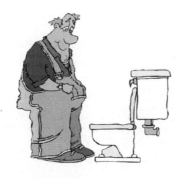

It's slightly more problematic if the customer is out. Whatever you do, don't be tempted to have a pee in the garden. We've all tried to get away with it at some point, but the temporary relief simply isn't worth the potential embarrassment of being spotted by a neighbour. Take a five minute walk and find a public convenience or pub or a secluded patch of wasteland.

Weather

Protecting yourself against the weather is pretty much commonsense. If you work in the rain till you're soaked to the skin, you'll make the garden messier than it was before and probably catch a nasty cold into the bargain. If you work unprotected on a hot day in the full glare of the sun, you risk dehydration, headaches, sunburn and possibly sunstroke or skin cancer. So carry some rudimentary protection from the rain. Find shelter during heavy showers and if the rain is heavy and persistent, pack up and go home. Try to find work to do in the shade when the sun's hot. Wear some protective head covering, such as a wide brimmed hat, and cover any exposed parts of your body with a high factor sun screen.

Health

Apart from pneumonia, sunstroke and fatal accidents, there are one or two other long term health issues you need to deal with. It's a good idea to make sure you've had an anti-tetanus jab. You should consider using a kneeling pad to avoid constant kneeling on wet ground, since I'm told that this can contribute to arthritis. And then of course there's the question of your back.

You won't believe the number of people who complain about their backs. You need to keep yours in good shape however, as it's your livelihood. I'm ashamed to say that the fact that my back has held up is due more to luck than good usage. I'm probably on borrowed time and definitely not the person to give advice about Pilates or Alexander technique. There are one or two rules that I try to stick to however.

1. When lifting heavy objects or doing heavy work, try not to put too much pressure on your back; let other parts of your body, such as your legs take some of the strain.

2. Try to avoid bending down too much. If you need to be close to the ground, simply work on your knees.

3. If you do strain your back, don't be tempted to carry on working. Take a few days off until it's recovered. If the problem persists, seek medical advice but also consider going to an osteopath or chiropractor. GPs don't always take the problem seriously enough.

Customers and Other People

Gardening involves getting on with customers. This isn't usually too difficult but there are a few fairly obvious rules of etiquette. It also helps if you are able to anticipate, understand and respond to your customers' concerns,

Money and Marketing Etiquette

Customers don't mind if you're eccentric, socially inept or have appalling dress sense; it just adds to your rustic charm. They do however; appreciate certain courtesies, most of which should be pretty obvious to anyone who's had dealings with the British public.

Don't be pushy when it comes to promoting your services or asking for money. Nobody likes a hard sell and in gardening, it's simply not necessary. There are plenty of people who want their gardens done. If they know you exist, and that you're half way competent, they will contact you when they are ready. You might get one or two jobs by using high pressure tactics but you will scare a lot more people away. Likewise, most people are happy to pay you fairly for your work, but they won't like it if you overcharge them, demand money before starting work or act like Del Boy from "Only Fools and Horses".

It's not a good idea to allow customers to haggle with you. Only a few customers will try, but my experience is that if you allow them to beat you down on the price, they lose respect and try to exploit you in other ways. By the same token, don't let customers owe you large sums of money until you're sure you can trust them. By all means make your rates competitive, or make concessions for genuinely hard up pensioners, but don't cheapen yourself in the process.

Good Manners Generally

As in most areas of life, good manners are mainly a matter of common sense. Should you have occasion to go into the house, take off your muddy boots. If you're going to be seriously late, give the customer a rung. Whatever you do, don't simply fail to turn up without cancelling or rescheduling the appointment. Don't take long tea breaks, unless you make it clear to the customer that you're doing this in your own time and don't expect to be paid for them. It's OK to answer your mobile phone at work – you have a business to run - but if you're kept talking a long time, then apologise to the customer and if appropriate, deduct the time spent talking from what you charge them. If you want to play music, ask if this is OK and keep the volume at a reasonable level. If you've found a way of working while using headphones, then please get in contact with me as I'd love to know about it.

Knowing Your Customers

A lot of your customers are pretty straightforward to deal with. They want you to do the garden because they lead busy lives. They'll tell you what they want, let you get on with it and pay you before you go. Provided you do a half decent job, you'll have no problems with them.

There are a few you should know about, however. There are the uncommunicative types to start with. Not being "hands on" is one thing, but you will get some customers who are so unresponsive that working for them can be quite soul destroying.

You: These forget me nots look very nice, do you want to keep them.

Customer: Yeah, OK.

You: Or would you prefer me to pull them out?

Customer: Yeah, OK

You: And do you want me to cut the grass?

Customer: You're the gardener.

You'll probably end up wondering why they called you in the first place. It's generally best to assume that they simply want

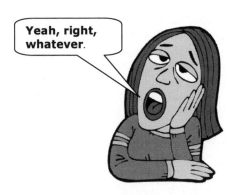

Yeah, right, whatever.

everything; lawn, bushes, hedges etc. cut back into neat shapes, all paved surfaces swept and everything that isn't officially a flower pulled out. I generally finish the job as quickly as I can and tell them to call me when they need me again. Few do; no doubt because they've decided to have everything concreted over.

The apathetics however, shouldn't be confused with a far larger category of people who do care how their garden looks, but have difficulty in telling you. Sometimes, they're worried you might come out on strike if they ask you to clear the brambles or scrape dog poo off the lawn. More often, they find it difficult to articulate what they want done or to think systematically about what is involved in doing it. Sometimes, they'll point to seemingly unimportant tasks like deadheading the roses or edging the lawn, simply because these are the only jobs they are able to describe.

When you're confronted with someone who can't express what they want it's up to you to take the lead. My approach is to think what the person probably wants done and suggest it to them, as in "shall I clear the back area, mow the lawn, trim the hedges, weed the herbaceous borders etc". Sometimes, when customers are getting really confused, I simply ask "shall I just use my common sense?" You only need to see the relief on their faces to know that they appreciate you taking the initiative.

Some customers take real delight in their gardens, and while it's not compulsory, they'll appreciate it if you do too. Don't worry if you don't know much; it's more than sufficient to be able to look and sound interested, and be patient while they keep changing their minds about where to stick a laurel bush. Always have a few complements of the "your Dahlias are looking lovely" variety to hand. Women like to be complimented, or didn't you know that?

A very small number of customers are simply not nice people. They may be bullying, pathologically mean, congenital liars or simply incapable of acknowledging, let alone returning, a good deed. Maybe they think you're someone they can exploit. Perhaps they were brought up to despise anyone who gets their hands dirty for a living. But provided they don't owe you any money, it isn't your problem. All you have to do is not work for them. Tell them you've broken your back or that you're booked six months ahead, or simply say you've had enough and walk off the job. There are plenty of people who will genuinely appreciate your services so why waste your energies on someone who is only gong to make a victim of you?

Often however, the most maddening customers are those with the best intentions; like the ones who want to help you. If you're anything like me, you like to do things in your own way without interference. Any helpful suggestions feel like personal criticism, especially if a job isn't going all that well. Of course if their advice is correct, that only makes it worse. Many such "hands on" customers are elderly, and I suspect that it often stems from a need to feel useful. It may not have been all that long since they were doing the garden themselves, and having to rely on other people could well make them feel helpless or redundant.

A lot of elderly people value your company almost as much as the work you do for them. I've found that even those with family and friends value having someone to talk to. If you can be a good listener, you'll not only provide a social service and learn something about gardening; many older customers have a lot of worthwhile things to say, and even discounting the war, their lives have generally been every bit as interesting and adventurous as yours and those of your contemporaries.

Working for elderly people does require patience though, as everything takes longer, from opening the door and finding the keys to the shed to getting paid at the end. All perfectly reasonable but it can be maddening when you're trying to get to the next job. Sometimes, it's better to think of yourself as the nice person who helps them out in the garden rather than as a professional gardener trying to run an efficient operation. If it's what the customer wants, then why worry if you haven't got as much work done as you might have if left to your own devices?

Some elderly people can be quite confused, and this can be very frustrating. They can't tell you clearly what they want done and you're sometimes not sure if they want you there at all. In such cases, I find it's best to make sure that the person has a relative, friend or carer present when you come. Not only will they be able to give you clear instructions, but it will also ensure that nobody suspects you of trying to defraud the customer, who may not fully understand the financial side of things.

Customers, of course, aren't the only people you will come into contact with.

Neighbours

If the neighbours are out in the garden socialising, eating a meal or engaging in romantic encounters, they probably want to be left alone. If they're out doing a bit of gardening however, then a casual remark about the weather or a cheery hello will usually be well received. It's basic suburban courtesy and it can be good for business, since it helps spread the message that you're the nice person who does everyone's garden in the area.

There are one or two things to be careful about though. Firstly, if a neighbour asks you to do something in the garden you are working in, like chopping down a branch or trimming a shrub, never, ever do it without first checking with the customer. I've only had two such requests in my career, and both of them were made with malicious intent.

A much more common dilemma is what to do when chopping down hedges or bushes that grow between the garden you are working in and the one next door. Generally speaking, if you're trimming something like a privet hedge, the neighbour will be grateful, especially if you trim the whole of the top, since that saves them having to do their side. But you could have all sorts of things growing there, like jasmine, clematis, passionflowers, climbing roses and the like. Generally, you can check with your customer on the best course of action, since it's his/her responsibility to negotiate these things with the people next door. If you're in doubt though, it's best to err on the side of caution. Some neighbours can be pretty upset if you cut away something they've grown attached to.

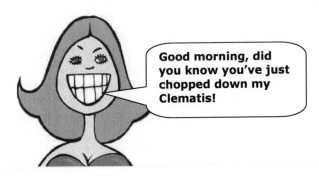

It's also a good idea, when chopping down branches on large bushes, to try and make sure they fall in the garden you're working in, rather than next door.

Other Workers

Sometimes, you will come into contact with other people working in the garden or house. Builders, decorators, window cleaners, domestics, pest controllers; they come in all shapes and sizes.

Again, an attempt at friendliness is appreciated; even expected; there's a certain amount of camaraderie between fellow workers. As with neighbours, you don't need to be a conversationalist. A simple remark about the weather is usually enough to ascertain whether they want to talk or not. Domestics, in particular, really appreciate your taking the trouble to be friendly to them. Workmen will occasionally offer you a cup of tea if they're putting on a brew. They're just as likely to take the mickey though, so have a bit of banter ready and be prepared to deflect questions about your sex life unless you're prepared to wildly exaggerate.

As you're working for lots of different people, some workmen will ask you to recommend them to your customers. There's nothing wrong with this, and some customers will ask if you can recommend a good decorator or tree surgeon. It's a good idea however, to check that the customer the tradesperson was working for was satisfied with them before passing on their details to other customers.

They say that Southern Californians are interested in money, health and sex, in that order. Gardening won't make you a Hollywood star, but in this chapter, I've tried to cover the financial side of gardening, as well as physical survival and human relationships.

Overall, I think I've told you pretty much everything I know. It's almost time to wish you luck in your new career and bid you farewell.

FINAL WORD

Well like I say, I've shared the benefits of my experience; the rest is up to you.

Perhaps gardening for you is a part time or day job, allowing you to earn a bit of money while you get your degree or pursue your career as a poet or professional footballer. There's nothing wrong with that, and when you're successful and famous in years to come, I hope you will still enjoy fond memories of glorious summer afternoons and raking up leaves in autumn mists.

You may however, want to make a career out of gardening. If so, there are lots of paths open, none of which I have explored myself.

If you want to make a good living, as opposed to merely wages, you might want to upgrade your operation, get a van and mechanical equipment and start employing people.

If you're a creative person, you might consider going in for garden design. There are numerous courses, and if you can get the custom, it can pay very well. The same is true of landscaping, though it's harder to find an appropriate course. Furthermore, if you don't have building experience and want to avoid serious financial risks, you'd be well advised to stick to "soft landscaping" jobs, such as creating rockeries, lawns or gravel paths, as opposed to "hard landscaping" such as putting up fences or laying patios.

There are lots of courses available that are intended to improve your knowledge of plants and horticulture, and there are plenty of occupations for the specialist, including teaching/lecturing, research and working in places like Kew or Chatsworth.

As for me, I'm going to carry on as I am for the foreseeable future. I can't say I've become an expert gardener or made much money, but I've kept body and soul together while having time for my other pursuits. Just as important; I've been happy at work, stayed healthy and often felt a degree of inner contentment that I'd never have experienced otherwise.

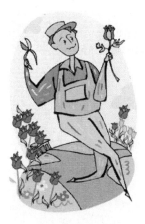

The End

4050561R00089

Printed in Great Britain
by Amazon.co.uk, Ltd.,
Marston Gate.